THE PLANT-BASED ATHLETE

ALSO BY MATT FRAZIER
The No Meat Athlete Cookbook

ALSO BY ROBERT CHEEKE
Shred It!

THE
PLANT-BASED
ATHLETE

A Game-Changing Approach
to Peak Performance

MATT FRAZIER and **ROBERT CHEEKE**

with Rachel Holtzman

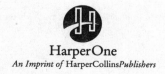

HarperOne

An Imprint of HarperCollinsPublishers

THE PLANT-BASED ATHLETE. Copyright © 2021 by Matt Frazier and Robert Cheeke. All rights reserved. Printed in the United States of America. No part of this book may be used or reproduced in any manner whatsoever without written permission except in the case of brief quotations embodied in critical articles and reviews. For information, address HarperCollins Publishers, 195 Broadway, New York, NY 10007.

HarperCollins books may be purchased for educational, business, or sales promotional use. For information, please email the Special Markets Department at SPsales@harpercollins.com.

FIRST EDITION

Designed by Terry McGrath

Library of Congress Cataloging-in-Publication Data is available upon request.

ISBN 978-0-06-304201-8

21 22 23 24 25 LSC 10 9 8 7 6 5 4 3 2 1

Generations of athletes have used exercise combined with animal protein diets to get bigger, stronger, and faster, all in the name of a competitive edge. Unknowingly to most, their efforts to achieve the short-term gain of athletic success have often resulted in the long-term pain of chronic disease. This book demonstrates that today's athletes, from the top stars to the weekend warriors, are embracing the fact that they can reach their short-term goals without sacrificing their long-term health. Replacing an animal protein diet with a plant-based diet not only protects the heart, battles cancer, defeats diabetes, and stomps out strokes, but it also decreases inflammation, improves recovery time, and can fuel an athlete's fire to win.

—Dr. Columbus Batiste, interventional cardiologist

CONTENTS

Foreword by Michael Greger, MD *ix*

1 Becoming a Plant-Based Athlete *1*

2 Understanding the Power Behind the Food: Macronutrients, Micronutrients, and Calorie Density *13*

3 It's Time to Have the Protein Talk *35*

4 Carbohydrates: The Body's Perfect Fuel *67*

5 Fat: It's Not All Bad *91*

6 Supplements: Should I or Shouldn't I? *107*

7 Putting It All Together *141*

8 Recover Better, Train More *175*

9 Unleashing Your Inner Athlete *203*

10 A Day in the Life of a Plant-Based Athlete *237*

11 Recipes *263*

Acknowledgments *329*
Notes *333*
About the Authors *337*

We'd like to thank all of the plant-based athletes
who contributed to this project:

James Wilks, Champion Mixed Martial Artist

Breana Wigley, IFBB Pro Bikini Competitor

Seychelle Webster, World Champion Athlete

Dustin Watten, Team USA Volleyball Player

Orla Walsh, National Champion Cyclist

Hulda Waage, National Champion Powerlifter

Andreas Vojta, Olympic Runner

David Verburg, Olympic Sprinter

Christine Vardaros, Professional Cyclist

Ebiye Jeremy Udo-Udoma, Team USA Beach Handball player

Korin Sutton, Champion Bodybuilder

Nick Squires, Champion Powerlifter

Rebecca Soni, Olympic Swimmer

Mary Schneider, Elite Marathoner

John Salley, 4-Time NBA Champion

David Rother, Professional Triathlete

Rich Roll, Champion Ultrarunner

Jeremy Reijnders, Netherlands' Fittest Man

Fiona Oakes, Guinness World Record Holding Marathoner

James Newbury, 4-time Australia's Fittest Man

Daniel Negreanu, World Series of Poker Champion

Julia Murray, Olympic Skier

Sophie Mullins, National Champion Ultrarunner

Heather Mitts, Olympic Soccer Player

Natalie Matthews, IFBB Pro Bikini Competitor

Jehina Malik, IFBB Pro Bodybuilder

Sonya Looney, World Champion Mountain Biker

Vera Levi, Strength Coach

Georges Laraque, Former NHL Player

Josh LaJaunie, Champion Ultrarunner

Kätlin Kukk, National Champion Cyclist

Vivian Kong, Elite Fencer

Laura Kline, World Champion Duathlete

Maggie Kattan, USA Track & Field Coach

Scott Jurek, World Champion Ultrarunner

John Joseph, Ironman Triathlete

Shanda Hill, Champion Ultrarunner

Kevin Hill, Olympic Snowboarder

Stephen Gray, Professional Football Freestyler

Darcy Gaechter, World Champion Kayaker

Yuri Foreman, World Champion Boxer

Sharon Fichman, WTA Professional Tennis Player

Rip Esselstyn, World Record Holding Swimmer

Vanessa Espinoza, Champion Boxer

Meagan Duhamel, Olympic Figure Skater

Alastair Dixon, Trail Runner

Yassine Diboun, Champion Ultrarunner

Patrick Delorenzi, Ironman Triathlete

Harriet Davis, IFBB Pro Bikini Competitor

Olessya Dadema, Elite Gymnast

Catra Corbett, Ultrarunner

David Carter, Former NFL Player

Brendan Brazier, Professional Ironman Triathlete

Tia Blanco, World Champion Surfer

Kim Best, World Record Holding Strongwoman

James Bebbington, World Champion Kayaker

Dotsie Bausch, Olympic Cyclist

Robbie Balenger, Ultra Endurance Athlete

Cam Awesome, Champion Boxer

Ünsal Arik, World Champion Boxer

Austin Aires, World Champion Pro Wrestler

FOREWORD

Being a plant-based athlete is not a new concept. History is rife with examples, from the Gladiators in ancient Rome to the Tarahumara tribe of Northern Mexico, who run 160-mile races fueled by plants purely for enjoyment. While the research supporting plant-based athletes isn't new either, it is more compelling than ever today. Take, for instance, the study "Is a Vegan Diet Detrimental to Endurance and Muscle Strength?" that was published in April 2020. Researchers followed two groups of healthy, young, lean, physically active women—a vegan group and the other omnivorous—over a two-year period. They evaluated body composition, estimated maximal oxygen consumption (VO2 Max), a submaximal endurance test, and muscle strength. The results revealed that both groups were comparable for physical activity levels, body mass index, percent body fat, lean body mass, and muscle strength. However, results also showed that the vegans had a significantly higher estimated VO2 Max and submaximal endurance time to exhaustion compared with the omnivores. The conclusion? A vegan diet is not detrimental to endurance and strength, and the vegan group achieved *greater* endurance. For those who follow the likes of legendary plant-based runners Fiona Oakes, Scott Jurek, and Brendan Brazier, these findings come as no surprise. It is, after all, the scientific evidence that explains the athletic success, not the other way around.

You'll get your share of success stories from plant-based athletes in this book, such as those of Olympic gold medalists and world champions from seemingly every sports background, and they are all truly inspiring. I'm most interested in the science behind their athletic performance, though. We know a lot of the fundamentals, such as you can get all the protein you need from plants; plant foods contain sixty-four times more antioxidants than animal foods; fiber is only found in plants, and dietary cholesterol is only found in animal foods; and plants have a far superior nutrient density ratio of nutrients per calorie than animal foods. But the story is much deeper than that. Whether we're discussing the way that nitric oxide in leafy green vegetables may increase blood flow, antioxidants may help muscle tissue repair, plants may improve resting metabolic rate, and avoidance of animal protein may lead to a decreased risk of obesity, the scientific literature makes it abundantly clear that plants have been our preferred fuel source for ages—and now they may be the solution to successful and prolonged active lifestyles.

Robert and Matt are the embodiment of these truths, as are the many athletes profiled in this book. What makes *The Plant-Based Athlete* a formidable and refreshingly unique resource is that it draws from not only decades of personal experience and world-class success stories, but also from both age-old and cutting-edge research. You would be wise to take heed of the advice in this book, as it is essential for creating a lifestyle—not a diet—to improve your athletic capabilities as well as your overall quality of life. Your opportunity to become your most healthful, happiest, and fittest self may very well be determined by what you choose to put on your plate. Choose thoughtfully and wisely, and discover your best athletic self along the way.

—Michael Greger, MD, FACLM, *New York Times* bestselling
   author of *How Not to Die* and *How Not to Diet* and founder
   of NutritionFacts.org

THE
PLANT-BASED
ATHLETE

1

BECOMING
A PLANT-BASED ATHLETE

Hidden behind the world-class performances of many of the planet's elite athletes—the biggest, strongest, and fastest humans on the planet—is a secret weapon. These competitors swear by it, affirming that it helps them work harder, play longer, move faster, perform better, prevent injuries, and recover faster. It's been credited for winning Olympic medals, World Cup championships, Wimbledon titles, and the Super Bowl, in addition to shattering world records. But it's not high-tech gear or a grueling training regimen, nor is it access to a dedicated team of trainers or even the athletes' DNA. On the contrary, it's something that's inexpensive, accessible, and available to anyone with the inclination to try it: *a plant-based diet*. Consider just a sampling of the evidence.

When **Alex Morgan** catapulted the US women's soccer team to a World Cup championship and into the limelight in the summer of 2019, she credited a plant-based diet for her strength and endurance. Also in the summer of 2019, **Novak Djokovic**, the world's number-one–ranked men's tennis player, outlasted Roger Federer in epic fashion to capture his fifth Wimbledon title. When asked about his performance, Djokovic was quick to proclaim the benefits of a plant-based diet for his energy, stamina, and overall performance. When professional tennis icon **Venus Williams** discovered she was suffering from Sjogren's syndrome, an autoimmune disease, which caused her to withdraw from the US Open (and later from competitive tennis entirely) because of fatigue and joint pain, she turned to a plant-based diet for help. The very next year, after adopting a plant-based diet, she won a Wimbledon title and an Olympic gold medal. Her sister **Serena**—who has dominated women's tennis for years—has at times embraced a fully plant-based diet and currently follows more of a plant-centered diet (mostly plants, some animal-based foods).

When National Basketball Association all-star **Kyrie Irving** was traded from Cleveland to Boston in 2017, it represented an opportunity for him to finally emerge from the shadow of LeBron James. After his new team got off to an unexpectedly slow start, he adopted a plant-based diet. The Celtics went on to win the next thirteen games and Irving never looked back, becoming the leader of his team and a perennial all-star. He is now one of the faces of the Brooklyn Nets franchise, where he has a fresh start for putting his plant-based stamp on the NBA. Kyrie set an NBA record in his first game of the 2019–2020 season by scoring 50 points in his debut with a new team. And he's not alone in looking to a plant-based diet as a competitive advantage in the NBA: fellow all-star **Damian Lillard**, also one of the NBA's top 10, adopted a plant-based diet to both drop weight and improve his speed. He accomplished those two goals and catapulted himself from a second-tier all-star to one of the league's very best players. NBA stars **Chris Paul**, **JaVale McGee**, **DeAndre Jordan**, **Wilson Chandler**, and others throughout the association have adopted a plant-based diet for improved performance. Chris Paul's renaissance season in 2019–2020 speaks volumes about the personal benefits he has experienced after more than a full year of following a plant-based diet, having had one of his best seasons relatively late in his career. In the Women's National Basketball Association, the plant-based diet is catching fire, and some of the greatest female basketball players in the world, including **Diana**

Taurasi—considered by many to be the greatest of all time—have embraced a plant-based diet for energy, performance, and longevity. Fellow WNBA stars **Liz Cambage**, **Rebekkah Brunson**, and **Nneka Ogwumike** have also leaned on plants to elevate their game.

In 2017, National Football League linebacker **Derrick Morgan** adopted a plant-based diet, along with the rest of the starting defensive line of the Tennessee Titans, and led his team to the playoffs for the first time in nine years. Not to be outdone, the starting offensive line for the Washington Football Team implemented a plant-based diet for part of their 2017 season as well. More recently, former NFL MVP **Cam Newton** adopted a plant-based diet for its athletic benefits. He has been featured in a Vegan Strong campaign on major media outlets, proclaiming the positive results he has experienced with a plant-based diet on his recovery after injuries, which helped him fuel his comeback as a starting quarterback in the NFL.

Mike Tyson's epic comeback to boxing at age fifty-four comes on the heels of a decade of following a plant-based diet, in which he reclaimed his health and his athletic youthfulness, power, and strength. Ultimate fighters **Nate Diaz**, **Nick Diaz**, **Mac Danzig**, **James Wilks**, and many others have embraced the power of plants to boost their endurance and aid their recovery in their grueling sport, just as renowned national and world champions in boxing **Timothy Bradley**, **David Haye**, **Cam Awesome**, **Ünsal Arik**, and **Yuri Foreman** incorporated a plant-based diet for endurance to last the intense rounds in one of the world's toughest sports and for the ability to recover quickly and have constant improvement.

Olympic medalists **Heather Mitts**, **Rebecca Soni**, **Meagan Duhamel**, and **Dotsie Bausch** know the healing and performance-enhancing power of plants and embrace a plant-based diet to this day while encouraging others to do the same. One of the greatest Olympic athletes in history, track-and-field legend **Carl Lewis**, credited his best all-time performances to a vegan lifestyle and plant-based diet. He won ten Olympic medals, including nine gold medals, paving the way for the amazing world-class plant-based athletes who would follow in his footsteps on their own way to Olympic glory.

Cricket icon **Virat Kohli** not only is one of the best cricketers in the world, with a massively impressive résumé of awards and titles, but also ranked seventh in ESPN's list of the one hundred most famous athletes, made the *Forbes* list of the top 100 highest-paid athletes, and was on *TIME* magazine's list of the 100 most influential people. He's in good company—among the top 21 most influential athletes in the world are these plant-based household names: **Lionel** and **Lewis Hamilton**.

Speaking of **Lewis Hamilton**, a six-time Formula One world champion and perhaps the most famous race-car driver in the world, he is one of the most outspoken about his plant-based diet, whereas some other leading plant-based athletes tend to keep their vegan lifestyle to themselves. Lewis not only follows a plant-based diet but also promotes the lifestyle frequently to his massive audience, encouraging his millions of followers to embrace a plant-based diet for their health and for the health of the environment. He set records in 2019 and 2020, making him one of the most consistent champions in any sport and one of the most recognized athletes in the world today.

And then there's **Arnold Schwarzenegger**, as synonymous with power, strength, and masculinity as it gets, who has acknowledged that you don't need meat to build muscle. In fact, he follows a mostly plant-based diet himself these days while encouraging others to do the same.

A plant-based diet isn't a fringe topic for athletes anymore. Consider the headlines in recent years:

USA Today: **Plant-Based Diets Take Over Sports World**
CNBC: **Why NFL Players and Other Athletes Are Going Vegan**
U.S. News & World Report: **Athletes Can Thrive on Plant-Based Diets**
Forbes: **Five Reasons Why Sport Is Going Vegan**
New York Times: **Lewis Hamilton Changed His Diet, and It's Been Off to the Races Since**

A growing group of decorated professional players, Olympians, and other elite athletes are embracing a plant-based approach to their fitness because they realize that it can not only improve their physical abilities in ways that they couldn't have dreamed possible but also add years to their careers *and* their lives. This is powerful proof that *the human body doesn't need meat, eggs, or dairy to be strong.* And if the NBA's brightest stars can thrive during their high-intensity eighty-two-game season, the NFL's biggest and best can do the same in the most physically demanding major US sport, and professional tennis players can make it through their taxing yearlong season while facing extreme elements and time-zone changes, imagine what the average athlete can experience by following a healthy plant-based diet. That's the message we've dedicated the past twenty years of our careers to sharing, and that's what *The Plant-Based Athlete* is all about: teaching you how you can adapt these strategies to your own life and unlock your own potential, then showing you firsthand how these exceptional athletes eat, train, and recover in real life.

It's no secret that veganism is one of the biggest lifestyle trends of our times. It makes sense: almost everyone who tries this diet—whether fully plant-based or more tentatively plant-curious—reaps the benefits from eating more plants and fewer animal products, including loss of excess body fat, stabilization of blood sugar (and in many cases reversal of a diabetes diagnosis), lowering of cholesterol, reversal of heart disease, alleviation of joint pain and other forms of inflammation, and an end to various chronic ailments.

Now it's time for the movement's next evolution: plant-based *fitness*. This isn't exactly a new idea in the plant-based world—and we should know, because between us we have a combined thirty years of experience as competitive vegan athletes. Robert Cheeke is considered the godfather of the vegan bodybuilding movement, having been a vegan athlete since the mid-1990s. And Matt Frazier is a competitive marathoner who has been leading the conversation about the plant-based athlete lifestyle since 2009 with perhaps the largest plant-based athlete platform in the world, No Meat Athlete (nomeatathlete.com). For years, the two of us have provided reassurance, backed by both research and firsthand experience, that athletes not only can get adequate protein and overall nutrition on a plant-based diet, but also can excel athletically and absolutely can achieve their highest physical goals. From experienced competitors to weekend warriors, die-hard vegans to plant-curious dabblers, we've helped many thousands of readers discover what's possible for them. But up until now, this conversation had not made the jump into the mainstream fitness dialogue. *The Plant-Based Athlete* will change that.

Picking Up Where the Trailblazers Left Off

Champion athletes in many sports were fueled by plants long before the internet came around, before there were books and documentaries on the subject, before it was cool to proclaim that you were a vegetarian or a vegan, and before social media influencers got paid to promote products or could make a living by being muscular and fit. In the ages that preceded these modern updates to the plant-based landscape, there were plant-based athletes winning Olympic medals while also speaking out against food injustices, government subsidies, environmental degradation, factory farming, and animal cruelty. Others simply made the case that they didn't need animal protein to compete at the highest level. Many, even decades ago, arrived at a plant-based diet in search of improved athletic performance and found what they were looking for. If it worked, why didn't it catch on way back then? As they say, old habits die hard, change takes time, and going against the grain isn't easy, even if it's worth it. But that was then, and a new day is dawning for the modern plant-based athlete, a theme we will visit throughout this book.

Plant-based athletes have been around since the time of the Roman gladiators, who ate a mostly plant-based diet, as forensic scientists determined after studying the composition of their bones.[1] While there are some records of plant-based Olympians in the early history of the competition, it was the 1970s and 1980s that saw the rise of legendary athletes who embraced a plant-based (either vegetarian or vegan) diet for sports performance benefits. This included track-and-field icons **Edwin Moses** and **Carl Lewis**, bodybuilding greats **Bill Pearl** and **Andreas Cahling**, and women's tennis champion **Martina Navratilova**. Moses won a mind-boggling 122 consecutive races from 1977 to 1987, which is especially impressive when you factor in that his sport was the 400-meter hurdle, where one slip or one scrape of a spike from his sprinter shoe on the crossbar of the hurdle could cause a fall and end a perfect winning streak. The fact that Moses went on to set four world records, win two Olympic gold medals, and win two world championship gold medals following a diet devoid of meat sent a message to anyone who was paying attention: If one of the world's greatest athletes, especially one in an explosive, powerful sport, can succeed at such a high level without consuming meat, what could the rest of us accomplish?

As Moses's career was winding down, another track-and-field star's career was in full bloom. Carl Lewis, a sprinter and long jumper who joined Moses as a gold medal winner in the 1984 Olympics in Los Angeles, set out to become one of the greatest Olympic champions of all time. He has said on multiple occasions that his best year in track and field was his first year as a vegan, and Lewis is still an advocate for a plant-based diet. Around that same time, Martina Navratilova was paving the way toward being considered one of the greatest, if not *the* greatest, female tennis players of all time. Her accomplishments and records seem to be endless, including being ranked the number one player in the world for hundreds of weeks during her career, in both singles and doubles. One notable attribute of her career was her longevity—she played at an elite level well into her forties. She once said in an interview that moving toward a more plant-based diet was the major reason she was able to continue playing professional tennis for so long. Though she wasn't fully vegan during her playing days, she was a vegetarian, and she has since adopted a fully plant-based diet.

In the 1990s, four-time NBA champion **John Salley** opened the door for many NBA players to embrace a plant-based diet when, near the end of his playing career, he began vocally espousing its benefits. He ended up opening a vegan café in Southern California, was an early investor in Beyond Meat, and has appeared in countless documentaries and articles on the topic. But it was the long-distance runners of the 1990s who gave plant-based athletes their biggest push, most notably **Brendan Brazier**, **Ruth Heidrich**, and **Scott Jurek**. All legends in the plant-based and running worlds, they showed that plants can fuel some of the most challenging human athletic achievements, including running 100-plus-mile ultramarathons. After that incredible and convincing demonstration, vegan bodybuilders such as Robert, **Kenneth Williams**, **Robbie Hazeley**, and **Alexander Dargatz** came onboard, as did mixed martial arts (MMA) fighters such as **Mac Danzig** and **Jake Shields**, paving the way for many more to follow in their footsteps.

When it became unequivocally clear that that you could achieve and succeed on a plant-based diet—whether you were an endurance, strength, or power athlete—the world took notice, and by the early 2000s, a movement was born. Robert's Vegan Bodybuilding & Fitness website launched in 2003, quickly becoming a popular destination for hundreds of thousands of plant-based athletes of all backgrounds to form a community. Matt's No Meat Athlete site arrived on the scene six years later and became the largest platform of its kind, the current leading voice in the plant-based athlete community that is now millions of people strong.

Together, we have witnessed our heroes pave the way and make good on what they started. From having posters of Carl Lewis on our bedroom wall as a kid (Robert)—not knowing he was plant-based at the time—to having Brendan Brazier write the foreword for his first book (Matt), it has been a rewarding journey to get to the point where a plant-based diet is truly mainstream in sports. What these incredible individuals have taught us is that if all athletes train essentially the same way and all have similar performance results, what would separate one athlete from the next? It would be the ability to recover more efficiently, train more often, and improve their overall speed, endurance, strength, and performance. The hypothesis began as "What if the difference is in nutrition?" Decade after decade, these athletes have proven that to be the case. And they've also proven that there's really no such thing as a specialized diet for each type of athlete. Instead, we now have ample evidence—from both experience and a number of scientific studies—that a well-planned, calorically sufficient plant-based diet in general is enough to boost energy, reduce inflammation, improve athletic recovery, minimize soreness, provide the most efficient pre- and post-workout fuel, improve gut health and digestion, reduce unwanted body fat, and even improve sleep—regardless of the sport. Add to that a robust collection of plant-based physicians, nutritionists, and other medical specialists who actively proclaim the health benefits of a plant-based diet in areas of cardiology, neurology, psychiatry, functional and lifestyle medicine, and autoimmune disease prevention and reversal.

Thanks to increasing awareness of the benefits of a plant-based diet, more and more prominent competitors are coming forward to share their experiences of how this dietary shift has improved their performance in unimaginable ways, from overcoming chronic illness to dramatically surpassing personal goals to extending the life of their careers well beyond what has been considered the norm. This has raised two very big, very important questions: What *exactly* are these athletes doing to get the most mileage out of their plant-based diets, and how *exactly* can you do it too?

We're going to tell you just that.

We learned from the most decorated, visible plant-based athletes in the world—including pro football, basketball, soccer, and tennis players; surfers, wrestlers, MMA fighters, cyclists, and triathletes; and long-distance runners, boxers, powerlifters, and bodybuilders—about the specific and nuanced elements of how they're eating and training to get maximum results with minimal injury. Then we set out to give you a step-by-step blueprint for how to build the best plant-based fitness regimen for *you*. We'll help you figure out what exactly you should be eating, how much, and when (depending on specific physiological factors such as your sex, age, height, weight, activity type, and fitness goals—endurance, agility, strength, or speed), as well as how to recover from intense training more quickly and effectively and how to get in the kitchen and make the most delicious, nutrient-packed food possible.

Along the way, beyond the first-person experiences shared by elite plant-based athletes, we'll include plenty of input from medical and nutritional experts, including doctors and registered dietitians. What they've seen in their research and in their patients confirms what we, and every single one of the athletes we've mentioned in this chapter, have seen in the gym: plants have the extraordinary power to increase circulation, oxygenate the blood, quell inflammation, flush out unwanted toxins, nourish the muscles, keep the heart robust, and feed the brain—all of which turbocharge athletic performance. Add in the specific knowledge of how to tailor this potent fuel specifically to your body and its needs—whether it's moving or resting—and you'll be taking your training to the next level as a plant-based athlete.

The truth is, *everyone*—not just athletes and those who lead an active lifestyle—can benefit from eating more whole-plant foods. What we're challenging you to do is to keep an open mind about what is possible when taking your fitness to a higher level and about what role plant-based nutrition can play in your health, athletic, and everyday performance. If you take our advice—and the advice of these elite athletes and medical experts—you'll have a significant set of tools to help in your training and performance, while at the same time profoundly benefiting your overall health.

As we've said before, we know this approach works. But you have to be willing to do the work and commit for the long haul, just as these athletes have. Our hope is that by following the advice outlined in this book, you'll feel confident embracing plants as you attack your new and improved fitness goals. As with any challenge worth taking on, there will be some tough days and there will be roadblocks. But the measure of success is in how you overcome them. And when you come out on the other side, joining the ranks of hundreds of thousands of athletes who have experienced the performance benefits of adopting a plant-based diet, you'll be stronger, faster, and more resilient. In the meantime, we'll be here for you, cheering you on every step of the way.

● ● ● ● ●

One of the biggest advantages of a plant-based diet for athletes and other active individuals is that it prevents the hypertension, inflammation, oxidative stress, lipotoxicity, and dysbiosis associated with Western-style diets. Eating plant-based seems to provide an advantage where fuel, function, and recovery are concerned. I am constantly inspired by elite plant-based athletes who are setting world records. I am equally inspired by plant-based individuals in their seventies, eighties, and beyond who are still fit, vibrant, and free of chronic disease. To me, this is the real acid test . . . nothing surpasses plant-based diets where long-term health is concerned.
—**Brenda Davis, RD, author, researcher, and speaker**

Recovery time is the number one benefit of a plant-based diet. I am able to train more, and therefore improve quicker. Since my cortisol levels have dropped because of the removal of nutritional stress, I'm also able to sleep better.
—**Brendan Brazier, ultramarathon champion**

The industry has accepted that athletes can survive on a plant-based diet for years, but now thanks to legends who paved the way, other health professionals see that we do more than survive on a plant-based diet; we thrive! I challenged my college education in kinesiology and dietetics and searched for truth. Within a week of eating a whole-foods plant-based diet (imperfectly) I was pushing more weight and breaking more personal records than I had in years. I was ready to compete the next day feeling almost no inflammatory response. The epiphany came while I was lifting and felt a deep intuition with my placement because for the first time, I had a mind-body control that I didn't know was possible.

—**Alyssa Strong, American College of Sports Medicine–certified exercise physiologist**

As I worked in hospitals through physical therapy school it became clear to me that I needed to change my diet to avoid the health problems I was seeing. It was definitely a long-term decision rather than one made for short-term performance gains. If [athletes] aren't fueled properly, they don't have great results.

—**Scott Jurek, seven-time consecutive winner of the Western States 100-Mile Endurance Run and two-time winner of the 135-mile Badwater Ultramarathon**

For me, the most significant change after switching to a whole-foods plant-based diet was that I had more energy and was less sore from my trainings. And because of that, I could add an extra training day into my week.

—**Jeremy Reijnders, 2018 Netherlands' Fittest Man**

UNDERSTANDING THE POWER BEHIND THE FOOD:
Macronutrients, Micronutrients, and Calorie Density

If you're reading this book, you've opened your mind to the possibility of leaving behind animal-based foods in favor of plant-based ones so that you can take your health and athleticism to the next level (even if it's level one). And that's a great thing, because as you'll see in every single chapter, there is ample evidence that such a switch could have huge effects on both your health and your athletic abilities. An athlete who exemplifies physical, mental, and overall athletic and lifestyle transformation as a result of switching to a plant-based diet during a critical period of his life is **Rich Roll**.

One of the most popular plant-based athletes in the world today, Rich Roll is an ultramarathon runner and host of *The Rich Roll Podcast*. Rich's popularity has grown so much that for many elite athletes and thought leaders, simply being a guest on his podcast is a form of "making it," much like landing on a magazine cover or making a major television appearance. He has an almost cultlike following, but it wasn't always that way. In fact, it's all fairly new. One of Rich's most famous quotes is as follows: "I didn't reach my athletic peak until I was 43. I didn't write my first book until I was 44. I didn't start my podcast until I was 45. At 30, I thought my life was over. At 52, I know it's just beginning. Keep running. Never give up. And watch your kite soar." He has completely transformed his life over the past decade, and a plant-based diet has been central to his personal growth.

Like many athletes we've interviewed, Rich has a complex story. Once a former standout swimmer at Stanford University, Rich saw his life crumble, even as a lawyer and perceived success story, as he succumbed to drugs and alcohol and ended up in jail and rehab. And like many people who create their own life transformations, Rich had a wake-up call. Though sober at the time of his fortieth birthday, as a husband and father of four, he was fifty pounds overweight and collapsed in pain while trying to ascend a staircase, fearing a heart attack was near. Though many years removed from being a competitive athlete, Rich felt compelled to take his life in a different direction and reclaim his health and vitality. It was a choice between remaining sick and depressed or becoming healthy and happy, and Rich chose to thrive. He adopted a plant-based diet, started swimming again, picked up running, and purchased a bike. This was the start of an ultrarunning career that would eventually see him featured on major magazine covers and proclaimed by *Men's Fitness* magazine as one of the 25 Fittest Men in the World. It was also the start of his discovery of Ultraman triathlons, where he would leave a strong imprint as an innovator and a world-class athlete. He eventually became one of the most successful in the sport as a top finisher at the Ultraman World Championships, setting records along the way. Though Rich had a background in swimming, he didn't even own a bike two years prior to competing in his first Ultraman triathlon, yet he cycled 170 miles in a single day during that three-day race.

In 2010, Rich and fellow ultra-endurance athlete Jason Lester completed what they called the EPIC5 Challenge. They finished five Ironman distance triathlons on five Hawaiian islands in under a week. Two years later, Rich released his number one bestselling memoir, *Finding Ultra,* and given his popular quote we mentioned earlier, you now know the rest of the story. Today, Rich is in his mid-fifties and still exercises daily. Much of his energy also goes to his award-winning podcast, sharing the stories of luminaries and thought leaders from around the world. To Rich, conversation is the key to improving the world. If we can talk about important issues, ask deeply meaningful questions, listen attentively without judgment, and have a respectful conversation about moving society forward, we can do just that. In fact, it was his quest for knowledge and thirst for self-improvement that brought him to a plant-based diet in the first place, which was the catalyst for everything he stands for and represents today.

A plant-based diet was the fuel that helped Rich discover his way as an athlete after drugs, alcohol, depression, stress, and poor eating habits engulfed his life. How exactly did a plant-based diet make a real impact on Rich's athletic performance? By eating foods that are nutrient rich but calorie poor, Rich discovered that with a whole-foods plant-based diet, you can eat more food while being able to lose weight. And you can consume more total nutrition with diversity in calorie sources from fruits, vegetables, legumes, grains, nuts, and seeds, all packed with nutrients, by eating the colors of the rainbow and by avoiding animal-based foods, which cause inflammation and promote disease. Losing weight made exercise easier, more efficient, and more enjoyable for Rich as he swam, cycled, and ran his way into a new passion for sports and life. A nutrient-dense smoothie became a staple of his diet, and the absence of animal protein, dietary cholesterol, copious amounts of saturated fats, and dense calories enabled Rich to fill up on much more health-promoting foods, those highest in vitamins, minerals, antioxidants, fiber, and phytonutrients. For Rich, the plant-based diet was transformative. Rather than wondering if a heart attack was imminent and feeling tired and sluggish as a result of being overweight, like most of the American population, Rich transformed his body into a plant-powered machine, capable of incredible athletic feats such as completing Ironman distance triathlons for numerous consecutive days.

It's fair to say that without the influence of a plant-based diet, and the direct impact it had on increasing his energy, expediting his recovery, and improving his overall athleticism and happiness, there wouldn't be *The Rich Roll Podcast*, and there wouldn't be this powerful story to tell. But like so many others, Rich invested his whole self into a diet and lifestyle that would forever change him, just as a plant-based diet might forever change so many of you.

Rich has been a particularly inspirational athlete for both of us. We have had the honor of learning from his wisdom over the years, which we hold in high regard, especially his mantra of "keep showing up," which reminds all of us to keep going even in the face of adversity and struggle. It's deceptively simple, but if you indeed do show up, day after day, and do what you love to do, you will find happiness in the process, and you may even discover your best self.

As you've seen in Rich Roll's profile, and as you'll see in the stories of the other world-class athletes in this book, there's plenty of evidence that choosing plants over animal-based foods is a game changer in the performance department. As elite athletes fueled exclusively by plants, this is not only something we can attest to firsthand—the fact that plants are optimal athlete fuel is confirmed by the medical and scientific communities. We can now say with certainty that plants are the preferred energy source, thanks to recent scientific study conclusions such as the following:

- A vegan diet is not detrimental to endurance or muscle strength. In fact, submaximal endurance might be better in vegans than in omnivores.[1]
- Adhering to vegetarian kinds of diets, but in particular to a vegan dietary pattern, is compatible with ambitious endurance running and is a healthy alternative to an omnivorous diet for athletes.[2]
- The possibility that a plant-based diet contributes to improved performance and accelerated recovery in endurance sports is raised by its effects on blood flow, body composition, antioxidant

capacity, systemic inflammation, and glycogen storage. These attributes provide a scientific foundation for the increased use of plant-based diets by athletes.[3]

In the next few chapters, we'll help you answer the common, and crucial, question "But what the heck do I eat?!" Because when it comes to plant-based athletes, the answer is more nuanced than "not animal products" or "only plants, mostly whole." In this chapter we'll break it down, giving you an essential introduction to how to fuel the plant-based body—especially one that's being pushed to its limits.

The place to begin is with understanding **macro- and micronutrients** and **calorie density**. These concepts will influence not just which plant-based foods you eat but also how much and in what ratio. Learning how to calibrate your diet with regard to these factors will ensure that you get the most out of your fuel, whether your fitness goals are to lose weight, gain weight, improve endurance, build strength, or cultivate explosive agility. We'll eventually get to creating your unique meal plans, but first we're going to break down the universal ins and outs of what you're eating so you won't have to take our word for it—you'll understand how to create a balanced plant-based diet, one that will deliver everything you need to be both an athlete and an all-around healthy person. (And yes, that includes plenty of protein—but more on that in a bit!)

To give you a sense of the power of harnessing the nutritional and caloric makeup of your daily diet, here are a few examples of how athletes implement this in real life.

First, we'll start close to home. When Robert—who has been a vegan since his early teens—got into the sport of bodybuilding, coming off a long-distance running career, he had his sights set on building lots of muscle quickly. At twenty years of age, with optimal testosterone to grow muscle and armed with an exceptional level of enthusiasm, he embraced the pursuit of muscle building with a passion . . . but failed miserably. What happened was that Robert was still thinking like a runner. He had been a competitive runner since childhood and had run cross-country for one year in college, so his workouts entailed burning large amounts of calories while consuming a modest amount of food. This enabled him to maintain his light 150-pound weight on a six-foot-tall frame, which was beneficial to running. When he embraced weight lifting, he was still running to stay fit—and for the pure joy of it—while also cycling, doing daily calisthenics such as push-ups and crunches, and lifting weights—but without significantly increasing his calorie intake. So rather than building muscle and adding mass to his frame, after an entire year of training he hadn't gained a single pound. He even documented his daily workouts in a journal, hoping for and expecting change, but came up short.

Robert's problem wasn't that his plant-based diet prevented him from building muscle—it was simply that he did not understand the role of calorie density and total calorie intake in relation to his calorie expenditure. In essence, he was burning far more calories than he was consuming with the goal of building muscle. His diet and his goals were at odds with each other. It was only after frustration set in and he nearly gave up entirely that he stumbled upon the Body for Life program (a weight-training program that was incredibly popular at the time), which encouraged him to follow a six-days-per-week exercise program and document his exercise and calorie intake. The program also encouraged him to consume six meals a day, eating every three hours, which meant he was consuming adequate calories on a regular basis. He also removed cycling and reduced the amount he was running, while incorporating a structured weight-training routine, which finally made his program sustainable. And this time around, he had the documentation, which he took the time to evaluate each day and determine what was working and what wasn't.

The results spoke for themselves. After adding no mass and having no change in weight over an entire year, Robert gained 19 pounds in twelve weeks and a total of 28 pounds over a ten-month period. He added another 10 pounds the following year, became a competitive bodybuilder the year after that, and became a champion bodybuilder a couple of years later. With his new 200-pound frame, he helped establish that the concept of vegan bodybuilding was viable. That simple body transformation did more than just add muscle to Robert's frame. It gave him confidence and permission to believe in himself and to believe in the power of a plant-based diet. He had become a vegan to reduce animal cruelty, and he had accepted the idea that it might hinder his athletic performance—or so he had been told by almost every friend, teammate, and coach when he was a five-sport high school vegan athlete in the 1990s. And when he struggled to build muscle as a weight lifter, he started to wonder if they were right. But Robert proved—to himself and to others—that it was possible not only to build plant-based muscle but also to become a champion in a sport he was told he had no business competing in.

He would later gain an even better understanding of nutrient density and calorie density, which enabled him to select the foods that provided the best return on investment for his muscle-building goals and reach a body weight of approximately 220 pounds by age forty, up a full 100 pounds from when he adopted a plant-based diet a quarter century earlier. Valuable lessons are often etched deeply in experience. Failing numerous times, learning from those experiences, and having the persistence to try again with an open mind changed Robert from someone who tried and failed to someone who tried again and succeeded.

Matt also got his start by thinking big . . . and failing bigger.

Having grown up like most kids—playing sports and eating the standard American diet—Matt didn't get serious about his diet or fitness until he was in college. He and some friends decided they were going to not just run a marathon (despite having barely run more than three miles at a time, ever) but qualify for the prestigious Boston Marathon. At that time, qualifying for Boston meant running a marathon in 3 hours, 10 minutes—about a 7:15 mile pace. Ignoring that this was closer to his *one*-mile personal record time, a far cry from a marathon pace, Matt began logging miles and fumbling his way through the process of becoming a runner. Six months later, he and his friends crossed the finish line of the San Diego Rock 'n' Roll Marathon . . . after 4 hours and 52 of the most painful minutes they'd ever experienced, missing the Boston qualifying goal by more than 100 minutes.

This could have been the end of Matt's running career, but instead it was the beginning. Rather than getting down about his disappointing result, he got inspired by the possibilities: *If the shape I'm in now is enough to complete a marathon, what kind of shape would I have to be in to run one* 100 *minutes faster? How disciplined about my workouts, nutrition, and recovery would I have to be? How rock-solid a mindset would I have to develop?*

Matt spent the next seven years working toward the Boston goal, failing over and over but all the while getting better at avoiding injuries, training efficiently, and, perhaps most important, eating for optimal performance. A few years into the process, Matt decided (mostly for ethical reasons) to stop eating cows and pigs. He wanted to go vegetarian, but like a lot of athletes, he worried about not getting enough protein. So he started by giving up meat from four-legged animals and gradually eliminated poultry and fish over the next couple of years. Having searched for information about how to fuel for endurance sports with a vegetarian diet but finding almost nothing helpful, Matt decided to detail his experiment with a blog, which he called No Meat Athlete.

Even though performance hadn't been his motivating factor, Matt was surprised by how well the workouts—and, just as important, the subsequent recovery after each one—were going after he ditched meat. He lost a few pounds but maintained his strength, and the most surprising part was that once his marathon training hit peak mileage, with long runs topping 20 miles and unrelenting midweek speed and tempo workouts, Matt didn't slow down. In the past, this level of training had always led to an injury, but this time . . . nothing. And after a summer of the most consistent and intense training of his life, Matt crossed the finish line of the Wineglass Marathon in Corning, New York, in a time of 3:09:59—enough to quality for the race of his dreams by one second.

(Well, not quite one second; the official qualifying standard was 3:10:59, so he actually qualified by 1 minute and 1 second.)

After finally qualifying for Boston, Matt shifted his focus to ultra-running goals. He started running 50-kilometer (50K) and 50-mile races and experimenting with a vegan diet. By the time Matt ran his first 100-mile race, he had been 100 percent vegan for two full years. Prior to that, running two marathons in three months would have been a sure way to get injured. But now Matt was routinely putting in 60 miles per week, with 30 of those miles coming within twenty-four hours of each other on weekends, not to mention that he was able to run a 50K, a 50-miler, and the 100-mile race all in the short span of a few months. Injury never became a factor, which Matt credits to the nutrient density and anti-inflammatory properties of his plant-based diet.

Making a Plant-Based Diet Work for You

We'll be getting into the specifics of how to tailor your diet to your unique physiology, athletic endeavors, and goals, but for now let's cover the basic building blocks that make up every single successful plant-based diet.

First up, **macronutrients**. These are the components of every food you eat that give your body its required fuel, and they're a massive factor for athletic performance—in addition to overall health and wellness. Eating a diet with optimally calibrated macronutrients and plenty of micronutrients is crucial for using your food as fuel. If you are eating too much of one macronutrient and not enough of another, there could be consequences ranging from excess calorie intake and increased body fat to not having adequate energy for workouts, to not taking in enough vitamins and minerals that help your body repair after a workout. And beyond your training, your overall health can suffer if you're not getting enough of a certain macronutrient.

Macronutrients are the three main nutrients in your diet. They comprise the calories (or energy) that you consume and fall into three categories: **protein**, **carbohydrates**, and **fat**. Each of these supplies its own unique benefits, which is why each macronutrient comes with its own general recommendations. Once they have been digested, absorbed by the intestines, transmitted into the bloodstream, and then metabolized by the liver, macronutrients fuel many specialized biological functions.

Protein
- Aids growth (especially important for children, teens, and pregnant women)
- Encourages tissue repair
- Strengthens immune function
- Makes essential hormones and enzymes
- Provides energy when carbohydrates are not available
- Preserves lean muscle mass

Carbohydrates
- Provide fuel for the body (all of the tissues and cells in our body can use glucose, a component of many carbohydrates, for energy)
- Are necessary for the functioning of the central nervous system, kidneys, brain, and muscles (including the heart)
- Can be stored in the muscles and liver and later used for energy
- Are important in intestinal health and waste elimination

Fat
- Assists normal growth and development
- Provides energy (fat is the most concentrated source we have)
- Encourages the absorption of certain vitamins (such as vitamins A, D, E, and K and carotenoids, or "fat-soluble vitamins")
- Provides cushioning for the organs
- Maintains cell membranes
- Contributes to the taste, consistency, and shelf stability of foods[4]

Micronutrients: Small but Mighty

Even though macronutrients are usually the star of the show when we talk about the makeup of a diet, we can't overlook the absolute power of micronutrients, the vitamins and minerals that provide the deep nutrition delivered by plants. Micronutrients are essential to keeping our bodies healthy. They play a vital role in energy production, immune function, protection of the body from oxidative damage and stress, creation of neurotransmitters, and generation and repair of muscles, tendons, ligaments, and cartilage. These vitamins and minerals keep our blood oxygenated, our bones strong, and our electrolytes replenished— all integral components of excelling in physical fitness.

Since our bodies can't make most micronutrients, it is crucial that we get them from our diet. There are some exceptions, such as vitamins D and B_{12}, which often need to be supplemented regardless of whether or not you're eating a plant-based diet (more on this in chapter 6). All other micronutrients should come from the foods we eat. However, while it's good to know where these sources of nutrition come from naturally, in order to make a conscious effort to consume the foods that provide the most nutrition (e.g., kale versus iceberg lettuce or potatoes versus potato chips), you're never going to set out to hit your individual vitamin and mineral levels for the day. Instead, eating a wide variety of plant-based foods helps ensure that you're getting adequate nutrition, including a diversity of micronutrients. The goal is not to think about vitamin C when eating fruits, or B_2 when eating leafy greens, or B_7 when eating sweet potatoes, or any other vitamin or mineral as we eat specific foods known to contain them.

Unless you have a medical condition that requires it, there is simply no need to consume 1,000 percent of your recommended daily allowance (RDA) of a specific micronutrient. You wouldn't easily find numbers of that scale in nature, and there is rarely ever a need for such an extreme level of consumption. So be wary of the thousands of food products that have isolated nutrients injected into them in order to reach RDA scores in the hundreds or even thousands of percent. Rather, a balanced diet of fruits, vegetables, nuts, grains, seeds, and legumes will provide sufficient micronutrient diversity and quantities, assuming you have adequate calorie intake; more on that in a moment. (Note: For as rich as a plant-based diet is in most nutrients, certain vitamins and minerals, most notably vitamin B_{12}, are hard to get from plants. We'll cover supplementation options in chapter 6.)

Plant-Based Sources of Water-Soluble Vitamins

Vitamin B_1: soy milk, watermelon, acorn squash

Vitamin B_2: whole and enriched grains and cereals

Vitamin B_3: fortified and whole grains, mushrooms, potatoes

Vitamin B_5: whole grains, broccoli, avocados, mushrooms

Vitamin B_6: legumes, tofu, bananas

Vitamin B_7: whole grains, soybeans

Vitamin B_9: asparagus, spinach, black-eyed peas

Vitamin C: citrus fruit, potatoes, bell peppers, tomatoes

Plant-Based Sources of Fat-Soluble Vitamins

Vitamin A: sweet potatoes, carrots, mangoes

Vitamin E: leafy green vegetables, nuts

Vitamin K_1: kale, spinach, broccoli, asparagus, green beans

Plant-Based Sources of Major Minerals

Calcium: leafy green vegetables

Chloride: salt

Magnesium: spinach, broccoli, legumes, seeds

Potassium: fruits, vegetables, grains, legumes

Sodium: salt, soy sauce, vegetables

Plant-Based Sources of Trace Minerals

Chromium: nuts

Copper: nuts, seeds, whole grains, beans, prunes

Fluoride: teas
Iodine: iodized salt
Iron: fruits, green vegetables
Manganese: nuts, legumes, whole grains, teas
Selenium: Brazil nuts
Zinc: legumes, whole grains

Calorie Density

Let's set aside micronutrients for a moment and swing back to the macros. We'll look at what it means to eat carbohydrates versus fat versus protein in a bit, but for now, we're going to use them as the foundation for understanding a just-as-crucial piece of nutrition: **calorie density**.

Calorie density is the *number of calories a food item contains per unit of measurement*—calories per gram, calories per pound, calories per serving, and so forth. The calorie density of foods that you most likely have in your fridge or pantry varies widely—nonstarchy vegetables (spinach, kale, green beans, cauliflower, broccoli, and so on) are significantly lower than options such as oils, other processed foods, and, especially, animal-based foods.

Calorie density is a measure of the macronutrient content of a given food, because different macronutrients have different calorie densities. Here's how it breaks down:

Fat: 9 calories per gram
Alcohol: 7 calories per gram
Protein: 4 calories per gram
Carbohydrates: 4 calories per gram

You can see that a food high in fat will be more calorie dense than a food high in carbohydrates, which is why a serving of peanut butter contains far more calories than a serving of lettuce of the same size. This is also why junk foods are more calorie dense than fruit: they are loaded with fat, oils, and other processed ingredients that boost their total calories per serving. Calorie density also has a dramatic impact on satiety—how full you feel after you eat. Your stomach has stretch receptors to let it know that a certain volume of food has been consumed. But calorie-rich, low-volume foods, such as oil—at 4,000 calories per pound of pure fat—take up very little space in your stomach and don't signal to your brain that your stomach is "full." As a result, you eat more to feel satisfied, leading to overconsumption of calories. Alternatively, eating foods that are high in volume but low in calories, such as cruciferous vegetables, fruits, and legumes, will fill up your stomach—not to mention deliver high levels of nutrients—even though you have consumed a smaller amount of calories.

Here's a list of calorie density for common food groups:

Food Calorie Density Chart
Vegetables: 200 calories per pound
Fruits: 300 calories per pound
Unrefined complex carbohydrates: 500 calories per pound
Legumes: 600 calories per pound
Animal protein: 1,000 calories per pound
Refined carbohydrates: 1,400 calories per pound
Junk food: 2,300 calories per pound
Nuts and seeds: 2,800 calories per pound
Oils and other pure fats: 4,000 calories per pound

There are a few reasons why this is important.

- Understanding calorie density means that you won't over- or undereat. If you require 3,000 calories a day to maintain your current ideal weight but are eating whatever you feel like without regard for calorie density, chances are you're going to either overshoot that number and gain weight over time or undershoot and lose weight over time (which prevents you from building quality muscle).

- Calorie density sheds light on just how much food you can get away with eating when you're sticking with plant-based options. For example, you're going to get a lot more caloric mileage out of a huge bowl of grains, greens, and beans than you are out of a steak. And since you'll ultimately be aiming to eat a mostly carbohydrate diet (which we'll get to in chapter 4), that means rarely feeling deprived while also hitting your intake goals—no matter how frequently you need to fuel throughout the day.

- Calorie density plays a practical role in your meal planning because it helps you compare one food with another given the same serving size. For example, from a calorie-density perspective, 16 ounces of fruit is far different from 16 ounces of nuts. (As you saw in the preceding chart, the fruit contains about 300 calories, while the nuts pack *2,800* calories.) That's why we'll also talk about how to strategically build a meal so that you can still enjoy more calorie-dense foods without their needing to take up the majority of your plate.

Label Libel

It's particularly important to know the calorie density per gram of macronutrients when reading food labels. For example, when looking at the back of an energy or protein bar package, you may read something like "7 g fat." That may not mean a whole lot to you, but if you know that fat is 9 calories per gram, and can do some quick math, you'll recognize that the 200-calorie "protein bar" or "energy bar" could just as aptly be called a "fat bar," since nearly one-third of its calories are coming from fat, while the rest of the calories are split between carbohydrates and protein. Furthermore, this "protein bar" could have 12 grams of protein, which may sound sufficient, but also contain 30 grams of carbohydrates. And since you know that protein and carbohydrates both contain 4 calories per gram, you will instantly realize you are not eating a protein bar; you have been marketed a carbohydrate bar in a protein bar's clothing.

Similarly, if you see a cooking spray that is composed of 100 percent fat but claims to be fat-free, it is cause for a pause and raise of the eyebrow. A deeper dig may reveal that the serving size is a "one-third-of-a-second spray," which is essentially impossible to perform. And since the serving size is so low, it is not subject to the same food-labeling standards as larger serving sizes are. Therefore, you could load up a pan for some stir-fried vegetables thinking you are putting a fat-free spray all over your food, only to realize that 100 percent of the calories added are indeed from fat, at 9 calories per gram.

Calorie Density at a Glance

Let's take a look at the calorie density of common foods.

High Calorie Density	Medium Calorie Density	Low Calorie Density
1,400–4,000 cal./lb.	350–750 cal./lb.	100–300 cal./lb.
Oils	Lentils	Kale
Processed foods	Kidney beans	Spinach
Almonds	Chickpeas	Broccoli
Walnuts	Pinto beans	Carrots
Cashews	Black beans	Cauliflower
Peanut butter	Brown rice	Peas
Almond butter	Split peas	Mangoes
Cashew butter	Potatoes	Bananas
Sunflower butter	Sweet potatoes	Blueberries
Pumpkin seeds	Yams	Strawberries
Hempseeds	Tofu	Cherries
Sunflower seeds	Tempeh	Apples
Sesame seeds	Oats	Oranges

Calorie Density Versus Nutrient Density

It's important to note that calorie density and *nutrient* density are completely different things. Calorie density measures how many calories a food or beverage contains in a unit of measurement, while nutrient density is about how many nutrients per calorie a food or beverage contains. For example, vegetable oil provides 4,000 calories per pound, making it (along with all oils and pure fat sources) the most calorie-dense food on the planet, but it has very little nutrient density (nutrition per calorie). Conversely, a vegetable such as kale—at only about 100 calories per pound—is incredibly low in calorie density but has the highest level of nutrients per calorie of any food, making it far more nutrient dense and a much better nutritional return on investment than oil in terms of your health.

With such a big impact on your health, it's clear that calorie and nutrient density should play a large role in your meal planning. Let's start with dispelling a very common misconception: the fact that a food has lots of calories does not mean it should be the centerpiece of your plate. As established, oils and other forms of pure fat are the most calorie-dense foods available, but you shouldn't plan your dinner around a bowl of olive oil. You would also not plan your dinner around sesame seeds, even though they are a food, because they're so calorie dense. Instead, choose a hearty, less calorie-dense option around which to build a meal—such as oats, beans, tofu, tempeh, potatoes, brown rice, lentils, or yams. The lower calorie density of these foods will allow you to enjoy a substantial *volume* of these foods without exceeding your calorie considerations.

The point here is that some foods are great for anchoring a meal, while others are better as accessories (side dishes) and still others as ancillaries (condiments to be drizzled, sprinkled, and dabbed on top). The role each food plays in your meal planning should be informed primarily by its calorie and nutrient density.

Here are some examples of mains, sides, and condiment foods. We've included the full list on page 153.

Mains	Sides	Condiments
Legumes	**Greens**	**Herbs**
Lentils	Kale	Basil
Pinto beans	Spinach	Thyme
Chickpeas	Romaine lettuce	Dill
Black beans	Swiss chard	Oregano
Kidney beans	Arugula	Parsley

Grains	Cruciferous vegetables	Spices
Rice	Broccoli	Turmeric
Quinoa	Cauliflower	Cinnamon
Wheat	Cabbage	Black pepper
Barley	Brussels sprouts	Ginger
Oats	Radishes	Peppermint
Millet	Turnips	Nutmeg

Starchy Vegetables	Nonstarchy Vegetables	Seeds
Potatoes	Carrots	Flaxseeds
Sweet potatoes	Asparagus	Sesame seeds
Plantains	Eggplant	Hempseeds
Butternut squash	Peppers	Sunflower seeds
Acorn squash	Cucumber	Pumpkin seeds
Yams	Green beans	Chia seeds
Parsnips	Mushrooms	Pomegranate seeds
Corn	Zucchini	Poppy seeds
Cassava	Onions	Watermelon seeds

Heavy Proteins	High Water-Content Fruits	Nuts
Tofu	Watermelon	Cashews
Tempeh	Berries	Almonds
Seitan (vital wheat gluten)	Oranges	Walnuts
Nut butters	Cantaloupe	Pistachios
Seed butters	Grapefruit	Hazelnuts
Textured Vegetable Protein (TVP)	Pineapple	Pecans
Soy foods	Peaches	Brazil nuts

Dense Fruits	Condiments
Avocados	Salsas
Bananas	Dressings
Jackfruit	Hummus
Plums	Guacamole
Apricots	Ketchup
Persimmons	Mustard
Pears	Tahini
Papayas	Jams

Common Snacks	Common Beverages
Crackers	Nondairy milks
Applesauce	Fruit or vegetable juice
Trail mix	Coffee
Granola	Tea
Dried fruit	Coconut water
Snack/energy/protein bars	Sparkling water
Energy gels/chews	Freshly squeezed juice
Rice cakes	Dairy-free kefir
Dairy-free yogurt	Fermented drink (kombucha)

From a nutritional perspective, the basic objective for each of your meals is to include one or two foods from each category, such as a burrito bowl with rice, beans, avocado, lettuce, and tomato. Then you can add big-flavor ingredients (especially herbs, spices, and condiments) to bring your meal to life. In chapter 7, we'll go into more detail about how to build a successful meal plan based on your true calorie needs. That way, you'll know what to load up your oatmeal with, which ingredients to toss into a green smoothie, or how to assemble a balanced bowl or wrap. (Our recipes in chapter 11 are another great place to go for guidance.) But the bottom line is: so long as there are optimal calories represented in your meal (which our calorie density system is designed to help with), in addition to snacks and beverages consumed throughout the day, then it's going to deliver adequate nutritional benefits.

Now let's bring this conversation back to macronutrients. While on one hand they help to explain calorie density (carbohydrates and plant-based proteins are lower in calories, while fats are higher), macronutrients are the *nutritional* building blocks of your diet—which we'd argue is a healthier, more sustainable way of looking at your food (versus just considering the calories).

As you saw earlier with the "main," "side," and "condiment" foods, you could eat 3,000 calories a day's worth of fat, but you'd be consistently hungry because the serving size for that amount of calories is relatively small and would not sufficiently fill your stomach. It's also important to know that fat is a secondary energy source, behind carbohydrates, the body's preferred energy source. Though fat is a very concentrated source of energy and can be used when carbohydrate are not available, the body wants to run on carbohydrate fuel as often as possible. So eliminating that entire macronutrient group would be leaving your body without its preferred energy source, as well as all the vitamins, minerals, antioxidants, fiber, and water it provides. The same goes for consuming exclusively high protein as a source for energy and nourishment—a controversial fact to be sure, since high-protein diets tend to be popular among certain communities, but protein is the least efficient source of energy of all macronutrients, and one we'll unpack in greater detail in chapter 3. That's not to say that any one macronutrient is bad—as you read earlier, they're all essential. But knowing how to use each one as you would a tool in your toolbox (or an iron in your golf bag) and combining that with your knowledge of calorie and nutrient density is the difference between eating a diet that simply doesn't include animal-based foods (ignoring other aspects of health) and eating one that truly harnesses the power of plants. Over the next few chapters, we'll spend some time looking at carbohydrates, protein, and fat and what they contribute to your diet, as well as how to build meals that perfectly highlight their unique benefits.

Macronutrient Cheat Sheet

Worried about nailing your macros on a plant-based diet? Worry no more! We've put together a Macronutrient Cheat Sheet, complete with macronutrient breakdowns for 80 of our favorite plant-based foods, along with simple meal blueprints you can use to build easy meals that hit your numbers. Download it at No Meat Athlete (nomeatathlete.com/book-bonus) to get started now.

• • • • •

Eating a plant-based diet has improved my ability to read labels and understand what's in my food. I've learned to maintain my weight with ease, and it has given me tons of energy. I spend less energy cutting weight and more energy working on knocking people out!
—**Cam Awesome, US amateur boxing champion**

People questioned my choice to eat plant-based, but they never questioned the fact that I had more energy than most anyone else they knew. I learned in the early years to stop trying to educate people on my decision and to simply lead by example. When you are healthy, fit, active, and thriving, people want to know what you are doing right.
—**Seychelle Webster, world-class stand-up paddleboarder and coach**

My strength and endurance improved immediately when I switched to a plant-based diet while playing in the National Hockey League. I even did medical testing with a doctor the day I decided to become vegan, and six months after adopting a plant-based diet, my strength, endurance, blood levels, and everything were much better. I never looked back.
—**Georges Laraque, former NHL hockey player**

I have more energy now than twenty years ago, when I first went from vegetarian to vegan. I no longer bonk in the middle of the day. My mental energy has also increased, which comes in handy when the races require intense concentration, such as a high-intensity cyclo-cross or when I need to be extremely aware of micromovements in the Peloton during a road race for up to five hours straight.
—**Christine Vardaros, professional cyclist**

IT'S TIME TO HAVE THE PROTEIN TALK

Having broadly covered macronutrients and unpacked calorie density, it's now time to figure out how exactly to divide all those calories you consume in a day among the macros. And of the three macros, it's fair to say that protein is usually foremost on the mind of nearly every athlete, particularly those who are plant-based. After all, the most common question every vegan—especially an athlete—gets asked is "But how will you get enough protein?"

There are literally hundreds of thousands (if not millions) of plant-based athletes—which we know just by scrolling through social media platforms—who go about their day eating their favorite foods in the right calorie ratios, completely unfettered by concerns about protein needs. One of those athletes is former NFL football player **David Carter**. David played for five teams in the NFL over the course of four years, and even though he was only in his midtwenties at the time, the wear and tear of being a 300-pound defensive lineman was taking a toll. His pain had become so severe that he'd started losing feeling in his hands and fingers, and there were some days when he could barely push himself out of the bathtub because of the pain in his elbows. He relied on pain medication to keep playing. In search of a solution, he watched the groundbreaking documentary *Forks Over Knives*, which examines the claim that most, if not all, degenerative diseases can be controlled or even reversed by eliminating animal-based and processed foods from one's diet. David poured out his milkshake and went vegan overnight. When he learned that consuming dairy products can contribute to tendinitis, one of his chief complaints, it was a wake-up call he desperately needed. Add cheese to the six double hamburgers he could eat in a single meal, and staples such as chicken breasts and pork chops, and you get a fairly typical NFL diet, which left his body ravaged with inflammation, excess body fat, and high blood pressure—as a twenty-five-year-old star athlete.

David's overnight transition to a plant-based diet produced immediate measurable results. In the first month, he dropped 40 pounds. And within two months, all his pain went away. He became stronger and faster than ever before, and he shared his amazing results with teammates who were intrigued by his new diet and newfound boost in athletic performance. With his lighter frame, he was faster, running longer distances, and pain free. But as a defensive lineman in the NFL, he needed to maintain a body mass of roughly 300 pounds. So he enlisted the help of some vegan bodybuilding coaches, who created a 10,000-calorie plant-based meal plan for him, and he was able to bulk back up to 300 pounds, fueled entirely by plants. Even after regaining the weight, he was leaner, faster, and stronger than he had ever been when eating animal protein all day long for years.

To gain and maintain his optimal body mass, David put a strong emphasis on consuming large quantities of plant-based protein, up to 1.2 grams per pound of body weight per day, which added up to a whopping *360 grams* of protein each day. Instead of getting that from cheeseburgers, he made protein shakes using white beans as the base, with added fruit for color and flavor. He loaded up on rice and beans, oats, cashews (especially cashew cheese, his favorite), greens, and lots of fruit. Eating every two hours, grazing between meals, and being prepared by making large batches of smoothies to drink throughout the day enabled him to amass an astonishing 10,000-calorie intake as a plant-based athlete.

When David retired from the NFL, he no longer needed to maintain the often unhealthy and unsustainable mass of 300 pounds in body weight. Once again, he adjusted the ratio of foods he was eating along with his calorie intake, and he dropped 40 pounds fairly quickly. He still trains hard and maintains an even more efficient athletic body than he had in his days in the NFL, even though he still loves comfort food—but these days, it's chickpea burgers, cashew mac and cheese, and plant-based protein waffles. David's passion for the diet that helped prolong his career and ultimately saved his life is palpable. And as a result, he has dedicated his life to educating athletes—especially in minority groups—about the benefits of a plant-based diet.

David isn't alone in exemplifying how an athlete who needs mass, strength, and speed can get enough protein from plants. Nearly a decade before David began his plant-based journey, the greatest tight end in NFL history, **Tony Gonzalez**, went through a similar transformation. Like David, he initially lost weight quickly, dropping fifteen pounds in a matter of weeks. Though Tony was a strict vegan for only about a month, he followed a plant-centered diet for years, and he credits this diet with prolonging his career by *seven* years. **Arian Foster** was another NFL star who adopted a plant-based diet during his prime, leaving animals off his plate even when he needed to fuel one of football's toughest positions. He went on to be the number one running back in the league the next season, leading in rushing attempts and rushing touchdowns. **Derrick Morgan** of the NFL's Tennessee Titans adopted a plant-based diet, inspiring his defensive line and ten other players on the team to do the same. In 2017, they powered their way into the playoffs for the first time in a decade. **Griff Whalen** played his final seasons in the NFL on a purely plant-based diet as a wide receiver for multiple teams, including four seasons with the Indianapolis Colts. **Cam Newton**'s revitalized and rejuvenated career came on the heels of a switch to a plant-based diet to overcome injuries and boost his recovery and performance. The former NFL MVP is probably the most outspoken plant-based football player in the league today. If NFL players such as these can get enough plant protein in their diet, it's a pretty good bet that you can too.

But in case you're not convinced that plants can fuel serious muscle gains, consider **Jehina Malik**, a professional bodybuilder and a vegan since birth. Becoming a pro bodybuilder is hard enough as it is—there's an immense pressure to both put on and maintain a significant amount of lean muscle of a specific size and shape. Some athletes believe the solution is piling on the animal protein, eating up to six chickens and dozens of eggs per day. Many rely on anabolic drugs such as steroids and hormones. Enter Jehina.

As Jehina likes to say, "My five siblings and I have all been vegan since the womb." (In fact, it's worth noting that all of Jehina's siblings are athletes.) She grew up onstage, performing in dance recitals from the time she was three. But when she first started sharing with people that she wanted to be a professional bodybuilder, she got laughed at. People said it wasn't possible for her to achieve that kind of muscle without eating meat. But year after year, she trained hard, and eventually she starting winning shows. In 2014, she made history as the first vegan-since-birth International Federation of Bodybuilding and Fitness (IFBB) pro. "I shut everyone up when I earned an IFBB pro card in my first national show! I let the work do all the talking. Now who gets the last laugh?"

Naturally, some of the most common questions Jehina gets about her vegan bodybuilding lifestyle revolve around what she eats, whether she cooks, what kind of supplements she takes, and how she gets enough protein to fuel a plant-based professional bodybuilding career. Jehina says protein is very important for a bodybuilder, but she never worries about how much she gets because "protein is in everything," and she eats throughout the day, aware of her intake. She also points out that these days, it's a lot easier to reach her protein goals because, thanks to growing market demand for nutrient-dense plant-based foods, she has plenty of delicious options, whether she's cooking or buying something premade. Some of her favorites are plant-based burgers and sausages, vegan chicken, vegan pho, plant-based protein drinks and protein cookies, and, of course, whole-plant foods such as oats, cashews, sautéed kale, salad greens, vegetables, fruits, and nuts. She takes some supplements as well, uses a sauna to relax and stretch, and follows a typical bodybuilding training routine.

But what makes Jehina feel that the work has paid off—perhaps as much as her national titles—are all the mothers who reach out to let her know that they are raising their children vegan because of her, as well as the other athletes she's inspired to adopt a plant-based diet. She feels honored knowing that she can make a difference and have a positive impact on people's lives.

Okay, so it's pretty clear that plants have strength athletes covered in the protein department, but what about endurance athletes? Meet **Mary Schneider**. Mary is a long-distance runner who qualified for the 2020 United States Olympic Trials in the marathon, with a personal best time of 2:42:01 (which is a scorching 6-minute, 11-second mile pace for 26.2 miles). She has been a key member of the Prado Racing Team in San Diego, California, and has won races across the country. But Mary wasn't always a plant-based athlete. And she didn't always feel all that well, even as a competitive athlete. She had chronically low iron levels her whole life, typically falling barely within the parameters that are considered normal, and significantly lower than optimum for athletic performance. That changed dramatically after she adopted a plant-based diet—a fact that shocks people, mainly because iron is associated with red meat. Two months before she adopted a plant-based diet, Mary's iron levels were 46 micrograms per deciliter (mcg/dL); normal is 40 to 190 mcg/dL. She would get so fatigued that she couldn't work out and train as regularly as she wanted to. In fact, some days, she just couldn't train at all because of soreness and feeling worn out. It got to the point where she was training and racing in a state of chronic fatigue.

When Mary switched to a plant-based diet, she was hyperfixated on protein because she was used to eating a meat-heavy diet. Some type of meat would be the centerpiece of each meal, accompanied by starchy carbohydrates or vegetables as a side. She worried about the clichéd question anyone who has ever adopted a plant-based diet has heard ad nauseam: "Where do you get your protein?" Those concerns were reinforced by her low iron levels. But after just four months on a plant-based diet, her iron levels had almost doubled, to 76 mcg/dL. And it wasn't just the blood work results that confirmed she had made an improvement; she had also started noticing some fairly significant changes in her body. Before she chose to stop eating animal products, she would get knots in her legs, but that completely dissipated. And far from not having enough energy because of the perceived lack of protein, Mary had *more* energy on a plant-based diet. Before adopting a plant-based diet, she felt lethargic after meals and "needed an afternoon nap or coffee to get through the day." But with her new diet, she had high energy consistently throughout the day. Even after an especially long, hard workout or race (including a marathon), she didn't need to spend the remainder of the day recovering on the couch. The change had been *that* profound and impactful for her. Mary also credits a plant-based diet for her substantially improved recovery time. In her own words, "I used to be sore for days after a workout. Now, the vast majority of the time, I feel completely recovered later that day or by the next morning. After a marathon, I am not sore and fatigued for weeks (like I used to be), but only for a few days—if that." She is able to run more miles during training, run more quickly than ever before, and race more often because her recovery is more efficient. Mary also noticed that she was able to change her body composition after changing her diet, putting on more muscle and decreasing her body fat without consciously making the effort to do so.

What she learned firsthand is what we'll be unpacking in this chapter: protein is found in almost all plant foods, and it adds up throughout the day. So a diet high in carbohydrates will still deliver that protein while also keeping the body's tank topped off with plenty of fuel. These days,

Mary powers her long-distance training and competitive marathons with plenty of carbohydrates, though she makes sure to include foods that are known for their substantial protein content—beans, lentils, tofu, and tempeh. To sum up her plant-based running success, Mary puts it this way: "I used to have people question me as to whether this was a way of eating that was sustainable long-term. I put myself out there as an example of a plant-based athlete competing at a high level, and I know people were watching to see how I would do, and if I could excel while eating this way. After racing five marathons within fourteen months, running personal bests in four out of the five, and placing fifty-first in the United States at the Olympic Trials Women's Marathon in February 2020, with no injuries or chronic fatigue during that time, the critics and skeptics have stopped."

What we hope you take away from these examples is that whether you are a strength athlete, an endurance athlete, a recreational athlete, or a weekend warrior, consuming adequate protein on a plant-based diet is an easily attainable goal. And plant protein is in no way inferior to animal protein when it comes to delivering nutrients or building muscle. There's a lot of baggage that comes along with animal protein—cholesterol, excess calories, carcinogens, lack of fiber, and saturated fat, not to mention the devastating environmental impacts and cruelty concerns. Instead, you can go straight to the source of amino acids in their plant form, reaping all the nutrients and benefits that come with them.

The Protein Basics: Plant Versus Animal

While most people ask, "Am I getting enough protein?"—which we'll definitely address—we think the better question to address first is "Why are we so obsessed with protein?" Let's finally break it down.

As we've already established, protein is a macronutrient made up of 4 calories per gram that plays an important role in building and repairing muscle tissue and making essential hormones and enzymes, and it is involved in preserving lean muscle mass and aiding immune function. Its primary function is related to growth, from infancy to childhood through adulthood, and muscle maintenance and repair after exercise. *But even though protein is absolutely important, it is dramatically overhyped.*

Huge numbers of athletes, including those who have lots of body mass to begin with, fear that they will shrivel up and die if they don't consume "enough" protein, and as a result they are constantly in search of it—in the form of animal products, protein drinks, and foods supplemented with additional protein. Then there are the millions of people who do no additional exercise beyond their sedentary lifestyle but also consume protein drinks and bars for "health" because that's what marketers and advertisers have told them to do. And on top of that, you have the fearmongering that uninformed health-care professionals have perpetuated—promoting the idea that someone on a plant-based diet just won't get enough of the stuff.

Why did we develop an obsession with protein, particularly animal protein and protein isolates? (Protein isolates are supplements or foods that have had carbohydrates, fats, and often fiber and water removed to isolate a specific nutrient for concentrated consumption, in this case protein.) As is often the case with health-related fads, the answer is in marketing and advertising. If there is money in it, people will find a way to exploit a claim and get customers hooked on the idea of necessity. In this way, protein and meat companies often resemble alcohol, tobacco, and pharmaceutical companies, making use of clever and effective strategies to convince populations, often from childhood, that their products are not only desirable but *required* for health, even if that is not actually the case.

Meat and animal products became synonymous with health and fitness during the rise of widespread television viewing in the 1930s. That coincided with expanded farming efforts and marketing of animal-based food products to consumers by any means necessary. After viewing ads positioning meat as healthy, manly, and essential, Americans—and citizens of many other nations around the world—

turned to meat, milk, and eggs for nourishment. It soon became the norm to consume large quantities of animal protein, from bacon and eggs at breakfast to a roast beef, ham, or turkey sandwich at lunch to steak and potatoes for dinner.

In the world of sports, animal-based protein really took off in the 1970s, when sports-nutrition-related products were coming of age, particularly those targeted at bodybuilders. The milk proteins casein and whey—which would otherwise have been wasted by-products of cheese making—were extracted, powdered into isolated protein supplements, and marketed to athletes as the magical protein solution. When Joe Weider and Arnold Schwarzenegger put bodybuilding on the map in the 1970s with their muscle magazine covers and advertisements for casein and whey supplements, consumers bought in and created what is now a multibillion-dollar sports nutrition industry. Protein powders led to protein bars and meal-replacement powders, branched-chain amino acid powders, essential fatty acids, and many, many more supplements that are now available not just in "health food" stores but in supermarkets around the world. A rapidly increasing number of products with different blends, formulas, and promises fed the collective desire to achieve the muscle mass, strength, and athletic prowess portrayed in advertisements and modeled by athletes who were vocal spokespeople for these products. Already protein-obsessed Americans couldn't get enough, and as a result, high-protein diets, particularly those high in animal proteins, became as American as apple pie. And here we are today—with fat and carbohydrates each having undergone periods during which they were villainized as the cause of our health problems—still obsessed with protein, trying to find more of it anywhere we can.

But here's the deal: *not only do you not need that much protein, but you also can get everything you need from plants.* We'll get into the specifics later in the chapter about how to make sure you're getting a healthy amount of protein, but to put it into context, consider this: consensus among nutrition experts, dietitians, and sports scientists is that it is advised—for both men and women—to consume **0.8 grams of protein**

per kilogram of body weight (or 0.8 grams per 0.36 pound of body weight)—which comes out to **56 grams per day for men engaged in modest physical activity** and **46 grams per day for women engaged in modest physical activity**. That's really not a whole lot of protein, especially when many protein drinks contain 20 to 30 grams of protein per serving. Combined with just a small amount of additional calories, a protein drink and a little food would hit your entire daily protein requirements if you're not active. While these numbers are higher for active individuals, they don't differ that dramatically.

Now stay with us for just a little math. There are 20 different amino acids that combine to form proteins. Your body can make 11 of them (called nonessential amino acids), which means it needs to get the 9 essential amino acids from your diet. And you can obtain all 9 by eating a variety of plant foods. In fact, *all plant proteins have, in various amounts, some of each and every essential amino acid*. And your body, being the amazing machine that it is, does the work of making "complete" proteins for you as you hand it the raw materials throughout the day. So your oats in the morning, salad at lunch, and legumes at dinner all collectively provide the protein that you need. That's why **there is no specific nutritional requirement to consume protein from animals or animal-based foods such as meat, milk, and eggs—or a need to get it from supplements**—*because the amino acids that form proteins are found in all plant foods to begin with*.

A recent study published in the *American Journal of Clinical Nutrition* compared the muscle mass and strength of 2,986 men and women between nineteen and seventy-two years of age who ate a plant-based diet with that of omnivores. They found that as long as people were eating enough protein, it didn't matter whether it was plant- or animal-based.[1] But a study by the National Center for Biotechnology Information found that instead of focusing on increasing overall protein consumption, simply increasing the number of calories consumed in a day from plant-based sources was enough to satisfy the protein needs of 97 percent of their cases. The researchers concluded that vegan and vegetarian athletes should concentrate on increasing calories when required, thereby hitting their optimal protein intake.[2]

Okay, so you know that you don't need as much protein as you might have thought. And you know that you can get enough protein from plants. But before we get into how to put that to work in your daily diet, we want to unpack not just why plants have your back when it comes to your health and training but also how animal proteins really don't.

Animal Protein Does Not Do a Body Good

We now know that the consumption of animal protein can be associated with many of the top killers of Americans, from obesity and diabetes to hypertension and organ failure. In fact, the number one killer of Americans is heart disease, which is directly linked to a diet rich in animal protein, including meat, milk, and eggs, and the often large amounts of dietary cholesterol (which is found only in animal-based foods) and saturated fat they bring with them. That is because of how dietary cholesterol and animal fat create plaque buildup in arteries, which restricts blood flow to vital organs. This decreased blood flow is what leads to conditions such as erectile dysfunction, heart disease, heart attack, and stroke. And, as you can imagine, it's also going to work against you as an athlete because proper circulation and blood flow are required for optimal endurance, strength, and recovery.

And then there's the issue of inflammation and oxidative stress. Inflammation isn't necessarily a bad thing; in fact, it's a useful tool that your immune system uses to help combat outside invaders. However, when your immune system is repeatedly triggered by "alerts" that it's under attack, that leads to constant or chronic inflammation. This is essentially a state in which your body is attacking itself and, as a result, creating damage to your tissues—or oxidative stress. Inflammation can be caused by a number of things and can be short-term (acute) or long-term (chronic). Infection and injury typically create acute inflammation, while repeated exposure to irritants, most notably stress, as well as certain foods, causes chronic inflammation. And studies have definitely linked the consumption of red meat and processed meat with an increase in inflammation and oxidative stress.[3] The consequence of chronic inflammation is stark: it is the most significant cause of death in the world today. It is the underlying culprit behind obesity and asthma, and 50 percent of all deaths can be linked to inflammation-related diseases, such as heart disease, stroke, cancer, diabetes, chronic kidney disease, and nonalcoholic fatty liver disease, and autoimmune and neurodegenerative conditions such as Alzheimer's disease.[4] On the less severe end of the spectrum—though no less relevant to an athlete—you have the impact of inflammation and oxidative stress on your training. Namely, the more you exercise, the more difficult it is to recover, and the more downtime you'll need between workouts—something we'll explore in more detail in chapter 8.

Understanding Inflammation

Inflammation is the foundation of the body's healing response because it brings nourishment and immune system activity to a site of injury or infection. In many cases, inflammation is beneficial and essential for healing. The problem arises when inflammation stops serving a purpose and becomes chronic or delays recovery. Our modern lifestyles present many potential inflammatory triggers, such as environmental toxins, cigarette smoking, carrying excess weight, chronic stress, poor sleep, being sedentary . . . and our diets.

—Linda Plowright, MD, integrative practitioner

Most foods can be considered more or less pro-inflammatory or anti-inflammatory on the basis of their composition. The goal is to make changes to our diet to decrease pro-inflammatory foods and emphasize anti-inflammatory foods. The standard American diet is exceedingly high in pro-inflammatory foods. For example:

- It often has an unhealthy ratio of omega fatty acids, with a high intake of omega-6 fatty acids. Our bodies synthesize hormones from omega-6 fatty acids that promote inflammation, whereas omega-3 fatty acids tend to be more anti-inflammatory.

- As opposed to a whole-foods plant-based diet, which centers on foods that have a lower glycemic index, the standard American diet contains an abundance of foods that are high on the glycemic index, consumption of which leads to a sharp rise in blood sugar. This causes abnormal reactions between sugar and proteins in the body, called glycation reactions, which produce pro-inflammatory compounds called advanced glycation end products. These compounds can damage DNA, disrupt cell membranes, and promote the aging process.
- Animal-based foods (meat, dairy products, and eggs) are considered pro-inflammatory, especially when they come from an animal that has been fed an unnatural, grain-rich diet, because this results in the meat, dairy, or eggs being higher in inflammatory fats, especially saturated fat.

A whole-foods plant-based diet is much more anti-inflammatory and therefore better able to combat exercise-induced inflammation for many reasons, which include the following:

- The natural pigments that color fruits and vegetables have potent anti-inflammatory properties.
- Whole or cracked grains are less inflammatory because they cause a gentler rise in blood sugar.
- A whole-foods plant-based diet tends to have a better ratio of omega-6 to omega-3 fatty acids.
- A whole-foods plant-based diet tends to be higher in foods that have specific, potent anti-inflammatory antioxidants, which can reduce oxidative stress and resulting free radicals. Examples include olives, green tea, and dark chocolate; some herbs and spices, such as ginger and turmeric, especially when combined with black pepper; and cruciferous vegetables such as kale, broccoli, cauliflower, brussels sprouts, and cabbage.

We also know, thanks to many studies and the World Health Organization, that meat (especially beef, pork, and lamb) and particularly processed meat (e.g., hot dogs and lunch meats), has been linked to the development of certain cancers—particularly colorectal, pancreatic, and prostate—a link just as strong as that between smoking and lung cancer, to the point that processed meat is now classified as a Class 1 carcinogen. And researchers have discovered that not only is intake of dairy milk associated with a greater risk—up to 80 percent—of breast cancer in women,[5] but also the milk protein casein can promote the proliferation of prostate cancer cells.[6]

The connection between high consumption of animal-based food and chronic disease has been well documented in the sports world, particularly in professional football, bodybuilding, and other sports focused on body mass, in which athletes consume as much animal protein as possible in order to bulk up. These athletes consistently have the shortest life spans and, almost like clockwork, develop heart disease, cancer, diabetes, obesity, and other adverse health conditions. Many of these athletes who had a high animal protein intake, including numerous bodybuilders we have known personally, died from heart disease and organ failure in their early forties, a trend that unfortunately is pervasive across the board.

If meat is so bad for us, according to the leading health, wellness, and nutrition authorities—a fact supported by scientific studies proving the relationship between consumption of animal products and the likelihood of developing chronic disease—why isn't this a bigger topic in the public conversation?

Dr. Michael Greger, author of the bestselling book *How Not to Die*, asserts that it's because it is "normal" to eat meat. Essentially, most people eat meat because most people eat meat. It's not too much more complicated than that, but it is a bit more sinister than that when you compare the modern meat industry with the tobacco industry of a couple of generations ago. Seven thousand studies showed the relationship between smoking and the likelihood of developing lung cancer before the surgeon general reported that smoking was dangerous and could cause cancer. Why did it take seven thousand studies for anyone to take action to deter people from smoking to save lives?

Because smoking was normal. Even doctors smoked, and encouraging patients to do something they themselves were unwilling to do (quit smoking) was not a recommendation many were comfortable making. Smoking cigarettes was just part of life—in restaurants, at work, at sporting events, at home, at bars, at parties, and yes, at the doctor's office. So if we know that eating meat is generally bad for us, possibly fatal, why hasn't someone said something? Well, the World Health Organization is saying something, and it has been for years. Doctors who know the science have also been speaking up, writing books, starring in documentaries, writing and publishing papers and studies, touring, and even educating university staff and students about the dangers of consuming animal protein. The primary reasons why the plant-based (or simply no-meat) message is not penetrating the public media as a national topic of conversation are as follows:

1. Eating meat has become normalized.
2. A lot of big-business and federal money is riding on people continuing to eat meat.
3. Many people are unwilling to change their lifestyle, even if it could literally cost them their life.

That's quite a barrier, but it's something many plant-based athletes, experts, chefs, doctors, and authors have been more vocal about in recent years, and it seems now, more than ever, that it's time to get this message out to the masses.

What About Fish?

While there are some documented health benefits from eating fish (mostly involving omega-3 fatty acids), doctors who advocate a plant-based diet agree that any potential upside is far outweighed by the risks posed by animal protein in general, as well as some issues specific to seafood. Most notably, fish contain mercury, which can harm the brain, heart, kidneys, lungs, and immune system. Even though smaller fish, and seafood such as salmon, cod, shrimp, and trout, have lower levels of mercury than notorious sources such as tilefish, swordfish, mackerel, and tuna, they contain high enough levels to prompt many health-care professionals to advise against eating them. Another issue is microplastics, the remnants of plastic items deteriorating in lakes and oceans. These particles are consumed by small plankton-eating fish, which are in turn eaten by fish higher up the food chain and then by people. Ingested microplastic particles not only damage organs but also leach toxic chemicals (most notably hormone-disrupting bisphenol A, or BPA), which can compromise immune function and reproductive health.[7]

Eating farm-raised fish isn't much better because they're frequently raised with antibiotics, and studies have found that even farmed salmon had concerning levels of industrial toxins called polychlorinated biphenyls (PCBs), most likely because they were fed ground-up fish that was wild-caught.[8]

Save the World: Don't Eat Meat

It's impossible to build a complete case against meat without also talking about the negative impact it has on the planet. Aside from causing extensive harm to your body, meat is one of the biggest offenders when it comes to harming the environment—with the meat-production industry accounting for *50 percent* of global warming. This is owing mainly to livestock and their greenhouse gas emissions, the fossil fuel used and emissions generated by planes and trucks to distribute meat products, water pollution from toxic factory farm runoff, clear-cutting to make room for larger factory farms and the growing of crops to feed livestock (most notably in the Amazon rain forest, the lungs of our planet, thanks to Brazil being the world's largest beef exporter). Then there's the overwhelming amount of water that's required to raise livestock—for example, it takes 1,910 gallons of water per pound of beef to raise a cow from birth to burger, largely because of the water that is required to grow its feed.[9]

And now, we've seen in no uncertain terms that meat production is one of the main culprits behind the COVID-19 pandemic. A majority of pandemic diseases are those that have been passed from animals to humans, also called zoonotic diseases. COVID-19 isn't the first; it was preceded by the bubonic plague, Spanish flu, the Ebola virus, the human immunodeficiency virus (HIV), the H1N1 virus (swine flu), the H7N9 virus (avian flu), and the virus causing SARS, or severe acute respiratory syndrome. Unfortunately, it won't be the last. The Centers for Disease Control and Prevention (CDC) has warned that three out of four new or emerging diseases in people come from animals, and we've created the perfect conditions for this to happen. Thanks to the meat-processing industry, the global warming it creates, and the destruction of natural habitats that result from its expansion, we've forced animals to live not only in close proximity to one another but also in closer proximity to us. Before this most recent health crisis, it seemed easy to believe that this was an issue only in places such as Asia or the Amazon. But the swine flu outbreak in 2009 was a result of industrial pig farming in Iowa. And COVID-19 has shown us that these pandemics have no borders. Many experts agree that the most important change we can all make to help prevent future pandemics is to stop eating meat.

Another reason to consider not eating meat is ethical concerns. Arguments for this run the gamut from not wanting to harm living creatures for food to the fact that factory-farmed animals—those raised on industrial feedlots—have a subpar quality of life. Often these animals are crowded together, are not allowed to roam and graze, are separated from their mothers at an early age, and experience high amounts of stress.

Fortunately, there is a healthier and more sustainable alternative to a diet of animal-based food: a diet rich in plant-based whole foods. Plant-based proteins, even when consumed in large quantities, do not have the same adverse health implications as animal proteins do. These proteins—in the form of whole-plant foods, especially legumes and whole grains—are just as bioavailable as animal-based sources and come with the additional benefits of naturally occurring vitamins, minerals, antioxidants, phytonutrients, water content, and, most important, fiber, which animal protein does not contain. Also, unlike animal-based foods, which can contain anywhere from 1,000 to 2,000 calories per pound, plants hover around 200 to 600 calories per pound, meaning you can consume a higher volume of plant foods while staying within your target calorie intake. This all adds up to a food source that is not only *not* making you sick, it's actively making you *less* sick. Plants and their antioxidants fight inflammation and oxidative stress, which when combined with no longer eating animal foods, has the power to reverse certain conditions, particularly obesity, diabetes, and heart disease. As you shed excess weight, relieve your arteries and improve blood flow, flood your body with micronutrients, and quell inflammation, you'll not only perform better and recover more quickly; you'll also be able to live a longer, more satisfying life.

And more to the point: **plant proteins are just as effective as animal proteins for building strength and muscle**. A 2015 double-blind study published in the *Journal of the International Society of Sports Nutrition* found that participants taking a pea protein supplement during twelve weeks of resistance training gained just as much muscle mass as the group taking whey protein (and more muscle mass than those taking a placebo).[10] Similarly, a 2013 *Nutrition Journal* study established that a group of athletes taking rice protein over the course of eight weeks reaped the same strength and recovery benefits as the group taking whey protein and undergoing the same training regimen.[11]

So, if you can experience the same gains without the adverse effects of animal protein consumption on your health and the planet, why not pass the peas and rice?

Vegans and Paleos: Can't We All Just Get Along?

In recent years, many people have turned to a Paleo diet—one modeled after what our caveman ancestors supposedly ate—in order to make gains in the gym or lose weight. Instead of writing off those who have embraced this diet or giving you a litany of reasons why it's wrong, we want to highlight the common ground that Paleo and plant-based eating share.

The fact is, most of the foods in a typical healthy vegan diet are Paleo. Sure, the seeds are iffy. And beans and wheat products are out for Paleo. But beyond that, the foods we plant-based athletes eat could have, by and large, been eaten by a caveman. The converse is true, too. Most (yes, most) of a Paleo dieter's foods are vegan. They're whole plants, including a ton of vegetables and nuts, a fair amount of fruits, and no dairy. So it's safe to say that the healthy versions of these diets look an awful lot alike.

Here are just a few of the things we agree on:

- Vegetables are good, and organic vegetables are better.
- Nuts are good.
- Fruits are good (with some qualifications).
- Fast food is awful.
- It isn't natural or healthy for adult humans to drink milk meant for baby cows.
- Whole foods are crucial; we should eat food as close to its natural state as possible.
- Processed food is evil, and there's something very wrong with the system that is foisting it upon us.

Do you realize what a small minority these shared beliefs put us in? Those of us who avoid fast food, pass on milk, and choose whole foods versus processed are the weirdos in a world of processed food and rapidly expanding waistlines.

Even when it comes to meat—the "staple" of the Paleo diet—we think most Paleos would agree that what our factory-farm system produces, whether because of the way the animals are confined or what they're fed or what's injected into them, is not healthy.

So why the beef with one another?

We get that the ethical issues muddy things up a bit. Vegans hate that Paleos so proudly eat meat; Paleos hate that vegans try to tell them that something humans have done throughout our history is suddenly wrong.

We can argue forever over which diet is better. Guess what? Nobody is going to convince anyone to switch sides. And in the face of the chronic disease epidemic our processed-food society faces, it doesn't matter. In that way, the distinction between Paleo and vegan is completely insignificant. We both agree: *eat whole foods*. That's what will make the difference in people's health and in our food system, and it's neither Paleo nor vegan. Whole foods are both, and that common ground, along with the tremendous passion we all have for healthy eating, is something we should leverage if we want to make a real difference.

Now back to the original question: "How much protein do I actually need?"

Protein and amino acid needs are the same for women as for men, and the amount is based on body weight in kilograms. For the general adult population (ages nineteen to fifty-nine), the recommended daily allowance is 0.8 grams (g) of protein per kilogram (kg) of body weight per day.[12] So if you weigh 60 kg (132 pounds), you need 48 g of protein per day. What does that look like in real life? One cup of cooked oatmeal contains about 6 g of protein, plus a tablespoon of peanut butter is another 4 g, and ½ cup of soy milk is 4 g. That's 14 g of protein, 30 percent of your daily goal, and it's only breakfast.

For athletes, however, the recommendations look a little different.

In a 2016 joint position paper[13] on nutrition and athletic performance, the American College of Sports Medicine, the Academy of Nutrition and Dietetics, and the Dietitians of Canada recommended higher protein intakes for athletes. Current data suggest that dietary protein intake necessary to support metabolic adaptation, repair, remodeling, and for protein turnover generally ranges from 1.2–2.0 g/kg/day.

In other words, if you're a vegan endurance athlete who weighs 60 kg (132 pounds), you need roughly 70 to 120 g of protein per day. This is about 40 percent more than nonvegan nonathletes—again, not too difficult if you're eating a well-rounded diet and hitting your daily calorie goal. Furthermore, a February 2021 paper titled "High-Protein Plant-Based Diet Versus a Protein-Matched Omnivorous Diet to Support Resistance Training Adaptations: A Comparison Between Habitual Vegans and Omnivores"[14] concluded that a high-protein (1.6 g/kg/day) exclusively plant-based diet (plant-based whole foods + soy protein isolate supplementation) is not different than a protein-matched mixed diet (whole foods + whey protein supplementation) in supporting muscle strength and mass accrual. It suggests that a protein source does not affect resistance training-induced adaptations when adequate amounts of protein are consumed. But before we give you a sample menu to show what that could look like, we need to address another piece of the puzzle that will affect how you track your protein intake: lysine.

Lysine: The Limiting Amino Acid in Vegan Diets

All right, so when it comes to protein, there is one aspect in particular vegans need to consider more than others. Lysine is an essential amino acid that plays an important role in producing carnitine—a nutrient that helps convert fatty acids into energy and helps lower cholesterol. It also helps produce collagen, a fibrous protein found in bone, cartilage, and skin. Lysine is considered a limiting amino acid because plant foods generally contain only a small amount of it. So some plant-based nutritionists argue that meeting your daily lysine need is more important than meeting your overall daily protein need. That way, if you hit your lysine requirements, you'll certainly also meet your overall protein requirements.

The recommended daily allowance of lysine is 38 milligrams (mg) per kg of body weight. So if you weigh 60 kg (132 pounds), you need 2,280 mg of lysine.

Luckily, many of the plant foods that are rich in lysine are also great "mains" and would otherwise be taking up a lot of real estate on your plate. Here's a chart that illustrates where you can get your fill of this amino acid.

Food	Serving	Lysine (mg)
Tempeh	½ cup	754
Seitan	3 oz.	656
Lentils	½ cup	624
Tofu	½ cup	582
Amaranth	1 cup	515
Quinoa	1 cup	442
Pistachios	¼ cup	367
Pumpkin seeds	¼ cup	360

Aminos in Action

To better illustrate how to keep tabs on your protein intake—and how easy it is to hit your optimal numbers—here are sample menus for two vegan athletes.

Troy

Troy is 5'10" tall and weighs 155 pounds (70.3 kg). He's training to run the Boston Marathon.

His daily protein requirement is 70.3 kg × 1.3 g = **91 g**.

His daily lysine requirement is 70.3 kg × 38 mg = **2,671 mg**.

He meets his daily protein (including lysine) needs by eating
the following.

Meal	Food	Protein	Lysine
Breakfast	2 slices whole-grain bread	7.3 g	93 mg
	2 tbsp. peanut butter	8.0 g	290 mg
	8 oz. soy milk	9.2 g	439 mg
	1 banana	1.3 g	59 mg
Snack	½ cup hummus	4.0 g	291 mg
	2 lavash crackers	4.0 g	144 mg
	1 cup veggie sticks	1.3 g	102 mg
Lunch	1 cup vegetarian baked beans	12.0 g	488 mg
	1 medium baked potato	4.3 g	263 mg
	1 cup broccoli	3.6 g	234 mg
Snack	1 orange	1.2 g	62 mg
	⅓ cup pistachios	8.2 g	489 mg
Dinner	5 oz. firm tofu	12.0 g	651 mg
	1 cup quinoa	8.1 g	442 mg
	½ cup peas	3.9 g	463 mg
	½ cup corn	2.3 g	272 mg
Snack	¼ cup dry-roasted chickpeas	3.6 g	243 mg
	1 cup strawberries	1.0 g	37 mg
	TOTAL	**95.3 g**	**5,062 mg**

Sarah

Sarah is 5'2" tall and weighs 125 pounds (56.8 kg). She's a
powerlifter.

Her daily protein requirement is 56.8 kg × 1.6 g = **91 g**.

Her daily lysine requirement is 56.8 kg × 38 mg = **2,158 mg**.

Here's her sample menu.

Meal	Food	Protein	Lysine
Breakfast	¾ cup steel-cut oats	7.5 g	501 mg
	1 tbsp. chia seeds	2.0 g	150 mg
	1 tbsp. cocoa nibs	1.0 g	70 mg
	1 kiwifruit	1.1 g	200 mg
Snack	6 oz. soy yogurt	6.0 g	439 mg
	3 tbsp. pumpkin seeds	6.6 g	270 mg
Lunch	1 medium whole-grain bagel	10.0 g	186 mg
	2 tbsp. peanut butter	8.0 g	290 mg
	8 oz. soy milk	9.2 g	439 mg
Snack	⅓ cup roasted soybeans	22.6 g	427 mg
	1 orange	1.2 g	62 mg
Dinner	1 cup cooked amaranth	9.3 g	515 mg
	½ cup black beans	7.6 g	523 mg
	½ cup lentils	8.9 g	624 mg
	½ cup cooked spinach	3.0 g	115 mg
	TOTAL	**104 g**	**4,811 mg**

Looking deeper at these two examples, you'll notice they both include a well-rounded mix of the following:

- Fruits
- Veggies
- Legumes
- Nuts

And they don't include any of these:

- Protein powders
- Fake meats
- Mega protein-loaded meals

The point is: it's really not hard to hit your dietary requirements as a plant-based athlete, even without resorting to processed foods and protein powders, as so many athletes assume you need to.

You would have to put in quite an effort to eat a calorically sufficient diet that was deficient in protein. Without even trying, many Americans consume three to four times their true protein intake needs daily. And remember, more protein doesn't just make more muscle. Protein consumption beyond what your body needs is either eliminated or stored as fat. So while you want to get enough protein, you still want to make sure that carbohydrates are the primary player on your plate. We'll dig deeper into what that split looks like—and how fat fits into the equation—but for now, suffice to say that if you're eating whole, high-nutrient plants and a variety of them, you're off to a great start.

If you still have concerns about how to get enough protein in your diet, use this list of plant-based protein sources the next time you're grocery shopping.

Nuts and Seeds

Almonds	Cashew butter	Hempseeds
Almond butter	Pistachios	Sunflower seeds
Peanuts	Walnuts	Flaxseeds
Peanut butter	Hazelnuts	Chia seeds
Cashews	Pumpkin seeds	

Legumes

Adzuki beans	White beans	Black beans
Soybeans	Split peas	Navy beans
Chickpeas	Kidney beans	Green peas
Lentils	Lima beans	

Grains

Quinoa	Buckwheat	Cornmeal
Amaranth	Oats	Bulgur
Wild rice	Kamut	
Millet	Teff	

Vegetables

Brussels sprouts	Potatoes	Broccoli
Spinach	Asparagus	Broccoli rabe
Alfalfa sprouts	Portobello	Kale
Watercress	mushrooms	Collard greens

Minimally processed plant-based protein foods

Tofu

Tempeh

Seitan

Bread made with sprouted grains

Plant-based protein drinks

Plant-based protein bars

Plant-based protein pudding

Smoothies with nuts, seeds, and leafy greens

Soy: Fact over Fear

Soy is a frequently misunderstood food, and because it has been a big, beneficial part of our diets, and of many other plant-based athletes' diets, for decades—and part of some Asian diets for thousands of years—we want to clear a few things up. "Soy" refers to products made from soybeans, a member of the legume family. This includes *whole-soy products* such as edamame (mature soybeans), soy milk (emulsified soybeans), tofu (soy milk curds), and tempeh (fermented soybeans), in addition to many *processed soy products* (a.k.a. soy protein isolate): soybean oil and soy flours (found in many packaged goods), textured vegetable protein (used in meat alternatives), and dairy substitutes such as yogurts and cheeses.

Soy in its most natural state is a complete, high-quality, nutrient-dense form of protein. It is naturally cholesterol-free, low in saturated fat, and high in polyunsaturated fats (the kind we want, which includes omega-3s), and it also delivers fiber, B vitamins, iron, zinc, and a variety of antioxidants. Eating whole-soy products has been linked to lowered cholesterol, improved fertility, reduced menopause symptoms, and decreased risk of osteoporosis, diabetes, heart disease, and breast cancer. That's because, contrary to popular belief, soy does not contain estrogen; rather, it contains a beneficial class of phytoestrogens called isoflavones. In a nutshell, these natural compounds found in plants act as selective estrogen receptor modulators. Translation: they deliver the positive effects of estrogen to the tissues that benefit from it while having an antiestrogenic effect on those that don't.[15] So no, those phytoestrogens are not making you less of a man. And yes, soy is just as effective as animal-based protein sources for building lean muscle mass, if not more so because of its additional health benefits, particularly its cardiometabolic advantages.[16]

However, that depends on how you eat soy. We've already put forth that a whole plant is better than a processed one, and the same holds true for soy. While minimally processed forms such as tofu, tempeh, and soy milk actively contribute to your health, stripped-down protein isolates don't deliver any of the fiber or nutrients that whole soy does, and they typically come along with other nutritionally inferior ingredients such as refined sugar and trans fats.

Instead, opt not only for whole-soy products but also for organic and non-GMO whole-soy forms whenever possible. ("Organic" implies non-GMO, so if you see that on the label, you're good.) Conventional soybeans are frequently grown using genetically modified material that has been artificially manipulated in a laboratory. While there are no credible independent long-term studies about the potential health detriments of genetically modified organisms (GMOs), many health experts advise against eating these foods out of concern for how such genetic modifications may affect the human body. In the United States, there is no law requiring companies to disclose whether their products are genetically modified; however, you can't get an organic certification for GMOs. So buying organic, or products labeled as non-GMO, is the safest bet.

To give you an idea of the wonderful variety of amazing, tasty, and protein-filled dishes that await you, here are thirty-five plant-based, protein-rich meal ideas:

- Burrito bowl with grains, beans, and greens
- Curry bowl with rice, tofu, bell peppers, and carrots
- Tofu scramble with tofu, spinach, mushrooms, and tomatoes
- Tempeh Reuben with rye bread, sauerkraut, and plant-based cheese
- Thai curry with tofu, coconut milk, mushrooms, peppers, and broccoli
- Lentil soup with vegetables and barley
- Veggie burger with lettuce, tomato, pickle, and plant-based cheese
- Tempeh or tofu sandwich with lettuce, tomato, pickles, and plant-based cheese
- Chili with beans and vegetables
- Lentil loaf with vegetables, herbs, and spices
- Black bean soup with corn, tomatoes, carrots, and onions
- Tacos with seitan, cabbage, tomatoes, and salsa
- Burrito with rice, beans, avocado, lettuce, and tomato
- Wrap with tempeh, greens, sprouts, and dressing
- Salad with tofu, assorted sliced vegetables, leafy greens, and dressing
- Seitan skewers with a glaze or dipping sauce
- Chickpea and fava bean falafel with herbs and spices
- Peanut butter sandwich with sprouted bread and jam
- Sweet-and-sour tofu with peas, green peppers, and red peppers
- Chickpea stew with lentils, barley, celery, onions, and corn
- Fried rice with tofu, cucumbers, broccoli, and carrots
- BBQ seitan strips with mixed vegetables
- Fresh tofu spring rolls with peanut sauce, noodles, radishes, and carrots
- Oatmeal with nuts, fruits, and seeds

- White bean and kale soup with vegetable broth
- Almond butter and spelt pancakes with berries and maple syrup
- Tofu Bolognese with pasta
- Tempeh sushi with brown rice, seaweed, avocado, cucumber, and carrots
- Korean tofu bowl with seasoned tofu, brown rice, vegetables, and hot sauce
- Whole-grain cereal with soy milk, mixed berries, and nuts
- Mediterranean quinoa bowl with olives, avocado, roasted red peppers, olive oil, and red wine vinegar
- Spinach and tofu lasagna with marinara sauce and olives
- Sweet potato and chickpea patties with onion, flaxseed meal, and chili powder
- Lentil pasta with spinach, plant-based meat, and marinara sauce
- Pizza with mushrooms, olives, spinach, sun-dried tomatoes, and green peppers

The bottom line is this: you're going to get enough protein without breaking a sweat. And you definitely don't need to make sacrifices in order to reach your macronutrient intake needs—you can still enjoy the foods you love most. The mouthwatering protein-rich, plant-based meal ideas are endless. For more ideas, check out the recipes in chapter 11.

Printable Protein Grocery List

It's true, you probably don't need to worry about protein as much as most people think. But just in case it's still a concern for you, we've got you covered: download our Plant-Based Protein Grocery List, which lists our favorite sources of plant-based protein and provides some extra info about amino acids to make sure you're getting everything you need. Grab it at nomeatathlete.com/book-bonus.

• • • • •

In powerlifting particularly, protein is king. I spend hours a week in the gym pushing my body to its breaking point and have to be able to recover in time to do it again forty-eight hours later. As a 220- to 250-pound powerlifter, I'm consuming 200 to 260 grams of protein a day. Believe it or not, I don't find this any more or less challenging than anyone else, considering the current availability of high-protein vegan foods.

—**Nick Squires, international powerlifting champion, California state powerlifting record holder**

As a cath lab nurse, I am seeing more and more athletes in their thirties and forties come in after suffering a heart attack during their workouts. It is still eye-opening to see so many clogged arteries on people who are not over fifty; heart disease and heart attacks used to be a "disease of the old," but not so much anymore. I am also seeing more and more athletes question their dietary choices after a heart attack. The interventional cardiologist does not discuss diet, and these patients—athletes or not—are hungry for more than just medications. They want to know if their diets contributed and whether they should stop eating, or start eating, certain foods. This is where the plant-based fairy nurse (a.k.a. me) whispers in their ear about consuming less animal products.

—**Alba Mendez, RN, BSN**

As a gastroenterologist, I have firsthand experience in how diet can make or break our health. Animal products may be "digested well," but in our gut they give rise to inflammatory by-products. On the other hand, fiber-rich whole foods do the opposite and lower inflammation and are associated with improved digestive, renal, and cardiovascular health and increased longevity. There's no doubt that our bodies thrive on whole-plant foods, as this is the fuel that our gut and our gut microbiome need to work efficiently and be effective in keeping our gut healthy, our immune system in top shape, and our fitness at its optimal level!

—Vanessa Méndez, MD, board-certified gastroenterologist and internist and director of telehealth, Institute of Plant-Based Medicine

As a doctor of acupuncture and Chinese medicine specializing in sports acupuncture, I treat athletes daily. My number one recommendation when supporting athletes through their training is to adopt a plant-based diet as soon as possible.

—Hilda A. Gonzalez, DACM, L.Ac

Children and young athletes can absolutely thrive on a plant-based diet. In fact, in my office I often counsel young athletes to be mindful about their nutrition if they want to improve their performance. Eating a diet that includes fiber and antioxidants and is hydrating will benefit active individuals, including children. It's one of the best things that we can do for our health and well-being.

—Yami Cazorla-Lancaster, DO, MPH, MS, FAAP, DipABLM, pediatrician, coach, author, and speaker

As an athlete and a rabbi, I find that nutrition is of paramount importance to achieve your goals on body and soul levels. I believe that for the ultimate fitness "achievement," it's necessary to have food with as little "violence" in it as possible.

Ever since I switched to a plant-based diet, I have felt much more energy.

—Yuri Foreman, Israel's first world boxing champion

4

CARBOHYDRATES:
THE BODY'S PERFECT FUEL

By now, we hope we've made it pretty clear that protein is no longer going to be the main event on your plate. But then what should take its place? The answer might surprise you. When we tell athletes, particularly strength athletes, what *should* be at the foundation of their diet, they're often surprised. After all, it's not every day that people in the mainstream fitness community are told to fill up on this food group, especially when it comes to building muscle. And yet there's no doubt about it in our minds: **carbohydrates** should be what it's all about.

We both have experience in endurance and strength sports and have both discovered our best results with a nutrition program that is high in carbohydrate intake, even when it comes to building muscle. We believe that the reason for our success comes down to the fact that carbohydrate-rich foods contain the most nutrients. They have the highest ANDI score (Aggregate Nutrient Density Index, which scores foods based on their ratio of nutrients to calories) of any food, and they do so much more than supply calories for energy. They help to reduce inflammation, aid in recovery after exercise, assist in hydration, and facilitate the distribution of electrolytes, vitamins, and minerals into your system. And most carbohydrate-rich whole foods contain low levels of fat and modest levels of protein, which is what our bodies require, making them the perfect fuel for athletes. Nutrition is like exercise: you get out of it what you put into it. But the most powerful way to drive that point home is to see it in action. Here to testify to that are some elite professional, Olympic, and world-class athletes who follow our mantra that when it comes to an optimal diet, carbohydrates are king.

Speaking of kings, if you were to ask us to name the most accomplished plant-based athlete in history, **Scott Jurek** would be near the top of the list. A brief snapshot of his accomplishments will show you why. He may not be an Olympic medalist like some of the other plant-based athletes we've written about, but his career spanning the past two decades reveals that Scott is one of the greatest ultrarunners in history. And he's not just an amazing ultrarunner; he was named by *Runner's World* as one of the Top Ten Greatest Runners of All Time. After switching to a plant-based diet in 1999 at the start of his storied professional running career, Scott went on to win accolades including *National Geographic* Adventurer of the Year, *UltraRunning* magazine's UltraRunner of the Year (four times), and one of *Men's Health* magazine's 100 Fittest Men of All Time.

More impressive than his accolades are the accomplishments that earned him those accolades, and his multidecade plant-based diet made Scott a pioneer in the plant-based athlete community. You could say he paved the way for others who would follow his example, running thousands upon thousands of miles on paved roads and dirt trails all over the world and into endurance running record books. Scott won the Western States 100-Mile Endurance Run for seven consecutive years, from 1999 to 2005. He also twice won the most grueling footrace in the world, the Badwater 135 ultramarathon, a 135-mile race through Death Valley, California, during mid-July, when temperatures reach 130°F, with an elevation climb of more than 8,500 feet. It's hard to even comprehend running that distance in those conditions, let alone at a championship pace. Scott also set the Appalachian Trail thru-hike speed record in 2015, making massive elevation ascents and descents in constantly changing weather, some of it incredibly harsh, as he navigated the 2,189-mile trail in forty-six days, eight hours, and seven minutes. The journey was so profound that he wrote a book about the experience, titled *North*, a memoir about his transformative expedition to self-discovery on the Appalachian Trail. Not to be overlooked is the US speed record Scott holds for the most miles run in a road race during a twenty-four-hour period; at 165.7 miles, it is equivalent to running six and one-half marathons in a single day. Again, these kinds of feats are unfathomable for most of us, and they are precisely what makes the stories of world-class plant-based athletes such as Scott so compelling. And the fact that he has been fueled by plants for decades—opening doors for other athletes, instilling confidence in others that they too can achieve meaningful athletic goals by trusting in the power of plant-based nutrition—has been a gift to the world.

Scott claims that his plant-based diet has contributed to his success as a runner, enabling him to have faster recovery times and better overall endurance. So, what fuels Scott's record-setting ultraruns? For starters, he's big on green drinks—smoothies and juice blends with kale, spinach, barley grass, arugula, spirulina, and chlorella. Like most of us, he blends in fruit to mask the strong green flavors, and to add carbohydrate fuel, electrolytes, antioxidants, and overall nutrition, along with all the flavors that come from berries, pineapples, bananas, and mangoes. Scott's focus on sports nutrition is imperative for an athlete of his caliber. He uses brown rice and pea protein, essential fatty acids, and whole-food sources of good fats from avocado and coconut to round out his diet, which also includes starchy vegetables, legumes, grains, nuts, and seeds. Scott said, "Some people assume that you can't get full with a plant-based diet, but it really comes down to the amount of foods you eat, and getting enough quality fats. I'm someone who likes to eat. That's the beauty of a plant-based diet: unless you're filling up on junk foods, you can eat a lot of volume of [real] food."

When it comes to fueling an ultrarunner, Scott says that you have to find the foods that are easiest for you to digest, consuming twenty-five grams of carbohydrates every twenty to thirty minutes and washing it down with lots of water and electrolytes. Scott is hyperfocused on eating sports-specific foods, which is of paramount importance in a sport such as his. It is a high priority to consume the right ratios of carbohydrates, proteins, and fats to propel his body to perform more than one hundred miles of running at a time. Macronutrient ratios, meal timing, sports supplementation, and total calorie intake would be less essential (though still important) for a recreational athlete exercising for thirty or sixty minutes per day, a few days per week, but for Scott, it can make or break a performance. Scott says, "As an athlete, I pay close attention to how I fuel my body, but it's also really fun." He enjoys shopping at farmers markets in Colorado, where he resides, cooking food at home, and eating a variety of foods that always make his plant-based diet feel abundant. He even said that he consumes solid foods such as burritos during races (yes, you read that correctly) and that part of his nutrition approach during long runs is eating heavy, solid foods to fuel many hours on the road or trails. Whether it's burritos, sandwiches, plant-based sushi, or pizza, Scott has a varied plant-based diet on and off the trail. He spends so many hours running, sometimes twenty-four hours in super-long races, that his body has adapted to eating "meals" while he runs rather than relying only on gels or drinks. His body requires something much more substantial, and over the years he has learned through trial and error what works best for him. He says that there is really no one-size-fits-all approach, since every body is different, but adequate fuel is paramount, and through experimentation and practice, you'll find what best fuels your long workouts.

Why a plant-based diet in the first place? While growing up in Minnesota, Scott was a hunter and fisherman—a real meat-and-potatoes guy, as he says. But when he entered the health-care industry, going to physical therapy school and then working in the medical profession, he saw a lot of chronic disease. He sought out alternative ways to achieve good health, intrigued by what impact diet could have on total health.

Scott was inspired by the long-term health benefits of a plant-based diet, which he learned about by reading books by experts in natural health such as Dr. Andrew Weil. He then read *Mad Cowboy* by former cattle rancher turned outspoken animal rights activist Howard Lyman, and those authors were his inspirations for a complete dietary overhaul and lifestyle switch to become a vegan athlete. Though Scott had already run a number of ultramarathons, he was still very early into his twenty-plus-year career when he switched to plants in his first year of competitive ultramarathon running. But what about performance results when he abandoned his meat-and-potato diet in favor of smoothies, fruits, vegetables, vegan burritos, and plant-based sushi? Scott said this when describing his switch to a plant-based diet: "I just started noticing the recovery benefits, the ability of my body to be consistent for workouts and for races. And that's so critical [for performance]." He added, "On a vegan diet, I was not only improving my body composition but also increasing muscle mass. A lot of people assume that one needs to eat animal products to gain a lot of muscle mass, or sufficient muscle mass for power sports, and that has been proven false time and time again." And, of course, Scott shattered that myth on the road to becoming one of the most dominant runners in his sport for decades, all fueled by plants.

We know the historic legacy Scott leaves behind—a trail of inspiration uplifting the next generation of plant-based ultrarunners—and it all started with curiosity about how to help bring health to others. That is precisely what Scott's Hall of Fame running career has done for so many who have changed their lives for the better because of the example he has set.

Darcy Gaechter is the first and only woman to kayak the entire length of the Amazon River—the longest river in the world, at 4,200 miles from source to sea. When she was twenty-one years old, she adopted a plant-based diet, and right about that same time, she got serious about whitewater and expedition kayaking. With an athletic background playing volleyball and other organized sports growing up, and eventually venturing into climbing and mountaineering, she was looking for her next adventure, and it was kayaking that spoke to her the loudest.

Darcy's chosen sport is challenging on pretty much all levels. First, there's concern for her safety, whether it's dangerous conditions on the water, native wildlife, or, in the case of the Amazon, the constant risk of encountering pirates and illegal loggers. (In fact, before beginning her trek, she cut her hair to disguise her gender from a distance.) And then there's the fact that she often has to carry her 50-pound kayak for miles, along with another 30 pounds of camping gear and food. And at just five feet, four inches tall and 120 pounds, she needs to call on every bit of strength to literally carry her through her sport.

To fuel herself, Darcy looks to two main contributors: her diet and her mental state. In order to make sure she has enough energy to keep moving, she relies on a varied menu high in plant carbohydrates. Here's a sample day, both at home and in the kayak.

A typical day at home:
Breakfast: Granola and hemp milk
Lunch: Veggie burger (based on adzuki beans)
Dinner: Burrito bowl with rice, pinto beans, tofu, crushed
red pepper, olive oil, liquid aminos, avocado, tomato,
onion, and bell pepper, served with tortilla chips and
hot sauce

A typical day in the kayak:
Breakfast: Bagel, avocado, hot sauce
Lunch: Not always an option on the river, so energy bars do
the trick
Dinner: Dehydrated black bean or lentil soup

What also helps her get through extreme outdoor conditions and long stretches of time away from the comforts of home is her strong mental outlook. As she says about facing challenges and obstacles: "If you let these things become a point of focus in your mind, it's going to turn into an unbearable situation. But if you can keep a positive mental attitude, focus on the amazing things you are seeing and the amazing things your body is doing, you will undoubtedly feel a lot better about staying in your situation." And she doesn't let being on the road—or river—discourage her from her commitment to a plant-based diet. "When I get off a weeklong river trip and my entire crew goes into a restaurant to eat hamburgers, it takes real dedication to sit in the parking lot and cook myself a meal. But it's always been worth it over the past two decades."

More than five years after conquering the Amazon—and many other challenges in between—Darcy wanted to take on something equally inspiring. So in honor of her fortieth birthday, she decided to run forty miles in the Elk Mountains in Colorado, covering 16,000 feet of vertical gain—which she accomplished after just six weeks of training to be a runner in the first place. As she described it, "This sort of thing was 100 percent unimaginable to me before my plant-based days."

It's not just endurance athletes who can benefit from the power and fuel provided by a high-carbohydrate diet. It may surprise you to learn that many team-sport athletes and even many bodybuilders and pow-erlifters follow a diet relatively high in carbohydrates. That's why we'd like to introduce you to one of the pound-for-pound strongest athletes in the world, a twenty-year plant-based veteran who has dominated every sports discipline she has ever engaged in: **Vanessa Espinoza**.

Vanessa adopted a plant-based diet in the early 2000s as an all-American high school basketball player. She went on to play for the then number seven–ranked Colorado State University women's bas-ketball team on a full scholarship before graduating from Colorado State with a bachelor of science degree in exercise science. From there, she was drafted into the Women's National Basketball Association (WNBA) by the Indiana Fever. However, she never set foot on the bas-ketball court wearing a WNBA jersey. After the passing of her father, a former professional boxer, she opted to skip the WNBA to stay home with her mother, and then she dedicated her life to boxing as a way to honor her late father. She quickly became a three-time Colorado Golden Gloves state boxing champion before committing the rest of her athletic career to weight lifting and her mission to become as strong as possible. Vanessa packed on more muscle and strength than many thought was possible. After years of weight training, she decided to dabble in competitive powerlifting. At her very first meet, she nearly set a world record, and she went on to win every meet she competed in, going all the way to the Olympia stage, the most prestigious bodybuilding event in the world.

As an elite basketball player, boxer, weight lifter, and competitive powerlifter, with a formal education in exercise science, Vanessa knows that it's not just protein that builds a body capable of such feats, and that the micronutrients found in complex carbohydrates are critical for the elevated athletic performance, robust immunity, and high levels of health that keep an athlete performing in top form on a daily basis. Though proteins and fats are integral parts of her daily nutritional program, carbohydrates stand at the foundation.

When you look at the nutritional breakdown of Vanessa's carefully calculated meals made from real, whole foods over the course of a week, you can see that her calorie consumption favors carbohydrates, followed by fat, followed by protein, and is always high in fiber and water. Though she does have an emotional preference for protein-rich foods—as many strength athletes do—it is important to point out that many of those protein-rich foods are also carbohydrate rich, with some containing more carbohydrates than protein. Beans are a great example. Though we often think of beans as a protein-rich plant-based food, nearly three-quarters of their calories come from carbohydrates. (Soybeans are the exception, which is what makes tofu and tempeh much more concentrated protein sources than most other beans. The high protein content of soybeans—and even higher protein content of minimally processed tofu and tempeh—is what makes those foods so versatile as replacements for animal protein.) Other protein sources in Vanessa's diet, such as quinoa and lentils, are also high in carbohydrates, as are all the vegetables, leafy greens, and fruits that pack her menu with loads of micronutrients.

Taken from a collection of her meal plans and recipes, with nutritional information calculated over a full week, Vanessa's average intake is as follows:

Calories per day: 2,270
Calories from carbohydrates per day: 1,100
Calories from protein per day: 540
Calories from fat per day: 630
Percentage of macronutrient intake: 48 percent
     carbohydrate, 28 percent fat, 24 percent protein
Average daily fiber intake: 74 g

Here is a summary in the most common method of reporting numbers:

Calories: 2,270
Carbohydrates: 275 g
Protein: 135 g
Fat: 70 g
Fiber: 74 g

If you were to quickly look at those numbers listed in grams, without accounting for calorie density, you would likely conclude that after carbohydrates, Vanessa gets the majority of her remaining calories from protein, followed by fat. But that's not the case. As we established earlier, there are only 4 calories per gram of carbohydrates and protein, but 9 calories per gram of fat. So even though the number of grams of protein is nearly twice the number of grams of fat, there are actually more calories coming from fat in her diet (approximately 630 per day) than from protein (approximately 540 per day). This is why it is helpful to know both the percentage of your macronutrient averages (around 50/25/25 in Vanessa's case, a common number for strength athletes) and the number of grams of each macronutrient, since most nutrition information is written in the language of grams.

Looking at her bio as a champion basketball player, boxer, and powerlifter, one might assume that Vanessa would stand tall and weigh 150 to 200 pounds. But at just five feet, three inches tall and 130 pounds, Vanessa can deadlift more than 400 pounds, squat 365 pounds, and bench-press an amazing 245 pounds. And it is because of her size and her short-duration, explosive exercise routine of weight lifting, boxing, and sprinting that her calorie intake averages out to just under 2,300 calories per day, rather than the 3,000 or more required by many larger athletes and those who train for longer durations. Though Vanessa is incredibly muscular, carrying more muscle size on her frame than most athletic men of her weight, she maintains a low level of body fat and doesn't consume excess calories just for the sake of eating more— especially because she doesn't want to hinder her performance by carrying extra mass in the form of stored fat.

Fueling with Plants

Our brains as well as our muscles *prefer* to run on carbohydrate fuel (followed by fats, and then protein as a last resort—more on that later). When we consume carbohydrates, they are first converted to glucose, then stored in our liver and in our muscles as glycogen to be used as energy later on. When we exercise, our bodies call upon that stored glycogen for fuel. Then, when we burn through those glycogen stores, our bodies use stored fat as a secondary fuel source. (As we mentioned in the previous chapter, and will reiterate throughout the book, protein is rarely used as energy, despite the popularity of mistaken notions to the contrary.)

You may have heard the argument for following a low-carb diet, including a ketogenic diet, which suggests that by not eating carbohydrates, you're forcing your body to dip into its fat stores for energy. The idea is that by using fatty acids and amino acids instead of glucose, the body can burn fat while also prompting your pancreas to reduce insulin production, helping to reduce your blood glucose. But this physiological state (called ketosis) is not sustainable in the long term. Remember how we told you that your brain needs glucose as its fuel? In ketosis, your liver starts to make ketone bodies as emergency backup for glucose, but that's still not your brain's preferred source of energy. As a result, keeping your body in a perpetual state of ketosis can have a negative effect on your health and eventually lead to chronic disease. While this may work for some individuals, it's not something we want to stake our health on. Carbohydrates, on the other hand, offer an immediately available source of energy, allow you to keep a balanced macronutrient profile, and support optimal physiological function.

So let's get you eating more carbohydrates, shall we? First, it's important to understand that not all carbohydrates are created equal; they come in simple and complex forms. Think of **complex carbohydrates** as whole, unprocessed foods with their fiber and starch still intact—whole grains, legumes, vegetables, and fruits. In contrast, **simple carbohydrates** are *processed*—think apple juice versus apples, for example, and, of course, refined foods such as sugar, brown sugar, corn syrup, and processed grains including white flour, as well as any food or beverage with added sugars that are not naturally occurring, such as cake and soda.

The main difference between these two is that simple carbohydrates are digested quickly and cause a sharp and temporary spike in your blood sugar followed by an equally quick drop, while complex carbohydrates take longer to break down. Think of the quick-hit, quick-peaking energy you get from simple carbohydrates such as fruit juice, candy, energy drinks, energy gels, and sweetened foods, as opposed to the slower-releasing fuel that lentils, corn, squash, and yams provide. Celebrity trainer John Pierre, an expert on plant-based nutrition and fitness, describes the difference between these carbohydrates in a memorable way. Simple carbohydrates are like a newspaper burning in the fireplace, while complex carbohydrates are like a slow-burning log on the fire. One is used up quickly, and the other provides energy for the long haul.

The Complex Case
Against Simple Carbohydrates

One of the primary reasons to limit simple carbohydrates is the sheer amount of sugar they contain. In 2014, the World Health Organization halved its recommendation for daily sugar intake, decreasing it from 10 percent of total daily calorie intake to 5 percent. For an adult with a normal body mass index (BMI), that equates to six teaspoons, or 25 g, of sugar per day. A common sports drink may have more than 35 g of sugar in a single 20-ounce bottle! A 32-ounce bottle, which is one of the most popular sizes to purchase and is sold for a dollar or less, can contain upward of 50 g of sugar, or twice the total daily intake recommendation.

Many people don't realize that much of the sugars they take in are "hidden" in processed foods. Examples:

- A can of soda may contain up to 10 teaspoons (40 g) of sugar.
- One tablespoon of ketchup contains 1 teaspoon of sugar.
- A typical bowl of cereal contains 20 g of added sugar.
- Fruit juice may contain up to 40 g of sugar per serving.
- Store-bought granola often contains 6 teaspoons of sugar per serving.
- Iced tea can pack 33 g of sugar into a 12-ounce serving.
- Protein bars contain up to 30 g of added sugars.
- Canned fruit is preserved in sugary syrup.
- Bottled smoothies can contain up to 24 teaspoons of sugar in a single serving.
- BBQ sauce, pasta sauce, and other sauces and condiments are often loaded with sugar, containing multiple teaspoons of sugar per serving.

Unless used strategically to replace calories lost during exercise, intake of additional simple sugars often leads to excess calorie consumption, and according to the National Institutes of Health it has been linked to an increased risk of obesity, type 2 diabetes, heart disease, and cancer.

And then there's the issue of artificial sweeteners such as aspartame, saccharine, and sucralose, which can be found in products including NutraSweet, Equal, Sweet'N Low, and Splenda. These synthetic substitutes are derived from naturally occurring substances, but they've been chemically altered and have been linked to weight gain, weight-loss resistance, upset bacterial balance in the digestive tract, increased sugar cravings, and blood sugar disturbances.

To reclaim control of your nutrition, start by becoming aware of the processed foods in your diet—the refined sugars and flours, sugary beverages, chocolate-covered energy and protein bars, and other unnecessary simple carbohydrates that have crept into your daily routine. You can start to eliminate them, either one by one or all together. It's a challenge, but it's one worth accepting to position yourself for nutritional intake that is in line with both your health and your athletic goals. It is also incredibly empowering to develop the ability to reject the foods that have adversely affected your health while embracing the ones that will help you become your very best.

As for sugars in whole foods—no need to fear! Many foods are designed by nature to contain sugars, and we are designed by nature to eat them. Fruits and vegetables also contain water and fiber, which mitigate the adverse effects, such as insulin spikes, that their naturally occurring sugars would otherwise have on the body. But when sugar is extracted, concentrated, and added to other foods—or consumed on its own—it becomes problematic because of its impact on blood sugar and the fact that it is essentially devoid of micronutrients. Foods with lots of simple sugars are also often loaded with fat (think pastries and other sweets).

Whole plants, on the other hand—particularly fruits and vegetables—are very low in calories, and the body uses their sugar content as fuel or stores it as glycogen for future use. (In contrast, the energy in fatty, sugary, calorie-rich foods is stored as fat if it is not entirely burned as fuel.) Much of the processed food we eat gets stored as fat, unless small amounts of simple sugars—as in an energy gel or a sports drink—are consumed immediately before or during an athletic event and burned as fuel through exercise. Fruit, therefore, is nature's perfect short-term energy source, packaged so precisely with water, fiber, antioxidants, vitamins, and minerals. It's one of the best pre-workout foods available, which we will expand on later in this chapter. And certain foods, such as fruits as they ripen, will release even more sugar (energy), essentially transitioning from complex carbohydrates to simple carbohydrates as far as their impact on energy is concerned, as is the case with ripening bananas. Dried fruit, though no longer in a whole state containing water, is also rich in fiber and simple carbohydrates, making it another exception to the simple carbohydrate rule that is primarily reserved for isolated, processed, or extracted sugars added to other foods.

Which carbohydrates should you reach for on a regular basis? It probably comes as no surprise that the answer is complex carbohydrates, most of the time. Whole-food carbohydrates such as leafy green vegetables, cruciferous vegetables, fruits, and legumes are the healthiest foods on the planet on the basis of their nutrient density, the truest measurement of nutrition they provide. And while minimally processed grains aren't quite as nutrient rich as fruits, vegetables, and legumes, they are head and shoulders above non-plant-based foods in their energy-producing qualities and nutritional yield. Wheat, oats, rice, barley, quinoa, buckwheat, and spelt are cornerstones of diets for populations around the world, and they are typically some of the carbohydrate sources that you will consume most in following a plant-based diet. For many of the Olympic and professional athletes featured in this book, grains are a dominant feature of their daily meal plan, particularly combined with legumes and vegetables, making for a calorie-rich, nutrient-dense, energy-producing menu to fuel their athletic endeavors.

Nothing illustrates the nutrient bang for the buck that complex carbohydrates deliver (as well as the evidence that plant-based foods far outweigh their animal counterparts in this department) than the Aggregate Nutrient Density Index (ANDI) score created by Dr. Joel Fuhrman. The ANDI score "grades" foods on the basis of the micronutrition they provide per calorie using thirty-four important nutritional parameters, ranging from 1 (least nutrient dense) to 1,000 (most nutrient dense). Any guesses as to which foods top the ANDI scorecard with scores of 1,000? Yep, leafy green vegetables, particularly those in the cruciferous family. Here's a sampling of results, so you can see how different types of foods stack up:

ANDI Scorecard for Common Foods

Kale: 1,000

Collard greens: 1,000

Mustard greens: 1,000

Watercress: 1,000

Swiss chard: 895

Spinach: 707

Arugula: 604

Romaine lettuce: 510

Brussels sprouts: 490

Carrots: 458

Cabbage: 434

Broccoli: 340

Cauliflower: 315

Bell peppers: 265

Mushrooms: 238

Asparagus: 205

Tomatoes: 186

Strawberries: 182

Sweet potatoes: 181

Zucchini: 164

Artichokes: 145

Blueberries: 132

Iceberg lettuce: 127

Grapes: 119

Cantaloupe: 118

Onions: 109

Flaxseeds: 103

Oranges: 98

Cucumbers: 87

Tofu: 82

Sesame seeds: 74

Lentils: 72

Peaches: 65

Sunflower seeds: 64

Kidney beans: 64

Green peas: 63

Cherries: 55

Pineapple: 54

Apples: 53

Mangoes: 53

Peanut butter: 51

Corn: 45

Pistachios: 37

Oatmeal: 36

Shrimp: 36 (highest-ranking animal product)

Eggs: 31

Walnuts: 30

Bananas: 30

Almonds: 28

Avocados: 28

White potatoes: 28

Chicken breast: 24

Ground beef: 21

French fries: 12

Cheddar cheese: 11

Apple juice: 11

Olive oil: 10

White bread: 9

Corn chips: 7

Cola: 1

Notice that kale scores twenty-seven times higher than the highest-ranking animal-based food, and tofu is two times more nutrient dense than any meat, milk, or eggs. (As we explained in chapter 3, tofu is, in fact, a good, clean way to get your protein, despite the bad rap that soy gets.) But here's the catch: leafy green vegetables don't provide a lot of calories. So even though they earn the highest ANDI scores by delivering the most nutrients per calorie, you couldn't possibly eat enough leafy greens to get any substantial calorie intake from them. This is where diversity in nutrition plays a role in your total calorie intake. Foods such as kale, collard greens, spinach, and brussels sprouts are some of the most nutrient-dense foods, but in order to eat enough calories to thrive as an athlete, you'll need to pair them with more calorie-dense foods, such as sweet potatoes, tofu, lentils, beans, tempeh, avocados, nut butters, oats, and rice.

Feeding the Gut

Yet another reason to embrace whole-plant carbohydrates as the foundation of your diet is that they are also the preferred food source for your gut. Your gut, part of your digestive system, contains trillions of microorganisms that are mainly bacteria. Some of the bacteria are beneficial and promote health, while some cause inflammation. The goal is to keep the balance tipped in favor of the good guys, which is where whole plants come in. The fiber you get from plants—especially leafy greens—feeds beneficial bacteria and keeps the disease-causing bacteria at bay. And keeping the good guys stocked with plant fiber has powerful effects. It can heal inflammation, balance your pH, mend digestive issues such as irritable bowel syndrome (IBS) and diverticulitis, reduce your risk of colon cancer, increase your energy, and diminish bloating. Also, because your gut can directly communicate with your brain, your hormones, and your immune system, taking care of this vital powerhouse is the key to keeping your moods balanced, your metabolism stoked, your stress response on an even keel, and your immune response regulated.

The Sweet Exceptions

There are some scenarios in which complex carbohydrates aren't the plants to get the job done—specifically, when you need a quick shot of energy without slowing down your digestion. For example, in the middle of a marathon, an electrolyte drink with simple sugars can provide an energy boost in a way that lentils—with their starches and more complex carbohydrates—can't. This is why endurance athletes use gels, fruit chews, energy and snack bars, and sports drinks despite their apparent lack of nutrition: these products are packaged in convenient forms to consume quickly, even in the middle of a run or on a bike. Trying to do the same with a banana, apple, or other whole fruit, vegetable, legume, or grain sometimes won't cut it (though you will occasionally see things such as potatoes on offer at ultramarathon aid stations because the intensity of exertion is low enough that your body can afford to digest some extra fiber). So when transporting, chewing, or digesting whole foods isn't an option, that's when fuel in the form of simple carbohydrates can help more than hurt.

It's also worth noting that you can make your own sports nutrition products using real foods, such as by pitting dates and blending them with coconut water for a supercharged boost of the naturally occurring sugar from dates and the natural electrolytes in coconut water. This has been aptly referred to as "Datorade" in the plant-based endurance community for years.

Another (small) exception to the no refined sugar or artificial sweetener rule is *natural* sweeteners. These are minimally processed, plant-based sugars that you can use every so often to sweeten your meals, such as your overnight oats, or maybe a batch of Sweet Potato Brownies (page 319). These better-for-you sweeteners include coconut palm sugar, maple syrup, yacón syrup, sorghum syrup, and stevia. Stevia, a sweetener derived from the plant species *Stevia rebaudiana*, is particularly worth highlighting because it has a glycemic index of zero. That means that it won't cause a spike in your blood sugar or insulin level.

The Carbohydrates on Your Plate

Since carbohydrates are the body's preferred energy source, it makes sense to eat a lot of them—about **50 to 70 percent of your total calories**, depending on your activity level. Exactly how many carbohydrates to eat depends on the type of sport you participate in. In general, more endurance-focused sports rely on a higher percentage of total calories coming from carbohydrates, whereas strength and power sports tend to rely on a lower percentage of total carbohydrate intake, while their protein and fat intake may be increased.

The best way to find out what works for you is to **first try out a 70 percent carbohydrate intake and then try a 50 percent carbohydrate intake for a couple of weeks each**, documenting your food intake as well as how you feel, and then work toward the most ideal and practical combination for you. For most endurance athletes, the optimum will be somewhere around a 60/20/20 percentage of carbohydrates/fat/protein, with some athletes doing better at 70/15/15, and a 50/25/25 split for most strength athletes. Using a food calculator app such as MyFitnessPal or Cronometer will help you keep tabs on these percentages.

Once you settle on the ranges of carbohydrates, proteins, and fats that work best for you, you may choose to think of them in terms of grams rather than as percentages of calories. For the first few days or even a week, it may be helpful to write down (or input into an app) everything you eat and calculate the macros so you can see how that breakdown compares with your ideal. The more you become aware of the calorie and macronutrient content of whole plant-based foods, the easier it will become to gauge your intake without having to rely on tedious logging, instead looking at how you feel and the results you're getting.

As far as deciding *what* to eat, high-carbohydrate foods are almost limitless because they encompass just about all fruits, vegetables, grains, and legumes—and the more the better, so long as you're eating a variety and so long as they fit into your daily calorie allowance based on your specific athletic goals. That's because not all complex carbohydrates work the same way. As we discussed earlier, foods such as oats, potatoes, brown rice, lentils, yams, beans, and other starchy carbohydrates provide energy for a long period of time, whereas carbohydrates from fruits and less starchy vegetables typically burn more quickly. Therefore, if you have a workout coming up within ten to thirty minutes, fruit would be a great option for quickly digested carbohydrate energy. But if your workout is a couple of hours away, more calorie-dense foods, such as potatoes, oats, rice, or beans, would be a better option, providing slow-releasing, longer-lasting carbohydrate fuel. Similarly, if you start to lose steam during workouts that are longer than an hour—for example, losing strength while lifting weights or feeling like you've hit a wall while running or cycling—faster-acting complex carbohydrates can be beneficial. Eating a banana or a couple of handfuls of berries near the start of your workout can help you finish strong. After the workout, starchier, heartier carbohydrates such as yams, squash, lentils, and rice are great for recovery.

Fortunately, the choice of foods in the carbohydrate category are plentiful and diverse. The following is a list of ideal carbohydrate sources for athletes and the best times to consume them.

Fruits
(excellent fuel for before and during workouts)

Apples	Melons	Tomatoes
Oranges	Pineapple	Grapefruit
Bananas	Plums	Dates
Blueberries	Peaches	Jackfruit
Blackberries	Nectarines	Passion fruit
Raspberries	Apricots	Figs
Strawberries	Cherries	Kiwifruit
Cranberries	Grapes	Pomegranates
Mangoes		

Starchy Vegetables
(great for advanced pre-workout energy, an hour or two before training, and post-workout nutrition)

Potatoes	Acorn squash	Plantains
Yams	Butternut squash	Peas
Sweet potatoes		

Low-Starch and Nonstarchy Vegetables
(great for post-workout nutrition)

Beets	Lettuce	Artichokes
Carrots	Brussels sprouts	Cucumbers
Corn	Broccoli	Onions
Green beans	Cauliflower	Radishes
Kale	Asparagus	Zucchini

Legumes
(great for post-workout nourishment and satiety)

Lentils	Pinto beans	Black-eyed peas
Kidney beans	Black beans	Adzuki beans
Garbanzo beans	Split peas	Lima beans
Soybeans	Fava beans	

Grains and Pseudograins

(great for pre-workout energy and post-workout nutrition)

Brown rice	Buckwheat*	Millet*
White rice	Barley	Spelt
Oats	Amaranth*	Bulgur
Quinoa*	Wild rice*	

*Quinoa, buckwheat, amaranth, and millet are technically seeds known as "pseudograins"—they resemble grains, are enjoyed as grains, and deliver many of the same benefits as grains. Similarly, we put wild rice in the grain category, even though it's technically an aquatic plant and is considered to be a vegetable in some parts of the world. Similarly, the tomato is actually a fruit and peanuts are legumes, but we tend to classify tomatoes as vegetables because of the way we use them and classify peanuts as nuts.

Keep in mind that eating for improved athletic performance doesn't have to be boring. You can be as creative as you like when constructing your meal plans using the foods listed here—and many others that aren't listed—as well as protein-rich tofu, tempeh, and other dense protein foods and quality fat sources such as avocados, coconut, nuts, seeds, and nut butters. When these are combined and cooked with sauces, herbs, and spices that pull inspiration from cuisines around the globe, eating whole, plant-based foods starts to feel much more pleasurable than functional.

What you won't see on this list are simple carbohydrates, since they should be limited in your diet. You should aim to keep your use of simple carbohydrates from processed foods to a minimum. Save pre-workout drinks for when you really need them and electrolyte drinks for exceptionally grueling workouts, especially in hot weather. Leave the chocolate-covered "energy bar" on the shelf at the grocery store, and eat some blueberries or some trail mix instead. As often as possible, rely on whole-plant foods before, during, and after workouts, but if your sport calls for it, use gels, drinks, and simple sugars when necessary—just don't lean on them for actual nourishment, and be sure to replenish nutrients lost from exercise with whole-plant foods and water.

• • • • •

When I switched to a plant-based diet, I noticed that I had a lot more energy and that my body toned up. I have been vegan for seven years now, and I feel amazing! I work out almost every day, and it takes a very intense workout to make me feel sore post-workout. I feel lighter on my feet, and I feel stronger during workouts.
—**Tia Blanco, world champion professional surfer**

I feel lighter, not just weight-wise but in terms of light on my feet and less sluggish. My energy levels are more even-keeled throughout the day, and my recovery times are much quicker.
—**Yassine Diboun, ultrarunner**

After I went plant-based, I got stronger; my weight room numbers increased. Overall, physically I've been in the best shape of my life.
—**David Verburg, Olympic gold medal–winning sprinter**

I have so much energy on a plant-based diet that I twice ran the full Montreal Marathon at a body weight of 300 pounds. Running 42 km (26.2 miles) is something I would have never thought possible before adopting a plant-based diet.
—**Georges Laraque, former thirteen-year NHL hockey player**

Exercise is one of the most powerful ways to increase blood flow to tissues and promote oxygen delivery. When placed under a significant challenge, the mitochondria in muscle tissue replicate, creating a collection of profound metabolic effects. One of the most important effects of mitochondrial biogenesis in muscle tissue is increased insulin sensitivity. This allows muscles to uptake large quantities of glucose from the blood using small amounts of insulin, either to be used immediately for energy or to be stored for later use as glycogen. Insulin-sensitive muscles operate extremely efficiently, prioritizing glucose as a fuel. Eating a wide variety of plant-based whole foods including fruits, starchy vegetables, legumes, and whole grains provides athletes with a significant quantity of glucose from carbohydrate energy, providing insulin-sensitive muscles the exact fuel they require to manufacture ATP efficiently, using very small amounts of insulin. Research indicates that insulin-sensitive individuals are at a dramatically lower risk for many chronic diseases, including type 2 diabetes, cardiovascular disease, and cancer. Therefore, being insulin sensitive improves muscle function during exercise and dramatically reduces your long-term chronic disease risk simultaneously.

—**Cyrus Khambatta, PhD,** *New York Times*–**bestselling author of** ***Mastering Diabetes***

People have heard of the brain-gut connection, which is the way our gut microbes can affect our mood, our brain function, even our cravings. But did you realize there is a gut-muscle connection too? Research suggests our gut microbiome helps preserve muscle size, strength, and function as we age. New research suggests our gut microbes may actually enhance our exercise performance. You can look like a Greek god or goddess on the outside yet be absolutely rotting on the inside. Too many bodybuilders sacrifice their long-term health in the interest of their short-term physique. This compromise is completely unneeded. With a plant-based diet, you can have that optimal physique and simultaneously enhance your health, rather than giving it up. The gut microbiota are connected to inflammation and our immune system, both of which are critical for muscle gain and recovery from exercise. When we optimize our gut, we will see gains in the gym and recover faster. The way to optimize the gut microbiome is clear—eat an abundance and variety of plants.

—**Will Bulsiewicz, MD, MSCI,** *New York Times*–**bestselling author of** ***Fiber Fueled***

FAT: IT'S NOT ALL BAD

Fat, as strange as it may sound, is an essential part of your diet. As one of the three macronutrients, it's a requirement for sustaining life, no matter how taboo it has at times become in the areas of health, fitness, athletic performance, and weight loss. But before we get into it, let's first acknowledge that we all *have* fat. Even if you're tempted to describe yourself as *being* fat, let's just keep it at the healthier observation that we all have fat. Once again: Fat is necessary. It protects your organs, helps your body absorb nutrients, produces important hormones, supports cell growth, and provides your body with energy. In fact, it's your body's second preferred source of fuel, after carbohydrates. Fats, not proteins, are what get used as energy when your carbohydrate stores run out, especially after a long workout or training session. We'd also like you to accept that *eating fat does not necessarily make you become fat.* So instead of learning to avoid fat, we recommend learning how to consume the best possible sources of it, in the best amounts, in order to produce the best results.

So what do athletes do to improve their athletic performance when it comes to calibrating their fat intake? We talked with a number of elite competitors who embrace fat and make a point of consuming it in its most natural, healthiest state as often as possible.

Austin Aries is a world champion pro wrestler. Before we go any further, we want to acknowledge that, yes, we realize pro wrestling is choreographed sports entertainment, not based on a particular athletic skill or on the technique of one competitor versus another, as in collegiate or Olympic wrestling. But even though the wrestling is staged, the wrestlers build their bodies to have the muscle size, strength, endurance, and flexibility to perform difficult acts of power and agility in front of live audiences. Austin is one of those guys. Pro wrestling is about as macho as it gets, perhaps even more so than professional football, rugby, or boxing, rivaling mixed martial arts for the title of the "manliest" sports to follow on weeknight television. So it comes as a surprise to many that a growing number of pro wrestlers are leaving animal proteins off their plates.

Austin challenged the status quo back in 2002 when he rejected all forms of animal protein and became a dedicated vegan athlete. He went on to build his body with plants and became a leaner, more efficient, and more aesthetic (read: ripped) pro wrestler. He worked his way up the ranks, winning championships in independent wrestling leagues all over the world, and eventually landed a job with the biggest company in the industry, World Wrestling Entertainment (WWE). And not only that, he was selected to perform at WrestleMania, the Super Bowl of professional wrestling, watched by millions of viewers around the globe.

We've known Austin for years, and when we talked with him about his plant-based nutrition approach, he unequivocally embraced a fat intake of nearly one-third of his calories, unabashed by critics who may suggest it is a little high. In reality, Austin's fat intake is (albeit just barely) within the general guidelines we recommend, coming in at the high end at just around 30 percent of his 3,000-calorie diet. Austin achieves this fat intake by eating mostly whole foods, focusing on nuts and nut butters, and by eating foods known to have high fat content, such as avocados, seeds, and various kinds of nuts. The rest of his calorie intake is relatively similar to that of many strength athletes, with about 50 percent of his calories coming from carbohydrates and the remaining 20 percent from protein. Austin knows that fats are one of the best sources of energy, second only to carbohydrates as the body's preferred fuel. And because it is the most concentrated energy source, having more than twice the calorie density of carbohydrates and protein, he doesn't fear this macronutrient. He also knows that maintaining an optimal diet isn't about total fat intake but about the types of fats he eats.

To maintain his weight, Austin eats about six times per day, mostly whole foods, but with some processed foods from favorite plant-based restaurants in Las Vegas. He aims to consume 20 to 30 grams of fat with every full meal (he has three full meals a day), which adds up to over 100 grams of daily fat intake. He exercises about four days per week to maintain his muscle mass, preferring free weight exercises such as dumbbell and barbell movements to build and maintain muscle and strength. He is also as laid back as it gets when it comes to professional athletes. He doesn't take himself too seriously and doesn't allow stress to negatively influence his health. Along with his relaxed demeanor, he gets good-quality sleep, which supports his high-quality plant-based diet and exercise routine.

Even in the testosterone-rich industry of pro wrestling, Austin has not met much resistance to his plant-based diet. The most difficult part is getting the catering staff to understand and embrace plant-based options on the menu for the wrestlers when he is on tour, but the other athletes have been supportive of Austin's "different way of eating." In fact, many have been intrigued. And wouldn't you know it, years after Austin made his debut in the WWE, some of the top pro wrestlers in the world adopted a plant-based diet too—at least for a period of time—most notably multiple-time WWE champion Daniel Bryan (**Brian Danielson**), WWE Champion CM Punk (**Phillip Brooks**), WWE Intercontinental Champion Ryback (**Ryan Allen Reeves**), and Allie (**Laura Dennis**), who has continued to be plant-based. At the time of this writing, it's estimated that there are dozens of plant-based athletes on the professional wrestling circuit. Sometimes it takes just one person to lead by example and pave the way for others to feel inspired that they too can achieve great athletic results on a plant-based diet.

It is common for strength athletes such as Austin to follow a relatively high-fat plant-based diet—especially with a 3,000-calorie intake—but they're not the only ones who are embracing fat. Long-distance runners, triathletes, and ultramarathoners know a thing or two about depending on high calorie intake to fuel their many hours of training and competitive races, and many don't shy away from the concentrated energy source that fat calories provide. **Laura Kline**, an elite athlete in multiple endurance sports disciplines, knows that fat is her kind of fuel.

Laura is a world champion duathlete, earning the title of best in the world in a sport that consists of running and cycling. Duathlons are similar to triathlons, but with running replacing the swimming (run and bike and run). She is also a national champion triathlete (representing Team USA in 2008), was selected as the 2013 Ironman All World Athlete in her age bracket, has spent time as the number one nationally ranked female duathlete in her age group, and has pretty much dominated the racing scene. And we should point out that even though these races have some commonalities (namely endurance), it's straight-up impressive that she has reached such distinction in these different disciplines. And she's done it all while following a plant-based diet for the past fifteen years.

Healthy fats are an important part of that diet. "As a female endurance athlete, my main focus is always on the amount of healthy fat I am consuming," she says. "This is the most important to me for maintaining healthy bones and joints. While I am easily obtaining sufficient protein and carbohydrates from all of my plant-based meals, I always make sure to add a healthy fat source such as nuts, seeds, avocado, or coconut milk. Both protein and carbohydrate intake are important to athletes, but as long as I am eating a healthy whole-foods diet, and consuming the proper amount of calories I need each day, the necessary carbohydrates and proteins are there." Like many elite athletes, Laura plans ahead and travels with fruit, sliced vegetables, and hummus and one of her favorite go-to travel foods—trail mix. Even as prepared as she is, though, there is always a chance that international travel will throw her for a loop. "When traveling abroad, I'll bring some packaged precooked rice and other options just in case. I once ate a package of precooked rice mixed with a container of hummus I found at the store the night before a world championship race overseas, and I won a gold medal!"

Far from weighing her down, these healthy fats, eaten in moderation, are what help her really fly. "When you eliminate the unnecessary animal products from your diet, your body doesn't have to work as hard to process and digest them, which leaves more energy for your body to perform," she notes. "You can skip right past the postmeal sluggishness and keep your engine burning long and strong throughout the entire day."

Instead of sweating the minutiae of each meal, she embraces the overall philosophy of "real food, real results." She knows that if she fills her plate with whole, plant-based foods, she'll be able to hit her nutrient requirements, including protein. In fact, her favorite response when people ask where she gets her protein is "From the same place the animals you eat get theirs!"

Nutrition aside, there are other important aspects to her journey to become a world champion, an endeavor that healthy plant-based whole foods support, but that must be supported by an iron will. For Laura, her drive to achieve runs deep, as it was instilled in her at a young age. "I have been a dedicated athlete since the age of eight," she told us. "Some of it is in my blood, but I was also raised in a competitive environment—my father always pushed me to work harder than my peers and never allowed me to give anything under a 100 percent effort. He must have seen that drive in me because I embraced the hard work and never backed down from a challenge. When you want something so bad, you have to be willing to dig deep into the well to achieve it. To be a world-class athlete, you have to be all in. You have to learn to thrive in tough conditions. You have to embrace the failures so you can learn from them, and acknowledge the successes only so that you can build upon them. You have to stay grounded, consistent, and intrinsically motivated. You have to put your head down and do the work with confidence and determination. Most of all, you have to absolutely love it—the journey, the victories, and the defeats."

But that kind of determination also has to be tempered by listening to your body's needs, as Laura learned the hard way earlier in her career. After some dark and challenging phases in her personal life, running was an escape that also gave her a feeling of being in control. She could be in control of her own pain, pushing her body to its limits. And it seemingly paid off, delivering results. But that came with a costly lesson that many of the world's greatest athletes know all too well. Instead of listening to what her body was asking of her and respecting its limits, she pushed through the warning signals, ignored injuries, and didn't get adequate rest. This led to a series of setbacks, including a collapse and hospitalization from heat stroke during a race, a DNF (did not finish) result at both a world championship and a national championship race, and an injury that she allowed to progress until she could barely walk, requiring her to take seventeen months off. That was when she realized she needed to change her mental approach to her sport. It can still sometimes be a challenge for her to ratchet things down when she wants to keep pushing, but she now has a much better handle on her relationship with her sport.

Laura loves the fact that she can still compete at a high level, even after fifteen years of racing among the world's best, but she knows that it can't last forever. But even though she, like any athlete, can't avoid the inevitable future when she won't be able to compete the way she once did, she is hopeful about the future of plant-based athletes: "Seeing the explosion of athletes switching to a plant-based diet is so exciting to me! The fact that we are seeing well-known plant-based athletes across the whole spectrum of sports is very telling—you can be successful and dominate as a vegan athlete no matter what your sport. The visibility of vegan athletes is breaking the old stereotypes that many people had— that you can't get enough protein and will be weak, malnourished, and unhealthy. Normalizing the plant-based diet in sports allows the next generation of athletes to easily transition, without some of the roadblocks vegan athlete pioneers have faced along the way. As a fifteen-year vegan athlete, I am proud to be able to squash the idea that you cannot have longevity as an athlete eating only plants, and I am honored to pass along my experience and knowledge to younger athletes."

Like Laura, **John Joseph** knows that it takes a balance of foods to fuel his Ironman distance triathlons. The challenge of swimming 2.4 miles, cycling 112 miles, and running 26.2 miles is not easy for anyone—even the athletes who rigorously train to do it. But when you factor in the fact that John is in his late fifties and is still living a late-night, hard-rock life as a touring musician with the hard-core punk band Cro-Mags, it adds another level of difficulty. But John has an edge. He has been plant-based for forty years, specifically focusing on organic and locally sourced food.

For John, it all began back in 1980 when he was a singer in a hard-core punk band, hanging out with other bands whose members were Rastafarians and into health, fitness, and plant-based eating. Inspired by them, the yoga community, and the Hippocrates Health Institute, he became a vegan. What motivated him most was the idea of ahimsa— that we don't have the right to inflict violence on other living entities for our food. For John, this idea of nonviolence was like an antidote to experiences earlier in his life. He came from an abusive household, spent time in jail and on the streets, was shot and stabbed, and bore witness to the violence on the streets of 1970s New York. Embracing a way of life free of animal cruelty was one way to escape to a more positive, peaceful place.

Around that same time, while spending time with his late uncle, who was a cycling enthusiast, John watched the Ironman triathlon on television. He was moved to tears by the stories of the athletes who were competing, some overcoming cancer or other major obstacles in their lives. Finishing the Ironman was their personal victory, and at that moment, John swore that some day he would compete too. And he did—almost thirty years later, at the age of fifty. It was just as humbling and invigorating as he expected. "Everybody's got their reason to show up and beat down their demons. That's what it's all about, because we all have them. We're all carrying baggage, and athletics, the world of sports, brings people together." For John, the countless hours of training and competing are a way to deal with life's challenges in a positive way. "I don't think there's been a race where I didn't have tears in my eyes when I finished because of everything I've been through in my life. To have that gift to be able to cross the finish line, to test yourself and what you're made of, that you never quit, you never give up. That's what it teaches you, that you have to be persistent and disciplined, and you have to have that determination, and it carries over into every other aspect of your life, the work ethic that comes with it."

John is now fifty-eight and has competed in Ironman events around the world, from Taiwan to Mexico. His plan is to continue competing in triathlons into his seventies, and he asserts that what some might dismiss as crazy is actually possible thanks to his plant-based diet. "Many of my peers who subscribe to a false belief of 'protein, protein, protein' and follow an animal-based diet are having a bunch of health issues that I don't have to deal with." John truly feels that he performs athletically now as he did when he was in his twenties—four decades ago—and he credits his diet, his positive mental attitude (what he terms a PMA), and his teachers along the way for helping him find his purpose. When it comes to nutrition, John doesn't count macronutrients. He eats by intuition but says he keeps his nutrition "dialed in" because he knows what works for his body. He uses sports gels when he's on the bike and organic plant-based protein drinks after a workout, and he loves to prepare his own foods, which naturally have a balance of protein, carbohydrates, and fats. He doesn't completely avoid added oils, but he keeps them to a minimum during cooking when possible. His primary focus is on consuming whole-plant foods, with an emphasis on leafy greens, lots of water, and performance-enhancing foods such as fruit, hempseeds, nut butters, and oats. "Depending on the activity I am doing, it's going to determine when I fuel, how I fuel, and what I am going to do to recover," which will vary according to the exercise—such as fruit before a run or oatmeal or quinoa before a longer training session such as a long bike ride.

John says that people notice what he's accomplishing as a plant-based athlete at his age, and they often ask him for insight. His advice is simple: "Give it a try." He said that among people for whom he recommends a plant-based diet, nine out of ten report that they're sticking with it because they feel so great. He also acknowledges that most people don't care what you say, but they're looking at what you do. When it comes to walking your talk, and truly leading by example, few do it better than the rugged, perpetually positive Ironman triathlete from the mean streets of New York.

Eat Fat, Stay Lean

As we discussed in chapter 2, fat contains 9 calories per gram, making it by far the most calorie-dense macronutrient—packing more than twice the calorie density of carbohydrates and proteins. What that means is that if a food has 10 grams of fat per serving, 90 calories in that serving are from fat. If you were to consume 100 grams of fat in a day (not difficult to do if you're eating animal products), that would be 900 calories coming purely from fat—nearly 50 percent of an entire day's 2,000-calorie diet. Of course, most athletes consume well over 2,000 calories per day, but the example is to show how dietary fat can easily make its way into the diet in high volume because of its unique calorie density. This can be problematic for two reasons. First, many fat sources have little to no nutritional value (especially oils and hydrogenated fats lurking in processed foods). Second, taking in too much fat can counteract the efforts you're putting in at the gym, especially if your goal is to lose weight. And even though your goal may be to put on mass, and therefore take in more calories to couple with your strength-training regimen—something we'll talk more about in chapter 7—you still don't want a majority of your calories to come from fat because fat crowds out the nutritional benefits you'd get from carbohydrate-rich foods. So understanding how fat fits into the macronutrient pie is crucial for keeping your fat intake within optimal range.

Back in chapter 2, where we recommended that you devote 50 to 75 percent of your total calories to carbohydrates, we also advised limiting your fat intake to 15 to 25 percent, depending on which ratio works best for you. While finding that sweet spot does take some trial and error and will depend on your sport and your goals, the rule of thumb stays consistent: fat should be only a supporting character on your plate and is what we call a "condiment" food. You need it in your meals, just not a lot of it.

This raises the next important point about fats: **they are not all created equal**. In addition to monitoring how much total fat you're including in your diet each day, it's important to know what kinds of fats you're eating. There are four main types of dietary fat:

Monounsaturated fat
Polyunsaturated fat
Saturated fat
Trans fat

Monounsaturated fats contain omega-9 essential fatty acids (EFAs). Omega-9 EFAs can be produced by the body, so you don't need to get them from dietary intake. But there are still benefits to consuming dietary sources of omega-9. Monounsaturated fats have been proven to decrease inflammation, improve insulin sensitivity, increase "good" HDL cholesterol, decrease "bad" LDL cholesterol, and help eliminate heart attack- and stroke-causing plaque in the arteries. Great sources of monounsaturated fats include nuts such as almonds, cashews, and walnuts; avocados; chia seeds; and coconut. While some vegetable oils, such as sunflower and olive oils, are rich in omega-9 EFAs, choosing the whole-food versions (nuts themselves rather than oils from nuts or seeds) will provide the most nutrition and contain micronutrients that are lost during the pressing and concentration of processed oils.

Polyunsaturated fats are made up of omega-3 and omega-6 EFAs. Unlike omega-9s, these are completely essential, meaning we must get them from our diet, since our bodies cannot make them, and they deliver so many benefits. But there's a catch: we tend to get too many omega-6 EFAs and not enough omega-3s.

Omega-6 EFAs are primarily used for energy and are crucial for our biological functioning, but because they're found in oil and other processed foods, most Americans tend to take in too much, which can have detrimental health effects. Omega-3s, on the other hand, are harder to come by through our food and therefore are deficient in most people's diets. This too has detrimental health effects because omega-3s are critical building blocks for our cell membranes and can also improve heart health, boost mental health and mood stability, aid weight loss, and contribute to brain development. They also fight inflammation, aid in preventing dementia, reduce the symptoms of asthma, promote bone health, and decrease liver fat.

The ideal ratio of omega-6 to omega-3 fatty acids is around 4:1, or even 3:1. But most people take in an omega-6 to omega-3 ratio that ranges from 10:1 to 20:1 to 50:1! The risks of eating too many omega-6s and too few omega-3s include increased likelihood of developing cardiovascular disease, inflammatory and autoimmune diseases, and cancer, whereas low ratios suppress those risks. That said, if you're eating primarily whole-plant foods—and therefore largely avoiding oils and other processed foods—your risk of taking in too many omega-6s is relatively low. However, you do still need to focus on making sure your omega-3 intake is optimal. The best plant-based sources of omega-3s include walnuts, hempseeds, chia seeds, and flaxseeds. Some people choose to supplement omega-3s as an "insurance policy" if they don't think they're getting a good variety of foods that naturally contain this essential fatty acid, or if their body has a hard time absorbing and utilizing essential fats. We'll talk more about that, as well as other supplements you may want to consider, in chapter 6. But for now, consider incorporating more omega-3-rich foods into your diet.

Saturated fats are the type of fats you don't want to add to your diet. Eating foods that contain them raises the level of harmful LDL cholesterol in your blood, which increases your risk of heart attack and stroke. The American Heart Association recommends an intake of just 5 to 6 percent of total calories from saturated fats, and this will take some vigilance, even if you're avoiding animal products. While saturated fats are frequently found in such things as butter, lard, cheese, ice cream, and other dairy products, some baked goods and even energy bars can contain saturated fats in the form of processed oils. That said, a *small* amount of saturated fat in your diet—roughly 5 percent of your total intake—is not only acceptable but also advised. A great healthy source of saturated fat is coconut, which also delivers medium-chain triglycerides (MCTs). These shorter chains of fats are easily digested and deliver many health benefits, such as improving brain and memory function, increasing energy and endurance, lowering blood sugar and cholesterol levels, and encouraging weight loss.

Trans fats are found in two forms, naturally occurring (in some animal foods, particularly processed meats and dairy) and artificial (partially hydrogenated vegetable oils). Artificial sources make up the majority of the trans fats we consume and are created by adding hydrogen to liquid vegetable oils, which makes a semisolid, semiliquid oil that is commonly used in baked goods and heavily processed foods such as pizza, chips, cookies, and anything with butter. Studies have linked consumption of trans fats to heart disease, inflammation, high LDL cholesterol, and low HDL cholesterol. Consumption of trans fats also leads to an increase in triglycerides, which can cause stroke and heart disease. Perhaps it's needless to say, but we recommend avoiding trans fats entirely. That should be relatively easy if you're following a whole-foods plant-based diet.

Daily Fat Guidelines

To ensure that you're keeping your fat intake in check and you're not including too many unhealthy fats in your diet, our recommendations are that you try to do the following:

- Keep your fat-derived calories to 15 to 25 percent of your daily diet.
- Limit saturated fats to less than 5 percent of those calories.
- Limit trans fats to as close to zero as possible.
- Try to include more sources of omega-3 and omega-9 while being vigilant about not overdoing it on omega-6 (especially from oils and processed foods). The optimal ratio of omega-6 to omega-3 ranges from 4:1 to 3:1. Note that some foods naturally contain omega-3 and omega-6 essential fats, such as walnuts and hemp seeds.

High-fat plant-based foods include the following:

Omega-3

Flaxseeds	Navy beans	Flaxseed oil
Chia seeds	Brussels sprouts	Fortified foods such
Walnuts	Avocados	as soy beverages
Tofu		

Omega-6

Tofu	Hempseeds	Olive oil
Walnuts	Pumpkin seeds	Palm oil
Almonds	Hulled sesame seeds	Hempseed oil
Cashews	Whole-grain breads	Grapeseed oil
Peanut butter	Cereals	Safflower oil
Sunflower seeds	Olives	Avocado oil

Omega-9

Olive oil	Macadamia oil
Sunflower oil	Almonds

Saturated Fat

Coconut (meat, yogurt, butter, oil)

Still Not Convinced That Fat Can Be Good?

Dietary fats often get a bad reputation because they are commonly associated with donuts, butter, ice cream, and animal foods that we are told to avoid because of their implications for weight gain and poor health. But that's where science comes in. Rarely do we acknowledge that there are fats in chia seeds, likely because chia seeds are far less common than jelly-filled donuts. Yet plant-based fats are abundant in foods such as avocado and coconut, peanut butter and almond butter, and nuts and seeds of all types—foods that most people have access to, even if they aren't on our radar as much as pizza and milkshakes are. And plant-based fats have benefits we should be aware of. Nutritional science doesn't care which ideas about fats are popular; it cares about what the evidence says is helpful or hurtful to human health.

What Evidence-Based Science Says About Plant-Based Fats Versus Animal-Based Fats

In 2018, researchers at the Harvard T.H. Chan School of Public Health published their findings from a study they conducted over twenty-two years with more than ninety thousand participants. Men and women were asked to record their food intake to the best of their ability and accuracy, which was then collected every four years. The researchers were particularly interested in the impact on coronary heart disease (CHD) of plant-based monounsaturated fatty acids (MUFA-Ps) compared with that of animal-based monounsaturated fatty acids (MUFA-As). Their conclusions were as follows.

Heart disease risk was lower when unhealthy saturated fats, refined carbohydrates, or trans fats were replaced by plant-based monounsaturated fat but not by animal-based monounsaturated fat. Higher intake of the plant-based fats was associated with a 16 percent lower risk of dying from any cause. In contrast, higher intake of animal-based fat was linked to a 21 percent higher risk of dying from any cause.[1]

Our observations from this study go a bit deeper. It was reported that the number one most eaten source of plant-based monounsaturated fat was olive oil. Even though it can deliver myriad health benefits, when compared with other whole-food sources of fat, olive oil is pretty low in nutritional value. It has an ANDI score of only 10 out of 1,000, and it is made up of 4,000 calories per pound of fat (a tablespoon alone has 14 grams and 120 calories). Also, foods such as French fries, salad dressings, margarine, and baked goods were counted as "plant-based sources" of these fats. Imagine what the results might have been had they studied the effects of *whole-food* plant-based fat sources. If more processed types of plant-based fats can contribute to a 16 percent decrease in any cause of mortality, just think of what a diet of fat sources from avocados, walnuts, almonds, cashews, flaxseeds, hempseeds, chia seeds, and coconuts could have produced!

Of course, that is just one aspect of one particular source of fat, but it tells a compelling story that is consistent with the theme of elevated nutrition and improved athletic performance through better nutritional intake: real, whole-plant foods supply the greatest nutritional return on investment, from carbohydrates to proteins to fats.

Don't worry, though—even serious plant-based athletes make exceptions sometimes. When they travel, go out to restaurants, or attend celebrations or holiday gatherings, they sometimes consume processed forms of fats (which are pretty much unavoidable in all restaurant foods and baked goods). But because they make a point of consuming healthy fats most of the time, they have a strong foundation of health rooted in real-food nutrition.

The point is, we don't want you to fear fats, or even to fear oils, but to be aware of the necessary balance of such foods.

At this point you have all the insight you need to start constructing your optimal diet to support your training—one that's balanced between the three macronutrients, calorically in range, and rich in nutritional value. That said, no matter how hard we try, there are some nutrients and essential compounds that we don't get from our food, or at least not enough of them. And some athletes swear by additional supplementation to boost their training or gain a competitive edge. In the next chapter, we'll break down the whys and whats of supplementation and help you figure out what kind of regimen might be right for you.

• • • • •

Since I transitioned to a plant-based diet after I retired from competitive swimming, the biggest thing I noted was how my body felt and looked. I had struggled with postathletic weight gain (despite still working out three-plus hours a day), and after incorporating a plant-based diet, I finally felt like myself in my body . . . perhaps for the first time.
—**Rebecca Soni, three-time Olympic gold medal-winning swimmer**

Though heavyweight boxers don't need to make weight, maintaining my weight is important. I've learned to almost hear my body's needs.
—**Cam Awesome, US amateur boxing champion**

The impact my lifelong vegan diet has had on me as an athlete is the ability to keep my body in shape 365 days a year, by sticking to a healthy vegan lifestyle. I've been blessed with two Olympic Games, gold and silver X Games medals, and gold at the US and Canadian championships, and I will give credit to the healthy lifestyle and diet that I've chosen to live by.
—**Kevin Hill, two-time Canadian Olympic snowboarder, X Games gold and silver medalist, vegan since birth**

6

SUPPLEMENTS:
SHOULD I OR SHOULDN'T I?

Perhaps the most controversial and most popular topic regarding a plant-based diet—outside of protein consumption—is dietary and sports supplementation. Specifically:

1. Do I need to supplement in order to get the nutrition I need?
2. Do I need to supplement in order to excel as an athlete?

While there's not a simple yes-or-no answer, there is some crucial information you can arm yourself with in order to make the most informed decision for yourself. So while we will eventually share the experiences of elite athletes and how they choose to supplement (or not), we first want to examine some of the major myths surrounding supplementation, nutrition, and sports training; which supplements are just marketing noise; and how some supplements can round out your plant-based diet. Let's break it down even more.

Do You Need to Supplement a Plant-Based Diet?

The answer to this often-asked question is complicated for a reason: it's rooted in long-standing misconceptions about diet and nutrition in general. The confusion around this topic stems from two major sources:

1. **The reductionist tendency to look to solve food problems by supplementing**

2. **The incorrect notion that a plant-based diet is lacking in nutrition**

For decades, we've been told to "take our vitamins." Remember those Flintstones chewables? Households across America had their pill cabinets stocked with them because doctors and drug companies were hawkish about the idea that everyone needed more vitamins in their diet. They weren't necessarily wrong—thanks to our obsession with fast food and convenient packaged foods, the vitamins, minerals, and other phytonutrients that we'd normally get from whole plants was pretty much going out the window. Selling these vitamins has also become a big-time moneymaker. Nutritional supplements—meaning products in liquid, pill, or powder form that provide one or more specific nutrients—are a multibillion-dollar global industry, totaling $130 billion in 2019, with projections of being north of $250 billion by 2025. According to the Council for Responsible Nutrition (CRN), 77 percent of adults take dietary supplements. While some of this reflects the number of individuals who take what we believe to be essential supplements, which we'll talk about in a moment, many people are taking supplements for nutrients that they could otherwise be getting from their diets.

Which leads us to the second piece of the puzzle: Can you get all the nutrition you need from a plant-based diet? As we discussed in depth in chapter 2, we know in no uncertain terms that plants have all the essential amino acids you need, and that a diverse plant-based diet that meets your daily calorie needs provides all the essential amino acids your body requires. It is also universally understood that plants represent the *origin* of vitamins and minerals in nutrition and therefore deliver ample levels of what you rely on to live a healthy life. A well-planned nutrition approach does not (largely) require additional multivitamins, fiber, or antioxidant pills because the diet itself contains large amounts of all of those nutrients. Nor does it require additional supplemental protein, since most people, including nonathletes, often consume two to three times the amount of protein they actually need—which is either eliminated or stored as fat. While there are a few exceptions that we'll touch on, in general, taking vitamin supplements is like playing catch-up with your diet. It serves only to fill in the holes that exist because of the plant foods that you don't eat. Supplements should be used as their name suggests: to *supplement* your nutrition program, not to be your nutrition.

When to Take Out a Nutritional Supplementation Insurance Policy

While a plant-based diet covers a majority of your nutritional bases, there are some elements that can elude even the healthiest vegan (and many omnivores). The fact is that not all nutrients come from plants. Rather, there are essential nutrients that aren't abundantly available from plants (such as vitamins B_{12} and D); others that may not be adequately absorbed from plant sources (zinc); and still others that may exist as part of certain plant foods but are not commonly consumed as part of a Western plant-based diet (iodine, vitamin K_2, and certain omega-3 fatty acids). Again, we're not encouraging you to use supplements as a nutritional crutch. Rather, we're encouraging you to *complement* your plant-based diet with a handful of essential nutrients that are critical for your health. The difference lies in the idea that you should continue to focus on reaping most of your essential nutrients from plants, while filling in the blanks left by the nutrients that are not found in the most commonly consumed plants or are not adequately absorbed from those plant sources. These include vitamin B_{12}, vitamin D, omega-3s, iodine, vitamin K_2, and zinc.

Vitamin B_{12}

This vitamin isn't made by plants or animals; rather, it's manufactured by microbes. These microbes can technically be found in soil as well as in our water; however, owing to modern farming practices and water filtration, we don't get many microbes anymore if we eat only plants, whereas meat-eaters do typically get more (only a tiny benefit when you factor in the cholesterol, saturated fat, and inflammation that come with the package deal). So because we've come a long way from our ape forefathers, who got their B_{12} fill by eating bugs, dirt, and feces, we may need to pop a daily supplement.

B_{12} is essential for your health, particularly to help make DNA, which is the blueprint your body uses to make new cells. Low levels of B_{12} can lead to fatigue, weakness, constipation, brain fog, difficulty with coordination and balance, depression, and neurological issues. It can be hard to detect a B_{12} deficiency, so it's a safer bet to preemptively supplement with it as an added measure of protection.

There are two primary potential sources of vitamin B_{12}: cyanocobalamin and methylcobalamin (along with its coenzyme, adenosylcobalamin, with which methylcobalamin should be combined for best results). They are nearly identical, but the primary difference is that methylcobalamin occurs naturally and can be obtained from food sources containing bacteria that house B_{12}, whereas cyanocobalamin is synthetic. There's currently no consensus as to which form is better, only that you should include B_{12} in your supplement lineup.

How Much You Need

You don't require large amounts of B_{12} in order to maintain optimal levels. That's because your body releases the vitamin in tiny amounts over long periods of time. So long as you consume around 2.4 micrograms (mcg) per day, you can rest assured that your body will be able to utilize ample stores of B_{12} for the foreseeable future, even if you miss a couple of days or even weeks. (Don't be alarmed if your supplement provides much more than 2.4 mcg. Because it's water-soluble, there is little risk of overloading to the point of toxicity.)

Vitamin D

This one is a little bit of a misnomer—vitamin D is not a vitamin at all; rather, it's a steroid with hormone-like attributes that helps influence the functions of pretty much all of our major systems, particularly immune, neurological, and cardiovascular. Vitamin D is not naturally part of any food source (some food manufacturers, namely in the dairy industry, fortify their products with it) and is produced by our own bodies when we are exposed to sunlight. However, because most of us spend a majority of our day under artificial light, combined with where we live (certain latitudes get less sun than others) and pollution (which blocks the rays we need from the sun in order to synthesize vitamin D), it's safe to say that most people not living in tropical climates need to supplement. This is particularly true if you figure in that a vitamin D deficiency can be the root of getting sick more often and more severely, and of depression, fatigue, muscle pain and weakness, bone loss, heart disease, high blood pressure, diabetes, and multiple sclerosis.

How Much You Need

It's possible you're already getting enough D from the sun. To find out, get a blood test and make sure that your doctor measures 25(OH)D or 25-hydroxy vitamin D. Most experts suggest that, for optimal health and even cancer prevention, blood levels of vitamin D should be greater than 30 milligrams per deciliter (mg/dL).

For low vitamin D levels, many experts, such as Dr. Michael Greger, suggest a supplemental dose of around 2,000 international units (IU) of vitamin D_3.

Omega-3 Fatty Acids

As we discussed in chapter 5, there are two kinds of "essential" omega fats: omega-3 and omega-6, and you want to aim for more of the former and fewer of the latter. Omega-3s consist of DHA, EPA, and ALA. While ALA is fairly easy to come by in a balanced plant-based diet (thanks to nuts and seeds), DHA and EPA can be more difficult. And research has shown that as many as two-thirds of people on a plant-based diet have low levels of omega-3 fatty acids. (It's worth mentioning that people who eat fish tend to have sufficient levels of DHA and EPA; however, those sources tend to be high in contaminants—so they're not exactly a great trade-off.) Also, some individuals have a difficult time converting ALA to DHA or EPA.

Omega-3s are particularly crucial for brain function and can quell depression and anxiety and contribute to better mental focus. And because they're also powerfully anti-inflammatory, omega-3s can help reduce risk factors for heart disease and metabolic syndrome.

How Much You Need

If you don't regularly consume food sources of DHA and EPA, you won't show signs of deficiency in the next year or two; the damage is more subtle and corrosive, the sort that is imperceptible until it manifests in a chronic disease later in life. But the potential benefits of increasing our intake of these compounds are considerable. For this reason, we recommend complementing your plant-based ALA with a purely produced, algae-derived source of DHA and EPA. The scientific community has not reached agreement in terms of a recommended daily intake for DHA and EPA, though Dr. Greger recommends taking 200 to 300 milligrams (mg) of an algae-based (fish-free) DHA/EPA supplement, two or three times per week.

Other supplements, beyond the Big 3 (vitamin B_{12}, vitamin D, and DHA/EPA), that some people on a plant-based diet may benefit from are **iodine, vitamin K_2, zinc, selenium,** and **magnesium**.

Iodine

Your body relies on iodine to create essential thyroid hormones. Without those, you would be unable to properly regulate metabolism and other vital functions. This process is even more important for pregnant women and for children because a growing human relies on thyroid hormones for skeletal and brain development. Iodine is similar to the omega-3s in that this mineral does exist as part of certain plants—

especially seaweeds such as kelp, hijiki, kombu, and wakame—but may not be adequately consumed as part of a Western plant-based diet. There are land-grown iodine sources, such as cranberries and potatoes, but their iodine content is largely dependent on cultivation practices and soil quality, including the iodine levels naturally present. So looking to those foods for sufficient iodine isn't a reliable avenue. And then there's iodized salt, or table salt that's fortified with iodine. But since we advise moving toward more natural forms of salt, such as sea salt or Himalayan rock or pink salt—which don't have added iodine—and doctors warn that too much sodium intake isn't great for blood pressure or cardiovascular health, that's not a viable source either. Oh, you could get iodine from consuming dairy, since small amounts are left over by the products used to clean the dairy-processing equipment, but we're going to take a pass. So in order to get enough iodine, you could make a point of eating more marine plants on a daily basis. Or you could look to a multivitamin or supplement.

How Much You Need

Whatever your chosen form, try to reach the recommended daily intake of 150 mcg for adult men and women.

Vitamin K$_2$

Most of us don't realize that vitamin K, like the omega-3s, comes in multiple forms. One of those, K$_2$, has only recently been understood to serve as a vital component of an optimal nutritional profile. If you take away only one thing about K$_2$, remember that it is critical for enabling your body to properly manage calcium. That means moving calcium away from soft tissues, such as your brain and your heart, and toward your bones and teeth. Vitamin K$_2$ also helps prevent coronary artery disease because it helps prevent calcification of arterial walls. And, like omega-3s, it can keep disease at bay by combating chronic inflammation.

Although it's easy to get enough vitamin K$_1$ from a typical plant-based diet (mainly thanks to leafy greens), K$_2$, typically found in animal-based foods such as butter and egg yolks, isn't as easy to come by. While fermented foods, such as natto, miso, and tempeh (all forms of fermented soybeans), contain K_2, it's not enough to be able to confidently say that you're getting everything you need.

How Much You Need

While there are general recommended intakes for vitamin K (120 mcg and 90 mcg for adult men and women, respectively), there are no official recommendations for K_2 specifically. Some experts, such as Dr. Andrew Weil, suggest a daily dose of 10 to 25 mcg.

Zinc

Zinc is an important nutrient with a complicated story. Our bodies utilize zinc in a variety of ways. In fact, the mineral helps stimulate the activity of more than one hundred enzymes. It also supports proper immune function, plays a role in ensuring normal growth, enables processes such as gene regulation, and even helps neurons communicate, thereby enabling memory formation and learning. Studies have even shown that zinc can help stave off age-related chronic illness by combating systemic inflammation.[1]

What makes zinc less than straightforward is the fact that while many vegetables contain zinc, we don't always absorb it. There are a number of variables that dictate how much of a substance actually enters your bloodstream: the amount of digestive juices available to break down a food and pull out the active components; the specific chemical form of those nutrients; and even the other items consumed at the same time. There are also blocking agents that inhibit the uptake of specific nutrients, which brings us back to zinc. Many vegan foods that are rich in zinc also contain phytates, which hinder our bodies' ability to absorb zinc. Some medical researchers suggest that, as a result, vegans and vegetarians may need to increase their zinc intake by as much as 50 percent in order to compensate for the diminished absorption.

To reiterate, zinc is available from a wide range of plant-based foods, including legumes, tempeh, and tofu, along with many nuts, seeds, and grains. It can also be derived from a variety of fortified products, such as plant-based milks, many cereals, and even certain meat substitutes. Just keep in mind, if you plan to get your zinc from the whole foods listed here, be sure to learn how to enhance zinc absorption by reducing phytates—such as by roasting nuts and soaking or sprouting beans and grains before cooking them.

How Much You Need

How can you tell if you're consuming and absorbing sufficient amounts of zinc?

The most accurate method is to simply ask your doctor to draw blood and check your serum zinc levels. Before you jump off the couch to schedule an appointment with your doctor, though, keep in mind that research suggests vegans do not have much lower zinc status than the general population. A 2013 meta-analysis found that zinc levels in vegans were only slightly lower than those of their nonvegetarian counterparts, and the difference was even less when comparing populations in developed nations.[2]

That should be heartening news. Nonetheless, given the importance of zinc in so many diverse bodily functions, and the potential complications with absorption, try to be mindful of the amount you consume each day. The recommended daily allowance for adults is 11 mg for men and 8 mg for women. If you think you might be consuming too little—or are diagnosed with a deficiency—the Academy of Nutrition and Dietetics suggests taking a supplement of 150 percent of the recommended daily allowance (RDA), though other experts suggest a more modest supplemental dose of 50 percent of the RDA. Since the upper tolerable limit is 40 mg per day, either dose is unlikely to pose a threat over time.

Other Minerals

Finally, other minerals may or may not be needed as supplements, depending on your definition of "supplement."

Selenium is important to help protect us from neurodegenerative disorders such as Alzheimer's disease, Parkinson's disease, mood changes, cardiovascular disease, and cancer, as well as reproductive problems in men and women. It's not in many plant foods (thanks, soil depletion!), but it is in one, and in abundance: Brazil nuts. If you want to get selenium this way, one nut a day is the right amount for most people.

Magnesium is another one that we can blame soil depletion for, and deficiency is a problem in vegans and omnivores alike. Magnesium also helps with the absorption of iodine, so if you're going to supplement with iodine, it makes sense to also include some magnesium, in the appropriate ratio.

What Supplements Do Vegans Need?

At a minimum, aim for the following per day:
- 300–1,000 mcg vitamin B_{12}
- 1,000–2,000 IU vitamin D_3
- 300 mg DHA
- 100–200 mg EPA

And if you want to cover all the bases, add the following per day:
- 100–150 mcg iodine
- 8–12 mg zinc
- 50–100 mcg vitamin K_2
- 30–50 mcg selenium
- 150–200 mg magnesium

These nutrients are so important for vegans, in our opinion, that one of us (Matt) started a company to produce a daily supplement that provides all of them. The goal is to make it easy for people following plant-based diets to get these nutrients without having to combine different pills or to take a typical multivitamin (since many of the nutrients most multivitamins provide are unnecessary or excessive when plant-based diets are so rich in them). You can learn more about the company's research and products at LoveComplement.com.

Busting the Iron Myth

Besides protein, iron is one of the biggest concerns of people coming off meat. After all, meat is the best source for the stuff, right? Nope. Not in the slightest. Here's what's up.

There are two types of iron: heme, which is found in animal foods, and nonheme, which is found in plants. It is a fact that heme is better absorbed than nonheme iron and that vegetarians and vegans may have lower iron stores than omnivores. But that said, **vegetarians and vegans do not have higher rates of anemia**. Studies point to the fact that a "low-normal" iron reading does not mean "less than ideal." In fact, there's some evidence that low-normal iron stores can actually be beneficial, contributing to better insulin function and lower rates of heart disease and cancer.[3] And what's more, vegans tend to have even better iron levels than vegetarians because they're replacing foods such as eggs and dairy products—which contain virtually no iron—with plant foods that have richer stores of the stuff. So experts, including our friend and dietitian Matt Ruscigno, agree: **iron doesn't have to be an issue in a plant-based diet**. A varied, well-rounded diet will most likely mean that you don't need to supplement. However, we encourage you to ask your health-care provider—ideally one who understands what healthy readings look like for someone following a plant-based diet—to test your levels, just to ensure you're within healthy range.

Here's how to ensure you get enough iron.

1. Start by making sure that you're eating foods that contain substantial amounts of iron. Some of the best plant sources include the following:
   —Legumes: lentils, soybeans, tofu, tempeh, lima beans
   —Grains: quinoa, fortified cereals, brown rice, oatmeal
   —Nuts and seeds: pumpkin, squash, pine, pistachio, sunflower, cashews, unhulled sesame
   —Vegetables: tomato sauce, swiss chard, collard greens
   —Other: blackstrap molasses, prune juice

2. Make sure that you're *absorbing* enough iron. This is just as important as eating enough iron-rich foods.

— **Eat a number of smaller "doses" throughout the day.** Iron isn't a one-and-done dose; in fact, the more you eat in one go, the less your body will absorb. The percentage of iron you'll absorb is higher when your meal contains only a few milligrams.

— **Eat iron-rich foods with foods higher in vitamin C.** The absorption of iron can increase by as much as five times when you combine nonheme sources with foods such as lemon, oranges, and tangerines. And some iron sources, such as leafy greens, broccoli, and tomato sauce, already contain vitamin C. We'll talk about this in more detail later in this chapter, starting on page 126.

— **Be mindful of coffee and tea.** These beverages contain tannins, which can block iron absorption. Experts recommend avoiding them an hour before or two hours after your meal.

When in Doubt, Check It Out

If you are unsure of whether you are deficient in any of these essential nutrients, or are curious about exactly how much to supplement, we recommend asking your primary care doctor about having blood work done and working with you to get your levels to where they should be. It may also shed light on whether you're able to absorb certain nutrients from your food, as some people have trouble doing (especially in the case of converting ALA to DHA/EPA). We particularly suggest working with a plant-based doctor, as they have a more nuanced sense of what optimal levels should look like and will be able to guide you with a food-first approach whenever possible. The website www.plantbaseddoctors.org/ is a great way to find someone in your area.

Sports Supplements

Whereas you don't need a ton of additional supplementation for optimal *health* when on a plant-based diet, some athletes choose to add supplements for optimal training and performance results. So should you?

If you were to ask whether sports supplements are *necessary* for success in athletics, the answer would be an emphatic no. There are many Olympic medalists, world-class athletes, and professional athletes at the highest level who do not use sports supplements to support their athletic achievements. We know this from our interviews with a huge number of elite athletes who don't use supplements, for example, Olympic medal–winning track cyclist Dotsie Bausch; Rebecca Soni, a six-time Olympic medal–winning swimmer who also set five world records; and three-time Olympic gold medal–winning soccer player Heather Mitts, along with former world-class triathlete and current world record holder in swimming for his age group Rip Esselstyn and Team USA heavyweight boxing champion Cam Awesome, who said, "I rarely use any supplements. Anything I've needed I've been able to get from my diet."

The Olympic athletes, Dotsie, Rebecca, Heather, and others, largely steered clear of supplements because they all feared failing drug tests. We heard this from almost all the Olympic athletes we spoke with. The fear of potentially failing a test and being disqualified from the Olympic Games outweighed the desire to try supplements with unknown risks. Many didn't even use protein powders because of feeling uncertain about what was in them. We also know that sports supplements are not necessary for success from our own experiences in sports—not needing supplements to gain significant amounts of muscle—and from learning about amazing athletes who don't have access to modern sports supplements, such as the famed long-distance running Tarahumara indigenous people of northwestern Mexico.

But can supplements provide an advantage? Likely so, especially at high levels of sports such as powerlifting and sprinting and other "explosive" sports that are brief and intense, where joint supplements and energy supplements in particular can help give a burst of energy, support tissue repair, and reduce inflammation. Supplements may also benefit endurance athletes who need to replenish electrolytes or need extra fuel during a sports competition, such as a marathon. But supplements tend to play a bigger role for more elite athletes than for amateurs. Does taking a protein powder daily make any measurable difference in performance for the average weekend warrior? Not a bit. But could protein powder help elite bodybuilders reach specific macronutrient intake goals in order to build their physique a certain way? Sure. That's because at the top levels of competition, even the slightest edge could put an athlete over the top of their competitors. But for most amateur athletes, these kinds of nuanced advantages tend to just be a drop in the bucket. By taking these supplements, it's not as though you will suddenly run significantly faster or lift substantially more weight (unless the supplementation in question is illegal anabolic steroids and growth hormones, which of course is not what we're advising here).

And don't be tempted to give too much credit to a supplement another athlete may be using. Sure, supplements may play a role in someone's ability to build muscle mass or burn fat, but it's a small role, and other aspects such as work ethic, consistency, diet, and attitude are the major determining factors. Also, what works for someone else may not necessarily work for you, since our bodies are so intricate and uniquely different. For example, creatine is a well-researched supplement shown to produce positive benefits, but for Robert, every time he used it, he had stomach pains that were so intense he couldn't even exercise. So that nullified any supposed benefits he would be getting. The same can be said for caffeine-based energy supplements, which have been proven to be fairly effective (and which we'll address more specifically in a moment). If you use a caffeine-based drink to prepare yourself for your evening workout, but then you are unable to sleep and you thereby disrupt your muscle recovery, the supplement is pretty useless for you.

But for someone who works out first thing in the morning, it could be helpful. So, there are plenty of ways to view the efficacy of supplements and determine whether they fit into your lifestyle.

The Exceptions

As they say, there's an exception to every rule. So even though supplements aren't to credit for most changes in athletic performance, there are a couple of secret weapons that have been scientifically proven to benefit some athletes.

Caffeine

Many people may not think of caffeine as a supplement, but it sure is one. In fact, caffeine can accurately be described as a drug because of the way it acts as a stimulant on the central nervous system. It is found naturally in plants, including coffee beans, tea leaves, and kola nuts, and it can have a significant impact on training and competition in sports that require a certain level of alertness or focus, such as tennis, table tennis, martial arts, and baseball, along with endurance sports such as distance running and triathlon. If you choose to give caffeine a try as a performance-enhancing tool, be mindful that many athletes report that the benefits are noticeable only if this is the only time you're taking in caffeine—as in, you may need to give up your morning (and afternoon) cup of coffee. Caffeine is also not recommended if you have any of the following: caffeine sensitivity, hypertension (high blood pressure), heart disease, rapid heart rate, or gastroesophageal reflux disease (GERD), and it should be omitted by pregnant women and women trying to get pregnant. We suggest using caffeine in low to moderate doses and as early in the day as possible so as not to disrupt all-important sleep, deep rest, and recovery. Also be mindful that caffeine is a substance that you can become addicted to or rely on just to get through the day. If you ever get to a point where you feel like caffeine has control over you, rather than you having control over it (can you go a day, or two or three, without any caffeinated stimulation?), then it may be time to evaluate whether it is enhancing your training or detracting from your life. Caffeinate with caution.

Creatine

Creatine is a substance that is found naturally in muscle cells and helps your muscles produce energy during heavy lifting or high-intensity exercise. Chemically, it shares many similarities with amino acids. Your body can produce its own creatine from the amino acids glycine and arginine, and it gets stored mainly in your muscles as phosphocreatine (the rest goes to your brain, kidneys, and liver), which is a form of stored energy that helps your body produce more of a high-energy molecule called ATP—the body's primary energy currency. Creatine also alters several cellular processes that lead to increased muscle mass, strength, and recovery.

Creatine has been shown to help build muscle in the following ways:

- Boosted workload
- Improved cell hormones
- Raised anabolic hormones
- Increased cell hydration
- Reduced protein breakdown
- Lower myostatin levels (which aids in muscle growth)

Creatine is one of the most well-researched supplements available, and studies thus far reveal no negative effects. Because of that, creatine has become one of the most popular and widely used supplements, particularly within the strength athlete community of bodybuilders, powerlifters, and football players.

Since creatine helps retain water in your body, you may notice that your weight will significantly increase by a few pounds or more. Don't get too excited—it's not all immediate muscle mass built overnight. But it is adding more total mass to your frame, which then allows you to lift, press, or pull more mass. That said, you will want to consume large quantities of water when using creatine, as recommended by creatine manufacturers.

Multiple studies also reveal that creatine has cognitive benefits for individuals who don't consume as much dietary creatine (which is found in meat), suggesting that creatine supplementation can help improve memory and brain function and that those following a plant-based diet may experience even more significant benefits or results from creatine supplementation than omnivores.

Adaptogens

This medicinal class of plants delivers exactly what their name sounds like: they help your body adapt, specifically to physical and mental stress. The term was first used by USSR scientists, who looked to these powerful plants to support the cosmonauts in their space program. What they saw was that adaptogens improved learning, memory, immune response, endurance, stamina, and recovery time. It's no wonder that elite athletes have embraced them as well. What makes adaptogens so effective is that they're "bidirectional," meaning they can energize you if you need a boost or help soothe your nervous system for a calming effect. And then they encourage your body to return to a healthy resting state once you've been recalibrated. Common adaptogens that you'll find in many athletes' pantries include ginseng, ashwagandha, cordyceps mushrooms, sea buckthorn, licorice root, goji berries, holy basil (tulsi), astragalus, reishi mushrooms, and rhodiola.

Beets

Not to state the obvious, but oxygen is important during exercise. As we breathe, our blood carries oxygen throughout our bodies to muscles that help us run, ride, or lift heavy things. Limit the oxygen and you limit your exercise performance. But reduce the physiological oxygen "cost"—or how quickly your body uses oxygen—by improving cardiovascular function and you perform better with the same level of effort. So how can you reduce your oxygen cost?

Studies show that beets can help. Beets contain high levels of nitrates, which help dilate your arteries and improve overall cardiovascular function, thus allowing for more oxygen delivery to your cells. A recent study found that a group of cyclists regularly drinking beet juice could perform an exercise task with 19 percent less oxygen than those in the placebo group.[4]

How to use it: Drink one to two glasses of raw beet juice forty-five minutes to an hour before a workout. Alternatively, you can eat cooked beets (three whole, to be exact) in a salad or stir-fry, or use a powdered version such as Healthy Skoop Ignite Performance Beet Blend.

Nutritional Yeast

Even though moderate exercise can strengthen immune function and even reduce risk of getting sick by up to 25 to 50 percent,[5] sometimes extreme physical exercise can have the opposite effect. The stress on your body from consecutive hours of exercise can impair immune function and increase your rate of upper respiratory infections. While a diverse whole-foods plant-based diet is one of the greatest ways to strengthen your immune system, sometimes you need an additional boost. You could wolf down Emergen-C drinks and hope for the best, or you can reach for nutrient-rich nutritional yeast. According to a study published in the *British Journal of Nutrition*, nutritional yeast can protect the body from an exercise-induced dip in immunity.[6] The study found that cyclists who endured a high-intensity bout of exercise showed a corresponding decrease in circulating white blood cells (the kind that fight off illness-causing viruses and bacteria). But when the same athletes added just three-quarters of a teaspoon of nutritional yeast per day to their diet and were tested again, they showed better immune function after the test than when they started. And a study published in the *Journal of Sports Science and Medicine* found that marathon runners who took roughly a spoonful of nutritional yeast per day were able to cut their rates of upper respiratory tract infections in *half*.[7] As an added bonus, those same runners also reported feeling less confusion, fatigue, tension, and anger and more vigor and energy.

How to use it: Luckily, nutritional yeast has a nutty, slightly cheesy flavor and is a delicious plant-based condiment on variety of dishes. Add three-quarters of a teaspoon of nutritional yeast per day to any food that would benefit from the addition of savory, Parmesan-type flavor: stir-fries, salads, grains, pasta dishes, potatoes, and the like.

Remember that supplements are designed to be the tip of your regimen's pyramid, not the foundation. They are potentially that little extra push that may help you get through a few more reps or shave a little time off your run, and if soreness prevents you from exercising as hard or as often as you like, targeted supplementation may alleviate some of that discomfort and allow for more productive workouts. If you are seeking particular results from specific supplements, start a nutrition journal and document your experiences, even just as audio or video recordings, in addition to tracking weight loss or weight gain. Use it to track otherwise imperceptible changes—are you bigger, stronger, or faster? Can you recover more quickly? Your experiences may be anecdotal, but you will have your own set of data to reflect back on.

No Whey, Man

Whey and casein are two of the most common types of protein to consume in supplement form. But though they might deliver results in muscle gain, they greatly lack in the health department.

Whey and casein are the two main proteins found in cow's milk. They're extracted during the cheese-making process, powdered, packaged, and then sold primarily to athletes. The problem with this is that cow's milk is unquestionably meant only for calves, just as all mammals' milk is meant for their specific offspring. There is no human nutritional requirement for cow's milk, just as there is no human nutritional requirement for giraffe's, zebra's, or cat's milk. Plus, cow's milk is designed to help a sixty-pound calf grow to six hundred pounds in a year, and by year two, double that weight. It's safe to say that milk protein is really good at helping things grow. And while whey and casein protein are great at growing muscle, they are also effective at growing cancer cells. When Dr. T. Colin Campbell, one of the most accomplished nutritional scientists in history, discovered that certain levels of casein were associated with cancer tumor cell growth in rats (and, conversely, decreasing the intake of casein protein stalled that growth), it became the foundation of his seminal work, *The China Study*. In his words, "Casein is the most relevant chemical carcinogen ever identified."[8] Recent studies on human cells second this finding, concluding that casein promotes the proliferation of prostate cancer cells.[9] Similarly, whey has been linked to "significantly" elevated prostate cancer mortality risks.[10]

So we say leave the milk to the cows and let the plants do the work.

The Next Level: Food Combining for Maximum Nutrient Absorption

While eating a diverse whole-foods plant-based diet is a strong baseline for getting ample nutrition, there are small "hacks" you can make in each meal to make sure your food is firing on all cylinders. No, there is no need to combine particular foods to get complete protein—a myth that was perpetuated in the 1970s and later corrected on the basis of nutritional science understanding of how our bodies use amino acids— but there are some benefits to intelligent and deliberate food pairing to maximize the absorption and utilization of vitamins and antioxidants.

Vitamin C Helps the Absorption of Plant-Based Iron

To better absorb plant-based (nonheme) iron, which both plant-based and animal eaters can be low on, add citrus fruits rich in vitamin C to iron-rich foods to aid in absorption. Orange or lemon juice drizzled on salad greens, such as kale, or grapefruit mixed with hempseeds and flaxseeds in a smoothie or toppings on oats or a plant-based yogurt, or slices of lime added to your lentil and rice dish topped with cashews are all strategies to aid in the absorption of plant-based iron. Here's a list of foods high in vitamin C and foods high in iron.

Foods Rich in Vitamin C

Lemons	Mandarins	Tangerines
Oranges	Pomelos	Tangelos
Limes	Kumquats	Blood oranges
Grapefruits	Clementines	

Foods Rich in Iron

Tofu	Hempseeds	Spinach
Tempeh	Flaxseeds	Broccoli
Lentils	Cashews	Brussels sprouts
Peas	Pine nuts	Potatoes
Chickpeas	Almonds	Mushrooms
Black-eyed peas	Macadamia nuts	Olives
Kidney beans	Kale	Amaranth
Lima beans	Swiss chard	Quinoa
Pumpkin seeds	Collard greens	Oats
Sesame seeds	Beet greens	

Increase the absorption of fat-soluble vitamins by eating them with healthy fats.

Consume unsaturated fat sources such as avocados, olives, nuts, and seeds with foods that are high in vitamin A, vitamin E, and vitamin K, such as yellow and orange vegetables, dark leafy green vegetables, and nuts and seeds. This could be as easy as adding a fat-based dressing to a salad—though we recommend limited oil intake in favor of whole-food sources such as olives, avocados, and sesame seeds, but since oil-based dressings are so common and readily available, using them is one easy way to increase the absorption of fat-soluble vitamins. Another, of course, is to just add nuts, seeds, or nut and seed butters to yellow and orange vegetables or to your salad greens. You can also effectively combine these foods in smoothies or smoothie bowls by adding leafy greens, nuts, and seeds to any recipe you prepare. We're particularly big fans of smoothies (especially Matt, who finds them an easy way to get lots of whole-food nutrients into his two athlete children), as they are one of the most universally effective ways of combining foods to maximize absorption and utilization, and they're also an efficient way to consume large amounts of calories in liquid form (if that is your goal), which can aid digestion. It's also a very cost-effective way to prepare meals packed full of nutrition. If drinking smoothies isn't your thing—for one of us, it's just not—you can make smoothie bowls, adding more whole foods such as berries and nuts on top of a thicker, more puddinglike smoothie in a bowl. A word of caution, though: if a smoothie is full of fruit, sip it rather than chug it to avoid spikes in blood sugar.

Foods Rich in Fat-Soluble Vitamins

Vitamin A:

Sweet potatoes	Other leafy greens	Cantaloupe
Kale	Carrots	Black-eyed peas
Spinach		

Vitamin E:

Sunflower seeds	Peanuts	Kiwifruit
Almonds	Spinach	Mango
Hazelnuts	Broccoli	

Vitamin K:

Kale	Parsley
Spinach	Fermented foods

Vitamin D:

Exposure to sunlight (a natural, non-food, non-supplement form of Vitamin D)

Vitamin D boosts calcium absorption.

As we talked about at the beginning of the chapter, since most of our vitamin D comes from exposure to the sun, and many people live where year-round sun exposure is not possible, supplementing with vitamin D is recommended. But rather than just supplementing with vitamin D at random, consider taking it at the same time you're eating calcium-rich foods, as vitamin D can increase the absorption of calcium in the body. So, if you're not eating a salad while shirtless in the sunshine, consider taking a vitamin D supplement at the same time you eat the following calcium-rich foods:

Collard greens	Oranges	Calcium-fortified
Broccoli	Orange juice	foods
Dried figs	Soymilk	

Turmeric and black pepper increase each other's anti-inflammatory and antioxidant properties.

You may be familiar with sunshine-yellow turmeric as a spice, which is ground from the root of the turmeric plant. Turmeric has been used for centuries in traditional healing practices thanks to its powerful anti-inflammatory properties, and athletes also love its performance-enhancing abilities, including its beneficial effects on recovery time. Black pepper is also known for its anti-inflammatory properties, and it specifically helps the absorption of curcumin, the most active compound in turmeric. When turmeric and black pepper are combined, they become a very powerful healing spice combo, compounding the absorption of curcumin by about *2,000 percent*. There are so many delicious ways to enjoy this pair, such as using them to season a tofu scramble, a curry, a smoothie, roasted vegetables, or your latte. This is one of the most common and most beneficial food pairings, especially for athletes seeking improved recovery through reduced inflammation.

Green Tea with Lemon

Green tea (especially matcha) is packed with health benefits, most notably its high antioxidant content, which helps improve brain function; support fat burning and weight loss; repair damage in the body; and prevent diseases including type 2 diabetes, cardiovascular disease, and some cancers. According to studies from universities such as Harvard and Purdue, citrus such as lemon helps increase the absorption of these antioxidants when paired with green tea.[11]

The Best Performance-Enhancing Drugs of All

Many successful athletes choose not to use any performance-enhancing supplements at all, opting instead for performance gains through an elite nutrition program, more consistent training, better hydration, clearer goals, or simply a stronger intrinsic motivation to succeed. You don't have to look much further for evidence than the careers and achievements of the following plant-based athletes.

Dotsie Bausch is an Olympic silver medalist in track cycling, landing on the podium in the 2012 London Summer Olympic Games. She is also a seven-time US national champion, a two-time Pan American champion, and a former world record holder, along with her teammates, in a three-kilometer standing-start sprint in track cycling. She adopted a plant-based diet three years before she earned an Olympic medal, and it was her plant-based nutrition program that fueled her six-hours-a-day, six-days-a-week training for the latter part of her career. Many Olympic athletes, if not most, started their careers young. We've all heard the stories, especially profiled on television during the Olympic Games, of athletes who began their Olympic pursuit when they were three years old, or who had five-hour practices at five years of age, hoping to some-day wave their country's flag as an Olympic athlete. Dotsie wasn't one of those athletes. She didn't even begin cycling until age twenty-six. That's almost unheard of for Olympic athletes. She was late to the game, but she made the most of it over a thirteen-year career that led her to becoming the oldest Olympic athlete in the history of her sport.

Why such a late start? Dotsie wasn't an athlete growing up. The Kentucky-born former fashion runway model rode horses and exercised at times throughout her life, but she was never a competitive athlete and didn't play on any sports teams while growing up as many eventual Olympic athletes do. Dotsie didn't get involved in any organized sport until she got to college, where she spent one season on the crew rowing team. She didn't like the early morning practices, however, and moved on after one season. Not only was Dotsie a nonathlete, but she also suffered from a near life-ending eating disorder and a cocaine addiction and survived multiple suicide attempts. In her midtwenties, after she spent three years in intensive therapy to address her anorexia and other disordered patterns and addictions, her therapist encouraged her to take up exercise to get her body moving again. She chose cycling because it sounded like a good idea to be out in nature. At first it was just an outlet for physical activity, but it didn't take long for Dotsie to realize that she had a natural talent for it. She went on to become an elite cyclist, excelling in road races, and then discovered track cycling. Track cycling takes place on a velodrome, an oval track with steep banks, and track bikes do not have any gears or brakes. With speeds as high as fifty miles per hour, it's a sport that relies on pure strength, endurance, skill, and bravery (as well as significant pain tolerance because lactic acid builds up in your muscles during an all-out sprint for three straight minutes).

Though Dotsie was already a national champion cyclist and one of the best in her sport in 2009, she had yet to unlock the upper bounds of her abilities. After turning on the television in a hotel while preparing for a race and seeing horrific undercover footage of animal cruelty, she decided to swear off meat for good. About a year later, she removed all animal-based foods and by-products from her diet. As a result, her joint and back pain disappeared, her premenstrual syndrome symptoms subsided, her mind cleared, and her recovery after training sped up so significantly that she was able to bounce back to training in half the time of her teammates, who were ten years her junior.

Dotsie's new approach to diet led to a dramatic change in how she was able to support herself nutritionally. Before adopting a plant-based diet, Dotsie was taking up to eight nutritional supplement pills a day and consuming protein drinks—though mainly because everyone else was having them. But once she started eating only whole, plant-based foods, she began eliminating those supplements, including the protein drinks (though she occasionally reaches for one but not out of necessity). Now the only supplements she's sure to include are for vitamins B_{12} and D and omega-3 fatty acids. She doesn't use sports-specific supplements either—nor did she during her quest for an Olympic medal—though she sometimes relies on a glycogen replenishment electrolyte hydration drink to help her recovery.

Dotsie is also a great example of how not all athletes need to follow a rigorously calibrated meal plan in order to maintain well-rounded nutrition. Even though it's something that the majority of athletes do, and it's what we recommend at the very least in the early days of being a plant-based athlete so you can ensure you're hitting all your macros and staying within bounds of your calorie intake, following a meal plan is not required. Dotsie chose not to go this route because it would likely trigger obsessive eating patterns. Instead, she's been eating mostly on the basis of her intuition and food preferences. She simply eats until satiated.

For individuals eating a diverse whole-foods plant-based diet, that's usually enough to get the fuel your body needs. And Dotsie is the perfect example of that. As she put it so well, "It's not that healthy to be an elite athlete. We are doing far too much damage—we damage, repair, damage, repair, all day long." But after she switched to plants—and her laid-back approach to eating with minimal supplemental support—her ability to contend with that recovery cycle was one of the keys to her success, or what she calls her "repeatability"—the ability to repeat intense training sessions over and over with limited rest periods in between. "The golden ticket is how much you can do, and do it over and over."

Dotsie retired from competitive cycling after her 2012 Olympic silver medal–winning performance, and she went on to found multiple nonprofit groups, including Compassion Champs and Switch4Good, of which she is also executive director, bringing plant-based Olympic athletes together to share their stories and to inspire people to leave animals off their plates. According to Dotsie, "Research shows that 96 percent of Americans say they are against animal cruelty, yet nearly 96 percent of Americans eat animals or animal by-products, being responsible for the direct cruelty and slaughter they claim to be against." Even though only a small percentage of Americans follow a purely plant-based diet, "it only takes one to make a difference in the life of another," meaning that every person who keeps animals off their plate saves dozens of animals each year, hundreds over the course of a decade, and thousands over the course of a lifetime.

Rip Esselstyn is a current swimming world record holder in the 200-meter backstroke for the men's fifty-five to fifty-nine age group, a former elite professional triathlete, and whole-foods plant-based devotee for more than thirty years. Rip was turned on to this way of eating during the late 1980s when his father, physician Caldwell B. Esselstyn Jr., was conducting groundbreaking research on how a plant-based diet could prevent and reverse heart disease. He was also inspired by Dave Scott, who won the Ironman World Championship a record six times— tied for the most of all time—and who was a vegetarian. Embracing the power of plants was a big shift for Rip, who grew up eating lots of animal protein and processed foods before his father's research made a compelling case against them and convinced the whole family to convert to a whole-foods plant-based diet.

This life-changing shift came at a pivotal time in Rip's athletic career. For Rip, sports were a way of life. His father won an Olympic gold medal as a member of the 1956 USA Olympic rowing team, and Rip continued this athletic legacy. He started swimming at a young age, which he enjoyed—mainly because he excelled at it. He eventually won a scholarship to swim at the University of Texas, where he was an all-American athlete. Despite his success, he never felt that he reached his true competitive potential in college, so after graduation he set out to become a professional triathlete. It was also at this point that he adopted a plant-based diet, motivated by the knowledge that there were triathletes having massive success in their sport while living a vegetarian or vegan lifestyle.

In 1987, he competed in his first professional triathlon in Chicago. There were four thousand racers, and he came in at ninth place. He recalled, "I won 900 bucks in prize money, and I was like 'I'm in!' I called my parents after the race and told them that my goal was to become one of the fittest people on the planet." He had finally found that spark.

Rip went on to have a storied career, competing in International distance triathlons, with each event requiring a 1.5K swim, a 40K bike ride, and a 10K run. He became one of the top 10 professional triathletes in the world—and the preeminent swimmer. And he rarely received any criticism from other triathletes about his diet because, in his words, "I blew their asses away in the water, and I could keep up with pretty much anyone on the bike. Among the guys that I trained with day in and day out, there was so much mutual respect that there wasn't much ribbing of one another over diet."

It also helped that triathlons were a sport ahead of their time when it came to how athletes fueled. According to Rip, almost all triathletes were consuming a high-carbohydrate, moderate-protein diet, since carbohydrates are the preferred energy source for endurance athletes. When it came to crafting his own nutritional approach, Rip's views echoed those of many of the other athletes in this book—don't get too caught up in the minutiae. "I was never fastidious with how many grams of protein, carbohydrates, or fats I was consuming. I never worried about protein. I just knew as long as I was getting enough calories, and my weight was where it needed to be, I was getting enough protein. I love (now) and loved (then) the simplicity of not making this a scientific experiment, and just basically eating until my body told me I had enough. Eating foods like breads, beans, and pasta, I easily hit my protein goals, even on a 4,000- to 5,000-calorie diet, easily getting 125 grams of protein a day, with roughly 15 percent of my calories coming from protein."

Rip was also only twenty-two years old when he went plant-based, and as many of us know from experience, we're almost invincible at that age, regardless of our diets. But while he doesn't recall a specific boost of energy or amazing recovery at the time he adopted the diet, now that he's in his late fifties, he is certain of the benefits. "I can't remember the last time I was sick or the last time I had the flu, or the last time I had a cold. I believe that is because I have such a fortress of an immune system that's been cultivated over the years as a result of this whole-foods plant-based diet, with all this diversity of fiber, and now I have a microbiome that is like this wonderful ecosystem that is just thriving. That's worth gold to me as an athlete, let alone as just a human that wants to go through each day with a higher quality of existence." He also continues to put his body through the paces, training as though he's still a competitive athlete. "I'm now fifty-seven years old, and I train six days a week. I still train basically like I did in my twenties, thirties, and forties. It's not like I think that because I'm in my fifties I've got to go easy or take two days off after a hard effort. I'm throwing it down every day. The whole-foods plant-based diet is doing what it's supposed to be doing as far as allowing me to recover faster, and reducing inflammation, and aiding in recovery. Whether it's the anthocyanins in blueberries, the beta-carotene in sweet potatoes, the lycopene in tomatoes, or the chlorophyll that's in the green leafy vegetables, they all have a purpose. And I seek them out deliberately. I seek out foods that allow for optimal performance, such as green leafy vegetables loaded with nitrates, which will turn into nitrites downstream and then allow your nitric oxide pool, your endothelial cells, to explode open, which leads to your blood vessels dilating, and then you're getting all this oxygen to working muscles, and that's what it's all about. I got a world record not too long ago, and I was throwing down the berries, the kale, and the beet greens, getting the nitric oxide benefits of whole plants, especially green vegetables."

To say that Rip believes in the healing, medicine-grade power of plants is an understatement. And what reflects that is the fact that he doesn't reach for supplements beyond essential nutrients. He doesn't take vitamin D because he knows he gets his fill from the hours of outdoor exercise he does per day in southern Texas. But he does take vitamin B_{12}, and he loads up on flaxseeds, chia seeds, hempseeds, and walnuts for omega-3 essential fats—something he emphasizes in his breakfast oatmeal or cereal. (Check out his recipe for the bowl he's been eating for the past twenty years on page 268.)

Though Rip spent a decade as a world-class triathlete, he is best known for his work as a firefighter in Austin, where he was part of Engine 2, the famed firehouse that adopted a plant-based diet as a show of camaraderie to improve their health after a number of their members were diagnosed with elevated levels of cholesterol from their animal-protein-heavy diets. This led to his slogan "Real men eat plants," as well as his Engine 2 brand of prepared plant-based foods, which are sold in grocery stores around the country. Rip now tours the country to teach people about the power that plants possess and their ability to prevent and reverse disease. Every year he shares the stage with his father at Plant-Stock, a weekend immersion program at the historic Esselstyn family farm in upstate New York that features many of the "rock stars" of the plant-based movement. People come from around the world to see powerful presentations about how they can change their health and their lives.

Olympic pairs figure skater **Meagan Duhamel** has won Olympic gold, silver, and bronze medals—all while being fueled exclusively by plants. When she first made the switch to plant-based eating almost a decade ago, she didn't have any specific expectations and she didn't necessarily plan on doing it long-term; she just wanted to be healthier in general. But the changes she experienced were significant. "When I became a vegan in 2008, I almost immediately noticed an improvement in my ability to recover. After that, I spent ten years at the elite level of Olympic sport and never once had an injury. I credit a lot of that to my diet, which allowed me to take care of my body on every level."

For Meagan, it wasn't a matter of *if* but only a matter of *when* she would be skating in the Olympics. "I always knew I was going to go to the Olympics. I started telling people when I was six years old that it was what I was going to do. I had a natural drive, and I was always the hardest worker in the room. I also faced every challenge with a positive attitude. Even after a tough defeat, I tried to find the positive so I could move forward even quicker." As a young girl, she studied famous figure skaters and tried to emulate their behaviors, strategies, and mental preparation. She describes it as creating a toolbox of skills to draw upon throughout her career. When she was fourteen years old, she told her parents that she wanted to move away from home to train with a more elite coach. That was the beginning of her junior career. And by twenty-one, she had moved to Montreal after feeling in her gut that it was where she'd find the right coach for her—whom she eventually found, along with a husband.

Even with her confidence in her lifelong dream, the Olympic Games nearly slipped from her grasp completely. She failed to qualify for the 2010 Olympics and almost walked away from the sport altogether. But her gut once again kicked in and told her to keep going, so she did. After being an alternate for the 2006 Olympics, she was ranked eighth in the world and second in Canada going into the 2010 Olympic qualifications, but she failed to make the team. "Everything kind of went black after that. I had my life planned out until the 2010 Olympics. I had no other plan. I felt like I had no purpose anymore and wasn't sure if I was going to continue my sport or stop and go back to school." Then she was offered the opportunity to skate with Eric Radford in the pairs category. She took it as an opportunity to rededicate her life to figure skating and become even more focused on her body's health and the quality of her training. Instead of leaning on sports supplements to give her an edge or aid recovery, she looked to whole-plant foods. She fueled with lots of high-protein oats—as warm oatmeal, cold overnight oats, or baked oatmeal casseroles, or blended into a smoothie—which were her pre- and post-workout go-to. Plenty of hydration and hard work rounded out her regimen.

With Eric as her new pairs partner, they went on to achieve a world #1 ranking for three consecutive years, including winning a 2015 World Championship in a year in which they won gold in every international competition they competed in. And in storied Olympic triumph fashion, after previously failing to qualify for the 2010 Olympics and then winning a silver medal at the 2014 Olympics, they eventually won the elusive Olympic gold as part of Team Canada at the 2018 Olympic Winter Games.

After retiring from figure skating in 2018, Meagan has continued to embrace the plant-based diet that fueled her standout career. She is so passionate about what this lifestyle has given her that she created a website where she shares tips and recipes for thousands of followers who also want to adopt this way of eating. And as the ultimate testament to the complete nutrition of plants, Meagan had an entirely vegan pregnancy when expecting her little girl. What she hopes to teach the next generation, especially athletes, is that they can't ignore their nutrition. "It's more than working hard in your field of play. They need to put more focus into the food they are eating and understand what that food is doing to help their performance and recovery."

• • • • •

I recommend that vegans who don't eat iodized salt or seaweed multiple times a week take an iodine supplement. A modest zinc supplement of about half the RDA is a good idea for active vegans. Vegans who aren't meeting the RDA for calcium through other foods should supplement their diets with calcium-fortified or calcium-added products, such as calcium-set tofu or calcium-fortified nondairy milks.
—**Jack Norris, RD, VeganHealth.org**

I first started on a whole-foods plant-based diet because I was looking for the competitive edge that athletes like Brendan Brazier and Rich Roll were talking about. One of the things that was important for me going into this new lifestyle was to thoroughly research the nutritional requirements for a plant-based athlete. Since the beginning, I've supplemented my diet with B_{12}, algae omega-3, vitamin D, and a multivitamin. I didn't want to set myself up for failure. Over the years, I have had extensive lab work done by my doctors out of concern that *a plant-based diet might not be sufficient for optimal health. To their surprise and mine, the lab results have always been excellent and have never shown any nutrient deficiency. At forty-eight years of age, I am full of energy and vitality. And I hope to be able to pursue all of my athletic interests into old age. My whole-foods plant-based diet is a key component in making it happen.*

—**Maggie Kattan, "the Fit Ninja," Ironman triathlete, USA Track & Field coach**

I don't use any sports supplements. I like to say I train on whole foods, water, and hard work! I do, however, make sure I am eating foods according to my needs. Post training, I love to load up on pineapples with hempseeds. The hemp gives me protein to repair and recover, and the bromelain in the pineapple helps with inflammation. So I am always mindful of what foods I eat at what time.

—**Meagan Duhamel, Olympic gold medal–winning figure skater**

7

PUTTING IT ALL TOGETHER

We've covered a lot of ground up until this point, from why a plant-based diet supports both health and athletic performance to which specific foods are truly best at providing the ideal fuel, to how much protein we need (and don't), to what supplements to take and why. Now, it's time to tie it all together in the name of figuring out what exactly to put on your plate at each meal.

Creating a meal plan that inspires you and compels you to stay on track is paramount for success as a plant-based athlete. First, it ensures that you're hitting your macronutrient goals—getting a majority of your fuel from carbohydrates, followed by healthy fats and protein—as well as your ideal caloric intake. Second, it helps you hold yourself accountable, as preplanned meals and snacks make it a lot easier to stick with your nutrition and fitness objectives than attempting to wing it. We can bet that if you wait until you are starving to search for something to eat, that something will most likely not be in line with your goals. Finally, a meal plan will help you cook and assemble meals that you love to eat. By giving some advance thought to what sounds tasty, having those foods in the house, and then knowing how exactly you want to combine them, you'll be a lot more likely to feel motivated to eat those meals. And when you do that, you'll be much more likely to stick with a program that will deliver results. Here's what that looks like in the life of an athlete.

When it comes to knowing how to build muscle, burn fat, improve athletic conditioning, and build strength, bodybuilders are naturally ahead of the pack because their entire career is based on their ability to build their physique. **Natalie Matthews** and **Harriet Davis** fall into this category—both are International Federation of Bodybuilding and Fitness (IFBB) pros at the highest level in the sport.

Natalie has been following a plant-based diet since 2012. As one of the top competitors in the world in the most competitive of all the divisions of bodybuilding, as well as in her work as a professional chef, Natalie has made a name for herself with the aptly titled social media nickname "Fit Vegan Chef." She is certainly fit, but even when she was competing as a professional surfer in her native Puerto Rico, she didn't have an abundance of muscle. She was unquestionably strong, but she was more lean than muscular. But once she made the leap to competing as a bodybuilder, her new objective for success was having balanced muscle on both her upper and lower body, as well as a low level of body fat. As a chef, Natalie knew what foods to eat in order to build muscle, but she had to learn about the increased volume it would take, combined with a rigorous weight-lifting routine and dedicated consistency in order to achieve her goals. Timing her meals precisely and measuring out every gram of protein, carbohydrate, and fat became part of her everyday routine to ensure that she was hitting specific amounts of macronutrients to reach a preferred ratio, with her total daily calorie intake being of utmost importance. It may sound tedious, but it is often the small, deliberate actions that separate world-class athletes from the rest of us. And the tracking of nutrients is unquestionably more important in the sport of bodybuilding than it is in other sports in which athletes are not scored on the basis of their body fat percentage or muscle mass or water retention.

Since you can't build mass without a calorie surplus, and since that calorie surplus will be stored as fat if you're not exercising, Natalie also created an exercise plan that enabled her to build muscle at a steady pace. Within a relatively short amount of time—over the course of a few years—Natalie transformed from a 100-pound professional surfer to a 110-pound champion bodybuilding competitor, at the height of five feet, three inches, increasing her total body mass by 10 percent.

They say that success leaves clues, and if we can glean any insight from Natalie, it's that setting a goal, creating a plan, developing habits, and being consistent with them is key. Even now, as she works toward competing on the Olympia stage and becoming the best bikini competitor in the world, she stands by these basic tenets of her training.

Harriet adopted a plant-based lifestyle to manage the digestive issues she experienced as a result of consuming animal products. She gradually transitioned from a standard American diet to a vegetarian diet and then ultimately to a 100 percent plant-based diet. She has now been plant-based for nearly a decade, but like many people who transition to a plant-based diet, Harriet's initial biggest challenge with her new lifestyle was finding dining options when traveling. As a bodybuilder who is accustomed to meal prepping and preparing foods for days at a time in order to stay on a specific nutrition program, Harriet overcame that challenge by preparing and freezing meals prior to travel. This isn't as out-there as it sounds—many bodybuilders travel with large coolers so they can have macronutrient-appropriate meals wherever they go. She also researched the locations she was traveling to, ensuring she would have markets close by at which to easily shop for perishable items. Beyond individual preparation and relying on standard grocery stores for produce, tofu, nuts, nondairy beverages, and other common plant-based bodybuilding foods, she uses the vegan restaurant finder app HappyCow to find plant-based restaurants nearby.

Harriet's dedication isn't just because of her commitment to her sport, it's also because she values leading by example. She is passionate about dispelling the myth that you need to eat animals in order to build muscle. "It gives me great joy to watch a new generation of plant-based athletes compete on all levels, amateur to elite. The compelling message emerging is that a plant-based diet is compatible with essentially any fitness goal you have, from building muscle to burning fat to increasing strength and endurance." This message is also at the center of her practice as a plant-based physician, which is her primary career when she's not competing onstage. The highlight of her career is when new patients select her as their primary care provider because she is plant-based. There are people who are genuinely looking for positive changes in their lives, and she feels privileged to help them as both a role model and a family medicine physician.

Christine Vardaros is a professional cyclist. She began her cycling career in 1996 as a mountain biker, turned pro in 2000, and transitioned to cyclo-cross racing in 2002. She represented USA Cycling at three UCI Cyclo-cross World Championships, along with more than thirty Cyclo-cross World Cup events over the past two decades, and she has been ranked as high as sixth in the world. Christine has fueled her success with a plant-based diet since 2000, but she had been steadily reducing her consumption of animal-based food for six years before she decided to become fully vegan.

Being a professional athlete was never a childhood dream of Christine's, that's for sure. "My dream was to become a neurosurgeon, which is what I studied at Columbia University. That is, until I discovered the bike!" Cycling began as a way for Christine to get out of Manhattan on the weekends. She'd ride with friends to the beautiful forests just outside the city; she'd just have to "suck it up and suffer for two to three hours on the bike." But truly, it was love at first sight with the bike, especially the moment she saw her first mountain bike, which showed up on her doorstep one day accompanied by her date. "It looked like something out of *Terminator* with its futuristic suspension. Eventually I ditched the guy, kept the bike, and we have never parted since." When it was just her third time on a bike, she entered a national championship mountain bike race at a ski resort. At that point, it was clear to her and everyone else that she had a knack for it. While her dad wasn't initially thrilled that she was giving up her neurosurgery education for this new dream, when she won her first internationally ranked events, he finally understood. "That day, when I crossed the line for the win, he was waiting for me, arms wide open, to embrace both me and my newfound career."

After her grandmother, who was living near her in New York, passed away, Christine left the Big Apple for California to join her first professional racing team. "I had one bike, a one-way ticket, and seven dollars to my name. I may have been homeless that first night, but for me, chasing a dream is priceless." Christine went on to embrace various modalities of cycling, eventually ending up in Belgium as a top cyclo-cross racer, in a country where cyclo-cross athletes are viewed as celebrities. Cyclo-cross is a form of bicycle racing that typically takes place in fall or winter (or year-round if there are fall- and winter-like conditions) and consists of many laps on a short course (usually 2.5 to 3.5 kilometers in length) that includes pavement, wooded trails, grass, steep hills, and obstacles requiring the rider to quickly dismount, carry the bike while navigating the obstruction, and then remount. Then you also have to factor in the weather conditions, which typically leave the athletes soaked and covered in mud—for a full hour. It's an enormously popular sport in Belgium, and Christine's name has become synonymous with both cyclo-cross and being the most prominent vegan cyclo-cross athlete.

Having been an elite cyclist for a few years before adopting a plant-based diet, and now having been a professional cyclist for twenty years on a plant-based diet, Christine has a unique opportunity to evaluate the impact her diet has had on her career. When we asked her about the biggest change she experienced in athletic performance when she first went plant-based, she said that with absolutely no other changes in her training, she quickly went from the back of the pro peloton (the pack of riders) to winning the races. She also noticed that she rode faster with the same perceived energy output and got more chiseled, especially after going from vegetarian to vegan.

To figure out the right macronutrient ratios for her training and performance, Christine experimented with a vegan ketogenic diet during her off season. The regimen was much higher in fat-derived calories than her usual carbohydrate-heavy fare. "What I found was that I lost my top-end speed and strength. Sprinting on the bike was pitiful. But what did improve was my endurance. I could go out for a six-hour bike ride and never feel tired. I also found that my concentration improved significantly. What I do now is eat more carbs on high-activity days and back it off on easy or recovery days." And she's faithfully stuck with it, even when faced with very few menu options. "I'll never forget competing in the women's Tour de France on nothing but French bread and green beans. Pasta without butter or sauce wasn't even an option in France at the time. I raced my heart out on that simple diet and even fared better than my teammates."

Christine was really onto something when she experimented with different types of plant-based diets to find what was optimal for her. She played around with her macronutrient ratios until she found that sweet spot that best supported her performance and athletic goals. Since maintaining that carbohydrate-focused stride, she reports having more energy than she did twenty years ago, with increased mental energy for concentrating on her high-intensity sport, and when it comes to her recovery, she describes it as "simply magic." That means more consecutive days when she can train hard and also a smoother time during multiday races such as the women's Tour de France. (She recalls waking up "fresh as a daisy" compared with her meat-eating teammates and competitors, who were slowly dwindling away as the days ticked by.)

But even though Christine has had incredible success following a plant-based diet, it wasn't a journey without its bumps. She recalls a moment after a particularly off race when she was in the supermarket shopping for ingredients to make dinner in preparation for the next day's race. A fellow competitor saw her and said, "You sucked today. Must be that broccoli diet of yours." Naturally, without any real plant-based role models back in 1999, she thought there might be some truth to what she said. Immediately she picked up her phone to reach out to her vegan coach for advice. He said, "Christine, step away from the fish aisle, go back home, make yourself some pancakes, get on the trainer for thirty minutes to loosen your legs, and go to sleep." She did exactly as instructed. The following day, she not only placed in the top 10 but also kicked the butt of the anti-broccoli woman, grinning as widely as she could as she left her in the dust. "The proof is in the (vegan) pudding, as they say. When you show to others that you are thriving on a plant-based diet, they take notice."

Christine is now in her fifties, still training and still racing, with no signs of slowing down. She says that when she eventually races competitively for the final time and reflects back on her career, the thing she will be most proud of is effecting change and saving lives through the example she set. She said, "As long as the upcoming generation of both female cyclists and vegan athletes continue to push for the generation to follow them, then I can be nothing but thrilled to help provide a base on which they can build."

Building Your Meal Plans

In this chapter you'll find all the tools you need to build the best meal plans for yourself, and we've divided these meal plans by objective: building muscle and burning fat. The difference is hitting a calorie surplus to put on muscle mass or a calorie deficit to burn fat. Both objectives share the goal of eating foods that will help you build strength while keeping excess fat at bay. Let's start with the basics.

The Basics

These are the true building blocks of your meal planning—they're the resources you should refer to again and again as you hone your own program, making sure that you're hitting your ideal numbers and filling your plate with the most nutrient-dense, calorically appropriate, macronutrient-balanced meals.

Calculate your daily calorie goal. First, you'll want to figure out your ideal calorie baseline. To do this, find a Harris-Benedict calculator online to evaluate your basal metabolic rate (BMR). This equation takes your gender, age, height, and current weight and computes how many calories you need simply to exist, not taking physical activity into account. Then factor in your true activity level by inputting whether you are sedentary, lightly active, moderately active, very active, or extremely active (the calculator will provide definitions of those options) to get your *real* calorie expenditure each day. Once you have your **calorie expenditure** determined, you can simply compare it with your actual **calorie intake**. You can figure out your average calorie intake by tracking your meals using an app such as Cronometer or MyFitnessPal. This is the formula for taking control of your muscle building or fat burning—knowing what you need to consume in relation to your expenditure. If you can clearly see that your daily calorie needs are 2,400 per day and you're trying to build muscle, but you're eating only 2,000 calories per day, you can easily determine that you are not going to have a surplus to add mass no matter how dedicated you are in the gym. Likewise, if you are trying to burn fat and lose weight but are consuming 2,800 calories per day, you can understand why that's not happening.

Remember that the calorie needs you determine are just estimates, and they don't factor in your lean body mass (the weight of your muscle and tissues once your weight in fat has been removed) or the truest, most objective reflection of you (things such as weight and true activity levels have a way of getting a little fuzzy sometimes). That's fine! What you're going for is a general range that will tell you how much food you're eating in a day and approximately how many calories you are burning, and this knowledge will put you in the driver's seat as you work toward your personal fitness goals. The Harris-Benedict calculator and the calorie-tracking apps are the best, most efficient and accurate technology we have to get a detailed look into our calorie intake versus expenditure, and these tools alone can help you make profound realizations about your habits, helping you course correct and get on the fast track to achieve your fitness goals. In our experience as athletes, this has been game-changing, enabling us to regain control of our muscle-building and fat-loss outcomes by being astutely aware of our daily actions and routines.

Mind your macros. When constructing the "perfect" meal (one that will deliver the cleanest, most efficient and long-lasting fuel), remember that it should contain the following:

1. Mostly **carbohydrates** (60 percent of calories)
2. Then a **relatively even split between protein and fats** (about 20 percent each)

That's because your body's preferred energy source is carbohydrates, which are stored as glycogen (or fuel) in your muscles and liver and are what the brain runs on. We can process and absorb only so much protein at a given time—usually about thirty grams per meal, with all protein consumption beyond that being eliminated or stored as energy reserves, that is, fat—and fats are so rich in calories that you need to consume them in moderation to get the best return on your investment (as in getting more mileage from your workouts by not having to work off all those excess calories).

These percentages vary from person to person depending on one's sport, such as carbohydrate loading for endurance athletes and carbohydrate depleting for competitive bodybuilders.

We're going to give you some numbers to find your ideal macro ratio. But, as we'll get to in just a moment, the ultimate goal is for you to step away from the food calculator and embrace a more intuitive approach to what and how much to eat based on how you feel. To begin to build that baseline, follow these guidelines:

• First, try out a 70 percent carbohydrate intake and then a 50 percent carbohydrate intake for a couple of weeks each, without changing your exercise routine.

- For most endurance athletes, the optimum will be somewhere around a 60/20/20 split (percentages of carbohydrates/fat/protein), with some athletes doing better at 70/15/15, and a 50/25/25 split for most strength athletes.

But in general, for good health, longevity, and support of your athletic pursuits, **we recommend getting the bulk of your calories from carbohydrate-rich foods**. This has been echoed by the athletes we've interviewed and has been supported by studies and by experts, and it is the approach that we have followed for many years. Complex carbohydrates are our best ally in the quest for athletic excellence, and, as it turns out, they are also the healthiest foods for us, making them the clear ideal choice for pre- and post-workout nutrition, staple meals, and the foundation of our daily calories. Our goal for you (as it is for ourselves) is eventually to get to a place where you don't need to track your calories on a daily or weekly basis, or even at all. The Harris-Benedict calculator and the meal-tracking apps are designed to help you gain awareness of your actual calorie intake versus expenditure. This is something most people are unaware of, which often leads to weight gain or muscle loss. But as you can see from one athlete's story to another (with the exception of highly competitive world-class bodybuilders), most athletes ease into more intuitive eating on the basis of routines they have developed over time, even as Olympic and world champions. The ultimate goal is to eat in an intuitive, stress-free environment as much as possible, but understanding where you are now is paramount to making any necessary shifts to get your nutrition plan working for you in the most beneficial ways.

In addition to following the sample meal plans we provide later in this chapter (or those contributed by top plant-based athletes, beginning on page 237), one of the best ways to make sure you're hitting your ideal macronutrient ratios is, again, to track your meals with an app such as MyFitnessPal or Cronometer. These allow you to input the calories you consume in exchange for a full breakdown of macro- and micronutrients. You also get many more details, including your percentage daily intake of vitamins and minerals, and other helpful metrics, all graphed out for you instantaneously. While it's not necessary to use these apps over the long term—many people start to get the hang of their macros after about a week of tracking—they're a very helpful resource as you begin this new approach to eating. The truth is, most people don't know what they're eating. By using some form of accountability food tracker, you remove the guesswork and reveal what your diet really looks like, which is the only accurate way to create the changes you seek.

Sample Plate for the Strength Athlete
- 50 percent carbohydrates
- 25 percent protein
- 25 percent fat
    - 1 large sweet potato
    - ½ cup steamed broccoli
    - ½ cup baked tofu
    - 2 tablespoons cashew cheese sauce

Sample Plate for the Endurance Athlete
- 70 percent carbohydrate
- 10 percent protein
- 20 percent fat
    - 1 large sweet potato
    - 1 cup steamed broccoli
    - ¼ cup baked tofu
    - 1 tablespoon cashew cheese sauce

Don't get too hung up on the math—just take a look at the noticeable differences between these two plates. The strength athlete, whose goal is to have a calorie surplus in order to build muscle, has a little bit less broccoli and a little more of the tofu and cashew cheese sauce—but there's still a lot of carbohydrates represented here. By comparison, the endurance athlete, whose goal is to stay relatively light and maximize strength-to-weight ratio, bumps up the broccoli (carbohydrates) and slightly decreases the amount of protein and fat (tofu and cashew cheese sauce). It's not a dramatic difference, but over time these shifts add up to calorie deficit or surplus. It's also important to note that in the scenario where staying lean is the goal, in no way is that plate sparse. It's still loaded up with food, just with an emphasis on foods with lower calorie density, which leads us to our next point.

Consider calorie density. In addition to being mindful of the macronutrient makeup of your meals, you'll also want to pay attention to their calorie density. This is like taking out an insurance policy against over- or undershooting your optimal calorie intake while also feeling satisfied at the end of your meal. Remember, some foods are great for anchoring a meal (mains), while others are better as accessories (side dishes), and still others are to be used more sparingly (condiments).

Get flexible. As in flexible dieting, a.k.a. IIFYM (if it fits your macros). Ideally, once you've figured out how many calories you should be aiming for and gained some experience assembling the "perfect plate" under your belt, you'll begin to move away from tracking every bite, calorie, and gram of carbohydrates and start eating more intuitively.

The first step toward doing that is to trust your food. Know that eating a diverse whole-foods plant-based diet in general is already moving you toward your goal because it naturally encourages lean muscle and discourages the accumulation of body fat. (Note the whole-foods element here—just eating plant-based but still eating processed foods isn't going to produce the same results.) Then maintain a general sense of how you're representing your macronutrients on your plate. Again, no calculator required. Look at your plate—is half or more filled with carbohydrates? Do you have some protein and a little fat represented there too? Then you're most likely on the right track. Look at how you feel and your results—that's ultimately the best metric you can use.

Of course, some people feel more successful having a more finely tuned approach, and that's okay too. In fact, some athletes require that kind of precision in order to hit their goals. But if you're looking to loosen the reins and not obsesses over numbers, you have our permission. Ultimately, we want you to realize that being a plant-based athlete means having food as your ally, not your foe.

Plant-Based Meal Builders at a Glance

Mains	Sides	Condiments
Legumes	**Greens**	**Herbs**
Lentils	Kale	Basil
Split peas	Spinach	Thyme
Pinto beans	Collard greens	Dill
Chickpeas	Mustard greens	Oregano
Lima beans	Romaine lettuce	Rosemary
Black beans	Swiss chard	Parsley
Navy beans	Arugula	Mint
Kidney beans	Butter lettuce	Cumin
Soybeans	Beet greens	Coriander
Adzuki beans	Bok choy	Cardamom

Grains	Cruciferous Vegetables	Spices
Rice	Broccoli	Turmeric
Quinoa	Cauliflower	Cinnamon
Wheat	Cabbage	Black pepper
Barley	Brussels sprouts	Ginger
Oats	Radishes	Peppermint
Millet	Turnips	Nutmeg
Rye	Rutabaga	Fennel
Bulgur	Watercress	Cloves
Buckwheat	Rapini	Paprika
Teff	Maca	Cayenne pepper

Starchy Vegetables	Nonstarchy Vegetables	Seeds
Potatoes	Carrots	Flaxseeds
Sweet potatoes	Asparagus	Sesame seeds
Acorn squash	Eggplant	Hempseeds
Butternut squash	Peppers	Sunflower seeds
Taro	Cucumber	Pumpkin seeds
Yams	Green beans	Mustard seeds
Parsnips	Mushrooms	Chia seeds
Corn	Zucchini	Poppy seeds
Plantains	Onions	Pine nuts
Pumpkin	Okra	Sorghum

Heavy Proteins	High Water-Content Fruits	Nuts
Tofu	Watermelon	Cashews
Tempeh	Strawberries	Almonds
Seitan	Oranges	Walnuts
Peanut butter	Cantaloupe	Hazelnuts
Almond butter	Grapefruit	Peanuts*
Cashew butter	Raspberries	Pistachios
Protein pudding	Pineapples	Pecans
Protein smoothies	Peaches	Brazil nuts
Plant-based jerky	Blackberries	Coconut
Bean chili or soup	Blueberries	Macadamias

*Technically a legume

Dense Fruits	Sauces and Spreads
Avocados	Salsas
Bananas	Dressings
Jackfruit	Hummus
Breadfruit	Guacamole
Passion fruit	Ketchup
Grapes	Mustard
Pears	Relishes
Mangoes	Tahini
Guavas	Chutney
Dragon fruit	Jams

Common Recipes	Common Snacks	Common Beverages
Vegan mac and cheese	Flaxseed crackers	Almond milk
Spinach quinoa pasta	Applesauce	Oat milk
BBQ tempeh bowl	Fig bars	Rice milk
Spaghetti squash	Trail mix	Soy milk
Curried lentil stew	Granola	Tea
Latin bowl	Dried fruit	Coconut water
Vegan queso	Protein pudding	Sparkling water
Mediterranean bowl	Snack bars	Freshly squeezed juice
Whole-wheat pizza	Rice cakes	Kombucha
Vegan lasagna	Dairy-free yogurt	Probiotic drink

Plant-Based Athlete Meal Plans
for Building Muscle

If your goal is to build muscle, then your guiding equation for your meal plans and training regimen will be this:

Calorie surplus + resistance/strength training =
mass added over time

But your meals not only have to deliver surplus calories; they also have to deliver *quality* surplus calories. Ice cream and processed foods will provide a different mass outcome from less calorie-dense plant-based foods such as potatoes, grains, and beans. It's the difference between adding fat and adding lean muscle.

How we recommend filling up your plate at each meal follows our general guideline of eating mostly carbohydrates followed by a pretty even split between protein and healthy fats. Keep in mind that you'll be adjusting the amounts of these foods to hit your specific optimal calorie intake. You'll also see that we recommend having five to six meals a day because you'll be better able to spread out your calorie intake.

Note that we haven't specifically noted condiments in the meal plan, but know that you can further tweak these meals and snacks to meet your calorie needs by either adding calorie-dense condiments (hummus, guacamole, nut-based salad dressing) to consume more calories or by skipping them and choosing lower-calorie options (mustard, vinegar, hot sauce, soy sauce) if you're looking to eat less.

Muscle-Building Meal Plan Template

Breakfast

2 mains	2 sides	1 condiment

Snack 1

2–3 sides

Lunch

2 mains	2 sides	1 condiment

Snack 2		
1–2 sides		

Dinner		
2 mains	2 sides	2 condiments

Snack 3/Dessert		
1 side	1 condiment	

Daily Totals		
6 mains	10–12 sides	5 condiments

Based on this template, a sample muscle-building meal plan might look like the following (remember to adjust for your own portion sizes, based on your individual caloric needs):

Breakfast		
1 large roasted sweet potato (main)	Bowl of oatmeal (main)	½ cup strawberries (side)
	½ cup blueberries (side)	Handful of walnuts (condiment)

Snack		
1 banana (side)	Handful of grapes (side)	
1 peach (side)		

Lunch		
Bowl of mashed cauliflower "potatoes" (main)	Veggie burger (main)	Cucumber (side)
	Romaine lettuce (side)	Optional side salad of leafy greens

Snack		
Handful of sliced carrots (side)	Handful of sliced bell peppers (side)	

Dinner		
Bowl of curry (main)	Bowl of brown rice (main)	Handful of sliced onions (side)

Handful of chopped zucchini (side)	Sprinkle of cashews (condiment)	Optional side salad of leafy greens*
	Black pepper (condiment)	

Snack/Dessert

½ cup pineapple (side)	Coconut flakes (condiment)

*Note that side salads can be added to any meal, since they are low in calories but add lots of nutrition with the addition of leafy green vegetables, and they are specifically recommended for lunch or dinner or both.

Fat-Burning Meal Plans

When it comes to burning fat, we're taking the opposite calorie approach from putting on mass:

**Fewer calories + more training =
decreased body weight**

However, when it comes to balancing your macronutrients, our advice stays exactly the same—more carbohydrates, followed by proteins and healthy fats. You'll see that, compared with the previous meal plan, these meals call for fewer foods represented at each meal, as well as slightly fewer meals, removing an after-dinner snack and dessert. You will also see sides taking up more room on the plate, providing high amounts of nutrition in fewer calories. But don't worry—if you're following this plan and filling your plate with lots of nutrient-dense but not calorie-dense foods, you will not feel deprived or as though you're running on empty.

Fat-Burning Meal Plan Template

Breakfast

1 main	2 sides	1 condiment

Snack 1

1 side

Lunch		
2 mains	1 condiment	Optional side salad
2 sides		of leafy greens

Snack 2	
1 side	1 condiment

Dinner		
2 mains	2 condiments	Optional side salad
2 sides		of leafy greens

Daily Totals		
5 mains	8 sides	5 condiments

Given this example, a sample fat-burning meal plan might look like the following (remember to adjust for your own portion sizes, based on your individual caloric needs):

Breakfast		
Green smoothie (main)	Handful of raspberries (side)	Sprinkle of flaxseeds (condiment)
Banana (side)		

Snack
Bowl of cubed watermelon (side)

Lunch	
1 baked potato (main)	Drizzle of tahini sauce (condiment)
½ cup lentils (main)	
½ cup green beans (side)	Optional side salad of leafy greens

Snack	
1 sliced cucumber (side)	Dollop of hummus (condiment)

Dinner		
Bowl of brown rice (main)	½ cup sliced eggplant (side)	Chutney (condiment)
½ cup cubed baked tofu	Sprinkle of pine nuts (condiment)	Optional side salad of leafy greens
1 cup broccoli (side)		

Three Meals That Make It Easy

To help you put it all together, we've devoted the next chapter to even more sample meal plans, along with a glimpse into the food journals of some elite plant-based athletes. But we also want you to see how easy it is to assemble meals that satisfy your macro needs and put a ton of nutrition on your plate. After all, it's one thing to learn how to eat, and it's quite another to actually do it. These "recipes" plus some strategic grocery shopping will guarantee that you'll pretty much always have something to reach for when you're hungry.

Smoothie or Oatmeal

With a smoothie you can get any (or all) of these high-micronutrient foods in a single meal:

- Berries and other fruits
- Flaxseeds and other nuts
- Greens
- Green or white tea leaves or matcha powder
- Turmeric (use a ¼-inch slice of the fresh root)
- Beans (People actually do this! White beans and silken tofu don't add much bean flavor but give smoothies rich creaminess.)

Giant Salad with Beans and Nut-Based Dressing

Start with a big bowl of greens, throw on beans, mix in a bunch of other veggies, and top it off with a creamy, satisfying healthy-fat-based dressing such as Cucumber Avocado Dressing (page 324) or Caesar Dressing (page 288). In a salad, you can include the following:

- Greens
- Cruciferous and other vegetables
- Onions (red, white, scallions, pickled, etc.)
- Beans

- Nuts and seeds
- Turmeric
- Fruits
- Whole grains or pseudograins (that's right—try tossing in some brown rice, farro, or quinoa for an extra-satisfying salad)

A Grain, a Green, and a Bean

It doesn't get simpler than this. When you structure your meal around these three foods, you not only hit your macros and optimal nutrient density; you also have a ton of variety to choose from. Just a few examples:

Stir-Fry
The grain: brown rice, rice noodles, or quinoa
The green: bok choy or broccoli
The bean: tofu, tempeh, black beans, or adzuki beans

Tacos
The grain: corn or whole-wheat tortillas
The green: lettuce or cabbage
The bean: crumbled tempeh or black beans

Pasta
The grain: whole-wheat, brown rice, or quinoa pasta
The green: arugula, basil (especially for pesto), or steamed kale
The bean: fava or cannellini beans

A Smoothie
The grain: oats
The green: baby spinach or kale (baby varieties tend to be the most tender and subtle in flavor)
The bean: silken tofu or even white beans

The Classic
The grain: up to you
The green: any!
The bean: whatever you've got

There's a Time and a Place for Packaged Food

It's time to address the elephant in the room. We know that whole, unprocessed plant-based foods are going to deliver the best possible nutrition. But we also know that these foods take time and effort to prepare. While we're big fans of doing a big batch cook once or twice a week in order to fill our refrigerators with things such as grains, legumes, marinated tofu, steamed or grilled vegetables, sliced fruit, and large quantities of oatmeal, we also get that life happens. If you're busy or traveling or both, sometimes you need a more efficient option. Or if you're aiming to eat 3,000 calories per day, that will require a lot of time, planning, coordinating, and scheduling in addition to buying a high volume of food. This is where packaged plant-based foods can be an option for you.

The reality is that even the most well-meaning among plant-based athletes are consuming processed plant-based foods, often on a daily basis. Yes, there are some athletes who eat only whole foods—and it's completely doable—but for the vast majority, being able to reach for a snack bar or prepared meal is a lifesaver. Luckily, with the growing number of companies now offering high-quality packaged foods at most grocery stores, that doesn't have to mean compromising on health or quality. The important thing is to be smart about what you're looking for in these products, as well as to not let them completely take over your meal plan.

Here's what to steer clear of in processed plant-based food:

- **MSG.** Monosodium glutamate is a flavor enhancer commonly found in savory foods such as fast foods, chips, instant noodles, frozen meals, and many soups and snacks. MSG consumption has been linked to obesity, liver damage, blood sugar fluctuations, and increased inflammation.
- **High-fructose corn syrup.** This sweetener made from corn is high in calories (57 calories per tablespoon) and is frequently found

in juice, soda, candy, snack foods, cereals, and sports drinks. Consuming high-fructose corn syrup increases your risk of obesity, type 2 diabetes, fatty liver disease, and inflammatory disease.

- **BHA and BHT.** These are petroleum-derived antioxidants used to preserve fat and are known carcinogens.
- **Partially hydrogenated vegetable oil.** This is a type of fat that's formed when liquid oils are made into solid fats, which are used to increase the shelf life and flavor stability of packaged foods (especially baked goods) and many fast foods. These oils contain trans fats, which upset the balance between good and bad cholesterol levels in your body, which in turn leads to lifestyle diseases such as heart disease, stroke, and type 2 diabetes.
- **Artificial sweeteners.** These synthetic substitutes are derived from naturally occurring substances, but they've been chemically altered. Examples include NutraSweet, Equal, Sweet'N Low, and Splenda. These substances have been linked to weight gain and weight-loss resistance, upset bacterial balance in the digestive tract, and increased sugar cravings, and they may cause blood sugar disturbances. Stick with natural alternatives such as stevia and maple syrup.
- **Artificial flavors.** Manufacturers use these chemical additives to boost the flavor of products that are meant to sit on the shelf for extended periods of time. Spotting them can be tricky because food companies are not required to be any more specific on the label than "artificial flavors." While it's almost impossible to know which specific chemicals are being used in an artificially flavored food or drink, it's safe to say that steering clear in general is the best way to preserve your health. It is known that in the case of diacetyl, which is used in microwave popcorn, potato chips, and crackers, there have been links to nausea, headaches, dizziness, fatigue, seizures, and Alzheimer's disease.
- **Artificial colors.** These are chemical dyes that are used to color food and drinks and have been linked to hyperactivity, behavioral

problems, and lowered IQ in some children and have been shown to cause cancer in laboratory animals.

- **Added sugars.** Keep added sugars to a minimum, aiming for less than 25 g per day.
- **Saturated fat.** Limit saturated fat intake to 5 g, or 45 calories, per day.
- **Sodium.** Aim to consume a sodium-to-calorie ratio of 1:1. If a package has 200 mg of sodium, it should have approximately 200 calories per serving. High sodium intake can increase blood pressure because it causes your body to hold excess fluid. It can also increase your risk of stroke, heart failure, osteoporosis, stomach cancer, and kidney disease.

Grocery Shopping Lists

As we wrap up this chapter, we want to leave you with some sample grocery lists so you will feel equipped to master the grocery store as a plant-based athlete. You can see from the lists that follow—curated from some of our featured athletes—how you can easily be prepared to make a green smoothie or a bowl of oatmeal covered in fruits and nuts without a lot of prior planning. Have the foods on hand for a dish featuring a grain, a green, and a bean, and have tasty whole-food options that will help you avoid the temptation of eating processed, packaged, or fast food when hunger strikes.

Robert's Grocery Shopping List

For Robert, the equation is simple: as his friend Chef AJ says, "If it's in your house, it's in your mouth." So one of the preemptive steps in creating a healthy nutrition program is to surround ourselves (our kitchen, pantry, cupboards, shelves) with the healthiest foods, so we're not tempted to eat chips and salsa and chocolate bars (Robert is guilty as charged) when taking a break from working at home. Robert has what he calls the Rule of 3, which includes three specific categories of foods making it onto his shopping list, to ensure a variety of fresh and frozen produce, canned and bulk goods, staple foods, seasonal foods, and some treats, since even athletes enjoy desserts and sweets. It's a healthy relationship to have with food to not exclude some of your favorite foods, so long as they are relatively harmless with just some added sugars or a higher concentration of calories for such treats. This shopping list is designed to last for a week or two; obviously, some foods such as dry bulk goods will last longer than others, such as fresh berries. When supplies start to get low, Robert simply replenishes his stock, not necessarily following the exact volume of grocery shopping each time but filling in gaps, where necessary, to keep ample options available at home. And he often swaps out some foods for others, such as getting different fruits, often depending on what's on sale or what meals are planned for the week ahead.

Robert's "Rule of 3" Grocery Shopping List

3 types of seasonal fruit (berries, cherries, nectarines)

3 types of annual fruit (bananas, apples, oranges)

3 types of green vegetables (romaine lettuce, broccoli, kale)

3 types of other vegetables (potatoes, sweet potatoes, carrots)

3 types of grains (rice, oats, quinoa)

3 types of grain-based foods (pasta, bread, crackers)

3 types of legumes (lentils, pinto beans, garbanzo beans)

3 types of canned legumes (kidney beans, black beans, refried pinto beans)

3 types of nuts (almonds, cashews, walnuts)

3 types of seeds (hempseeds, flaxseeds, chia seeds)

3 types of frozen foods (mixed berries, mixed vegetables, plant-based frozen entrees)

3 types of packaged foods (organic chips, plant-based meat, snack bars)

3 types of condiments (salsa, guacamole, hummus)

3 types of canned or jarred condiments (pickles, olives, artichoke
   hearts)

3 types of snacks and treats (chocolate bars, nondairy ice cream,
   fruit chews)

3 types of staples (tofu, avocado, prepackaged vegan meals)

3 types of beverages (almond milk, sparkling water, zero-calorie
   natural soda)

From this list, Robert can make many of his absolute favorite meals: burrito bowls; hearty soups with potatoes, beans, and kale; pasta dishes with olives and greens; oatmeal with fruit and nuts; tofu and vegetable stir-fries; plant-based burgers; seasonal fruit salads; green salads with beans, olives, and artichokes; plant-based pizza or lasagna; tofu scramble; and dozens or hundreds of other options. The point of the Rule of 3 is to have variety to give ourselves options so we don't get bored or end up eating the same things day after day. If you're just not in the mood for berries, it's nice to have other fruit on hand to choose from. If you've enjoyed way too many potatoes lately, maybe broccoli, brussels sprouts, or peppers are something you're in the mood for instead. If you're tired of rice and beans and vegetables, have some quinoa with lentils and herbs and spices. And if you simply can't decide what to make, don't make anything at all and just heat up a prepared vegan entrée such as a burrito or pizza, or enjoy a wrap or vegetable sushi. The objective, of course, is to have plentiful, delicious options and to select your own favorite foods. Robert's samples listed earlier reflect his favorites, and though he emphasizes a whole-foods diet, he still does have some frozen burritos, chocolate bars, fruit chews, and nondairy ice cream from time to time, and that's part of what makes a plant-based diet so practical, doable, and adventurous. There is no deprivation or sacrifice, but there is a world of possibilities out there, and Robert's sample grocery list is testament to that. Of course, many foods are omitted from this list because it's just a sample. One could easily swap in nut butters, ketchup, mustard, tempeh, seitan, sports supplements, bulk grains and legumes, nondairy cheeses and yogurts, and plenty of other foods. This is just a transparent sample of what Robert reaches for at the grocery store on a weekly or biweekly basis. It may seem like a lot of food—seventeen categories of three items for a total of fifty-one items—but we've all been there many times: at the grocery store with a full cart, or carts, and we've spent a little more than planned, but in this case the food lasts for a while, and the next trip is only a fraction of the purchase to fill in the gaps. And in Robert's scenarios, he's shopping for a family of two, himself and his wife (plus snacks for their little plant-based dogs, whose favorite food is tofu—true story).

Matt's Grocery Shopping List

Here's a basic vegan grocery list that covers all the general foods a plant-based athlete would need. If you're new to the plant-based diet, don't freak out. There's a lot of green here and maybe a few other ingredients you don't typically purchase, and that's totally fine. Maybe leave some of them off for now and try out just a few new items at a time. (Note: These include a few items you obviously don't buy at every trip to the store, but they're good to keep around for cooking.)

- **Fruit:** apples, oranges, bananas, pineapples, fresh berries, frozen mixed berries (for smoothies), lemons, limes, tomatoes, avocados, Medjool dates
- **Fresh vegetables:** romaine lettuce, spinach, broccoli, kale, celery, cucumbers, bell peppers, jalapeño peppers, onions, carrots, garlic, basil, parsley, cilantro
- **Starchy vegetables:** potatoes, sweet potatoes
- **Canned or dried fruits and vegetables:** diced tomatoes, raisins
- **Legumes:** lentils, chickpeas, black beans (preferably dry, but sometimes in BPA-free cans for convenience)
- **Nonwheat grains:** brown rice, quinoa (not technically a grain), granola, steel-cut oats

- **Wheat products:** whole-wheat bread, pasta, pitas, bagels, and wraps; low-sugar breakfast cereals
- **Nuts and seeds:** almonds, cashews, walnuts, flaxseeds, chia seeds
- **Spreads and pastes:** hummus, nut butters, tahini (sesame seed paste)
- **Oils:** olive oil, toasted sesame oil
- **Vinegars:** apple cider vinegar, balsamic vinegar, red wine vinegar
- **Protein powder:** if you're going to get one, be sure it's low in heavy metals (as is Complement Protein)
- **Plant-based milks:** almond is my favorite
- **Tea and coffee**
- **Soy products:** tofu, tempeh, tamari, or soy sauce
- **Other snacks (limited):** tortilla chips, salsa, popcorn kernels
- **Plant-based meat (optional and limited):** Amy's frozen veggie burgers, veggie meat slices
- **Miscellaneous:** maple syrup, dark chocolate, Miyoko's plant-based butter
- **Complement** (a daily supplement for the hard-to-find nutrients in a plant-based diet, available at www.lovecomplement.com)

Sonya Looney's Grocery Shopping List

Sonya Looney is a world champion mountain biker you'll read about soon.

When it comes to grocery shopping, I try to keep my pantry stocked with several types of whole grains and a few different types of canned beans, and I keep a variety of nuts and seeds in my freezer. You'll see these varieties in my grocery list, but I don't buy them every week. I also keep at least one loaf of bread and one block of tempeh in my freezer in case of emergencies. I always have at least one type of greens in my fridge. I opt to get locally grown fruits and vegetables as much as possible, but in the winter I get my produce at the grocery store. I use nuts and seeds in bowls, but I also use them to make sauces. I have a wide variety of spices in my cabinet and most frequently use turmeric, cumin, basil, chili powder, smoked paprika, and oregano.

From this list, I can easily make bowls, burritos, snacks, and pasta dishes.

Fruits and Veggies

Arugula

Mixed greens or power greens

Cherry tomatoes

Onions

Garlic

Broccoli

Red bell peppers

Avocados

Mushrooms, especially shiitake

Fresh berries

Apples, peaches, whatever fruit is in season

Green onions

Sweet potatoes

Olives

Grains and Breads

Sprouted spelt

Whole-grain farro

Steel-cut oats

Black rice

Silver Hills Bakery sprouted whole-grain bread

Mary's Gone Crackers seed-based crackers

I choose sprouted grains as much as possible because they have a much higher nutrient density. I also choose whole grains instead of fast-cooking grains because they have their shell intact—that also means more fiber!

Proteins

Smoked tofu

Regular tofu

Tempeh

Soft tofu (for sauces)

Black beans

Chickpeas

Lentils

Hemp hearts

Ground flaxseed

Walnuts

Cashews

Almonds

Cold Section

Soy milk

Almond milk

Vegan cheese as a treat

Other

Peanut or almond butter   Herbal teas

Coffee

Vanessa Espinoza's Grocery Shopping List

I like to eat as fresh as possible, so going to the grocery store is a twice-a-week event for me. My refrigerator is stocked mostly with fresh veggies and tofu and tempeh all the time. I really focus on putting foods together rather than eating a ton of recipe dishes. Recipes tend to have more ingredients and unwanted calories, full of oil, salt, and sugar. I never cook with oil but rather cook, roast, or steam my veggies in vegetable broth. This saves hundreds of calories weekly. With just tofu and veggies you can make so many different dishes. This is my meal prep a few times a week. I just change the flavor each day so I don't get tired of eating the same flavor. This a great way to mix things up. I will add salsa one day, BBQ sauce the next, or just a mix of spices to add different flavor.

I love to keep fresh and frozen fruit in my house at all times. Fruit is typically my midmorning snack after breakfast. It's quick and easy and very satisfying. Grains such as quinoa, millet, kamut, and spelt are some of my favorites for breakfast. I just add a scoop of peanut butter, banana, chia seed, hempseed, and cinnamon. This makes a very hearty and satisfying breakfast. It gives me energy to last all morning.

I'm on the go the entire day, so I always pack my lunch and snacks. I really try to keep it simple: fresh fruit, veggies, nuts, seeds, protein bars, and protein shakes. I always keep a huge bowl of raw nuts (no oil or salt) in the refrigerator. This is a great quick and easy snack to have on hand. My dinners vary weekly, but this is a meal that I prep a few times a week. My staple for dinner is always veggies and some type of tofu or tempeh or beans or bean pasta. I do enjoy veggie burgers and faux meats. I don't eat them every day, but I enjoy some of these foods a few times a week.

This is what I typically shop for when I go to the grocery store.

Veggies

Cabbage	Cauliflower	Spinach
Squash	Bok choy	Kale
Poblano peppers	Onions	Avocados
Zucchini	Garlic	Sweet potatoes
Peppers		

Fruit

Bananas	Wild blueberries	Mangoes
Watermelon	Strawberries	Apples
Pineapple	Raspberries	

Grains

Quinoa	Teff	Amaranth
Millet	Fonio	Wild rice
Spelt	Kamut	Oats

Proteins

Tofu	Seitan
Tempeh	Jackfruit
Textured vegetable protein	Red and green lentil pasta
Legumes	Faux meats, veggie burgers

Nuts and Seeds

Walnuts	Cashews	Sunflower seeds
Peanuts	Brazil nuts	Chia seeds
Almonds	Pumpkin seeds	Hempseeds
Pecans		

Teas and Coffee

Four Sigmatic coffee	Hibiscus tea	Moringa tea
Matcha green tea	Rooibos tea	

Plant-Based Milks

Soy	Almond
Oat	

Other

Veggie broth

Peanut butter

Nutritional yeast

Protein bars

Protein powder

BBQ sauce

Salsa

Sriracha sauce

Spices—Flavor God and Feast Mode seasonings, garlic and onion powders, garlic and onion salts, cumin, smoked paprika, marjoram, and dill

Julia Murray's Grocery Shopping List

When it comes to eating plant-based, it's all about the flavors, sauces, spices, and textures.

Condiment staples are something I have in my kitchen at all times. A combo of just a couple of these, or using one or two as the base of a sauce, can make any bland-tasting veggie into a delicious and extravagant gourmet-tasting dish with little effort.

Bragg Liquid Aminos or tamari (or coconut aminos)

Nutritional yeast

Maple syrup

Balsamic vinegar

Apple cider vinegar

Sriracha

Miso paste

Tahini

Pickle juice!

(When in doubt, add Bragg Liquid Aminos and nutritional yeast to anything savory to make it *delish*.)

Here are a few tips for when you're hitting the grocery store:

• Variety is key. If you want a healthy gut microbiome, remember to stock up on different plants, grains, and legumes that you've never tried before. Do this often and your gut bacteria will flourish (this is a good thing). The number one precursor to a healthy gut microbiome is the diversity of plants you eat. Simple hack? Pick up something new each time you're at the store, use your old friend Google, and cook it up.

- Get into buying frozen fruits and veggies! They are just as nutritious as fresh produce, sometimes even more so because they're frozen at the ripest stage, plus they're cheaper. Stock your freezer so your smoothies are packed to the brim with whole-plant goodness.
- Make friends with your produce manager for affordability. Usually there are "imperfect" fruits and veggies just behind the door of the warehouse in the grocery store. Ask someone who works there if there's anything in the back that can't be sold anymore. Typically they'll give it to you for half price or free! Take it home and freeze it for later use.
- Buy in bulk when you can, and bring your own jar (weigh it before filling) or bags to the store.
- Buy local if you can. Do you have farmers markets or any farms around you that do veggie boxes? Order up! Chances are these are the most nutritious veggies you'll ever eat—grown in organic soil with minimal traveling time.

Personalized Meal Plans

The meal plans in this chapter will help you to get started, but they're (obviously) not the only way to eat. Check out several other meal plans, including some that can be personalized to your particular body type, at nomeatathlete.com/book-bonus.

• • • • •

I have never recommended that people eat with a calculator. I think it is more important to recognize the superior nutrient density of vitamins, minerals, fiber, phytonutrients, and polyphenols contained in plant-based foods, which optimize all forms and phases of athleticism.
—**Caldwell B. Esselstyn Jr., MD, author of *Prevent and Reverse Heart Disease***

The leading edge of peak performance, fitness, and human potential resides not in the unfolding of technological advancements or scientific breakthroughs but rather in potentiating human form and function through lifestyle modification, most notably plant-based nutrition. Fundamental to the future of exercise prescriptions, an integrative approach to fitness is essential. Beyond the scope of adequate macronutrient intake and biomechanics, an emphasis on eating more whole plants, whose unique inherent constituents, such as polyphenols, terpenes, alkaloids, and sterols, work synergistically, modulating enzymatic reactions and reducing oxidative stress while optimizing molecular and biochemical reactions, will prove vital in optimizing and augmenting human potential in athleticism and in the totality of health.

—**Justyna Sanders, MD, public health researcher, international speaker**

RECOVER BETTER, TRAIN MORE

Aside from being able to burn cleaner, more efficient fuel for longer, more effective workouts and harder play on the field, one of the biggest upsides that athletes experience from a whole-foods plant-based diet is faster, more complete recovery. That means less muscle soreness and fatigue, which leads to shorter recovery time, which in turn leads to more training being possible. It also means more training without injury, which prolongs careers, increases income and opportunities for professional athletes, and improves the mental and physical feeling of wellness for any athlete.

Considering the enormous benefits, the reason why all this is true is astonishingly simple: whole plant-based foods have anti-inflammatory properties while also delivering high levels of vitamins, minerals, antioxidants, phytochemicals, fiber, and water. This directly contributes to helping the entire body repair and refresh after physical exertion.

Recreational and elite athletes alike stand to benefit from an increase in plant-based foods in their diet. Ask any elite plant-based or plant-forward athlete and they'll tell you that this diet has helped them recover from the stress of championship-level training that they put their bodies through, as well as helping them to prevent injuries, recover quickly after workouts, and reduce the aches and pains that most of them deal with on a regular basis.

Even the Best Take a Rest

Elite athletes often become elite athletes because of their dedication and attention to detail—not just with their training, nutrition, and goal-setting but also with how they take care of their bodies when they're not working out or competing.

Former Olympic track cyclist **Dotsie Bausch** relies on rest and mindfulness but also sports massage therapy and other bodywork, ice baths, and weight training to balance out her cycling and give her leg muscles a break from their usual routine of spinning for six hours a day. Professional bodybuilder **Jehina Malik** regularly uses a sauna to wind down and allow her muscles to relax following an intense weight-training workout. It's the perfect environment for deep stretching and encouraging her muscle fibers to expand and elongate while boosting circulation. The prolonged heat also prompts her to take in more hydration. World-record-holding 200-meter swimmer **Rip Esselstyn** takes an entire day off from training each week to rest. He also uses his evenings to wind down and relax. Professional bikini competitor **Natalie Matthews** spends months training seven days a week in preparation for a single competition, so once she gets off the stage, she takes as much as a whole week off to allow her body to recover and return to homeostasis. Plant-based world champions and Olympians know that there is no shame in taking a rest. In fact, they have a profound respect for it and therefore make it a priority as part of their holistic approach to athletic greatness.

Fiona Oakes, a Guinness World Record–holding ultrarunner, adopted a plant-based diet and vegan lifestyle when she was only six years old, becoming an animal rights activist at a young age in the United Kingdom. Becoming a vegan would later prove to be not just a compassionate decision but also an athletic performance–enhancing decision that has supported her elite sports career for decades. She holds four Guinness World Records and is the fastest woman in aggregate time to run a marathon on each continent and the North Pole. Now in her fifties, Fiona still runs about 100 miles per week—more than 14 miles per day, on average, as she trains for marathons that often take place in extreme climates or conditions. To fuel herself, Fiona follows a plant-based diet made up mostly of whole foods in meals that she largely makes from scratch. That fuel is consistently put to the test. To meet her race goals, Fiona trains a minimum of once a day, often training two to three times a day. And in addition to putting in her 100 miles a week, she cares for 600 animals at the animal sanctuary she founded while also working as a volunteer firefighter. To fit it all in, she begins her day at 3:30 a.m., as she has done for the past twenty years. She credits her plant-based diet with giving her the ability to recover so quickly and recognizes that as her racing "edge." As she points out, consistency is key to marathon training, which means there's a lot of pressure to get in the workouts every day, and so there's very little margin for injury. She strongly believes that it's because of her diet that she's able to keep this up into her fifties and that she's never had a running-related injury, despite her high-volume mileage.

Running didn't always come easily for Fiona. She had a major setback when she was a teenager that could have prevented her entire world-class athletic career from even happening: having multiple necessary surgeries that left her without a kneecap on her right leg. She was told that the procedures would make normal walking difficult and running impossible. "It has been an enormous challenge to prove them all wrong, but that is exactly what I have done and continue to do. I have achieved this by having 100 percent dedication, coupled with discipline and determination, and a mantra, which has made failure not an option." What's also propelled Fiona forward is the fact that she's running for a purpose, not for her own gain. Awards and accolades don't appeal to her ego but rather to her dedication to spreading the word about plant-based eating and its benefits for the well-being of animals. "The better I can run, and the more accomplished my achievements, the more successful and credible an ambassador I can be for what I believe in. I don't do it for any other reason than a love of animals and not wishing to harm them. And it's about being able to stand on any start line knowing no other creature has suffered for the performance I am about to deliver."

Some things have dramatically changed for Fiona through the years, such as her world renown as an athlete and as an animal-rights advocate. A documentary was made about her life, *Running for Good*, which was directed by Keegan Kuhn (the award-winning codirector of *Cowspiracy* and *What the Health*), narrated by plant-based royalty Rich Roll, and produced by Academy Award–nominated actor James Cromwell. But some things have remained the same. Fiona has observed that she maintains the same weight and muscle mass as when she started running. The years go by, but she still performs at the same high level. She recently qualified to run for England in the 10K, the half marathon, and the Elite Start in the London Marathon, acknowledging that "a vegan diet is obviously sustaining me very well after decades of pretty extreme and physically demanding living."

Brendan Brazier is another competitor who relies on his diet to help his body keep up with his training. He's an ultramarathon champion and professional Ironman triathlete who is considered one of the pioneers of the plant-based athlete movement. He went plant-based in 1990 after realizing that if all elite runners trained in basically the same way and ran at roughly the same pace, the difference between one runner and the next could come down to their ability to recover after workouts. His hypothesis was that if he could improve his recovery time, train more, and better adapt to a new workload or a faster pace, then he could produce better outcomes and find more success. So he put it to the test. As a result, he did find more success, going on to compete as a professional athlete in some of the most grueling races in the world, and he continues to be in top shape in his midforties.

To eat for performance and recovery, Brendan prioritizes eliminating "biological debt," or the energy-depleted state that many people find themselves in as a result of looking to substances such as coffee or refined sugar for fuel. It's the difference between getting your calories from stimulation or from nourishment. The former is short-term energy and only treats the symptoms of fatigue. By contrast, eating foods that are high in net-gain micronutrients eliminates the need for stimulation because a steady supply of energy is available thanks to nutritional needs having been met. As Brendan puts it: "In effect, sound nutrition is a preemptive strike against fatigue and the ensuing desire for stimulants. With nutrient-dense, whole food as the foundation of your diet, there's no need to ever get into biological debt."

Brendan also prioritizes foods that eliminate inflammation and acidity in the body—a.k.a. "alkaline-forming" foods—such as copious amounts of vegetables (especially leafy greens); fruits; pseudograins such as quinoa; healthy fats such as avocado; staples such as brown rice, lentils, potatoes, and squash; and nutrient-dense nuts and seeds. That is how you get a big nutritional return on investment from your diet, and according to Brendan, it's how you thrive as a plant-based athlete. Brendan came from humble beginnings, literally living in a shed as a pro athlete, without an income, but with a lot of passion and enthusiasm for the sport of triathlon and a quest to construct a plant-based diet to further his success in the sport. Fast-forward all these years later, and the brand that Brendan cocreated, Vega, was the title sponsor of the Ironman Triathlon World Championship in Kona, Hawaii, in 2019, and Brendan was there at the finish line to congratulate the competitors as they completed the race. The Ironman World Championship is considered by many to be the pinnacle of endurance racing, showcasing some of the best all-around athletes in the world, and things came full circle for Brendan, from being a competitor in the Ironman triathlon to sponsoring the event, which is viewed online by tens of millions of people each year.

These days, Brendan still trains six days per week, he still focuses on alkaline whole-plant-based foods including plenty of leafy greens, grains, legumes, vegetables, and fruits, and he has created multiple business ventures in the plant-based world, always innovating, a few steps ahead of the competition. Training is just part of life for Brendan. He says it is easier for him to train than not to train because "I've been doing it for so long, it's embedded in me." As authors and former and current runners, we can say with confidence that of all the plant-based athletes in the world, Brendan had the greatest impact on both of us when we were starting out as plant-based athletes. His legacy will be one of the most significant in the history of the plant-based athlete movement, and it has been an honor for us to consider Brendan a role model and friend for many years.

Kätlin Kukk is an Estonian national champion in road cycling, cyclo-cross, and BMX racing. Aside from how much success she's reached at the young age of nineteen, she's also noteworthy because she specifi-cally chose a plant-based diet to assist in her muscle recovery. She had been experiencing inflammation in her knee, and she learned that a plant-based diet might help relieve her joint pain and make racing more comfortable. She got relief almost immediately, and her career took off as a result.

As with many people, Kätlin's transition to a plant-based diet was a gradual one. The meat just gradually disappeared from her diet, and then the dairy. "It wasn't really hard for me. As soon as I realized what the animal products do to us, and how much suffering consuming those products causes the animals, it wasn't even a question for me. I don't see meat as food anymore, honestly." Once she made the complete switch to plants, she started filling her meals with foods such as avocados, sweet potatoes, roasted beets, zucchini, chia seeds, and hummus to go with plants she was already eating during her transition, including lentils, chickpeas, and salad greens. Her new diet fueled her sport better than she expected, and she even surprised herself by winning major races such as the Estonian National Championship in road cycling in the under-twenty-three age category. It was a major victory regardless of the circumstances, but for Kätlin it was also the ultimate reassurance that going plant-based had only benefited her cycling life.

As is the case for many Europeans, Kätlin's first sports love was soccer. She played for three years until her brother and father—who owned a bike shop—were heading to a bike race one day, and Kätlin said she wanted to race too. Her father selected a bike for her and gave her instructions for how to race. The next day, she got her first taste of a criterium, which is a race involving cycling around numerous laps on a closed course. She followed the racing technique and strategy instructions to the best of her ability and finished third in her age group. From that day on, she has been "stuck with bicycles."

In many ways Kätlin has become a role model for young athletes. She is the perfect example of what it takes to excel in a sport, particularly when it comes to overcoming the distractions of being a teenager. "Some people don't make it this far because around the ages of sixteen to eighteen, everyone is discovering what they want to do with their lives, and a lot of the time it's not being an athlete, because that would mean a lot of focus on one particular thing, and less time for 'fun stuff' that people that age are interested in (parties, socializing, and not being obsessed with improving their performance for their chosen craft). I've given up most of my friendships, all parties, and a lot of time with my family—it's a very time-consuming sport. But I've also made new friends all over the world and have had memorable moments and adventures." Kätlin also hopes that her success will encourage young or aspiring athletes to give a plant-based diet a try. "I hope I can show my generation and a newer generation of athletes and nonathletes alike how beneficial a plant-based lifestyle can be. A plant-based diet has so much potential to help with performance when done right, and plant-based whole foods are definitely something you can't go wrong with."

Professional women's tennis player **Sharon Fichman** developed chronic tendinitis in her Achilles tendon in 2013. She could manage it, but it became an ongoing issue that impacted her performance. By 2016, she had decided to walk away from the sport she'd been playing since she was six years old. The injuries and burnout were too much—she just wanted to be healthy and happy.

At trainer Marc Madilson's recommendation, she adopted a plant-based diet. Her initial expectations were simply to feel healthier and maybe lose some weight. But at first, she was nervous that she wouldn't have enough energy, so she didn't go all in right away. "I basically had things in my brain from former trainers, coaches, nutritionists, and others who were teaching me what they knew [about nutrition]. Once I gradually progressed into being fully plant-based, I realized that I functioned even better. I learned that I don't need the crazy-high amount of protein that people told me I needed. I felt light all the time, even after eating. I never again had that heavy feeling after I had eaten, like I needed a nap."

After just a few months, she was completely pain free. For the first time since her Achilles injury four years prior, she was able to go for a comfortable long-distance run. The inflammation around her muscles and joints was dramatically and visibly reduced. And she also saw improvements in her blood work. "As the changes to my body became more prevalent, I got more and more curious as to why it was happening. I learned that meat consumption and high cholesterol levels exacerbate inflammation, which can result in pain and impair athletic performance and recovery. I also read studies that showed that a plant-based diet can have an anti-inflammatory effect. I began to notice that my muscle fatigue decreased, my athletic performance improved, and my recovery accelerated. I discovered that this was largely due to free radicals being neutralized by the surplus of antioxidants my body was getting from my plant-based lifestyle. As well, my VO$_2$ max—the maximum amount of oxygen a person can use during intense exercise—had increased, which led to better endurance."

Sharon felt she was in better shape than she had ever been. So when her fiancé, Olympic silver medal–winning figure skater Dylan Moscovitch, suggested she return to professional tennis after a two-and-a-half-year hiatus, she was all in. And not just in—ready to start training for the Tokyo 2020 Olympics to compete for her native Canada.

Although the 2020 Olympic Games were postponed, Sharon's training has moved forward. In July 2019, after just ten months back on tour, she broke back into the top 100 in the world in doubles. In March 2020, she reached her career-high ranking of number 47 in the world in doubles on the WTA Tour. And by September 2020, she was competing in the US Open.

Not only is Sharon thriving as a plant-based athlete on the tennis court; she also inspired her fiancé to adopt a plant-based diet. Together, they consider themselves to be proud vegan athletes and ambassadors for the lifestyle. She continues to be grateful for Marc's support and his suggestion that she experiment with giving up animal foods. "He is one of those people who inspires you to become the best version of yourself, and the more time I spent working with him, the more motivated I became. I am so thankful that I made the switch, as it has played such a big part in helping me get back to doing what I love. While there are challenges, I find that the easiest way to stick to a plant-based lifestyle is to make sure I'm eating the things I enjoy. In addition to the benefits to my personal health and athletic performance, I am very happy I can live a healthy, happy, and prosperous life without the exploitation of animals."

Understanding Muscle Soreness and Inflammation

Whether you're trying to keep your training consistent, reach new athletic milestones, or just get started with a new regimen, muscle soreness can be a make-or-break situation. If you're sore after a workout to the point where you're in pain, that not only has a profound effect on whether you enjoy exercise; it also derails the best-laid plans to stick to a training plan. You probably see this played out every year around the New Year. People who have done little to no exercise walk into a gym expecting to get one step closer to their fitness goals, and after a day or two of working out with weights, machines, or a group cardio class, they are so sore that they can't go back to the gym for days. The momentum from their initial enthusiasm has been broken, along with their hopes of achieving their New Year's resolution. The stakes are even higher for athletes training for big games, competitions, and events. The more time they need to spend recovering, the less time they can spend training.

So it's safe to say that your ability to achieve many of your fitness-related goals is tied tightly to how efficiently you recover from your workouts. If soreness prevents you from being consistent, and lack of consistency prevents you from progressing, and lack of progress prevents you from finding joy or fulfillment in the process, then you'll likely find something else to pursue. That's why the ability to reduce or even prevent muscle soreness with a plant-based diet is a pretty big deal.

What Is Muscle Soreness?

Muscle soreness is a common side effect of the stress you put on your muscles during exercise. It can set in immediately after physical exertion or, more commonly, a few hours or up to twelve to twenty-four hours after exercise, the latter called delayed onset muscle soreness (DOMS). Most muscle soreness comes from changing the stress that's normally applied to your muscles to something they're not used to. (Note "most"—we'll talk about the other, equally preventable, causes in a bit.) Even if athletes are very experienced, perhaps professionals in their sport, and exercising up to seven days per week, a change in their muscular stress from uncommon movements could cause severe soreness. If an elite marathon runner were asked to participate in powerlifting movements at maximum effort, doing things such as barbell presses, squats, and deadlifts, he or she would likely barely be able to walk the next day. The same would happen if a powerlifter took on the challenge of long-distance running at an Olympics-qualifying pace. They likely would be out of commission for a few days, recovering from severe muscle soreness and fatigue.

Muscle soreness can also be categorized as inflammation. As we discussed in chapter 3, not all inflammation is bad. It's a vital part of your immune system's response to injury or infection. When inflammation occurs, chemicals from your white blood cells are released into the blood and affected tissues to protect your body from foreign substances and to expedite the repair process—the latter being exactly what is happening in the case of post-workout muscle tears. But unlike chronic inflammation, which is the result of your immune system being on high alert for an extended period of time because it is consistently under attack (and many times leads to white blood cells attacking healthy tissues and organs, leading to chronic diseases such as heart disease, diabetes, cancer, arthritis, and Crohn's disease—as you'll recall, unfortunate but frequent side effects of a diet high in animal-based foods), muscle soreness is an example of acute or temporary and localized inflammation.

Acute inflammation in the form of muscle soreness is a healthy, normal response that sometimes happens despite your best efforts. But what you can do is arm yourself with a diet that actively fights inflammation, which will lead to less soreness and a more efficient recovery after a tough workout.

Fueling Recovery

Reducing inflammation and improving recovery after exercise is not just about eating anti-inflammatory foods but also about avoiding the foods that cause inflammation in the first place. From Harvard University, a list of pro-inflammatory foods to **avoid** includes the following:[1]

- Red meat such as burgers and steaks
- Processed meat such as hot dogs and sausages
- Margarine, shortening, and lard
- Refined carbohydrates such as white bread and pastries
- French fries and other fried foods
- Soda and other sugar-sweetened beverages

And here's Harvard's list of foods to **include** in an anti-inflammatory diet. Look familiar? We'd certainly hope so—they are the cornerstone of a nutrient-dense plant-based diet!

- Tomatoes
- Olive oil
- Green leafy vegetables, such as spinach, kale, and collards
- Nuts such as almonds and walnuts
- Fruits such as strawberries, blueberries, cherries, and oranges

Even though research dictates that whole plants in general ease inflammation and support whole-body recovery after exercise, there are a few plants in particular that deserve special mention because of their supercharged abilities in this department. To get a feel for how and when to plug these foods into your diet, refer back to the muscle-building meal plan, which aids in recovery, in our meal-planning chapter on page 156.

Leafy Green Vegetables

Leafy green vegetables aren't just a regular-meal all-star with the highest-possible ANDI (Aggregate Nutrient Density Index) score; they're also a recovery meal standout. Thanks to their stores of vitamins A, C, E, B, and K, as well as their fiber, iron, magnesium, potassium, and calcium, foods such as kale, spinach, collard greens, and Swiss chard offer up potent inflammation fighting and recharging after a workout. Throw them into a smoothie or enjoy them raw in a salad or lightly sautéed for an extra boost. As we discussed in chapter 6, consider adding some citrus to help with iron absorption.

Dark-Pigmented Fruits

Dark-pigmented fruits—including most berries as well as tart cherries—contain robust amounts of antioxidants as well as vitamins, minerals, fiber, and water. And they do this within about 300 calories per pound, making dark-colored fruits and berries ideal post-workout foods to combat inflammation. They can be consumed whole, sprinkled on cereal or oatmeal, or blended into smoothies for even faster absorption and digestion. We recommend avoiding most fruit juice in order to sidestep the added sugar (not to mention the lack of fiber); also know that dried fruit will have a slightly different profile from fresh fruit, namely a different calorie density per portion.

Spotlight on Tart Cherry Juice

We're often skeptical of claims that a supplement can make a noticeable difference in your performance or recovery, but in the case of tart cherry juice, the data and the anecdotal evidence are there. Researchers found that athletes who drank tart cherry juice (specifically Montmorency juice—a type of cherry, not a brand) before and after long-distance races experienced faster recovery of strength and less muscle pain than did those who drank a different beverage.[2] In another study, sixteen well-trained male cyclists who drank Montmorency tart cherry juice concentrate twice a day for seven days experienced less inflammation and oxidative stress following a three-day simulated race than did those who drank another beverage.[3] Research has also found that the natural compounds in Montmorency tart cherries may help with soreness after a workout, as they simultaneously address inflammation, muscle damage, and oxidative stress.[4] Scott Jurek, one of the greatest long-distance runners of all time, who has claimed victories in nearly all of ultrarunning's elite trail and road events, uses tart cherry juice instead of pain-relief medication such as ibuprofen (which is so commonly used among long-distance runners that it's referred to as "vitamin I"). In Jurek's words, "All-natural tart cherry juice allows me to recover from tough races sooner, without taking needless chemicals that do more harm than good."

In matters of recovery, we usually think about what to eat after a workout to help our bodies begin the process of muscle repair. But with tart cherry juice, the recommendation is that you use it as a "precovery" drink, consuming it for several days before your big workout or race to help you feel better during and afterward.

Nuts

Nuts have long been associated with positive health benefits and are known for their unique nutritional properties that help boost athletic performance, namely their protein and fatty acid content, and their ability to help reduce inflammation. An article published in 2016 in the *American Journal of Clinical Nutrition* concluded that nut consumption was associated with reduced risk of cardiovascular disease and type 2 diabetes, as well as a healthy lipid profile. And frequent nut consumption by thousands of study participants was associated with a healthy profile of inflammatory biomarkers.[5]

Sweet Potatoes

It appears that sweet potatoes may do more than help replenish carbohydrates burned during exercise and provide anti-inflammatory benefits after workouts. Sweet potatoes are high in vitamins A and C and antioxidants with anti-inflammatory properties, which also help fight obesity, type 2 diabetes, heart disease, and cancer. They may even contribute to weight loss, since they contain resistant starch, a filling fiberlike substance that your body doesn't digest or absorb and therefore acts like a scrub brush on its way through your digestive system. Sweet potatoes also contain magnesium and potassium, which can help regulate blood pressure. On top of that, they are a versatile food that can be the centerpiece of a meal (breakfast, lunch, dinner, or post-workout snack) or a side dish and can even be served as a dessert, thanks to their sweet flavor. As one of very few foods that are both calorie dense and nutrient dense, sweet potatoes are one of the ultimate staple foods for athletes.

Turmeric

Turmeric is a spice that is packed with bioactive compounds called curcuminoids, which have powerful anti-inflammatory and antioxidant properties. Turmeric is also associated with better brain function and brain health, as well as lower risk of heart disease. It's easy to scoop a teaspoon or two of ground turmeric into your morning latte or smoothie or stir it into curries, soups, and sauces. There is evidence that combining turmeric with black pepper heightens its anti-inflammatory benefits, as we noted on page 129.

Everyone loves the post-workout meal. It serves as a reward, celebrates having worked your butt off, and is an opportunity to really feel nourished. But many athletes are mistaken or unsure about what to eat after a workout. We've covered which foods to reach for to actively combat post-workout inflammation, but here are a few more guidelines to use when figuring out how and when to replenish your nutrition after a workout.

Rules for Post-workout Nutrition to Enhance Recovery

What you are or are not prioritizing for your post-workout nutrition just might be the difference between falling short of your goals and achieving them. That is because there are particular nuances surrounding nutrition following exercise that, if adhered to, deliver superior results in muscle recovery, growth, and nutritional replenishment.

What to Eat After Your Workout

Post-workout nutrition is all about two things:

1. Timing
2. Ratio

Timing is important because after a workout your muscles are primed and ready to receive fuel to start the repair process. Try to consume your post-workout meal within an hour after your workout. This will replenish nutrients lost through exercise and expedite the repair and recovery process by giving your body what it needs to grow, leading to more efficient performance results.

If you're jumping in the car (or shower) and don't have time for a full meal, have a snack or smoothie on hand to eat within that window, and save the larger meal for later. This is what makes protein bars and powders so popular, because of their convenience and effectiveness at getting the recovery process started, but something as simple as fruit is packed full of nutrition and will contribute beneficial nutrients until you can get a larger meal. The key is to be prepared by keeping snacks in your car, gym bag, or backpack or within easy and quick access following exercise.

As for *ratio*, a 5:1 carbohydrate-to-protein plan is optimal after exercise. Carbohydrate-rich foods will replace energy, electrolytes, water, and other nutrients burned during your workout, while protein will help with muscle repair. After the toughest workouts or races, consume about 0.75 gram of carbohydrates per pound of body weight and protein accordingly. A little fat will also do you well. In your post-workout meal, aim for about half as much fat as protein.

Put It Together: Post-workout

For most of us, post-workout nutrition comes in the form of a real meal. Maybe that's a hearty lunch after a long morning run or dinner after a post-workout gym session. The good news is that a lot of standard plant-based meals are pretty close to that 5:1 carbohydrate-to-protein ratio, which makes designing the meal super easy. Think of foods such as a burrito bowl, salad, wrap, pasta, or grain bowl that is mostly carbohydrates with some quality proteins and fats, coming from primarily whole-food sources.

The Simple Formula for Better Workouts and Faster Recovery

We've offered a lot of information, and if you're new to workout nutrition, it probably feels overwhelming. But we're here to break it down into actionable steps to lead to desired results. At its core, workout nutrition can be distilled to a super-simple "3-4-5 Principle." If you remember nothing else from this section, this formula will take you far:

- **Before** your workout, aim for a **3:1** ratio of carbohydrate to protein.
- **During** your workout, aim for a **4:1** ratio of carbohydrate to protein.
- **After** your workout, aim for a **5:1** ratio of carbohydrate to protein (4:1 is okay too).

It's not about perfection or measuring every ounce of food. Most athletes are successful using the 3-4-5 Principle as a guide when making decisions about workout nutrition. Exactly what you eat during each phase depends on your body and needs, and as you experiment over time, you'll find your sweet spots.

To see these guidelines in action—along with great examples of post-workout replenishment—check out chapter 10 for a glimpse into the daily routines of elite plant-based athletes.

Recovery Beyond the Plate

A whole-foods plant-based diet is central to improved recovery, but it's not the only consideration. If you're serious about taking your training to the next level, you also need to be thinking about how you can best support your body as you push it further and further. The techniques that follow will multiply the recovery-boosting power of a plant-based diet.

Hydrating

Your body is made of up 70 percent water, and proper hydration nourishes your cells and muscles. It's an essential part of maintaining a high level of health and wellness, as well as insurance against muscle soreness. Dehydration can increase the discomfort caused by inflammation in the muscles, and being deficient in electrolytes—which water supplies—can also contribute. So drinking adequate water—every day, not just on the days you work out—is just about the simplest thing you can do to aid your post-workout recovery. Aim for a dozen cups of water a day. Don't worry about whether they're eight-ounce cups, twelve-ounce cups, or cups you don't measure. Just drink a dozen different cups of water a day, and that, combined with your high fruit and vegetable intake, should provide plenty of water to fuel your active lifestyle.

Also keep in mind that many fruits and vegetables are naturally high in water content. You may not want to count them toward your total daily water intake, but know that you're being completely covered in that department when you're eating whole plants all day long. That said, be mindful that if it's particularly hot or humid outside, if you consume caffeine (which is a natural diuretic), or if you take supplements or medications that are diuretics, you'll want to increase the amount of water you drink to make up for what you're losing in sweat or urine.

Warming Up, Stretching, and Cooling Down

Most people think that the intensity of their workout is to blame for their muscle soreness and stiffness the next day, but many times it's because they didn't take the time to warm up, cool down, stretch, or all of the above. These often overlooked activities are crucial parts of the recovery process and will help support your nutritional efforts. Failure to do them will almost guarantee some degree of muscle soreness. You can't just start sprinting at full speed without jogging first and expect to avoid a tough next day. The same can be said for weight training, especially when it involves strenuous movements such as deep squats with resistance. Without warming up and stretching throughout, you'll be in a world of hurt no matter how many anti-inflammatory foods you eat or supplements you take.

And as much as our culture associates soreness with progress or the efficacy of a given workout, make no mistake about it: muscle soreness slows you down, and it can potentially lead to injury. It's okay to be sore, but it's also okay to prevent that soreness in the first place by being proactive, being patient, and taking the time to invest in your muscle recovery, and muscle soreness prevention, just as you invest in your post-workout nutrition protocol.

Luckily, these activities don't cost anything but time.

Warming Up

Warming up before engaging in regular exercise prepares your body for the stress it is about to be subjected to. It engages your cardiovascular system by raising your body temperature and increasing blood flow to your muscles, which can help reduce your risk of injury while also improving athletic performance. In general, warming up means doing your activity at a slower pace and reduced intensity, such as walking before jogging and then jogging before running. Or it could be doing a bodyweight exercise before weight training, such as air squats before barbell squats. Whatever you choose, aim for five to ten minutes of warm-up before a more intense workout or, better yet, spend a few minutes stretching too. Warming up before stretching is particularly beneficial because it gets the blood flowing to your muscles, making them more flexible, supple, and ready to be stretched. Trying to stretch cold, tight muscles, on the other hand, is a fast track to injury.

Stretching

Stretching should be an integral part of your recovery and exercise program. In fact, this single habit can make one of the biggest differences in whether or not you will sustain muscle soreness after exercise. Case in point: if you spend just ten minutes jumping rope, where all of your impact is on your toes, engaging your calves with every single movement for that full duration, and you do not stretch your calves afterward— you will almost certainly experience prolonged muscle soreness that could even make it hard to walk for the next couple of days. We see this all the time, especially during leg training in the gym. Many weight lifters love the idea of doing heavy barbell squats, deep hip sled leg presses, and lunges without taking the time to stretch after the warm-up and before the workout, between sets, or after the workout, and then they wonder why they have severe cases of delayed onset muscle soreness (DOMS) that impede their ability to train their legs again for days. In fact, it's hard for them just to sit in a chair or climb into the seat of a car, all because they didn't take the time to stretch during their workout, which led to a debilitating amount of inflammation. And it's not just weight lifters who are affected by not stretching—runners, hikers, cyclists, and pretty much all athletes know this all too well: failure to stretch—before, during, and after a workout—can be a major flaw in an exercise program. Alternatively, following a sound dynamic stretching protocol can nearly eliminate soreness altogether.

There are many different styles of stretching: static stretching (holding a stationary stretch for fifteen to sixty seconds—think touching your toes), dynamic stretching (functional stretching accomplished by moving your limbs through a range of motion), ballistic stretching (involving momentum and bouncing into a stretch), and proprioceptive neuromuscular facilitation (or PNF, stretching muscles to their limits, often assisted by physical therapists and trainers). But the primary form of stretching we are referring to and advocating for is **dynamic stretching**. Evidence suggests that incorporating gentle movement into stretching is the most effective way to increase flexibility, improve muscle tone, and prevent injuries. We recommend adding dynamic stretches during your warm-up, periodically throughout your workout, and during your cooldown. Some examples include doing arm circles and brief cross-body and overhead stretches for your chest and triceps, grabbing your elbow and stretching muscles from origin to insertion between sets of bench presses, or doing some body-weight air squats to keep your groin, glutes, quads, and hamstrings loose between sets of squats or leg presses. (We've included a sample stretching routine in the next section.)

If you plan to do static stretches (such as touching your toes and holding the stretch for thirty seconds), you should do so after your workout, when your muscles are warm and more pliable. If you do no stretching at all, especially when performing resistance weight training, you will almost certainly get sore, often to a degree that will cause you to miss some future planned workouts due to severe DOMS.

If you want to try an experiment to see how much stretching plays a role in preventing muscle soreness, perform a simple test: Work out one day with your usual intensity and effort without stretching and note how sore you are the following day. When you've recovered, work out again with the same intensity and effort, but this time start out with a warm-up and stretching routine such as the one we outline in the section that follows. We're willing to bet you'll be happier with your results.

Stretch It Out

This basic warm-up and stretching routine will loosen the muscles that you're about to train, takes less than ten minutes, and will reduce the potential for post-workout muscle soreness.

First, warm up for five to ten minutes, doing some sort of cardiovascular exercise such as jogging, push-ups, crunches, or jumping jacks. Now briefly stretch the largest muscles in your body—your quads, hamstrings, glutes, calves, chest, back, abdominals, and fronts and backs of your arms to help loosen them up to be more flexible during your actual workout.

Here's a way to check all of these boxes quickly:

- Touch your toes to stretch your hamstrings.
- Stand on one leg, pulling on your foot to stretch your quads.
- Elevate your toe on a stair or wall or in a push-up position by pressing down on your heel to stretch your calves.
- From a plank position, get into an upward dog yoga pose to stretch your abdominals and then into a pigeon pose to stretch your glutes, adding a slight twist to stretch your back.
- From a standing position, stretch your arm across your chest to

stretch your shoulder and arm and then stretch from your arm overhead, pulling down on your elbow to stretch your triceps.

Each movement is held for only a few seconds, as it is designed to help create a greater range of motion, so one dynamic stretch can naturally flow into another one with ease, often with some jogging in place and arm circles thrown in to keep your body moving. These stretches can also be repeated during a workout as a natural way to keep your body loose during rest periods between sets, and you can choose the stretches depending on which muscle groups you are training. They take only a few seconds to perform, but they can prevent soreness for days.

Cooling Down

Like warming up, cooling down is an important part of the entire workout experience. Many of us rush this aspect and overlook it, eager to be finished. We complete a workout, and the main thing on our mind is our next meal or checking our social media notifications. This is where soreness can creep in, but a little patience here can go a long way. Cooling down allows for your heart rate to return to normal, for you to catch your breath, and for your muscles to gradually relax, rather than immediately going from sprinting or lifting to sitting for prolonged periods, such as sitting in your car on your drive home from the gym or sitting down for dinner and then crashing on the sofa for the evening.

After an intense cardio workout, consider going for a short walk while doing some arm circles or light stretching as you stroll, which will keep the blood circulating. Or, if you were performing weight-lifting exercises, you could finish with some machines or cables with light weights for twenty to twenty-five repetitions, which encourages more circulation as you stretch your muscles and move them through a wide range of motion with little resistance. If you just finished playing basketball at the community rec center or gym, you could finish with a little bit of light jogging, or shooting hoops and chasing rebounds if you have the time and the space. Regardless of how you choose to cool down, what you're going for is essentially the opposite of your warm-up—about five to ten minutes of movement that helps transition your muscles to resting.

Rest

Rest is not a four-letter word in sports. Although there used to be a stigma suggesting that if you were resting, you weren't working hard enough—and some athletes still feel that they need to push through in order to make gains—proper rest is crucial not only for preventing injury but also for seeing performance improvements. It's during rest that your muscles are repaired, strengthened, and built. Although you can adapt to a point where you can you push your body to greater and greater limits, like Robbie Balenger, who ran forty-plus miles every day for seventy-five consecutive days from California to New York (powered by a plant-based diet), you can bet that Robbie got plenty of rest after completing a marathon plus a half marathon of running each day so he could do it all over again the next day and continue that routine for months. Robbie also incorporated rest into his training regimen that prepared him to complete such a feat, which meant knowing when to allow his body to take a break from exerting in order to preserve his energy and to help his muscles and organs recover from the daily stress of performing at such intense and extreme levels.

We define rest as the **time that your body is not under physical stress**. This can be your entire body (taking a break during the day or a full day off from physical exercise), an isolated muscle group (giving your legs a rest day while you train your upper body), or even specific systems of the body (giving your cardiovascular system a break by not engaging in aerobic activity). Essentially, rest is relative to your sport and your level of training. For example, bodybuilders give their backs a rest by focusing on exercises that target chest muscles; ultrarunners may take some time off their feet during the course of a full-day or multiday endurance event. Many athletes take naps because they exert themselves far more than the average person, and napping can be rejuvenating for their athletic progress. And the most common form of rest, especially for athletes who aren't training for professional or elite events, is the rest day, which gives your entire body a full day to recover from physical stress.

It's worth noting that your regular night's sleep does not count toward rest, since that's already essential for sustaining your baseline of health. However, it's still a crucial contributor to recovery, as it's only when your body is in a deep state of rest that it can mend, repair, and refresh from a day's worth of effort.

How much rest do you need? The answer can depend on how many hours a day you're training, at what intensity you're training, and which other activities you're doing during the day (e.g., sitting at a desk versus being on your feet all day). But there are some rules of thumb that, if observed, will help you recover, repair, and rebound.

- **Limit your training to six days per week or less.** Give yourself at least one full day of physical rest, especially if you are active in your daily life aside from working out.
- **Change up your muscle groups.** If you're lifting weights, try not to work the same muscle groups every day, which can be too taxing on your muscles, joints, and ligaments. Believe it or not, many professional bodybuilders train specific muscle groups once a week, giving them each an entire week to recover. Vanessa Espinoza, for example, will train chest one day, her back the next, then legs, abs, and shoulders and arms, with each workout having its own focus and emphasis, while also giving each major muscle group nearly a week of rest before training it again.
- **Get plenty of rest at night.** Most people need a minimum of seven to nine hours of sleep per night. This is to ensure that your body properly powers down and performs the maintenance and repair that's required not only to recover from physical exertion

but also to keep your important systems (immune, nervous, cardiovascular, etc.) functioning optimally. Particularly if you're active most days of the week, we recommend aiming for the high end of that range. Because sleep is so important not just to your athletic performance but also to your overall health, be sure you're supporting that process at night by avoiding caffeinated beverages late in the day, not exposing yourself to bright light (including from your phone, computer, or television) one or two hours before bed, and sticking with a consistent waking and sleeping schedule, which will help your body fall into a better sleeping rhythm.

- **Take a nap.** Seriously. We've been told by bodybuilders, triathletes, and professional basketball players that they've incorporated napping into their training routines. This is because taking a well-timed short nap can help recharge your energy stores, giving your body an opportunity to rest while providing a boost the way caffeine normally would. If you're going to nap, make sure it's before 3:00 p.m., and nap for less than thirty minutes so it doesn't interfere with your night's sleep.

- **Incorporate other common practices to prevent and reduce muscle soreness.** These modalities help encourage circulation and repair, calm the central nervous system (which keeps inflammation in check), and keep muscles and tissues supple and flexible. Popular examples of these are as follows:
    — Massage therapy
    — Cryotherapy (cold or ice therapy)
    — Thermotherapy (heat therapy)
    — Chiropractic care
    — Restorative yoga and stretching
    — Muscle creams, gels, and pain-relief patches
    — Avoidance of prolonged sitting
    — Attention to posture
    — Positive attitude (yes, this can help!)

Whether we're talking about legendary ultrarunners, cyclists, NFL football players, a new crop of modern powerlifters and bodybuilders, or basketball players, it is becoming more and more clear that we are ushering in a new era of sports performance, and it is fueled by plants. As your athletic performance improves, energy increases, and muscle soreness is minimized, your body becomes healthier, reducing your risk of all-cause mortality and creating the greatest barrier we know of between you and the most common degenerative diseases. Being a plant-based athlete is not just about improving performance on the field or on the court; it's also about improving the quality of your life, one bite at a time.

Level Up Your Nutrition Around Workouts (Cheat Sheet)

Want to really nail your pre-, mid-, and post-workout meals? Download our free around-workout nutrition guide at nomeatathlete .com/book-bonus to get our favorite meals and tips for eating to optimize your workout.

• • • • •

I am able to bounce back from strenuous workouts in record time. Not to say I don't feel the fatigue; I just notice I am able to give the same percentage effort day in and day out.
—**David Verburg, Olympic gold medal–winning sprinter**

Recovery was one of the biggest differences I noticed by evolving to a plant-based diet. My body feels stronger and faster after tough workouts.
—**Rebecca Soni, six-time Olympic medal–winning swimmer and world record holder**

When I switched to a plant-based diet, the biggest difference was in my recovery. I would recover a lot faster from intense workouts, and my stamina was a lot better. And I had the speediest recoveries from both anterior cruciate ligament surgeries (I tore my ACL in 2017 and 2019). It took me only one month to get back to normal training and three months to compete again.
—**Vivian Kong, elite fencer**

The most impactful feeling I've had is less inflammation, and when I am inflamed from hard training, it doesn't last as long as before. In the past, DOMS could sometimes last six to seven days if I had taken a break from training, but now jumping back to routine I'm feeling normal after three to four days.
—**James Newbury, four-time winner of Australia's Fittest Man**

Initially after switching to a plant-based diet, I didn't expect any changes; I was just getting the same nutrients from different sources. But after more than two years being vegan, I'm now seeing my body recovering faster than ever. Hard workout? No problem! Competition? No problem! I need only a short time to recover before I'm 100 percent ready to go again, and that can make a big difference in professional sports!
—**Andreas Vojta, Olympic 1,500-meter runner**

My recovery improved dramatically on a plant-based diet. Most of my races are stage races, which means I race for seven days in a row. It's not only how fast and how technically savvy you are but also how well you recover. I went from chasing the last spot on the podium to standing on top of the podium at a lot of races! If you can recover faster, then you can go harder again sooner. Plant-based diets are incredibly anti-inflammatory, and endurance athletes tend to walk around with a lot of inflammation from training, and consuming animal products contributes to inflammation too. A notable marker

with inflammation for me is that I have way fewer overuse injuries than I used to get. If your body isn't working overtime trying to recover from the food you're eating, it can focus on helping you recover from exercise. The cleaner the fuel you put in the engine, the faster it can go.
—**Sonya Looney, world champion mountain biker**

UNLEASHING YOUR INNER ATHLETE

At this point, you have the tools you need to become your personal best. You know which foods to eat and which to avoid, how to build workout-fueling meals, the supplements to consider using, and how to properly recover. And you've read testimonials from some of the world's best plant-based athletes as part of your new blueprint to follow. But where do you go from here? How do you get to the core of what keeps these elite athletes striving to be the best at their game? How can you take all that good, clean fuel and really put the pedal to the metal? Nothing will happen if you just read the advice in this book—you have to do something with it. That's all about your *mental* game.

Your intentions, inspiration, and focus are just as big a part of your athletic performance as your nutrition and training. Even though there's no such thing as plant-based *thoughts*, it is possible to develop a mindset that sets you up for better success when following your new plant-based regimen. This is what unleashing your inner athlete is all about—discovering the potential you have, connecting with the fire burning deep within you, and creating results that you'll be proud of. And the tenets that we'll put forth in this chapter are the very same techniques that elite athletes credit for getting them where they are.

Korin Sutton knows a thing or two about creating a plant-based health and fitness program that works. After all, he is a professional bodybuilder in multiple federations, a nineteen-time champion, and a coach to hundreds of plant-based athletes. The secret to Korin's success is deceptively simple: have a plan and follow it. But no matter what that plan looks like, it's not going to work if you don't attack it with consistency, accountability, and giving 110 percent, all the time. Those are lessons ingrained in Korin from his eight years spent serving in the military—four as part of the United States Marine Corps and four in the United States Navy Reserve. "When it comes to me, I just never quit; because in the military you don't quit. You never quit. The definition of quitting isn't there. It's either you keep going, or you die. That's it. You don't just quit on something because it's hard or challenging. You just keep going until the mission is accomplished." And what keeps him motivated with that level of dedication—to his vegan lifestyle, to exercise, and to helping others—is his *why*. Having purpose behind his mission is the key that makes all the pieces work.

Korin connected with his why in college. After a well-known animal rights speaker gave a presentation at his school, Korin wasn't comfortable with the suffering and cruelty that is part of large-scale animal production. So he took a hard look at what he was eating and what kind of industry he was supporting when he bought animal products. Yet even though that speaker extolled the benefits of eating a plant-based diet, Korin wasn't convinced that he'd be able to build muscle without eating animal protein. But he was more convinced that he could no longer support abusive factory farming practices, so he put it to the test and left behind all animal protein except for fish. Not surprisingly (to us), he got more ripped and felt healthier; his skin cleared up; and his energy, stamina, and libido all increased. Then he thought, *If it's working this well just on a pescatarian diet, I can only imagine if I went fully vegan.* Sure enough, he put on even more muscle, got more lean, and has been the same super-ripped guy ever since. "I was very surprised when I saw the results. It's not just a noble act for animals, but it's something that is sustainable."

That kind of clarity and conviction is what's made Korin's career so noteworthy, but it's also made it more difficult of a climb. In a sport that's rampant with steroid use, and with some prestigious competitions not mandating drug tests, Korin is an all-natural, drug-free bodybuilder. He didn't want to subject his body to the kind of ravage that steroids can lead to, with many steroid-using bodybuilders having extremely short life spans (dying in their thirties and forties). As a natural athlete, he explains, you have to train really hard and be patient because your muscles aren't going to grow as quickly or get to the same size as someone who is using illegal drugs. But even though there are federations dedicated to the competition of all-natural athletes—in which Korin has won a number of times—the greatest prize has been winning in the largest, non-drug-tested federations. When that happens, he's not only debunking the need for steroids; he's also putting veganism on the map of mainstream bodybuilding. It didn't happen on his first try; in fact, it didn't happen in his first few attempts at trying to go pro in a nontesting federation. Instead of discouraging him, though, those setbacks pushed him to take his training up a few notches in order to go toe-to-toe with someone using anabolic steroids. The result was creating his best-ever bodybuilding physique and doing his all-time best on the national stage—something that definitely got people's attention and cemented his mission to raise awareness about the issues that matter most to him.

Orla Walsh is a record-holding track cyclist from Ireland. She won two gold medals and set a national record at the Cycling Ireland National Championship in August 2020. But she hadn't even been on a bike until 2015, at age twenty-six. Most athletes who set national records in any sport tend to start their careers at age six, not two decades later. To add to the uniqueness of her place in Irish track cycling history, she wasn't athletic growing up, and she didn't have a gym membership as an adult. Instead, she spent most of her twenties, in fact, nearly all of her twenties, as she says, as a heavy drinker and smoker, engaging in partying rather than healthy eating or exercise. Like many young people, she was focused on being social, and partying was a big part of that social experience. It wasn't until she started commuting to work by bike that she fell in love with cycling. She started cycling more and more, first for the enjoyment of it and later for the sport of it. And she gave up smoking entirely. She has mostly given up drinking too, and she has fully dedicated herself to being a full-time athlete.

Her rise to becoming a world-class athlete has been fast and impressive. Just a few years ago, she was still learning the ropes of track cycling, a sport that takes place in a velodrome with steep banks around an oval track built for speed and on bikes with no gears or brakes. With her newfound love of this fast and powerful form of indoor speed cycling, and her vastly healthier lifestyle, Orla questioned her diet as well. About her decision to adopt a plant-based diet, she said, "I had wanted to switch to a plant-based diet for ethical reasons for about a year before I switched, but I didn't think it was possible as an elite athlete at the time. I was still finding my feet in the athletic world, so I didn't want to take any risks with a drastic diet change. It just so happens that the Sport Ireland Institute is sponsored by the dairy council, so while they have been supportive (since I insisted this was what I wanted), there are definitely some conflicts of interest when it comes to dietary encouragement and advice. It was only when I had a consultation with a plant-based nutritionist that I felt confident I was making the right choice."

Orla's fears are common, ones we both had when we switched to a plant-based diet as competitive athletes. But as is true for so many others, Orla discovered firsthand the benefits of a plant-powered diet. Her results speak for themselves—not just her records, her medals, and her podium finishes, but results that really matter in the big picture of health. She said, "Originally, my favorite part of being plant-based *was* the belief that I was feeding my body with the best possible source of fuel. I felt that I had some sort of advantage as an athlete, and my blood test results indicated it was a great choice in terms of reducing my cholesterol, which was borderline too high before I switched (my LDL has reduced by over 30 percent). I felt more energetic, recovered faster, and overall felt 'cleaner' with the types of food I was consuming—I never had that sick, lethargic feeling after eating a meal that I would have from heavy meat and dairy meals. However, my favorite part of being plant-based *now* is feeling like I'm taking the most ethical and environmentally friendly approach too. This has extended from just my diet to all of my daily purchases, and I always try to make the most sustainable and harm-free choices when possible."

Sometimes the impact of a plant-based diet on our athletic performance catches us off guard too. There is often even a suspicion that perhaps moving away from animal protein will have detrimental effects, but a desire to live a compassionate lifestyle supersedes that worry, even if the potential for diminished performance is still present in our minds. In essence, it can be common for athletes to accept the possibility of perceived diminished returns in favor of following their hearts, embracing a more compassionate diet and lifestyle. The good news is that you can do both, live in line with your ethics and still perform at your very best, and Orla is testament to that. In fact, she is a phantasmagoric example of an athlete who completely changed her life, made evident by juxtaposed transformational photos of a nonathletic, fast-food-eating, drug-abusing partyer posed next to a national champion plant-based athlete with little resemblance to her prior self. Beyond feel-good photos of a life once derailed getting back on track, Orla has the results to validate her amazing transformation—both the blood labs and anecdotal observations in physical wellness, combined with amazing athletic achievements. She really is living a dream, made possible by self-realization and a shift in behavior and attitude to live in greater alignment with her authentic self.

In her own words: "I think a common belief is that you cannot be a powerful, strong athlete without eating meat. I've been surprised at how that is just not the case at all! Over the past year, I increased my max lift and max power output on isometric testing by over 20 percent. I also broke two national records and won two national titles as a track sprinter, which is a discipline that requires significant high power and speed. It has all been great with my energy and recovery since switching to a plant-based diet. If anything, I am recovering quicker and my immune system seems to be significantly improved! I haven't been sick once in the past year, and previously, I would have been regularly run down."

It's hard to ignore Orla's success as a plant-based athlete, and in the age of social media, she has become incredibly popular, with hundreds of thousands of followers who cheer her on and support her efforts, which include a quest to compete in the Olympic Games. When Orla cemented herself in Irish track cycling history at the Cycling Ireland National Championship in 2020, the official report from Cycling Ireland stated the following in its recap of the two-day championships. Day 1: "In the women's sprint, Orla Walsh was the red-hot favorite, having set multiple national records during her training for this event. While the conditions on the day were not favorable for setting fast times, there were to be no surprises when she won gold." Day 2: "Orla Walsh set the tone early as she powered around the track to set a new Irish record of 36.22 [seconds] in the women's 500 meter time trial, taking over a second off the previous mark. With a world class time on the board, Orla Walsh was unbeatable today."

You're probably wondering what Orla eats in order to achieve world-class status as a champion plant-based athlete. We were too. So we asked her. "Generally speaking, I eat four meals per day. I'll time my training around meals to give myself enough time to digest and be adequately fueled for my training sessions. A typical day might be breakfast (oats with all the toppings of nuts, seeds, and fruit, with a protein shake) about one and a half to two hours before a gym session. Gym workouts normally take about two hours, and directly after that, I'll have lunch, which could be a tempeh, bean, and rice burrito with a salad. I then might have a track session a few hours later in the afternoon, which I generally wouldn't eat during, since my efforts are very short and high-intensity. On some occasions, I'll have a smoothie or something high in natural sugars during a bike session, but light enough that I don't feel sick mid-training. I'll then have dinner, which could be toasted potatoes, seitan, and lots of vegetables. My final meal is usually quite late, at around 10:00 p.m., and I eat more oatmeal with fruits, nuts, and seeds again—I call it my 'evening breakfast.'" When it comes to the all-important protein question, she has it covered: "I always try to include a high-protein plant-based source in most of my meals, be it whole-food or supplement-based. In the morning with my oats (with nuts, seeds, and fruits), I will also have an organic pea protein shake from Nuzest brand with soy or oat milk. My go-to plant protein during the day is organic tempeh, which I bake for fifteen to twenty minutes with some Asian BBQ sauce. I do, of course, also include *lots* of slow-release, nonprocessed carbohydrates (I love potatoes!) and some fats."

Though now in her early thirties, Orla is often the oldest member of her cycling team, but she is determined that, much as with her experiences in her twenties, age is just a number, and she's a different person now—one who has dedicated her life to being the best plant-based athlete she can possibly be. We suspect there will be many more medals and records in her future, and perhaps Olympic glory will be hers to embrace.

Andreas Vojta is an Austrian Olympic runner who excels in track-and-field distances ranging from 800 to 10,000 meters. He's clinched thirty-six national titles, including recording the fastest 10,000-meter time in the world during the summer of 2020, which was the world-leading pace at the time. Andreas became vegan for ethical and environmental reasons, but he also reaped the athletic performance benefits, which paved the way for stellar track-and-field seasons in the years after his diet change. But his real success began after he combined that diet shift with the true grit it takes to make it to the Olympics. As he explains, "I always was a good runner in school, but having a hobby you're good at and actually performing professionally are two completely different pairs of shoes." First, most sports (except the major professional leagues) don't have a lot of money in them, especially in the beginning.

It's very hard to make it as a profession, and the sacrifices you have to make in the first years aren't easy. After seeing the 2008 Olympic Games on television, Andreas knew he wanted to be there. So he left behind his medical studies to attempt to go for a national title, and then an international one at the Olympics. The uncertainty of whether it was worth it and whether it would even happen was quite challenging. But Andreas believed in his dreams; he knew that it would take years before he'd see promising results; and he stuck with the incredibly hard and continuous work—what he believes stands between most people and their goals. "I've been in athletics professionally for more than ten years now," he says, "and I'm still learning and improving."

In addition to his work ethic, the other competitive edge Andreas has is the mindset that drives him. He's simply not satisfied unless he knows he's left everything he has on the track and given everything he has for his performance. "My greatest fear is always disappointing myself. I don't care what other people say; I want to be my best self and will be really unhappy if I know that I didn't give it all in the first place. If I did everything in my power and the result is not satisfying, that's okay for me. But I don't want to regret any chances I missed taking. I will always be my own hardest critic, and will always see room for improvement, even after my best performances. So in some way, I also fear stagnation, as you should always be improving in your life, no matter how old, successful, rich, or famous you are!" Andreas recognizes that it takes determination, persistence, resilience, and an unwavering belief in oneself and a dedication to self-improvement to make it to the Olympics, and that it also takes patience and time. In fact, that's how he sees the vegan movement growing too—with determination, persistence, resilience, and an unwavering belief in something you care deeply about. He described it this way: "Human progress takes time, and so does veganism. It is still a quite small but rapidly growing movement, which also found its way into performance-based nutrition in the last years. As more and more people start to realize the (ethical, environmental, and health) benefits, more and more people will follow. A plant-based diet is coming in hot, and it is always great to see if I can play my little part in getting people interested in it or helping them to change. It is a great feeling, but I also know it's not some kind of 'great act' but is the least I can do for myself and everyone else on the planet!"

What truly put Andreas's resolve to the test was when the 2020 Olympics were postponed as a result of the COVID-19 pandemic. As always, Andreas chose the path of positivity and saw the delay until 2021 as an opportunity to improve himself with an extra training year. "It felt good not having to rush the season, running every weekend and chasing times and standards. So, I found some time to focus on myself and my weaknesses. I could manage not only to get my national titles, numbers 34, 35, and 36, but also to run new personal bests for the 3,000 meters, the 5,000 meters, and the 10,000 meters, which was a world-leading time at the time of the performance. Even though I knew that [having less competition] was due to the coronavirus, it gave me a big boost to continue working hard and be even stronger in the 'new Olympic year,' 2021!"

Mental Strength Advice from a World Champion

World champion mountain biker Sonya Looney knows that you don't reach the mountaintop overnight and that it is not just the small, deliberate actions we take every day that help us ascend the mountain. Rather, much of our success depends on our mental strength and toughness. Take it from the world champion, who had to scrap and claw her way up the rankings to find her bliss as one of the best at her sport.

The most powerful voice is the one inside our own head. Becoming an elite athlete is not a straight path. There are ups and downs, and there are many moments of self-doubt and failure. Success and failure should both be acknowledged (success should be celebrated, and you should allow yourself to feel failure and then learn from it), but the highs and lows aren't what define you or your career. It's how you show up every day. It's the relentless commitment to the process. We don't learn who we are by staying comfortable and doing easy things. We learn who we are, and we gain self-confidence, which translates to everything in life, by doing hard things.

Learn self-awareness. Self-awareness and mindfulness are a practice for life. If you can learn to pay attention to what you are telling yourself—your self-talk—you are opening the door to something amazing: the ability to choose how you perceive the world and what you are capable of. People would ask me how I could stay so positive or how I didn't give up in these events. At first, I wasn't sure, and it set me on a path of exploration of my inner life to reverse engineer how I was actually doing it! Through that process, I've learned so much more about how I can get better and how to teach and coach others to do the same.

An interesting thing about my past is that my family didn't believe that I could become a professional cyclist. They thought it was just a hobby and could not understand the commitment and the things I chose to give up to pursue my dream. They couldn't understand that despite having my master's in electrical engineering and the security that offered, I continued to go the hard way. The hardest races in the world forced me to look inward. There's nowhere to hide from yourself when you're alone in the Sahara or the Himalayas—you have to figure out who you are, what your expectations are, and how to be resilient. Mountain bike racing has been a master class in positive psychology, mindfulness, and mental toughness. Becoming a world-class athlete has also taught me that there will always be people (even your closest family members) who will tell you it's impossible, it's stupid, and it's not worth it. Don't let someone put their own self-limiting beliefs on you, and surround yourself with people who *do* believe in you and believe in themselves.

Deal with failure and perfectionism. Elite athletes have failed more than most, and the reason is that they are *still* there giving it their all every day. To put yourself out there, to pursue a dream or do hard things, you are putting yourself in a position where things will eventually test you and go wrong. It's part of the work. What do you do when they go wrong? Do you give up? Do you think it's validation that you'll never get there? There have been plenty of days I wanted to give up, days I didn't want to show up, but overcoming that feeling of quitting over and over is empowering. It's a muscle. Choosing to stand back up every time you fall down gives you confidence and builds self-trust. Elite athletes and performers have failed more than most because they are still trying every day. It's what you do with those failures. Failure isn't proof that you aren't good; it's proof you're trying. Failure is an opportunity to learn something new; it doesn't mean that you aren't good enough. Failure doesn't feel good in the moment, and it's important to allow yourself to feel those feelings, but if you can view it as an opportunity to improve and learn (and believe that you *can* get better with effort and a curiosity for knowledge), it can be one of your best allies. Failure isn't a setback to the path; it *is* the path forward.

Learn to ask for help. No one does it alone. Putting your hand up and asking, "Can someone please help me?" requires vulnerability. It's scary to show one person or maybe even put on social media that you don't know how to do something. Everyone struggles with impostor syndrome—"They'll find out I'm not really as good as people think!" Asking for help and learning from others is what makes you stronger. Vulnerability is a superpower, but it's humbling to be honest with ourselves. Asking for help is what helps you get better. Not asking for help, coaching, etc., actually makes you weaker and more afraid of being yourself. It's hard for my ego, but I put it out for people to see when I'm trying to get help with something. I believe that showing people that they don't have to know everything, helping them see themselves in your story, and being able to help others while you help yourself is empowering.

In March 2019, plant-based endurance athlete **Robbie Balenger** took his first steps on the journey of a lifetime. He left the shores of Southern California on a quest to run across America to New York in seventy-five days, powered by plants and an iron will. Accompanied by plant-based ultrarunner Rich Roll, local media, family, and friends, Robbie set out on a mission to demonstrate to himself, and to the world, that a plant-based diet can sufficiently fuel a three-thousand-mile trek. His route would cover, on average, more than forty miles per day—the equivalent of running a marathon plus a half-marathon every day for two and a half months. NadaMoo!, a plant-based ice cream company, sponsored the endeavor, which made it financially possible.

Robbie hit the road with a plant-powered themed van, a small RV camper, and a multiperson crew trailing him to provide assistance, food, navigation, support, companionship, and a place to rest. He also had a plant-based nutritionist to help calibrate his daily meal plans. He documented his experiences with daily recap posts on Instagram so people could follow along, watching his beard grow as the days went on, connecting with him as he shared his feelings of both hope and despair at having to run an ultramarathon every day for months, cheering him on as he navigated setbacks and found the strength to persevere. He confided that by day four, his legs already felt thrashed, but he was rejuvenated when a friend drove two and a half hours to run alongside him for a number of miles. Days later, he described the eerie experience of running through the vast beauty of the Mojave Desert and surrounding ghost towns.

A couple weeks in, new realizations arose. "I never thought I would depend on my crew like I do, or that sleep would be so hard. I have learned to manage new physical sensations and aches that might have previously freaked me out a little. I didn't think consuming 7,500 plant-based calories a day would be so easy." He confided hardships: "Towards the end [of a fifty-one-mile day], I entered a new phase of darkness. The pain cave got real . . . I started to freak out a little and my mind raced to the what-ifs. I felt so fragile and vulnerable," and "The monotony is really setting in and putting me in a different head space." But there were also days like this: "Yesterday was perfect. It was a short day of only 31 miles. I was completely pain-free all day."

Robbie realized that little things he might have taken for granted made an enormous difference in his mental resilience. One day he and his crew drove thirty miles to Flagstaff, Arizona, to get some vegan pizza—an experience as energizing as it was surreal ("moving through space in a car going so quickly on the Interstate") and overstimulating ("I may need to just get take-out next time we splurge on town food"). And then there were the two nights of planned rest in a northern Arizona hotel to ensure some level of physical recovery. The warm nights' sleep in a bed he could actually sit up in, not to mention an indoor bathroom, were rejuvenating. Even a shower was cause for celebration at this (still early) point in his cross-country trek.

Robbie had many challenging days, physically and mentally. He continued to deal with aches and pains of the grueling daily mileage, painful blisters, and mental fatigue. He wrote, "Emotionally, I had some strong releases, and tears at times were uncontrollable. One of the main emotions I'm being confronted with is fear. As I march into uncharted emotional territory, my sensitivities, anxieties, euphoria, and calms are all heightened due to the extreme physical and mental fatigue." But he experienced elation when he was surprised by friends who showed up unannounced to run alongside him; when his fiancée, Shelley, joined him periodically; and when his mom came to cycle with him and later make him a spaghetti dinner. This feeling of community and connectedness was what helped him keep going as he ran through snow, storms, changing elevations and climates, strong headwinds, and mental exhaustion. He also felt extreme gratitude for what really allowed him to keep running—his diet. "I would not have made it this far in my run if it were not for a plant-based diet that allows me to consume the calories I need while also replenishing my body and keeping inflammation at bay. Animals are aware, have feelings, and are very observant of everything, especially a tall bearded man traversing by them at somewhere between a 10 and 15-minute mile pace." And the combination of all these factors added up to a deep sense of pride. "I feel more confident in myself as an individual than I ever have in my life."

Day by day, Robbie looked forward to the milestones that marked the progression of his journey—crossing the Mississippi River, leaving Missouri, and entering Illinois. He learned to take things one step at a time, one five-mile segment at a time, one day, one week, one month, and so on. If problems came up, he and his crew made adjustments. This kind of fortitude was a result of keeping their eyes on the larger goal of crossing the country in seventy-five days. Little by little, they just needed to keeping moving forward.

With fewer than ten days left, Robbie really started to sense the end was near, but that didn't mean it would be easy to get there. "Over this weekend the theme, without a doubt, was the hills and heat. Up until about four days ago, I really thought I was going to coast through the remaining portion of this run into NYC, but it has become clear that this is going to be a struggle until the end. With each passing day, these mountains just become more and more relentless, and the grade steeper and steeper. I originally thought I was in the Appalachians, but only as of last night I figured out I am actually in the Allegheny Mountains. We've not even yet reached the Appalachians. These mountains are their own beasts. They may not look as intimidating as the Rockies, but they're so much harder. They are unforgiving; climb after climb, descent after descent. The grade being so steep that I'm almost slower going down than going up. My body hurts. I'm tired and somewhat discouraged. I have more confidence today than in the beginning that I can persevere, but in no way does it make it any less daunting and painful."

And then it was over. On day seventy-five, in Central Park, the end of his journey "daily update" was as brief as the day he left the California coast. "It's over, Y'all. 75 days. 3,175 miles. 15 states. Lots of plant-based calories. Feeling all the feels." The next day, photographed with a haircut and a trimmed beard, he wrote, "I'm slowly starting to process the last 75 days and beginning to understand who this person is that has come out the other side. There are so many factors that have contributed to the success of this run across the United States. Some essential aspects include years of training, a clear and defined route, supportive sponsors like NadaMoo! and Switch4Good, and an amazing crew. But the one factor that stands out the most to me and cannot be overlooked or discredited is my diet. A plant-based diet, free of all animal products (meat, fish, dairy, honey, eggs, etc.) has allowed me to consume 8,000 calories a day without ever feeling weighed down by my food, bloated, or in any way uncomfortable because my body can't easily digest what I have put in it. The lack of animal proteins means less inflammation in my very much over-used joints. I haven't been sick, I haven't sustained any major injuries, and I feel as light and fresh as someone could who is running across the country. Despite being tired after 45 miles a day of continuous running, I actually experience little to no soreness. The fruits and vegetables that are present in essentially everything I eat provide the nutrients (antioxidants, flavonoids, etc.) for cellular repair and decreased oxidative stress. They say food is medicine, and in this particular setting, it is everything. Everything I consume is a positive, contributing to my nourishment instead of detracting from my total health."

We asked Robbie why he embarked on this journey to begin with, something you might be wondering too. His response shows just how human this real-life superhero really is. He said, "It was monumental. I couldn't think of anything bigger. If I could do this [cross-country run] plant-based, then I could put the 'you need meat for strength argument' to bed. I was doing this to show what was possible on a plant-based diet. If I failed, that would be a notch against the lifestyle, and I couldn't have that happen. Also, my suffering was voluntary. So many endure so much worse every day. The strength of others who are victims to whatever causes their suffering gives me strength. Who am I to quit? My run was a privilege, and to quit would be a slap in the face to all those who persevere through real adversity."

As for *how* he was able to accomplish such an amazing feat, his answer echoed his midrun realization: he needed to make his goal attainable throughout the day. It all came down to incremental goal setting, or breaking large goals down into smaller ones. As he put it, "I ran from LA to NYC, 3,175 miles, all in five-mile increments." He'd see his crew every five miles, so that was all that mattered until the next five. "We don't get to great things overnight. Big goals are merely a bunch of small goals accomplished in succession leading to the completion of something greater." Now, a year after completing his historic trek, Robbie still thinks about being back on the open road. He would do it all over again. And to anyone considering taking on a challenge that feels larger than life, he has this to say: "When you get the chance to do something bold, do it. Embrace the now, and breathe it in with everything you've got."

On a typical day while running across America, Robbie consumed approximately eight thousand calories. In addition to Skratch Labs hydration mix throughout the day to provide additional calories and replenish his salts, a sample meal plan looked something like this:

Breakfast—Coffee and oatmeal with peanut butter, chia
     seeds, maple syrup
Stop 1—Smoothie #1 with coconut milk, peanut butter,
     greens, carrots, bananas, chia seeds, Soylent
Stop 2—Bobo's Bar
Stop 3—Smoothie #2
Stop 4—Fruit, chocolate, nut butter
Stop 5—Smoothie #3
Stop 6—Boiled potatoes with salt
Stop 7—Smoothie #4
Stop 8—Spring Energy Gel, usually with caffeine
Dinner—Double portion of an Outdoor Herbivore camping
     meal cooked with coconut oil

When Goals Become Real Life

The pursuit of meaning and of happiness has been a critical component etched in the successful blueprint set forth by some amazing plant-based athletes who have overcome significant obstacles in order to feel fulfilled. Meet some plant-based athletes whose mental toughness set the stage for their physical transformational success.

Sonya Looney is a professional mountain biker who has won races around the world, powered by a plant-based diet. She has been following a whole-foods plant-based diet since 2013 and has racked up victories in her sport from Poland to Sri Lanka and from Argentina to Nepal as a true champion with a focus on goal setting, grit, and mental toughness. After switching to plants, she went from chasing the last spot on the podium to standing on the top tier. "The most notable accomplishment after changing my diet was becoming world champion in twenty-four-hour mountain biking. That means I raced my bike for twenty-four hours straight, and my only stops were bathroom breaks and to change batteries in my lights at night. Having the energy and trusting that my body could go hard for that long is due to my diet and the optimal health I had going into the race."

Though performing well, recovering efficiently, and staying healthy year-round are crucial elements of Sonya's success—and have all been aided by her plant-based diet—the foundation of her dominance in her sport is her mental toughness, or her grit, as she calls it. "I've competed in some of the world's hardest mountain bike races in places like the Sahara Desert and the Himalayas, where conditions are difficult. Unplanned things will happen; you won't want to get up the next morning to get started; and you'll want to give up. Just because you win a race doesn't mean you didn't want to quit the whole time; you just overcame that urge over and over. That's where grit comes from. It also comes from being stronger than your excuses every day when you say, 'I don't feel like doing it.' It takes mindfulness to realize when a negative thought pops in your head and starts creating all the feelings and stories that will make you perform worse. Racing has taught me how to apply mindfulness on race days, and now, on all days." Sonya shares a great example of how our mindset alone can end our competition before it even starts, or revitalize our careers when we thought they were over.

We've probably all been there at one time or another—feeling sorry for ourselves because of an injury or a setback or because we perceive our results as failure and it's just so much easier to give up and move on. Sonya reminds us there are other options than simply walking away when things get tough, and it starts with our own awareness of the incredible mental strength we can tap into. And when it comes to goal setting, especially for sports competition, she reminds us that it's not all about you and your results. She says, "Goal setting isn't about beating other people. In fact, having amazing people to compete against makes you better, and makes your results that much more meaningful." Sonya also has some advice about how to get started: "Showing up and getting started is often the momentum we need to keep going. When you stop showing up, when you start letting excuses swallow you up every day—that's when you start losing trust in yourself and in your grit. Make it easy to show up, or commit to doing just five minutes of exercise so you know whether you really are tired and need a break, or if it's just a struggle to overcome excuses."

Sonya credits her mental strength for her world championship success, and with that, she has a story to share: "The way we tell ourselves stories about what's happening around us is the key to a strong mindset. Dr. Martin Seligman names it our 'Explanatory Style.' A simple example would be looking outside on the morning of a 100-mile mountain bike race and seeing that it's cold and rainy. You could say, 'I'm going to be uncomfortable, I don't like riding in wet conditions, I hate being cold, etc.' Or you could say, 'I'm going to have an awesome adventure. I'm going to have fun today, and that will make me stronger. Today is an opportunity to get better on wet trails. I'm going to hoot and holler when I get more mud on my face.' Once you can learn to do that, you can do it anywhere in your life, and it's a practice." And that's not just a story of circumstances that might come up. These are conditions and scenarios that Sonya has faced throughout her career. She called upon her mental toughness and positive attitude on a particularly grueling race in the Himalayas. She recalls: "One of the more difficult moments in my career was one of my best teachers! I wanted to be the first woman to finish the Yak Attack, a ten-day mountain bike stage race across the Himalayas. You even have to hike in the dark (and snow) over one of the most hair-raising mountain passes with your bike strapped to your back. Thorong La Pass sits at 5,416 meters, or almost 18,000 feet, and you cross this pass on day nine of the ten-day race. I was leading the race and had survived the ascent. On the way down, I discovered my hydraulic brakes no longer worked and I had to walk my bike for eight hours to get to the finish for that day's stage of the race while people blew by me riding down. I had spent months preparing for the race, and showing up to that race was one of my most courageous acts at that point in time. I was going to fail on day nine, and I was going to have to quit the race because there are no bike shops or support in the middle of the Annapurna Circuit. I had to redefine what success meant to me in that moment. Success was having the courage to show up. Success was doing my best. Success was accepting things I couldn't change. Success was being brave enough to go for it. Spoiler alert—I was able to borrow brakes from a rider who dropped out, and still win the race! And I went back the next year to get another win under my belt!"

Josh LaJaunie's journey to becoming a champion plant-based athlete is one of the most remarkable we've shared, if not *the* most remarkable. If we told you that a guy who runs 100-mile races—which amount to nearly four consecutive marathons in a row—and wins ultramarathons used to weigh more than 400 pounds, you probably wouldn't believe us. It's one thing to lose a significant amount of weight, as many people are able to do, but to drop more than 200 pounds and then become an *elite* athlete, running marathons faster than many avid competitive marathoners, is quite another.

Josh was raised in the swamplands of Louisiana, where he grew up hunting, fishing, eating lots of fried food, and drinking beer—"Living the good life," as he describes it. As a huge fan of the New Orleans Saints, he dreamed of playing professional football, and as a six-foot-three, 320-pound lineman, he was awarded a scholarship to play at the University of Arkansas at Monticello. But in his very first semester, he slipped a disc in his back, ending his football career.

He moved back home to the bayou, where he put on another 100 pounds of body weight through a life of partying, drinking, and eating foods such as gumbo, jambalaya, and crawfish, plus rabbit, squirrel, and deer meat. He was about as far from being plant-based or, at this point, an athlete, as you could get, tipping the scale at 420 pounds. As his weight was getting out of control, a friend suggested that they work out together. So Josh started going to the gym, initially focusing on the strength-training exercises he had been doing as a football player. Then he thought he might give running a try, since he heard it was a good fat-burning workout. Unknowingly at the time, he had begun his journey toward becoming an ultramarathoner. He eventually built up the stamina and confidence to run a 10K, his first-ever race, in 2011. He still weighed 320 pounds, and it took him nearly two hours to complete it, but he finished. Inspired by when the New Orleans Saints won the Super Bowl back in 2010, Josh started to believe that anything was possible.

Shortly after, he was inspired by his wife to cut out all processed food from their diet for Lent. During those forty days he read Scott Jurek's book *Born to Run* and was amazed that the accomplishments of one of the world's greatest endurance athletes were fueled entirely by plants. It was a big change from the fried fish and boiled animals he grew up eating, but leaving animals off his plate, combined with a fascination with long-distance running, got the ball rolling for the former morbidly obese small-town Louisiana boy from Chackbay.

He decided to give a plant-based athlete lifestyle a try, and a year after his first race, he was down to 285 pounds and shaved almost an hour off his 10K time. Two years later, in 2014, he weighed less than 200 pounds and ran his first full marathon, followed by four full marathons over the next year and a half. By the time 2016 came around, he had won the Bear Bait Ultra 50-miler, finished second at the Gamelands Ultra 50K, and finished third at the Wildcat Ultras 100-miler. He even ran a

UNLEASHING YOUR INNER ATHLETE

three-hour and twenty-four-minute marathon and eventually finished a 10K in under forty minutes.

Josh's inspirational and unlikely story from obesity to ultramarathon champion landed him on the cover of *Runner's World* magazine and led to appearances on the *Today Show* and *Good Morning America*. He wrote a manifesto on his website, sharing his journey, and eventually wrote a book, *Sick to Fit*.

Today, Josh feels like a new person, inside and out. The emotional changes were some of the most dramatic that he went through during his transformation—letting go of old feelings about how he viewed himself and who he used to be while embracing who he is today and what he wants to achieve. There is a physical weight off his shoulders but also an emotional and mental weight off his lifestyle. He knows he is on a healthier path, one that allowed him to become an athlete again, a champion athlete at that, and is following a lifestyle that will support greater longevity to spend quality time with his wife and family down in the bayou. Josh is also as down to earth as it gets, not falling prey to the inflated ego that often comes with being on a major magazine cover and making appearances on the most popular television shows in America. In one of his many appearances on *The Rich Roll Podcast*, episode 404, he said, "There's nothing really special about me. Results are typical if you apply the power of plants to your life, and the power of bipedal locomotion, and getting outside and getting some sunshine, and using the body the way it was intended to be used." After never leaving his home state of Louisiana before that one semester in college in neighboring Arkansas, he is still in awe of his trips to make public speaking appearances today in our nation's capital, in major cities such as New York City, and at other locations where he's invited to share his story. We met Josh in Arizona when he was on a speaking tour in 2017, and we continue to be inspired by his accomplishments and by how grounded he is, with a sense of urgency to help others, not boost his own reputation.

The boy from Bayou Lafourche now makes it a point to help others discover the power of plants and empower themselves to reclaim their health, lose weight, and improve the quality of their lives. He has helped his family, including his parents, siblings, grandfather, wife, and mother-in-law, adopt a plant-based diet and get more active, including running, and collectively they have lost more than 1,000 pounds. Friends from his small Louisiana town have also lost more than 100 pounds each in some cases, inspired by Josh's example. He's somewhat of a celebrity in the bayou, but he takes it all in stride and doesn't even take credit for the countless people he's inspired. He says in an interview with Rich Roll, "It's happening, and I'm along for the ride, and I'm okay with it."

When we asked Josh about the major differences in physical fitness and in health that he experienced when making the switch to a plant-based diet, he acknowledged: "Everyone talks about recovery. That's a given. But feeling lighter inside my body, like I didn't have heavy insides anymore, was huge. I felt lighter and more energetic. I've been heavy all my life, so losing weight itself was a huge help to energy. But even after I had lost 100 pounds, while still following a low-carbohydrate/Paleo diet at the time, I struggled with energy. After going plant-based, before I even lost the rest of the weight, I noticed a massive energy boost, and that really helped my running take off." He said that once he made the permanent switch to a plant-based diet, his endurance was boosted so much that it helped ignite the inspiration to run his first ultramarathon. He's not as sore as he used to be following a workout, and his recovery is so efficient that running marathons, 50-milers, and even 100-mile races just seemed like the next thing to do in pursuit of running down his dreams of being a healthy, competitive athlete, sparking change in the world around him.

Though squirrel, rabbit, deer, and beer have gone by the wayside, his new Louisiana bayou diet consists of foods such as tofu scrambles with red beans and mushrooms, sautéed mushrooms with onions cooked with red sauce and spread over whole-wheat pasta, rice and beans, and tempeh bacon mushroom wraps using tofu sour cream with dill, garlic powder, salt, pepper, and lemon juice to create a ranch dressing flavor.

Forget the crawfish; he says he can eat about six to eight of those tempeh bacon mushroom wraps with ranch sauce in a single sitting. After all, you need a lot of fuel to go out on a twenty-mile training run. Despite the character-building level of humidity in the swamplands, Josh uses only a vitamin B_{12} supplement; the rest of his pre-, mid-, and post-workout nutrition comes from food. For a while he used an electrolyte and hydration sports drink on long runs, but now he lets food and water be his workout and recovery fuel. Even with his six-foot-three 190-pound frame, Josh doesn't worry about his protein intake, and after discovering that all plants have protein, he finds it to be "very liberating knowledge, especially when giving up your 'only' source of protein." Now that Josh finds himself traveling a lot more than ever before, for races or to make appearances and give speeches about his weight-loss and running success story, he finds airports to be a bit tricky when looking for plant-based options, but he says there's always an option—like a sushi restaurant that will have edamame, avocado rolls, vegetable sushi, seaweed salads, and other plant-based fare they are known for. And if he's driving to get from one place to another, as he was when we caught up with him through voice mail while he was driving to Houston, he stops at grocery stores, loading up on foods such as apples and potatoes, which he can prepare and even microwave in a motel or hotel room.

What we love most about Josh's story is his humble beginnings and his sincere desire to help the health and happiness of those he cares most about in his small town. Certain levels of fame can come from being a major magazine cover model, a three-time guest on *The Rich Roll Podcast*, and multiple national television appearances, but they have not changed the optimistic and cheerful boy from the bayou. He's the same guy he's always been, spending quality time with his family and friends in the swampland he is proud to call home. These days, Josh and his family just fry up a little different food on game day to tune in and cheer for their beloved Saints.

When former professional mixed martial arts (MMA) fighter **James Wilks** was a young boy growing up in his native England, he was inspired by martial artist Bruce Lee to one day become a champion fighter himself. So he started studying martial arts, fighting Bruce Lee's style, Jeet Kune Do, as well as Tae Kwon Do Brazilian Jiu-Jitsu (earning a black belt or its equivalent in kickboxing and combat submissive wrestling). He made a splash on the sports scene when he won *The Ultimate Fighter Season 9*, which jumpstarted his MMA career in the Ultimate Fighting Championship (UFC). He went on to fight with a record of ten wins and four losses before announcing his retirement in 2012 after doctors warned him that he would face a significantly high risk of paralysis if he continued to fight due to a severe neck injury.

But while Wilks's goal of becoming a successful professional MMA fighter is an excellent example of setting your sights high, it's what happened after he retired that took some major self-motivation and stepping outside his comfort zone. While training with future heavyweight champion Fabrício Werdum, Wilks tore ligaments in both his knees. Not wanting to resign himself to a sedentary life, and wanting to continue training athletes as well as members of the military and law enforcement as his primary professional work as a combative instructor, he looked into how a nutritional approach might help his recovery. That was when he discovered a paper detailing the plant-based diet of Roman gladiators. He realized that not only did he not need animal products to be strong and healthy but there was also an advantage to getting nutrition from plants. This became the jumping-off point for his exploration of a plant-based diet for athletes, which was detailed in the 2019 documentary *The Game Changers*. James became fully plant-based, experienced incredible increases in endurance and strength, and became one of the most influential plant-based athletes, literally overnight, when the film was released around the world to rave reviews. The film was screened in more than twenty countries on the night of its premiere in September 2019, and within a matter of weeks, *The Game Changers* became the number one documentary in iTunes history. It continues to set viewership records and influence millions of people (if not tens of millions by now) around the world to shift their diets toward plants. It was claimed in late 2020 that *The Game Changers* might be the most-watched documentary of all time, largely owing to its massive global success on Netflix and a Netflix equivalent in China with five times the audience. What started with a used camera James bought on Craigslist years ago to interview plant-based athletes about their experiences on a plant-based diet has become a game-changing phenomenon that has significantly influenced how many people view protein, food, and nutrition. It took a lot of mental strength, persistence, and persever-ance to complete the film, which was a multiyear project of filming and assembling the right team. There's no doubt that James's martial arts background and discipline helped him on his course to history-making success as a filmmaker and as a retired athlete who learned to fuel better and return to training. Now a plant-based athlete, he works as a combat instructor for US Navy Sea, Air, and Land (SEAL) Teams and the US Marshals Service.

After meeting and interviewing many of the greatest plant-based athletes on the planet and learning from some of the world's most knowledgeable medical practitioners why this diet is superior for ath-letes, Wilks has continued training with confidence that a plant-based diet provides the right fuel for the job. After the release of *The Game Changers*, he traveled the world and was a regular on popular podcasts, such as *The Joe Rogan Experience*, and television shows such as *Good Morning Britain*, cohosted by Piers Morgan. He was recognized daily when he was out and about, but with the COVID-19 pandemic, he set-tled into a routine devoid of travels and in-person media appearances. But the film and his plant-based athlete message are still going strong, resonating with audiences around the world. James is back to working out and enjoying plant-based meals, lower stress, and more family time.

James's success story, on and off camera, is a reminder to all of us to follow our passions, reach for our dreams, and keep pursuing them until we achieve them.

The reality is that the mental game may be the toughest of all to master in your quest for improved athletic performance. Anyone can

follow a meal plan, at least for a while, and anyone can follow an exercise program, at least for a while, but that's the key issue: How long
does "a while" last? What are the factors that impact the length of your
commitment to a nutrition or exercise program? It depends on you, how
clear you are on your goal, and why you want to get there. To arrive at
the answer for yourself, you'll need to be able to answer these questions:

1. WHAT goal do you want to achieve?
2. WHY does it matter to you?
3. HOW will it change your life?
4. WHEN will you get started?

Let's break it down. First up: goals.

Plain and simple—what's your ideal end game? If time, money, or
other obstacles were not factors, what would you want to achieve? Iden-
tifying this is the first step toward making the gains you want—namely
because after you identify *where* exactly you want to go, you can come
up with a plan of *how* to get there.

There are lots of different of types of goals, but they can neatly be
summed up as Okay Goals, Not-Okay Goals, and Great Goals. In other
words, there are goals that might pique your curiosity but do nothing to
motivate you (Okay Goals); there are goals that move you in the opposite
direction of what you really want (Not-Okay Goals); and then there are
the goals so spot-on, so exciting, so terrifying (as in, what if it actually
happened?!) that they're enough to keep you amped throughout your
journey of getting there (you guessed it, Great Goals). While you definitely
want to avoid goals that are counterproductive (for example, bulking up
at all costs, eating as much nondairy ice cream as possible because it is a
source of dense calories), you also want to be careful of adopting goals that
you *think* are great but wouldn't create any change in your life or feelings
of achievement if you attained them—such as losing or gaining just a few
pounds. Instead, you need to reach a little further, think a little harder,
dig a little deeper, and discover what really moves you.

Ultimately, a really great goal has a clear objective—what you're trying to achieve—along with an understanding of why it matters to you and how your life may be different as a result of achieving it. To move toward that kind of clarity, close your eyes and think of the things in your life that make you smile more than anything else. We're talking about deep, heartfelt joy: the kind of smile that comes from a moment that you don't want to end. As you let that moment linger in your mind, consider what kind of accomplishment would yield that kind of feeling. Similarly, think about all the attributes that you admire in other athletes—their talent, skill, strength, confidence, compassion, leadership, work ethic, passion, and so forth. What would you need to accomplish in order to feel you'd reached similar heights? How would it feel to elicit that same reaction from others?

Now Put a Little Fire Behind It

You have your goal and you know where you're going, but before you figure out your next steps toward reaching that goal, it's time to get clear on why that goal matters so much to you. We can try to motivate you all day (or book) long with our nutrition facts and exercise stories, sharing the journeys of those who have found the greatest fulfillment in their lives as champion plant-based athletes, but unless you come up with your own reason for standing at the starting line, you won't have the immediate connection with your goal that you need in order to be successful. So ask yourself: *Why did I pick up this book in the first place? What did I hope to get out of it?* Our guess is that you didn't just want to learn which vegetables to eat to lose weight, or to discover how to refuel after your strength-training workout. We suspect there's something a little bit deeper. After all, you could have just asked Google about plant-based protein. No, we think you picked up this book because you want to feel more alive, you want to boost your energy and vitality, and, ultimately, you want to smile more and feel prouder of what you can achieve when you give yourself permission to really crank the dial.

Ask yourself: *Why does my goal matter to me?* And *How will it change my life?* Your reason can be big and lofty and idealistic or simple and straightforward. Just pick something that's honest and feels right. We'll wait.

Finding Your "Why"

I became a pescatarian in 1990 at age nine. I didn't know anyone else who didn't eat meat, but I decided that I liked animals too much to want them to die for my pleasure. As it became clear that fish also think and feel deeply, I stopped eating fish. Then I learned about the atrocities in the egg industry and the cruelty of the dairy industries, and became vegan. The environmental impact of consuming animal products helped push me to take this step, but it wasn't really a hard choice. I know that all animals have complex social lives and feel as deeply as we do; I am not prepared to contribute to their suffering. I find that a plant-based diet works really well for me. It keeps me focused on quality nutrition, and getting the right nutrition at the right time, to help my body perform.
—Sophie Mullins, British 100K ultramarathon champion

I adopted a totally plant-based diet at the age of six after being vegetarian since age three. I didn't do it for any other reason than a love of animals and not wishing to harm them, but it has proven to be the best decision of my life from both a sporting and nonsporting perspective. My longevity of career, versatility of event range—still representing my country, from 5K road events to ultras—recovery rate, injury-free status, and mental motivation are just some of the many benefits of decades of vegan living.
—Fiona Oakes, Guinness World Record-holding marathoner

My reason to go vegan was for ethical and environmental aspects. I accumulated a lot of impressions about the industry on social media and couldn't justify it for myself anymore. Performance or health deliberations didn't play any role for me. I just wanted to be a better version of myself and bring my actions into alignment with my morals. Changing to a plant-based diet fully met my expectations and was the best decision I ever made!

—Andreas Vojta, Olympic 1,500-meter runner

I actually became a vegetarian a bit by accident. I was sitting with a girlfriend at lunch when she turned to me and said, "Let's be vegetarians. If everyone were vegetarian, we could feed the world four times over . . . and save the environment." I enthusiastically responded, "Sounds great. Let's do it! But . . . what's a vegetarian?" This was back in 1990, in Manhattan, New York City. After she explained it to me, we both looked at our plates of spaghetti and meatballs and, with long faces, plucked our meatballs out one by one. While becoming vegetarian was not exactly thought through, becoming vegan was a precisely calculated move that I made ten years later, in the year 2000. I had just upgraded to the professional ranks in cycling and was in search of that magic edge over the competition. What I found through thorough research was that all evidence pointed to a plant-based diet. Shortly after I turned vegan, I went from the back of the pack to the front— even winning international races and placing top 10 in world cups. It was only after I'd switched to a plant-based diet that I learned about the moral ramifications of my choice. Since that moment I have been a strict vegan so that I can state with a clear conscience that no creature had to suffer for my results.

—Christine Vardaros, professional cyclist

In the Words of the Great One . . .

Hockey legend Wayne Gretzky said it best: "You miss 100 percent of the shots you don't take." *You'll never know if you don't try.* It's been said many times, in many different ways, that your first step toward a new goal is always the hardest. Heck, sometimes just making the goal and committing to it is the hardest. There's a world of uncertainty that comes with this kind of undertaking: *What if my goal is too big? What will others think of me if I fail? What will I think of myself if I quit? What if my achievement isn't what I expected?* And so, what if you fail? Michael Jordan summed it up perfectly: "I've failed over and over and over again in my life. And that is why I succeed."

Time to Get Started

That's all that's left. You've planned, you've dreamed, you've read, you've made notes, you've grocery shopped, you've prepped, you've watched inspiring videos—you get the idea. You've done everything you can do up until the point of gearing up and digging in. Now is when you need a plan of action.

The most helpful tool to keep yourself accountable, focused, and on track is a timeline. First, figure out how long it will realistically take to achieve your goal. Be sure that your timeline isn't so short that your goal is unattainable (as is the case with many New Year's resolutions—you need longer than one month to lose twenty pounds) or so long that you lose interest or momentum (it doesn't take a year to train for a 5K). If it's helpful, do a little research online—or ask friends, if they've gone after the same goal—to see what is a reasonable amount of time to dedicate to this accomplishment.

Next, fill in the blanks. Come up with a training regimen that tracks with hitting that goal. That could be going to the gym X amount of times per week for Y period of time. It could be new daily habits that you'd like to add, such as waking up early to get in a workout or sticking to a meal plan. Consistently hitting a series of smaller goals is a lot more satisfying (and effective) than just keeping your eye on that one—seemingly—far-off goal. A big reason why this is important is that it will help you develop a routine, which in turn will keep you consistently on track to attain your goals and, beyond those, bigger and bigger goals.

It often also helps to have a support network. You don't necessarily need to make your goals public, but telling a few close and supportive friends what you plan to achieve not only will keep you accountable (a very powerful motivator) but also will create a cheering section to be there for you when you need it. These should be people you can lean on when times get tough, to talk to when things seem challenging, and to learn from if you need advice. Never underestimate the power of surrounding yourself with positive people.

Let Some Happiness into the Hard Work

No matter how hard you're trying to reach your goals, if you don't let a little joy into the equation, you're going to burn out. Weight loss is a classic example—you can "succeed" with a smaller number on the scale, but if that is the result of misery-making calorie restriction, deprivation of favorite foods, and agonizing cardiovascular training, it's not really a goal worth pursuing. That scenario is devoid of any happiness, and in our opinion would not qualify as successful. (Unless there is a critical health issue that needs to be resolved quickly, but even in that situation, there could be a more fulfilling way to reach that weight-loss goal.) So don't forget to smile along the way, even in the face of obstacles or setbacks.

We believe that every moment when success and happiness collide is a moment to be celebrated. That can look a number of different ways: It can be as simple as finding plant-based foods that you love and making sure to include them in many of your meals. It can be setting reminders for yourself to appreciate how far you've come and how building a stronger, more robust body is helping you to appreciate more of whatever brings happiness into your life. It can be being more mindful of those sweet-spot moments when, even for a second, there's an ease to your effort—you can't miss a shot, every lift feels manageable, that extra mile doesn't seem so hard. As you work toward your goal, remember that if you remain open to finding joy in the pursuit of whatever it is that moves you, you'll likely find your bliss.

Before we turn you loose into the world to carry the torch as part of the next generation of plant-based athletes, we want to let you know that we believe in you. We know how hard it can be to go against the grain, and to stand out in a world that hasn't fully embraced your lifestyle, but we know that the rewards of following your heart outweigh the fears and the challenges of the unknown. May you always be reminded of why you started out on your journey in the first place. When you're tempted to give up, quit, or throw in the towel on your plant-based diet, your nutrition plan, your exercise program, or your health and fitness goals, go back to your what, why, when, and how, and keep going. The most direct path to achievement is forward progress. It's often a winding one, sometimes with roadblocks, potholes, U-turns, and even detours, but if followed correctly, it will lead you where you want to go. There is no shame in falling off the wagon; your power comes from getting right back on it. Being a plant-based athlete is all about becoming your healthiest, fittest, happiest self. So go out there and change the world, one bite, one lift, one step, and one smile at a time.

Goal-Setting to Become Your Personal Best

It was a talk Robert gave about goal-setting, which Matt attended over a decade ago, that brought us together and ultimately resulted in the book you're holding now. Thinking big and setting goals is the secret weapon behind so much of what we've accomplished (and still plan to), and we want to share that power with you to help you realize your dreams as a plant-based athlete. Download our bonus Goal-Setting Workshop—the very process we've both used for years—at nomeatathlete.com/book-bonus and start creating a magnificent future today.

• • • • •

Mindfulness and goal setting are extremely important in my sport and in any sport. Sport is 90 percent mental. I spent a lot of time focusing on meditation and working with my mental trainer. I read a lot of sports psychology books and loved to listen to podcasts along those lines as well.
—**Meagan Duhamel, Olympic gold medal–winning figure skater**

All of those mindfulness and goal-setting techniques are really important in this sport. Whether it's in a training or competition environment, you have to be extremely focused and set yourself the right kind of goals. It's a very small margin between successfully landing a trick or not, so in competitions it really is high pressure and you've got to be so present and mindful in the moment to block out other factors and be at the top of your game mentally.
—**Stephen Gray, professional football freestyler,**
   two-time Guinness World Record holder

I felt it straightaway in my strength journey that getting stronger physically meant I became stronger mentally. The difference was huge. I controlled my emotions better and I was more capable to stand up for myself and others in situations where I had just felt unworthy before. The same thing happened when I went vegan. I felt so aligned with my emotions. Standing my ground and living my beliefs made me mentally stronger. Being true to myself. The mental aspect of strength is the biggest part of it all. To be stronger you have to believe you can and that you are. The only regret that I have is not going vegan sooner.
—**Hulda B. Waage, Icelandic national powerlifting record holder**

Journaling is a big part of my day, always starting the day with intention and purpose and making sure I have a clear path in regard to my growth day by day.
—**Dustin Watten, Team USA volleyball player**

When you're put in a position of having to dig deeper and you choose to—I think it's so incredible what we're capable of with our human bodies.
—**Shanda Hill, world champion ultratriathlete,**
   vegan since birth

10

A DAY IN THE LIFE
OF A PLANT-BASED ATHLETE

We've spent the previous nine chapters giving you all the basics you need to add some rocket fuel to your athletic training—namely the plants and how to use them, but also how to make sure your body is ready to receive the highest level of training you ask of it. Now we want to turn it over to the athletes and let them show you firsthand how they're putting all the pieces together. From how they schedule their workouts to how they're eating throughout the day to their favorite recovery methods, this chapter is a coveted glimpse inside the minds of the people who are putting a plant-based diet to the test.

Robert Cheeke, Bodybuilder

MORNING

Morning routine: I start my day by going outside in the backyard with our dogs, getting sunshine, fresh air, and checking email while eating fruit and drinking water or hibiscus tea. Having dogs helps develop routines, including daily dog walks. During winter months, I still go outside with our dogs to start my day, but just for brief periods, and then have breakfast and check email indoors.

Breakfast: Oatmeal or overnight oats, sometimes a breakfast burrito or fruit, such as seasonal berries, cherries, or sliced stone fruit. Occasionally I'll have a breakfast cereal, or something like bagels or muffins, but my breakfast mainly consists of oats and fruit.

Snack: Fruit, such as bananas, applesauce, berries, or a snack bar.

AFTERNOON

Lunch: Burrito bowl with brown rice, pinto beans, avocado, lettuce, tomato, and salsa. A burrito bowl is probably the meal I have the most often, and when I have ingredients prepared in bulk, such as batches of brown rice and beans, I can simply add in the toppings, which sometimes also include olives, peppers, and different varieties of beans and salsas.

Snacks: Fruit, such as berries, bananas, apple slices, and oranges, or a snack bar.

Workout 1: A thirty- to sixty-minute dog walk. In addition to time in the backyard with our dogs, I go on a dog walk every afternoon, often just before heading to the gym, making the dog walk part of my warm-up for a weight-training workout.

EVENING

Pre-workout fuel: Two bananas and water.

Workout 2: One-hour weight-training workout, typically focused on two muscle groups per workout, such as biceps and triceps, back and shoulders, or legs and abs. I often complete about 20–30 total sets, depending on the muscle groups trained and the length of the workout, often aiming for about 4–5 sets per exercise, completing 8–12 reps per set. I often do a bit of warm-up or cooldown, which may include using the StairMaster, elliptical trainer, stationary bike, and foam roller and sometimes stretching in a steam room or sauna.

Post-workout replenishment: Usually fruit for immediate replenishment, and then dinner, since I work out in the evenings. That often includes snacking on some berries or clementine or mandarin oranges while dinner is being prepared.

Dinner: Pad Thai or Thai fried rice. Thai food and Mexican food are my favorite international cuisines and the types of food I eat the most, when not having soup, pasta, plant-based burgers, burritos, or other common dinner themes. Thai food makes its way into my diet every month, if not every week, in one form or another— fresh rolls, Thai salad, fried rice, curry, pad Thai.

Dessert: I often enjoy a popsicle at the end of the day, especially during summer, occasionally some nondairy ice cream or something chocolate, but my favorite desserts are typically fruit (sliced nectarines or orange slices before bed).

Recovery routine: With a history of lower back soreness related to sports injuries sustained over the decades of being an athlete, I often take a hot shower after my evening workout to put heat on my lower back. I'm also a massive fan of basketball, so when I'm not writing late into the night, I take relaxation time after my workout, shower, and dinner to rest while watching my favorite sport on television as a way to destress and wind down.

Matt Frazier, Marathoner and Ultrarunner

MORNING

Morning routine: I have a cup of coffee within an hour of waking up; I typically don't have anything else until 11:00 a.m. or so, unless I'm trying to build muscle and gain weight. Sometimes I do a forty-minute yoga and meditation routine, but not always.

Breakfast: A twenty-four-ounce smoothie with frozen berries, cherries, mangoes, bananas, walnuts, and flaxseeds.

AFTERNOON

Lunch: Big salad with a cup of chickpeas. I usually make my salad with one part green leaf lettuce and one part cruciferous or bitter greens such as baby kale, plus red cabbage, carrots, and celery and cashew ranch dressing, tahini garlic dressing, or oil and vinegar. (If I have leftovers available from the previous night's dinner, I usually eat those instead of a salad and then eat a salad with dinner.)

Snack: Bananas or oranges, trail mix, hummus with cabbage or broccoli.

Pre-workout fuel: One or two Medjool dates, or eight ounces of fruit juice mixed with eight ounces of water, or one rice cake.

Workout: If I'm not training for anything in particular but want to maintain or improve general fitness, I alternate days between workouts A and B:

—Workout A: Two to three four-minute hill repeats with five-minute rest intervals and five-minute warmup and cooldown.

—Workout B: Six to eight one-minute "sprint" repeats with two-minute rest intervals and five-minute warmup and cooldown.

After each A or B workout day, I do an easy run or walk for thirty minutes.

For strength and more cardio, I do a simple, 20-minute kettlebell routine of 100 one-armed swings (in sets of 10) and 10 Turkish get-ups, alternating sides.

Post-workout replenishment: Rice cake and an eight-ounce glass of tart cherry juice immediately following my workout. Then a larger meal an hour or two later.

EVENING

Dinner: Most often some variation of "a grain, a green, and a bean." It can take the form of chickpea-pasta stew with kale; BBQ tempeh tacos with cabbage; tofu stir-fry with bok choy and brown rice; pasta with red sauce, chickpeas, and broccoli; and many other variations.

Dessert: None, unless you count a beer or glass of wine after dinner. Before bed, I take supplements (Complement and turmeric).

Recovery routine: Lots of good sleep due to blackout curtains, no screens in bed, and no food or alcohol near bedtime. I do active recovery only during heavy training periods. When I do, it's twenty minutes of foam rolling and mobility exercises in front of the TV.

Korin Sutton, Nineteen-Time Champion Bodybuilder

MORNING

Breakfast: Vegan Omelet (see recipe on page 275).

Morning routine: Yoga once or twice a week.

AFTERNOON

Lunch: Protein shake with Clean Machine brand Clean Green Protein and pea protein.

Snack: Mango, strawberries, avocados, dates, and peanut butter.

Pre-workout fuel: Coffee and Clean Machine brand Clean BCAA, Cell Block 80, and Ahiflower Oil; maca powder, L-arginine, L-citrulline, American ginseng, L-tryptophan, and tribulus.

Workout: High-intensity interval training (HIIT) and hypertrophy training five times per week doing a split routine—for example, chest and triceps, legs, push or pull days.

Post-workout replenishment: Tofu scramble made with tofu, bell peppers, kale, mushrooms, onions, garlic, turmeric, black salt, and liquid aminos.

EVENING

Dinner: Soup with seitan, vegetables, nutritional yeast, and vegetable broth.

Dessert: Strawberry ice cream made with frozen strawberries, almond milk, stevia, and vegan cream cheese. (Just once in a while.)

Recovery routine: Yoga twice per week, fifteen to thirty minutes of meditation every day, ten minutes of stretching four to five days per week, and ten to thirty minutes of walking three to four times per week.

James Wilks, Mixed Martial Arts Champion

MORNING

Breakfast and Pre-workout fuel: Overnight oats.

Workout: Weight training, martial arts, swimming, or sprint repeats.

Post-workout replenishment: Green smoothie or homemade protein bar.

AFTERNOON

Lunch: Hummus and vegetables on whole wheat pita or leftovers from dinner the night before.

EVENING

Dinner: Lentil pasta with vegetables, lentil cottage pie, or vegetable lasagna.

Recovery routine: Myofascial release on a foam roller or lacrosse ball.

Dotsie Bausch,
Olympic Silver Medal–Winning Track Cyclist

MORNING

Breakfast: Seven-grain sprouted toast with smashed avocado, chili flakes, and a sprinkle of salt and lemon juice.

AFTERNOON

Lunch: A big salad made with chopped kale, creamy dairy-free dressing (such as Annie's Goddess Dressing), a handful of roasted or plain chickpeas, shredded carrots, and diced onions.

Snacks: Raw veggies (carrots, jicama, celery, cucumber, mushrooms, peppers, etc.) and hummus or tahini and edamame with sea salt.

Pre-workout fuel: Water and half of my "epic" smoothie with oat milk, ice, loads of blueberries and raspberries, one banana, a scoop of almond butter, cacao nibs, and chia seeds. (The other half is my primary post-workout meal.)

Workout: One of the following, in no particular order, depending on my mood: lifting in my garage gym, spin class, hot yoga, power walk with the dogs, or an intense mountain bike ride with my very fast hubby :-).

Post-workout replenishment: The other half of my epic smoothie.

EVENING

Dinner: Quick curry made by simmering veggies (broccoli, bell peppers, onion, carrots, etc.) and chickpeas, tofu, or tempeh in a store-bought curry sauce (try Maya Kaimal brand) and tossing in spinach at the end. Served over black or brown rice.

Dessert: Pinot noir with dark chocolate.

Kätlin Kukk, Estonian National Champion Cyclist

MORNING

Breakfast: Raw buckwheat with molasses, nuts, and fruit, or a protein smoothie.

Pre-workout fuel: Banana and dates.

Workout: Three-hour endurance ride or three-hour gym session, sprint session, or technical abilities session.

Post-workout replenishment: Protein smoothie.

AFTERNOON

Lunch: Veggies (boiled or raw), hummus, mixed legumes with a lot of different spices.

Snacks: Frozen or fresh fruit, berries, or dates.

EVENING

Dinner: Veggie soup (I love vegan Tom Kha and beetroot soup).

Dessert: I usually don't have dessert, but if I want to, I will make chocolate pudding with avocados and dates or "nice" cream.

Recovery routine: Massage, stretching, yoga, swimming, sauna, napping, walking in fresh air.

John Joseph, Ironman Triathlete

MORNING

Water upon waking, plus E3Live blue-green algae supplement.

Breakfast: On days when a run follows, it's an acai bowl with organic fruit and berries, hempseeds, and nut butter. If a bike ride follows, it's oatmeal, berries, and nuts.

Workout 1: One-hour run.

Post-workout replenishment: Organic plant-based protein powder with some organic greens to boost the alkalinity, plus organic berries in a recovery shake, along with an organic iron supplement and an omega 3-6-9 supplement for essential fats.

Snack: Raw chia seed pudding with coconut cream and hempseeds, or something like avocado toast with nutritional yeast, organic raw food snack bars, or even a raw salad with avocado or fruit.

AFTERNOON

Lunch: Protein power bowl with brown rice, greens, avocado, BBQ tempeh, nutritional yeast, coconut aminos, and soaked almonds.

Pre-workout fuel: Two bananas, a tube of nut butter, and one or two organic raw food bars.

Workout 2: Three- to four-hour bike ride, using sports gels for additional fuel along with water.

Post-workout replenishment: Cooldown followed by meditation, bringing the heart rate down, and a shower; dinner within an hour of finishing on the bike.

EVENING

Dinner: Big bowl of organic rice and organic red lentils with spices and a bunch of vegetables, or a burrito, an organic plant-based pizza, or BBQ tofu or a lentil chili with homemade cornbread and steamed broccoli.

Dessert: Raw organic mousse with avocado, coconut, and cacao.

Recovery routine: Myofascial release, trigger point therapy, cooldown stretching, foam rolling, and using a rebounder to flush the lymphatic fluid through my system. Additional recovery techniques include hot tub to cold shower routine, Epsom salts, infrared sauna, compression boots, and working with trainers to help recover from hours of training.

Darcy Gaechter, World Record–Holding Kayaker

MORNING

Warm-up: I try to do a routine of sit-ups, push-ups, and pull-ups first thing every morning. This is not a hard-core workout, more like maintenance. I do 10 pull-ups, 200 sit-ups (I mix up the variety every day), and usually three sets of 20 push-ups. I find if I don't do it right when I wake up, I won't do it.

Breakfast: Granola with banana, berries, and hemp milk.

Pre-workout fuel: Breakfast (granola with fruit and hemp milk) or a snack bar.

Workout: Being self-employed, I feel like I always have an overwhelming amount of work to do, but it's also super important for me to get out every single day. I usually go kayaking. Class V kayaking is always a good workout, so I don't have to plan too much on training objectives if I'm paddling a hard river! But if I'm paddling on an easier river, I'll make sure to catch tons of eddies and work on my technique and strength throughout the day. Kayaking workouts during the week are usually just one or two hours long; on full days out they can be six to eight hours. If I can't kayak, I mountain bike or trail run.

Post-workout replenishment: I'm always starving after a big workout, and a big bowl of beans and rice usually makes me feel good. If I don't have time to cook, I'll eat a Crunchy Peanut Butter Clif Builder's Protein Bar or a big handful of nuts or dried fruit.

AFTERNOON

Lunch: Veggie burger—love the fake meat trend and how successful they've been in getting their products into fast-food chains, but I still prefer the grain- and bean-based veggie burgers.

Snacks: Dried figs, sunflower seeds, apples.

EVENING

Dinner: Burrito bowl with lightly fried tofu, Bragg Liquid Aminos, crushed red pepper flakes, pinto beans, brown rice, avocado, tomato, onion, bell pepper, and blue corn tortilla chips.

Recovery routine: I'm pretty bad about all of this . . . I continually try to work a stretching routine into my daily schedule, but so far, I've failed to make it a habit!

David Rother, Professional Triathlete

MORNING

Workout 1: Light 10K run or swimming, maybe followed by a stability workout.

Breakfast: Overnight oats with sprouted cereals and fresh fruits. Lots of it!

Workout 2: If it's a "heavy" training day, I'll also bike ride, two to four hours, at different intensities.

AFTERNOON

Lunch: Easily digestible carbs like quinoa or rice with fried vegetables.

Power nap: 20 to 40 minutes.

Snack: Double Espresso with a little sweetness like banana bread

Workout 3: Running. Either a long run (up to 35K) or a speed or interval session.

Post-workout replenishment: A shake with crushed ice, water, a little bit of almond milk, and vegan protein powder.

EVENING

Dinner: Mixed baked vegetables with lots of legumes, plus a large salad and tofu, topped with seeds.

Snack: Handful of nuts and a bit of dark (80%) chocolate.

Dessert: On a really hard day: Vegan Ben and Jerry's on the couch!;)

Recovery routine: One hour of physical therapy and stretching. On a cold day, 30 to 45 minutes of sauna.

Christine Vardaros, Professional Cyclist

MORNING

Breakfast: Chopped Granny Smith apple and banana, ¼–2 cups oats (depending on training day), 1 tablespoon flaxseeds, 1 tablespoon chia seeds, lukewarm water.

Snack: Seasonal fruit.

Pre-workout fuel: PB&J or oatmeal with spoonful coconut oil.

Workout: Anywhere from 2 to 6 hours training on the bike.

Nutrition during workout: Hammer bars or gels or drinks or dried figs, mangos.

Post-workout replenishment: PB&J or oatmeal.

AFTERNOON

Lunch: Veggie or lentil soup with hummus and/or avocado on corn cakes.

EVENING

Dinner: Vegetable stir-fry or curry with black rice.

Dessert: "Nice" cream: 2 frozen bananas, handful frozen cherries, 1 tablespoon lemon juice. Blend well, then add some crushed walnuts and dark chocolate chips.

Recovery routine: Lying on the floor, legs in the air against the wall, for ten to twenty minutes.

Julia Murray, Former Olympic Skier and Plant-Based Nutritionist

MORNING

Pre-morning workout fuel: Water and medicinal mushrooms (Stay Wyld Cordyceps and Lion's Mane and Turkey Tail).

Workout: 5-minute yoga and 10-minute circuit and 30- to 45-minute run

Post-workout replenishment: Overnight oats (oats, buckwheat, raisins, cinnamon, chia or hemp or ground flaxseeds, oat milk), a dollop of coconut yogurt, berries, and banana. Complement brand supplements.

AFTERNOON

Lunch: I'm usually still full from my late breakfast! Maybe some hummus and veggies, or apple and dates.

Snacks: Green Smoothie (greens to the brim, 1 to 2 frozen bananas, cup of berries, turmeric and ginger root, pinch of pepper, medicinal mushroom blend, Complement Protein powder.

Pre-afternoon workout fuel: Smoothie!

Afternoon workout: It varies between a one- to two-hour mountain bike ride, another run, paddleboard, or in the winter, ski touring.

Post-workout replenishment: snack bites made with oats and dates, or leftover smoothie.

EVENING

Dinner: Big salad (romaine, spinach, tomato, avocado, green onions, sunflower seeds, plus my pickle dressing). Then it varies—brown rice pasta or quinoa noodles with veggies and tempeh, a roasted veggie and tofu bowl with miso-tahini dressing, a loaded baked potato, veggie curry, or veggie burgers.

Dessert: vegan cookie, dark chocolate, banana "ice cream," an apple, or some frozen grapes.

Recovery routine: Stretching.

Jehina Malik, IFBB Professional Bodybuilder

MORNING

Breakfast: Rolled oats with 1½ tablespoons crunchy peanut butter.

AFTERNOON

Lunch: Two Gardein brand vegan chick'n cutlets and brown rice.

Snack: Fruit bowl and cashews.

EVENING

Pre-workout fuel: Handful of cashews.

Workout: One hour of weight training, three to four sets of fifteen to twenty reps (leg days are closer to one hour and thirty minutes).

Post-workout replenishment: Handful of cashews, followed by dinner.

Dinner: Large chickpea salad with romaine lettuce, arugula, parsley, onions, different-colored peppers, cucumbers, and spinach.

Dessert: None usually, but a treat would be vegan Ben and Jerry's ice cream in a cone.

Recovery routine: Stretching in the sauna or in the hot tub.

Vanessa Espinoza, Professional Powerlifter, Champion Boxer

MORNING

Breakfast: Quinoa with peanut butter, banana, chia seeds, hemp-seeds, and cinnamon.

Snack: Peanut butter and jelly sandwich, fruit, or a fruit smoothie.

Pre-workout fuel: A cup of mushroom coffee or TRU Supplements pre-workout drink.

Workout 1: I strength train for one hour and thirty minutes. I focus on one body part a day. I train with many rep ranges; some days it's very heavy for 1 to 5 reps, other days it's 10 to 20 reps, and other days it's 25-plus reps. I change up my routine often, but my volume is always high. During my workout I sip on BCAAs (branched-chain amino acids).

Post-workout replenishment (lunch): Protein shake.

Snack: Roasted peas.

EVENING

Dinner: Tofu or tempeh, roasted or steamed vegetables, wild rice with coconut aminos.

Dessert: Homemade protein brownies or protein cookies.

Workout 2: Some type of sprint workout. For example: ten 100-meter, ten 50-meter, ten 20-meter, and ten 10-meter sprints, or boxing/hitting the heavy bag.

Post-workout replenishment: Protein drink.

Recovery routine: Ice and stretching.

Robbie Balenger, Ultrarunner

MORNING

Pre-workout fuel: Water. I tend to eat dinner late in the evening, so I use that fuel to carry me through the first one and a half hours of my run.

Workout: Ten- to twenty-mile run.

Mid-workout replenishment: A whole-food bar such as Crafted Energy.

Post-workout replenishment: Muesli with fruit and berries and oat or cashew milk. And more water.

AFTERNOON

Lunch: Often a black bean and potato burrito with sautéed veggies, wrapped with fresh greens and topped with Valentina hot sauce—never forget the Valentina . . .

Snacks: I'm not much of a snacker, but sometimes nuts such as cashews, almonds, and pecans.

EVENING

Dinner: I'm a big fan of Asian noodle bowls with seared tofu, as well as rice and beans with fresh and cooked veggies.

Dessert: NadaMoo! vegan ice cream.

Nick Squires, International Champion Powerlifter

MORNING

Breakfast: Pancakes and Beyond Sausage with bananas and black coffee.

AFTERNOON

Lunch: Tofu or seitan with ancient grains and steamed broccoli or sautéed brussels sprouts.

Snacks: Protein cookie or bar (Munk Pack or Clif Builder's Protein Bar); cucumbers and hummus.

Pre-workout fuel: Protein bar or protein cookie.

Workout: Two to three hours of lifting centered on squat, bench, or deadlift and then accessories.

EVENING

Post-workout replenishment/dinner: Burger time! Of course I love Beyond Burgers, but I'm really into Trader Joe's Turkeyless Protein Patties right now too. If it's not burgers, it will be pasta with "meatballs" and a spinach salad.

Dessert: I'm not usually a dessert guy, but I've been known to take down a pint or two of vegan Ben and Jerry's ice cream, especially during bulking months.

Recovery routine: Hot baths, easy bike rides.

Sophie Mullins, British 100K Ultramarathon Champion

MORNING

Breakfast: Oats, chia seeds, turmeric, blueberries, and homemade oat or almond milk.

Pre-workout fuel: Apple and two small cookies (made from the left-over plant milk pulp and fruit and ginger).

Workout 1: Run: 5K easy warm-up, 12K surge run (twelve reps of one minute fast, four minutes focused effort (no recovery), easy cooldown.

AFTERNOON

Post-workout replenishment/lunch: Brown rice, beans, spring onions, butternut squash, broccoli, carrot, soy sauce.

Snack: Fruit such as a plum or nectarine.

Workout 2: A 5K to 10K recovery run; twenty minutes of body-weight exercise and foam rolling.

EVENING

Dinner: Lentils, leeks, parsnips, carrots, broccoli, homemade hummus, avocado, pine nuts.

Snack: If I'm hungry I'll have some air-popped popcorn or granola with homemade plant milk.

Recovery routine: Foam rolling.

Rip Esselstyn, Former Professional Triathlete, Swimming World Record Holder

MORNING

Workout 1: One-hour morning swim. I always have a better day when I can get a nice workout in in the morning. If I don't, I don't feel as grounded. I feel a little lethargic; I don't feel as sharp mentally; and I don't feel as lean and mean and ready to tackle the day.

Post-workout replenishment/breakfast: Rip's Big Bowl (recipe on page 268).

AFTERNOON

Lunch: Red lentil dal with onions, garlic, scallions, herbs, and spices such as turmeric over pearl barley with half an avocado, arugula, and spinach.

Workout 2: One hour of mountain biking.

EVENING

Workout 3: Some form of body-weight exercise at home, such as push-ups, pull-ups, planks, and sit-ups.

Post-workout replenishment/dinner: Rice and bean extravaganza, which includes brown rice, black beans, bell peppers, sliced tomatoes, water chestnuts, corn, salsa, mangoes, low-sodium tamari, and avocado.

Recovery routine: Relaxing, spending time with family.

Sonya Looney, World Champion Mountain Biker

MORNING

Breakfast: Steel-cut oats with hemp hearts, ground flaxseed, maple syrup, and berries.

Pre-workout fuel: Two pieces of sprouted whole-grain bread with almond butter or peanut butter.

Workout: My workouts are usually two- to three-hour mountain bike rides on weekdays and, if time allows (my time is a little different now that I'm a new mom), longer on weekends.

AFTERNOON

Post-workout replenishment/lunch: Instead of a recovery drink I have a meal, usually a bowl with whole grains, veggies, and legumes or leftovers from dinner the night before.

Snack: Fruit—I love apples and oranges. Sometimes I'll have avocado toast or a mini version of a meal.

EVENING

Dinner: Burritos, burrito bowls, quinoa/broccoli wraps, pasta dishes with veggies, homemade cashew-based sauce, and a legume.

Dessert: Chocolate bar or cookies I make at home.

Recovery routine: I like using compression boots, light yoga or foam rolling, and breathing and visualization for recovery. To be honest, I should spend more time on recovery, but it's really hard as a mom, pro athlete, and business owner!

Brendan Brazier, Ultramarathoner

MORNING

Workout 1: Thirty-minute run.

Breakfast: Banana-ginger-pear cereal with almond milk.

Morning snack: Energy bar.

AFTERNOON

Lunch: Spicy black-eyed pea quinoa pizza.

Afternoon snack: Smoothie.

Pre-workout fuel: Vega pre-workout energy drink.

Workout 2: One hour of weight training or one hour of cycling.

Post-workout replenishment: Vega recovery shake.

EVENING

Dinner: Cucumber pesto salad with tomato basil dressing.

Dessert: Crunchy cinnamon plantain strips.

Recovery routine: Foam rolling, ice baths, and stretching.

Natalie Matthews, IFBB Professional Bikini Competitor

MORNING

Breakfast: Overnight oats or granola with fruit.

Morning supplements: Vegan multivitamin (contains B_{12}, D_3, and

omegas), plus creatine monohydrate for strength and performance.

Pre-workout fuel: Coffee or a protein "Frappuccino" made with coffee,
a scoop of protein powder, and pea milk.

Workout 1: Sixty- to ninety-minute weight-training workout, focusing
on training one or two muscle groups such as back and shoulders.

Post-workout replenishment: Edamame or garbanzo beans or vegan
protein bar.

AFTERNOON

Lunch: Macro bowl with grilled tofu, greens, potato hash, sauerkraut,
tomatoes, sprouts, and Edamame-Spinach Hummus (recipe on
page 327).

Snack: Mushroom chips (store-bought; I get the Snaklins brand).

Pre-workout fuel: Fruit or a caffeinated energy drink, if needed.

Workout 2: Cardio workout, such as thirty to sixty minutes on the
treadmill, surfing, a functional fitness class, or hiking outside for
some fresh air.

EVENING

Dinner: A bowl of Sloppy Vegan Chili (recipe on page 305) topped
with a drizzle of vegan high-protein queso, avocado, and two small
corn tortillas; or homemade seitan with broccoli and queso.

Dessert: Blueberries and a piece of dark chocolate.

Recovery routine: Take nighttime supplements: ginger and turmeric
complex for recovery and ashwagandha and magnesium for sleep
and muscle recovery.

Laura Kline, World Champion Duathlete

MORNING

Pre-workout fuel: Banana and plenty of water.

Workout 1: Fifteen minutes of glute and hip activation exercises
before heading out for a ten-mile run with speed intervals on the
track.

Post-workout replenishment: Unived Elite Recovery drink (I enjoy it while I cool down with the foam roller).

Breakfast: I'll have muesli in the warmer months and oatmeal in the colder months. I start with rolled oats and add in all kinds of nutrient-dense toppings such as coconut shreds, dried and/or fresh fruits, nuts or nut butter, chia, flaxseeds or hempseeds, and dairy-free milk or hot water. It's basically a big hearty bowl with everything I need to refuel after my morning workout. I also like this breakfast because it is easy to find a healthy muesli or oatmeal while traveling, or the ingredients to make your own!

AFTERNOON

Lunch: I typically have a green and grain bowl. I'll start with a heaping base of romaine, spinach, or kale, then add a grain such as quinoa, rice, or farro. I'll top that with whatever veggies I have on hand, such as tomato, broccoli, cucumber, or beets. I'm a big fan of tempeh, so I'll usually add strips of sautéed tempeh, but I'll also sometimes use beans. Next is half an avocado—need those healthy fats! I'll top everything with a homemade tahini dressing or a healthy vinaigrette.

Pre-workout fuel: In the late afternoon I will have an apple with nut butter to fuel me for my afternoon workout.

Workout 2: Sixty minutes on the bike trainer with a few hard intervals mixed in followed by a sixty-minute strength and mobility routine at the gym.

Post-workout nourishment: If it's a light workout I'll have another piece of fruit along with a recovery drink—most often I'll have a kiwifruit or some watermelon, depending on the season. If my second workout is a long or intense one, I'll make a smoothie. This is my go-to: ¼ cup beet juice, ½ cup tart cherry juice, splash of apple cider vinegar, ½ tablespoon of hemp hearts, 1 scoop of chocolate protein powder with greens, 1 frozen banana, ½ cup frozen blueberries.

EVENING

Dinner: Once I've showered and completed my recovery protocol, it's time for a small dinner. I like to have a warm, hearty bowl like my coconut, quinoa, and sweet potato curry.

Dessert: Yes, I do sometimes enjoy a sweet treat when I'm in peak training. In the summer months, I'll make my own ice cream using coconut milk and dates and top that with some fresh fruit. Another favorite I like to keep on hand are the Healthy Fudge Bars I like to make (recipe on page 317).

Recovery routine: After my first workout, I spend time on the foam roller and follow a hip routine (Myrtl) to keep everything loose. After my second workout, I spend another half hour using rolling tools for deeper muscle recovery work, then spend fifteen to thirty minutes in compression boots.

Yassine Diboun, Record-Setting Ultrarunner

MORNING

Pre-workout fuel: Coffee, banana.

Workout 1: I do a forty-five-minute functional fitness workout: lunge variations, push-ups, squat variations, lots of core work, burpees.

Post-workout replenishment: Granola, banana, coconut milk yogurt, berries.

Supplement routine: I take a Complement B_{12}, D_3, EPA, DHA, calcium, and magnesium drink and sometimes a multivitamin or Immu-Core. Sometimes during heavy training, I take an amino acids supplement, omega supplement, and occasionally BeetElite before intense workouts. I usually just rely on whole foods, though.

AFTERNOON

Lunch: Rice and beans bowl that includes organic tempeh, onions, broccoli, shiitake mushrooms, zucchini, olive oil, and Swiss chard with Frank's RedHot sauce.

Workout 2: Afternoon run for an hour or two, followed by some sort of cross-training or mobility work.

Post-workout replenishment: Granola, banana, coconut milk yogurt, berries.

Snacks: Corn chips and Yumm! Sauce, grapefruit. I also drink a lot of the Circulatory Blend Tea from Brew Dr. In the summer, I brew it and chill it in the fridge to make iced tea. I add vanilla stevia to it. It's spicy and sweet!

EVENING

Dinner: Brown rice pasta with roasted garlic marinara sauce and vegetables such as peppers, onions, mushrooms, and broccoli and nutritional yeast.

Meagan Duhamel, Olympic Gold Medal–Winning Figure Skater

Note: After winning the gold medal in the 2018 Olympics, Meagan retired and started a family. This is what her routine was like for a decade as an elite world-class athlete.

MORNING

Before breakfast: Upon waking, I walked my dogs and did a short yoga movement session. I needed this to get my back mobile; otherwise it would be stuck all day long.

Pre-workout fuel: Overnight oats with blueberries.

Workout 1: Two hours on the ice with my pairs skating partner, Eric Radford. We worked on technical elements, choreography, and basic skating skills.

Post-workout replenishment: In between my two hours of morning training, I had a fifteen-minute break. I would usually have a green smoothie during this time. My favorite was spinach, bananas, mango, chia seeds, and omega fatty acid oils.

AFTERNOON

Lunch: Something simple, like crackers and hummus, trail mix, and a homemade muffin or bar.

Workout 2: My workouts changed every day. On Mondays and Wednesdays, I had one hour of strength and conditioning. Tuesdays, one hour of Pilates; Thursdays, one hour of eccentrics; and Fridays, thirty minutes of cardio.

Post-workout replenishment: Pineapples with hempseeds.

EVENING

Dinner: My favorite dinner options were lasagna with spinach and tofu ricotta cheese, shepherd's pie with sweet potatoes and lentils, and a quinoa casserole.

Recovery routine: In the afternoon, massage, osteopathic work, acupuncture, or physical therapy with my sports therapist. In the evening, a warm bath with Epsom salts.

Mary Schneider, Marathoner

MORNING

Breakfast: One cup of coffee with oat milk creamer. Oatmeal: oats, one banana, 1 tablespoon nut butter, 1 tablespoon hemp hearts, ¼ cup blueberries.

Pre-workout fuel: Breakfast, as just described.

Workout: One- to two-hour run.

Post-workout replenishment: Large Ultimate Green Smoothie for recovery (see page 264).

AFTERNOON

Lunch: Large salad, bowl, or soup. For a bowl, I have a carbohydrate-heavy source as the base, such as quinoa, millet, rice, potatoes, or some combination, and then I add a combination of greens and other vegetables, tossing it with a sauce.

EVENING

Dinner: Spaghetti Squash with Tempeh Bolognese Sauce (recipe on page 303)—I eat that one all the time, and I sometimes sub in gluten-free pasta. Or I could make a deconstructed burrito bowl, as that is another favorite—rice, beans, and sautéed veggies with avocado and salsa. I do the same thing with a loaded sweet potato.

Dessert: None (occasionally dark chocolate, but I go months without dessert, as I don't have much of a sweet tooth).

Recovery routine: My recovery routine is my Ultimate Green "recovery" Smoothie, which contains bananas, mixed berries, spinach or kale, hemp hearts, flaxseed meal, and chia seeds. I don't use any protein powder.

Andreas Vojta, Olympic Runner

MORNING

Workout 1 (fasted): For easy runs, I often train before breakfast if I don't feel really hungry. I just think it's a great energizer to wake up and train, and it feels good to start the day with breakfast after completing my workout.

Training times vary from 7:30 to 11:00 a.m., depending on when I wake up and how much sleep I need (I don't use an alarm; I just wake up naturally when my body is ready). I also try to get the important non-running-related stuff done in the morning, as I feel more concentrated and focused then.

Post-workout replenishment: I usually go for a quick snack, like a banana, an apple, or a slice of bread with a spread, such as peanut butter.

Breakfast: I keep my breakfast basically the same every morning. Therefore, it's kind of my ledger at the start of the day. The base of my breakfast is 100 grams of oats and 10 grams of ground flaxseed, soaked in soy milk overnight. In the morning, I top it up with berries, cocoa nibs, and cinnamon. A delicious breakfast that I look forward to every morning!

Workout 2 (Option A): I usually have about two additional strength sessions every week, which I execute after my easy morning run. On days I do not have a strength training session, I do a speed workout, or fast session.

Snack: Here, I also go with an easily prepared food, such as bread with peanut butter or jam or some cereal. These foods are not really healthy, but they get you some calories and carbs quickly and easily and are therefore perfect when you get a little hungry as an athlete.

AFTERNOON

Fast session: If I have an intense session ahead, in the morning I
  usually do a little thirty-minute warm-up with some strides and
  mobility exercises to get ready for the hard runs that I usually do
  in the afternoon.

Workout 2 (Option B): When there's an intense training session ahead,
  I try to eat three to four hours before my workout, which I usually
  do around 4:00 p.m. I try to relax a little bit after my lunch or even
  have a little power nap. That also gives me time to mentally focus
  on the workout ahead. Then I'm ready to go, and I leave my house
  about an hour before the start of the training to get to the track
  with public transport.

Post-workout replenishment: I try to get my nutrients in as quickly as
  possible, via either a meal or a chocolate shake on my way home
  from the track.

Lunch: I don't eat a similar dish every time but rather use what's
  available at the moment. But there's a guideline for which foods
  I always try to combine, which are grains, legumes, veggies, and
  some nuts and seeds. Grains fuel your carbohydrate storage, and
  combined with protein-rich legumes, they have a great amino acid
  profile. Vegetables add many important micronutrients, and nuts
  are a great source of unsaturated fat and protein.

EVENING

Dinner: This is pretty much the same as lunch, combining my main
  food groups, as just mentioned. I like to cook bigger portions so I
  have some food left and can just heat it up for dinner. This is important if I have an intense session in the afternoon and need to
  get my dinner in as fast as possible to ensure an optimal recovery.

Dessert: I'll be honest, I'm a dessert guy and like to try new stuff as
  often as possible. Whether it's a homemade dessert or a chocolate
  bar from the store, my body craves some sweet stuff after the
  main meal. I often just eat sweet cereal as a dessert in the evening.
  Many people think professional athletes are "not allowed" to eat

any dessert, but if you do it to the right extent, I don't think it impacts your performance. I would struggle mentally to completely kick sweet desserts out of my diet.

Recovery routine: When I'm back home from an intense session, I try to get into recovery mode as soon as possible. That means a lot of lying down and sleeping. I also go through the workout again in my head and try to recreate how it felt, what was good and what I should do better next time.

11

RECIPES

You've spent an entire book reading about how beneficial and health-promoting plants can be, and now you get to enjoy the fact that whole-plant-based meals are also incredibly delicious. Just as there's no shortage of plant foods to choose from when assembling your meals, there's no limit to how they can be paired with herbs, spices, and condiments. Whether it's to fuel your workouts or to enjoy as a relaxing meal with friends and family, you'll find that meals made with whole plants have the unique ability to feed both body and spirit.

This chapter is dedicated to some of our favorite recipes, as well as those of the athletes we've heard from throughout the book. These are the meals that they reach for again and again, and they range from hearty and nourishing to downright decadent. There are plenty of options to choose from as you begin assembling your new plant-based meal plans, so choose what sounds tastiest to you and feel free to customize to suit your preferences. (All of these recipes have ingredients that can be swapped out, especially the fruits and vegetables as the seasons change.) Go ahead—get inspired, get hungry, and fuel up.

BREAKFAST

Ultimate Green Smoothie

Contributed by **Mary Schneider**, *marathoner*
From her book Green Body Cookbook

This is my "kitchen sink" go-to smoothie for after the hardest of workouts to make sure I have the biggest anti-inflammatory kick start on recovery. A smoothie with the right combination of green leafy vegetables and fruits packed with vitamins, minerals, and antioxidants is the single best way to reduce inflammation in your body. And by replacing your glycogen stores with all of the fruit in the smoothie, you allow your body to recover faster. Each ingredient in this smoothie has a specific nutritional purpose, and they all come together for a delicious, dessert-like drink that you will never get tired of!

Serves 2

3 frozen bananas
1 cup frozen blueberries
1 cup frozen pineapple
1 cup frozen strawberries
2 large kale leaves, stems removed
1 large handful of spinach
2 cups water or nondairy milk of choice (use nondairy milk for a more calorie-dense option)
1 tablespoon hemp hearts
1 tablespoon flaxseed meal
½ teaspoon ground ginger (or thumb-sized piece of peeled fresh ginger)
¼ teaspoon ground turmeric (or thumb-sized piece of peeled fresh turmeric root)
Pinch of freshly ground black pepper

Add all ingredients to a high-speed blender and blend on high for 1 minute or until completely smooth.

Nutritional Totals per Serving:

Calories: 387	Fat: 7.7 g
Protein: 7.5 g	Fiber: 14.4 g
Carbohydrates: 80.7 g	

High-Energy Fruit Smoothie with Greens

Contributed by **Robert Cheeke**, *bodybuilder*

This is a supersized smoothie that's perfect for breakfast, especially if you're making it pre-workout and finishing it off post-workout. It delivers a potent combination of high-energy complex carbohydrates from fruit and leafy greens to fuel your training, along with antioxidants to help reduce inflammation afterward. This also makes a great snack during the day, especially when you're looking for something quick. Feel free to add even more fruits and greens—the goal is to get in the most nutrient-rich foods.

Serves 1

1 cup coconut water

1 ripe banana, plus 1 additional, if desired

1 cup frozen blueberries

1 cup frozen mangoes

1 cup frozen raspberries

1 cup leafy greens such as spinach

1 cup kale

½ cup ice, plus more, if desired

In a high-speed blender, combine the ingredients with 1 additional cup of water and blend until smooth. To make a creamier smoothie, add a second banana or more ice. To thin the consistency, add more water until the desired consistency is reached.

Nutritional Totals per Serving:

Calories: 564	Fat: 5.2 g
Protein: 8.5 g	Fiber: 25.2 g
Carbohydrates: 137.7 g	

Chia Seed Blueberry Maple Pudding

Contributed by **Brendan Brazier,** *ultramarathoner*

From his book Thrive Energy Cookbook

Easily digestible and packed with antioxidants, this energizing pudding is a beautiful start to any morning. It's also a great post-workout breakfast option. You can use frozen blueberries in a pinch, but fresh is preferred.

Serves 2

- 1 cup unsweetened almond milk
- 1 tablespoon maple syrup
- ½ teaspoon latte spice mix
- ¼ cup chia seeds
- 1 cup fresh blueberries, plus a few more for garnish
- 1 small handful slivered almonds

In a medium bowl or jar, combine the almond milk, maple syrup, latte spice mix, and chia seeds. Let the mixture sit for fifteen minutes, stirring once or twice. Garnish with fresh blueberries. Enjoy now or store in a lidded container in the fridge for up to two days.

Nutritional Totals per Serving:

Calories: 206	Fat: 9.4 g
Protein: 5.4 g	Fiber: 9.8 g
Carbohydrates: 28.2 g	

Farro Sweet Rice Bowl

Contributed by **Vanessa Espinoza,** *powerlifter*

I love farro because it is very nutrient dense, contains a ton of antioxidants, and is high in protein and fiber. It also has a slightly nutty flavor, which pairs well with a sweeter flavor profile. You could enjoy this rice pudding-like bowl for breakfast, a snack, or even dessert.

Serves 1

- 1 cup freshly cooked farro
- 1 cup unsweetened almond milk

1 tablespoon raisins

1 teaspoon ground cinnamon

When the farro has finished cooking (just follow the directions on the package), add the almond milk, raisins, and cinnamon. It's best to chill the mixture overnight before enjoying.

> Nutritional Totals per Serving:
> Calories: 250   Fat: 3 g
> Protein: 7 g   Fiber: 7 g
> Carbohydrates: 52 g

Finger-Lickin' Friggin' Good French Toast

Contributed by **John Joseph**, *triathlete*

I love the smell of French toast in the morning. The cinnamon and all the other good sh*t. What you won't find with this recipe are chicken periods (eggs), artery-clogging milk, or butter. This joint is 100 percent plant-based and f*cking delicious. There's also some protein, as we used silken tofu in the batter. So get down with this, but you still gotta work out like a beast. *One tip:* Use a very thick, sturdy bread or your joints will fall apart. Make the slices about ¾ inch thick. For a killer breakfast, you have my permission to serve this with some Field Roast brand morning sausages and some coconut yogurt and fruit.

Serves 2 hungry mofos

1½ cups silken tofu

½ cup full-fat coconut milk

½ cup almond milk

1 tablespoon millet flour

1 tablespoon ground flaxseed

¼ cup cornstarch

1 tablespoon pure maple syrup, plus more for serving

1 tablespoon nutritional yeast

1 teaspoon vanilla extract

1 teaspoon cinnamon

¼ teaspoon nutmeg

Pinch of Himalayan salt

8 slices of bread

Coconut oil, for the pan

Vegan butter, for serving

Fresh berries, for serving

Coconut yogurt, for serving

Field Roast or other plant-based sausages, for serving

In a high-speed blender combine everything but the bread and coconut oil. Blend thoroughly until smooth—get all the lumps out 'cause lumps are for chumps.

Heat a skillet over medium-low heat and add a teaspoonful of coconut oil. Dip a slice of your bread into the batter and place it in the skillet. Let it cook to a golden brown, with crispy edges. Flip and repeat. When all is said and done, serve these with vegan butter, maple syrup, fresh berries, sweetened coconut yogurt, and sausages. You're very f*cking welcome!

> Nutritional Totals per Serving (excluding optional extras such as butter, berries, yogurt, or sausages):
>
> Calories: 737.5   Fat: 23.4 g
>
> Protein: 33.1 g   Fiber: 12.3 g
>
> Carbohydrates: 97.1 g

Rip's Big Bowl

Contributed by **Rip Esselstyn**, *swimmer and firefighter*

From his book The Engine 2 Cookbook

This has been my mainstay breakfast for more than twenty years. I never get sick of it, and no two bowls are ever quite the same, depending on which fruits are in season and the milk substitute I have on hand. Let your appetite be your guide for the size of the bowl. If you don't have any nondairy milk, use water (the fruits blend with it and give the bowl a sweet taste). Add any fresh or frozen fruit such as peaches, cherries, mangoes, blueberries, or red grapes.

Serves 1

- ¼ cup old-fashioned oats
- ¼ cup Grape-Nuts or Ezekiel brand equivalent
- ¼ cup bite-size shredded wheat
- ¼ cup Uncle Sam Cereal
- 1 tablespoon ground flaxseed
- 2 tablespoons raisins
- ½ handful of walnuts
- 1 banana, sliced
- 1 kiwifruit, sliced
- 1 grapefruit
- ¾ cup nondairy milk of choice

In a medium bowl, toss all the ingredients together except the grapefruit and milk. After cutting the grapefruit in half, use a small, sharp knife to remove the segments. Add the segments to the top of the bowl and squeeze in the juice. Top with the milk.

Nutritional Totals per Serving:
Calories: 711   Fat: 15 g
Protein: 18.2 g   Fiber: 22.9 g
Carbohydrates: 142.1 g

Buckwheat Pancakes

Contributed by **James Newbury,** *CrossFit Athlete*

Not only are these free of dairy and refined sugar, but they're also grain free because buckwheat, unlike its name suggests, is a protein-packed pseudograin.

Makes about 8 pancakes

- 1 cup buckwheat flour
- 1 cup nondairy milk

1 teaspoon baking powder

1 teaspoon apple cider vinegar

½ teaspoon vanilla extract

¼ teaspoon ground cinnamon

Coconut oil for cooking

In a large bowl, combine the flour, milk, baking powder, apple cider vinegar, vanilla, and cinnamon and whisk until smooth.

Heat a pan or griddle over medium-high heat. Add a tablespoon of coconut oil and ladle ¼ cup batter into the pan. Cook until the edges begin to brown and the batter bubbles, about 2 minutes. Flip and repeat on the second side. Continue with the remaining batter.

Nutritional Totals per Serving (2 pancakes):

Calories: 122.5   Fat: 2.7 g

Protein: 4.15 g   Fiber: 3.1 g

Carbohydrates: 22.1 g

Champ Oatmeal

Contributed by **Sonya Looney,** *mountain biker*

This is my daily breakfast recipe, which keeps me fueled until lunch. Feel free to add other berries for boosted antioxidant power (I love dried goji berries for this) or walnuts for extra omega-3s.

Serves 2

1 cup steel-cut oats (I like Bob's Red Mill)

¼ cup ground flaxseed

1 cup blueberries

2 tablespoons hemp hearts

2 tablespoons pure maple syrup

In a small pot, combine the oats with 3 cups of water. Bring to a simmer over medium heat and cook for 10 minutes, stirring occasionally, until the water is absorbed. Top with the flaxseed, blueberries, hemp hearts, and maple syrup, and enjoy.

Nutritional Totals per Serving:

Calories: 601

Protein: 18.8 g

Carbohydrates: 89.1 g

Fat: 21 g

Fiber: 20.4 g

Overnight Oats

Contributed by **James Wilks**, *mixed martial artist*

Prep this the night before a busy morning when you know you won't have time to make a hot breakfast. Experiment with different fruits, nut butters, and plant milks to keep it fresh and exciting.

Serves 1

1 medium banana, mashed with a fork

1 cup soy milk, preferably unsweetened

½ cup rolled oats

1 tablespoon ground flaxseed

2 tablespoons hempseeds

1 tablespoon peanut butter

1 cup frozen mixed berries

Combine ingredients, stir, and place in the fridge overnight. Enjoy in the morning.

Nutritional Totals per Serving:

Calories: 639

Protein: 26.8 g

Carbohydrates: 82.8 g

Fat: 26.7 g

Fiber: 16.3 g

Banana Nut Protein Granola

Contributed by **Natalie Matthews**, *bikini competitor and fitness model*

The secret ingredient in this high-protein, no-oil granola is textured vegetable protein (TVP), which lends a hearty chewiness that gets dressed up in sweet, satisfying flavor. Use it to add crunch and protein to your favorite smoothie bowls, nondairy yogurt, or fruit bowls. Just be careful not to eat the whole batch before you know what hit you!

Makes 8 ½-cup servings

- **2 cups rice or kamut puffs**
- **1½ cups TVP**
- **1 cup rolled oats**
- **½ cup walnuts**
- **½ tablespoon ground cinnamon**
- **½ teaspoon sea salt**
- **2 ripe bananas, mashed into a puree**
- **½ cup baking stevia or sweetener of choice**
- **¼ cup pure maple syrup**

Preheat the oven to 350°F. Line a baking sheet with parchment paper and set aside.

In a large mixing bowl, combine the rice puffs, TVP, oats, walnuts, cinnamon, and salt. Stir until well combined. Using a spatula, fold in the mashed bananas, stevia, and maple syrup. Mix until well combined.

Spread the granola evenly over the baking sheet. Place it on the middle rack of the oven and bake for 35 minutes or until golden brown. Stir the granola every 10 minutes.

Before you start pounding it by the handful, let the granola cool completely. This is what gives the granola its crunch!

Nutritional Totals per Serving:
Calories: 205   Fat: 5 g
Protein: 12 g   Fiber: 8 g
Carbohydrates: 28 g

Kamut Peanut Butter Bowl

Contributed by **Vanessa Espinoza,** *powerlifter*

I typically have this breakfast kamut bowl after my morning lifting session because it provides so many nutrients including protein, fiber, and good complex carbohydrates. The chia seeds in particular are a very powerful antioxidant, have a ton of fiber, and are high in omega-3s. Hempseeds also deliver fiber, omega-3s, magnesium, zinc, and iron. And cinnamon is great for fighting inflammation and regulating blood sugar while adding nice flavor.

Serves 1

½ cup cooked kamut flakes
1 banana, sliced
1 tablespoon peanut butter
1 tablespoon chia seeds
1 tablespoon hempseeds
1 teaspoon ground cinnamon

Add the cooked kamut (just follow the directions on the package) to a bowl and top with the banana slices and peanut butter. Sprinkle with the chia seeds, hempseeds, and cinnamon.

Nutritional Totals per Serving:
Calories: 384   Fat: 17 g
Protein: 20 g   Fiber: 18 g
Carbohydrates: 59 g

Robert's Bodybuilding Trail Mix

Contributed by **Robert Cheeke**, *bodybuilder*

When I was twenty-one years old (twenty years ago), I was an enthusiastic vegan bodybuilder. I had transformed from a skinny farm kid to a soon-to-be champion bodybuilder, and I made my own trail mix to help me bulk up and build plant-based muscle. I would mix and match nuts, seeds, and fruits to get concentrated sources of nutrition for breakfast or a snack without the added sugars or other fillers and additives often found in energy and protein bars. I would go to my local co-op or grocery store that had bulk bins and select an assortment, which I could change up to make sure I was getting diverse nutrients while always keeping things interesting.

If you're someone who is focusing on building muscle, and especially if smoothies aren't really your thing, this trail mix is the perfect solution to boost your daily caloric intake. You can also pour it into a bowl, add fresh fruit and nondairy milk, and eat it as a cereal.

Serves 4

1 cup store-bought or homemade vegan granola (without honey)
½ cup almonds
½ cup walnuts
½ cup raisins
½ cup dried figs
¼ cup sunflower seeds
¼ cup pumpkin seeds
Fresh fruit, optional
Nondairy milk, optional

In a large bowl, combine the granola, almonds, walnuts, raisins, figs, sunflower seeds, and pumpkin seeds. Mix well, then transfer to a resealable bag or container. Enjoy as is or add it to a bowl with fruit and milk.

Nutritional Totals per Serving (without added fruit or nondairy milk):
Calories: 515   Fat: 32.4 g
Protein: 13.9 g   Fiber: 8.8 g
Carbohydrates: 51.1 g

Simple Tofu Scramble

Contributed by **Natalie Matthews**, *bikini competitor and fitness model*

The tofu scramble is perhaps the most iconic vegan breakfast recipe in existence. Whether it's made at home or enjoyed at a plant-based restaurant, for most vegans, this scramble is synonymous with brunch. And nothing says weekend relaxation like the smell of the peppers, onions, spices, and the sound of sizzling tofu in the pan. Topping this with salsa and serving with toast or tortillas is highly recommended, along with your favorite weekend beverage.

Serves 2

1 block extra-firm tofu, crumbled

1 medium red bell pepper, seeded and chopped

1 medium orange bell pepper, seeded and chopped

¼ cup chopped onion

1 cup raw spinach

2 tablespoons nutritional yeast

2 teaspoons adobo seasoning

1 tablespoon mild salsa, for serving (optional)

Toast or tortillas, for serving (optional)

Nut butter on bread, for serving (optional)

Heat a nonstick pan over medium-high heat. Add the crumbled tofu and cook for 5 minutes, stirring frequently to prevent sticking. Stir in the peppers, onion, spinach, nutritional yeast, and adobo seasoning. Cook until the spinach has wilted and turned dark green, 1 to 2 minutes.

If desired, top with salsa and serve with toast or tortillas.

Nutritional Totals per Serving (excluding optional sides):

Calories: 266

Protein: 28.9 g

Carbohydrates: 16 g

Fat: 12.9 g

Fiber: 6.3 g

Vegan Omelet

Contributed by **Korin Sutton**, *bodybuilder*

When I ate meat, I also consumed eggs pretty much every day. An omelet was one of my favorite breakfasts, but once I went vegan, I gave up omelets for good and never looked back. I tried egg replacements like tofu scrambles, but I was never able to replicate the taste and texture of an omelet . . . until now. I have officially made the ultimate vegan omelet! Now you can have your vegan egg omelet and eat it too. I hope you'll love it as much as I do.

Serves 1

Olive oil spray (1 second for each spray)

⅓ cup bell peppers, seeded and chopped

½ cup curly kale, chopped

¼ cup white onions, chopped

½ cup shiitake mushrooms, chopped

2 garlic cloves, minced

1 Field Roast sausage

½ cup plus 1 tablespoon JUST Egg brand vegan egg

1 slice smoked vegan Gouda-style cheese (I like Follow Your Heart)

Place a cast-iron skillet over medium heat and spray with the olive oil spray.

Add the peppers, kale, onions, mushrooms, and garlic to the skillet and sauté until the peppers are tender, about 7 minutes. Add the sausage and cook until warmed through, another 2 minutes. Set aside.

Place a nonstick skillet over medium heat and spray with the olive oil spray. Add the JUST Egg and cook until it just begins to brown around the edges, about 1 minute. Place the Gouda in the middle of the cooked JUST Egg along with the sauteed vegetables and sausage. Fold the edges of the omelet over the filling. Let the omelet cool slightly before eating.

Nutritional Totals per Serving:

Calories: 523   Fat: 31 g

Protein: 38.6 g   Fiber: 5.2 g

Carbohydrates: 22 g

LUNCH

Chickpea Salad Sandwich

Contributed by **Sonya Looney,** *mountain biker*

I like eating this for lunch after a ride or for a snack. The crunchy texture is one of my favorite things about it! The salad also keeps well in the fridge, so it's great for making in advance. I try to include as many servings of beans as I can because they are one of the healthiest foods on the planet and incredible for your gut flora too. This recipe is also super easy to make, which is a bonus for the time-crunched person!

Makes 1 sandwich

- 1 (15.5-ounce) can chickpeas, drained
- 3 celery stalks, chopped
- ½ cup chopped red bell pepper
- ½ cup chopped fresh dill
- ⅓ cup diced red onion
- ¼ avocado, smashed
- 3 tablespoons Dijon mustard
- 2 garlic cloves, minced
- Juice of ½ lemon
- 2 teaspoons fresh dill or ½ teaspoon dried
- 1 teaspoon white wine vinegar
- Sea salt and freshly ground black pepper to taste
- Fresh greens, for serving (optional)
- Sprouted whole-grain bread, for serving (optional)

In a medium bowl, mash the chickpeas with a fork until chunky. Add the remaining ingredients and stir, seasoning with salt and pepper to taste. Enjoy as a salad or on toasted sprouted whole-grain bread with greens.

Nutritional Totals per Serving (including two slices of
sprouted bread):
Calories: 553   Fat: 13 g
Protein: 27.1 g   Fiber: 23 g
Carbohydrates: 86.6 g

Vegan Bodybuilding Burrito Bowl

Contributed by **Robert Cheeke**, *bodybuilder*

This is one of the ultimate bodybuilding and muscle recovery meals, with an
ideal balance of carbohydrates, proteins, fats, and fiber. Prepare brown rice,
pinto beans, and black beans in batches so you can have the base of this
meal multiple times per week, adding toppings such as lettuce, tomato, and
avocado to make your burrito bowl take on unique flavor and texture every
time you eat it. It's perfect for lunch, dinner, or post-workout.

Serves 1

   1 cup cooked brown rice

   ½ cup cooked (or canned and rinsed) pinto beans

   ½ cup cooked (or canned and rinsed) black beans

   1 avocado, sliced

   1 tomato, sliced

   1 handful of romaine lettuce, chopped

   1 jalapeño, sliced (seeded if you prefer less heat, or omit altogether)

   1 pepperoncini, sliced (omit if you don't like spicy)

Combine the cooked rice and beans, then top with other ingredients as
desired.

Nutritional Totals per Serving:
Calories: 735   Fat: 25 g
Protein: 23.5 g   Fiber: 30 g
Carbohydrates: 112 g

Fiona's Feast

Contributed by **Fiona Oakes,** *marathoner*

I find this soup to be a wonderfully filling, simple-to-prepare, and satisfying meal, which is easily digestible and convenient after a long run or day outside with the animals. I have to say, I am a big fan of seasonal, locally sourced produce, so I will adapt recipes to suit availability. But I am an "all-year-round" eater when it comes to food, as my work and training regime never really change with the seasons or weather, and the demands on my body remain pretty constant.

Serves 1

  1 teaspoon extra-virgin olive oil
  1 medium onion, chopped
  1 cup lentils, washed and drained
  1 cup diced root vegetables, such as potatoes, carrots, or celeriac
  1 cup peas
  2 cups vegetable stock
  1 teaspoon ground turmeric
  Sea salt and pepper to taste
  Herbs or spices for serving, such as basil or coriander (optional)

Heat the olive oil in a medium pot over medium heat. Add the onions and sauté until tender, about 5 minutes. Add the lentils, root vegetables, peas, and stock and simmer until the vegetables are soft, about 20 minutes.

Transfer the mixture to a blender and blend until smooth. Return the soup to the pot, bring to a simmer, and season with salt and pepper to taste. Remove from the heat and serve with a garnish of your choice.

> Nutritional Totals per Serving:
> Calories: 618   Fat: 6.7 g
> Protein: 31.6 g   Fiber: 28.3 g
> Carbohydrates: 113.2 g

Western BBQ GoodBowl

Contributed by **Dotsie Bausch**, *cyclist*
Used with permission by chef Jason Wrobel

This hearty bowl is for the meat and potatoes lovers—though this version is made entirely from plants, doesn't require a barbecue, and won't leave you feeling weighed down afterward. Crispy barbecue-marinated tempeh provides protein along with savory baked beans, which sit on top of seasoned roasted potatoes and a bright, tangy, dairy-free cabbage slaw. This bowl is sure to be a hit with the pickiest of eaters—adults and children included.

Serves 2

For the Roasted Potatoes:
- 2 large white, russet, or red potatoes, diced
- ¼ cup low-sodium vegetable broth or 2 tablespoons olive or grapeseed oil
- 2 teaspoons dried rosemary or 1 tablespoon chopped fresh rosemary
- 1 teaspoon sea salt
- 1 pinch freshly ground black pepper

For the BBQ Baked Beans:
- 2½ cups store-bought vegetarian/vegan baked beans (such as Amy's, Sprouts, Pacific, or Bush's brand)

For the Coleslaw:
- 1 (9-ounce) bag store-bought preshredded coleslaw mix
- 2 teaspoons pure maple syrup
- 1 tablespoon apple cider vinegar
- 2 teaspoons fresh lemon juice
- ¼ cup dairy-free mayonnaise (such as Follow Your Heart Vegenaise, Sir Kensington's, or Thrive Market brand)
- 1 pinch sea salt
- 1 pinch freshly ground black pepper
- 2 teaspoons whole caraway or fennel seeds

For the BBQ Tempeh:

2 teaspoons avocado or coconut oil

1 package store-bought premarinated smoky tempeh bacon strips (such as Lightlife brand)

Make the roasted potatoes: Preheat the oven to 425°F. In a medium baking dish or roasting pan, combine the potatoes with the broth or oil, rosemary, salt, and pepper. Toss to coat the potatoes. Roast for 45 minutes, until the potatoes are golden brown and crispy around the edges. Set aside.

Make the coleslaw: While the potatoes are roasting, add the coleslaw mix to a medium bowl. In a small mixing bowl, whisk together the maple syrup, apple cider vinegar, lemon juice, dairy-free mayo, salt, and pepper. Pour the dressing over the coleslaw mix, add the caraway or fennel seeds, and toss well to combine. Set aside.

Make the BBQ tempeh: In a small sauté pan, warm the oil over medium-low heat and add the tempeh bacon strips. Cook on each side for 3 to 4 minutes, until crispy around the edges. Set aside.

Assemble: In a medium serving bowl, make a bed of the roasted potatoes and add a few heaping spoonfuls of baked beans, followed by the coleslaw and 2 to 3 strips of the BBQ tempeh.

Nutritional Totals per Serving:
Calories: 364   Fat: 11.1 g
Protein: 18.8 g   Fiber: 13.3 g
Carbohydrates: 50.3 g

Minestrone Soup

Contributed by **Meagan Duhamel,** *figure skater*

Making a creative, healthy lunch these days is getting harder and harder. Between work, playtime, day-care visits, training (or attempting to train) and an occasional crying baby, my hands seem tied. This minestrone soup can be prepped in advance, making it easy to store in the fridge or freezer and warm up for a hearty midday meal. Or if you want to make it fresh for dinner one night, you can prep the vegetables in advance, then cook off the rest of the soup before mealtime. Despite the effort, this minestrone soup recipe is absolutely amazing. I can't believe I only discovered it now. It is definitely going to be a staple in my household. Enjoy it with your favorite bread, or maybe a grilled vegan cheese sandwich!

Serves 4

1 tablespoon margarine (I like Becel Vegan)
2 tablespoons olive oil
1 small yellow onion, chopped
1 cup diced carrots
1 cup diced celery
2 chopped zucchini
1 (14.5-ounce) can petite diced tomatoes (not drained)
1 (15.5-ounce) can kidney beans, drained and rinsed
1 (14.5-ounce) can tomato sauce
5 cups vegetable broth
1 tablespoon dried basil
2 teaspoons dried parsley
1 teaspoon dried oregano
1 teaspoon sea salt
½ teaspoon freshly ground black pepper
1 cup spinach leaves (about two small handfuls)
1½ cups small shell pasta (I like GoGo quinoa pasta)
Bread or sandwich, for serving (optional)

In a large pot over medium heat, melt the margarine with the olive oil. Add the onion, carrots, celery, and zucchini and cook for 10 minutes, stirring occasionally, until tender.

Stir in the tomatoes, beans, tomato sauce, broth, and spices. Bring to a low boil, then reduce to a simmer and cook for 15 minutes.

Add the spinach and pasta and cook until the pasta is al dente, 10 to 15 minutes. Enjoy warm, or cool to room temperature and store in the fridge for up to 1 week or the freezer for up to 1 month.

Nutritional Totals per Serving:

Calories: 423

Protein: 16.8 g

Carbohydrates: 66.3 g

Fat: 12.3 g

Fiber: 13.6 g

Vegan Taco Bowl

Contributed by **Korin Sutton**, *bodybuilder*

With a macro-friendly balance of protein, carbohydrates, and fats, this epic taco bowl makes for a great post-workout meal any day of the week. It also makes a great lunch entrée any time of year, and you just can't go wrong with tacos. I especially like that it has six different vegetables in it for added nutrient density from superfoods such as garlic, onions, mushrooms, and leafy greens. And with two servings, I can enjoy all of it after a super-long workout or save some for dinner or the following day. With the meaty and cheesy texture, this makes a great meal to introduce to nonvegans as well, and it's sure to give them something to *taco bout*.

Serves 2

Olive oil spray

1 cup chopped shiitake mushrooms

1 cup seeded and chopped bell peppers, any color

2 large garlic cloves, chopped

⅔ cup chopped white onion

1 package Lightlife Smart Ground Crumbles

Dash of cayenne pepper (optional)

4 cups shredded romaine lettuce

12 grape tomatoes, chopped

2 tablespoons Tofutti Sour Cream

¼ cup shredded vegan cheese (I like Daiya)

Heat a large pan over medium heat and spray with the olive oil spray. Add the mushrooms, peppers, garlic, and onion and sauté until soft, about 7 minutes. Set aside.

In a nonstick pan over medium heat, brown the Smart Ground crumbles. Add the cayenne pepper if you want things spicier.

Build your taco bowl starting with the romaine, then the Smart Ground, sautéed veggies, tomatoes, sour cream, and cheese.

Nutritional Totals per Serving:

Calories: 368	Fat: 10.7 g
Protein: 36.7 g	Fiber: 16.7 g
Carbohydrates: 31.3 g	

Summer Pasta Salad

Contributed by **Robert Cheeke**, *bodybuilder*

This is one of my favorite summer meals, but the truth is, it can be enjoyed anytime. The nice thing about eating this pasta salad during warmer months is that it's so refreshing because it's enjoyable at room temperature or chilled. It's filled with vegetables such as tomatoes and spinach, along with some of my favorite toppings to put on anything, including black olives and artichoke hearts. By using red lentil pasta, which has only one ingredient (red lentil flour), this dish is naturally rich in carbohydrates and protein, and it also has heft and texture to make for a very satisfying and filling meal. After a midafternoon summer workout, I may eat two or three bowls of this pasta salad. This is also an excellent meal to serve at a gathering with people new to a plant-based diet because all ingredients are recognizable for vegans and nonvegans alike, as it contains only real foods, plus it's gluten free and really, really tasty.

Serves 6

1 (8-ounce) package red lentil pasta

2 cups spinach, chopped

1 pint of sweet cherry or grape tomatoes, cut into halves or thirds

1 (14-ounce) can artichoke hearts, drained and diced

½ large bell pepper, seeded and diced

1 (6-ounce) can black olives, drained and sliced

1 (15-ounce) can garbanzo beans, drained and rinsed
⅓ to ½ cup Italian dressing
Freshly ground black pepper to taste

Bring a large pot of water to a boil and cook the lentil pasta according to the package instructions.

While the pasta cooks, prep the remaining ingredients as directed.

Drain the pasta and rinse under cold water. Transfer to a large mixing bowl. Add the vegetables and beans. Pour enough dressing over the salad to coat, then toss to combine. Season with pepper to taste. Store any leftovers in the fridge for up to one week.

> Nutritional Totals per Serving:
> Calories: 346   Fat: 8.5 g
> Protein: 17.5 g   Fiber: 13.8 g
> Carbohydrates: 54 g

Latin GoodBowl

Contributed by **Dotsie Bausch**, *cyclist*
Used with permission by chef Jason Wrobel

Like a kick to your meal? This Latin-inspired GoodBowl brings the heat—along with robust nutrition to keep you fueled throughout your day. You can also turn down the spice level by going light on the jalapeño and chili peppers. Made with "meaty" cauliflower lentil taco filling, fresh romaine, crunchy plantain chips, and cool cashew sour cream, this bowl beats takeout by a long shot!

Serves 1

For the Sour Cream:
    1¾ cups store-bought dairy-free sour cream (such as Tofutti,
        Follow Your Heart, or Kite Hill brand)
    2 tablespoons fresh lemon juice
    2 teaspoons apple cider vinegar
    ¾ teaspoon sea salt

For the Quinoa:

- ⅓ cup low-sodium vegetable broth
- 2 tablespoons diced white onion
- ½ cup finely chopped red, green, or yellow bell peppers (or any combination)
- 1 small carrot, diced
- 1 cup store-bought precooked frozen or shelf-stable quinoa (such as Trader Joe's or Ancient Harvest brand)
- 2 tablespoons salsa or pico de gallo

For the Cauliflower Lentil Taco Filling:

- 2 teaspoons low-sodium vegetable broth or olive oil
- ¼ cup finely diced white onion
- 1 teaspoon seeded and finely minced jalapeño pepper
- 2 cups store-bought cauliflower rice (such as Sprouts, Trader Joe's, or Green Giant brand)
- 1 garlic clove, finely minced
- 1 teaspoon chili powder, divided
- ½ teaspoon ground cumin, divided
- ¼ teaspoon ground coriander, divided
- 3 tablespoons tomato paste
- ½ cup canned or shelf-stable lentils, drained and thoroughly rinsed (such as Trader Joe's brand)
- Sea salt and freshly ground black pepper to taste

For Assembly:

- ½ head romaine lettuce, chopped
- ½ avocado, diced
- 1 cup cherry tomatoes, halved
- 1 bag store-bought roasted plantain chips (such as Trader Joe's, Thrive Market, or Goya brand)
- ¼ cup chopped fresh cilantro

2 tablespoons store-bought preroasted pepitas (a.k.a. pumpkin
   seeds, such as Trader Joe's brand), toasted in a dry pan until
   fragrant
Salsa

Make the cashew sour cream: Combine all the ingredients in a small bowl
and whisk vigorously until well combined. Cover and store in the refrigerator
until ready to use, up to one week.

Make the quinoa: In a medium saucepan, combine the vegetable broth,
onion, bell pepper, and carrot and sauté over medium-low heat until onion
is translucent, about 5 minutes. Add the quinoa, cover the pan, and simmer
on low heat for an additional 3 to 4 minutes, until the water in the pan has
evaporated. Fluff with a fork, remove from the heat, and stir in the salsa or
pico de gallo. Set aside.

Make the Cauliflower Lentil Taco Filling: Add the vegetable broth or olive
oil to a medium skillet over medium heat. Sauté the onion and jalapeño until
the onion is translucent and the jalapeño has softened, 5 to 7 minutes. Add
the cauliflower rice, garlic, ½ teaspoon of the chili powder, ¼ teaspoon of the
cumin, and ⅛ teaspoon of the coriander and cook for 5 minutes. Stir in the
tomato paste and cook for another 4 to 5 minutes, until the cauliflower is
tender. Add the lentils and the remaining chili powder, cumin, and coriander.
Season with salt and pepper to taste. Reduce the heat to low and cook for
another 4 minutes, until the flavors have melded. Mash the lentils with a
fork to break them down into a "ground beef" consistency.

Assemble: In a medium serving bowl, make a bed of quinoa, and then add
the cauliflower lentil taco filling, shredded romaine lettuce, diced avocado,
cherry tomatoes, and a small handful of plantain chips. Garnish with fresh
cilantro and toasted pepitas. Add a dollop of sour cream and salsa.

Nutritional Totals per Serving:
Calories: 431   Fat: 10.4 g
Protein: 17 g   Fiber: 17 g
Carbohydrates: 72 g

Kale Yeah Caesar Salad

Contributed by **Mary Schneider,** *marathoner*
From her book Green Body Cookbook

Eat this salad when you are feeling like you really need to boost your intake of greens. Kale is a nutritional powerhouse. It is high in many nutrients, including iron; and iron absorption is increased when you pair it with vitamin C (in this case, lemon juice). And for those of you who aren't kale lovers quite yet, this salad with its plant-based take on Caesar dressing will get you there. One of the secrets is to "massage" the leaves with lemon juice fist, which makes them more tender.

This is a great lunch salad, or it can be served as a side with dinner.

Serves 2

For the Roasted Chickpeas:
    1 (15.5-ounce) can chickpeas
    2 tablespoons nutritional yeast
    ½ teaspoon onion powder
    ½ teaspoon garlic powder
    ½ teaspoon sea salt

For the Caesar Dressing:
    2 avocados
    2 teaspoons diced garlic (about 2 cloves)
    1 teaspoon Dijon mustard
    1 (7-ounce) container of capers, not drained
    2 tablespoons fresh lemon juice
    ¼ teaspoon sea salt
    ¼ teaspoon freshly ground black pepper

For Assembly:
    1 large bundle of kale (I prefer curly kale)
    2 tablespoons lemon juice
    2 tablespoons hemp hearts
    2 tablespoons nutritional yeast

Make the chickpeas: Preheat the oven to 400°F. Drain and rinse the chickpeas, but reserve 1 tablespoon of the liquid from the can. (This is also called aquafaba.) Add them to a medium bowl and toss them with the nutritional yeast, seasonings, and reserved aquafaba until well coated. Spread the seasoned chickpeas over a baking sheet in a single layer and bake for 30 minutes, or until they're browned and crisp. Set aside.

Make the dressing: Combine all the ingredients in a blender and blend until smooth, scraping down the sides as needed. If necessary, thin the dressing with 1 tablespoon of water at a time.

Assemble: In a large bowl, drizzle the lemon juice over the kale and use your hands to firmly squeeze the leaves until they are tender and beginning to give up their green juices. Toss the kale with the dressing, sprinkle with the hemp hearts and nutritional yeast, and top with roasted chickpeas.

Nutritional Totals per Serving:

Calories: 512

Protein: 17.5 g

Carbohydrates: 56.2 g

Fat: 29.4 g

Fiber: 26.1 g

Spinach-Tofu Quinoa Pasta Bowl

Contributed by **Vanessa Espinoza**, *powerlifter*

This dish checks all the boxes—it's quick to pull together for lunch; it's packed with nutrition; and it's got big flavor thanks to the simple dressing—though if you want a lower-calorie meal, you could make this dish without it.

Serves 4

For the Dressing:

¼ cup red wine vinegar

3 tablespoons extra-virgin olive oil

2 garlic cloves, minced

1 tablespoon dried oregano

1 teaspoon low-sodium soy sauce

For the Pasta:

2 cups quinoa pasta

¾ cup tofu

1 handful of spinach

1 handful of alfalfa sprouts

Make the dressing: In a medium bowl, whisk together the ingredients and set aside.

Make the pasta: Cook the pasta according to the package instructions. Rinse, drain, and return to the pot. Add the tofu, spinach, and alfalfa sprouts. Toss to combine, drizzle the dressing on top (if using), and toss again.

Nutritional Totals per Serving (without dressing):

Calories: 257   Fats: 4 g

Protein: 10 g   Fiber: 5 g

Carbohydrates: 51 g

Nutritional Totals per Serving (with dressing):

Calories: 357   Fat: 14 g

Protein: 10 g   Fiber: 5 g

Carbohydrates: 52 g

Acai Bowl

Contributed by **Korin Sutton**, *bodybuilder*

It doesn't get much better than an acai bowl. The tartness from berries and the fresh fruit goodness mixed with the crunch of granola makes me want to have this dish any time of day in the warm climate of Florida, where I live. Many people rely on smoothies to get a mix of lots of different fruits with high antioxidant content all in one meal. But smoothies can get old after a while, especially if you have one every single day. So a bowl with all the same fruits but with some added texture is the perfect replacement for your morning or afternoon smoothie. An acai bowl is also an excellent fuel source because of all the carbohydrates and fruit sugar, so working out within an hour of eating this bowl should leave you feeling powered up to tackle the challenge, as well as the rest of the day.

Serves 2

2 packets (198 g) unsweetened acai berries

1 frozen ripe banana

¼ cup unsweetened almond milk

2 cups granola

1 cup (144 g) strawberries, rinsed and sliced

1 cup (144 g) blueberries, rinsed

1 tablespoon stevia

1 tablespoon coconut flakes

Combine the acai, banana, and almond milk in a high-powered blender. Blend until smooth and thick. You may need to use your blender's tamper for this.

Transfer the mixture to a bowl and add toppings as desired.

Nutritional Totals per Serving:
Calories: 744   Fat: 34.2 g
Protein: 15.9 g   Fiber: 15.9 g
Carbohydrates: 103 g

Plant-Based Power Bowl

Contributed by **Pamela Fergusson**, *RD, PhD*

Try this hearty bowl after your next long ride, run, gym session, or swim. You'll be licking your lips and building muscle too. It uses kasha as a base, which is toasted buckwheat (you could just toast your buckwheat in a dry pan for a few minutes to get the same effect). I love buckwheat because, like quinoa, it is a complete protein (meaning it contains all of the essential amino acids) but is a domestic crop in North America and does not need to be imported. Buckwheat is also rich in fiber, magnesium, iron, and copper.

This bowl does call for the extra step of making your own sunflower seed sour cream, but I highly recommend you make a batch of it ahead of time (along with roasting the sweet potatoes and cooking the kasha) and keep it in your fridge to drizzle over bowls, baked potatoes, and vegan nachos.

Most people reach for cashews when they want to make a creamy sauce or dressing, but sunflower seeds make a great, lower-cost swap, are higher in protein, and are better for the environment because they require less water to grow.

Serves 1

For the Sunflower Seed Sour Cream:
    1 cup raw sunflower seeds, soaked overnight or boiled, then rinsed
    1 tablespoon fresh lemon juice
    2 teaspoons apple cider vinegar
    ½ teaspoon sea salt, plus more to taste

For the Bowl:
    1 sweet potato, diced into 1½-inch cubes (leave skin on)
    2 teaspoons extra-virgin olive oil (optional)
    1 cup kasha, or buckwheat toasted in a dry pan until fragrant
    2 cups vegetable stock, or water if preferred
    ½ cup cooked (or canned and rinsed) black beans
    ½ cup corn kernels
    ½ cup diced red peppers
    ½ small avocado, diced

Make the sour cream: In a blender, combine the ingredients with ½ cup water and blend for 2 minutes until completely smooth. You might need to scrape down the sides of the blender with a spatula. Adjust the seasoning with additional salt, if desired. Refrigerate until ready to use, up to 3 days.

Make the bowl: Preheat the oven to 440°F. Line a baking sheet with parchment paper.

Either toss the sweet potato with the oil, or place it directly on the lined baking sheet if you prefer cooking with no oil. Bake for 25 to 30 minutes, stirring halfway through.

In a small saucepan, combine the kasha or toasted buckwheat with 2 cups of vegetable stock or water. Bring to a boil, reduce to a simmer, and cover. Cook until all the liquid is absorbed, about 12 minutes.

Make a layer of ½ cup kasha in a bowl and add the beans, corn, peppers, and avocado, along with ½ cup of the roasted sweet potatoes. Drizzle ¼ cup sunflower seed sour cream over the top. Store leftover sweet potatoes and kasha in the fridge in a covered container for up to 5 days.

Nutritional Totals per Serving:

Calories: 1,501   Fat: 94.8 g

Protein: 49.1 g   Fiber: 37 g

Carbohydrates: 138.5 g

Ayurvedic Mosh-Down Meal

Contributed by **John Joseph**, *triathlete*

The best things about this dish, which is traditionally called kichiri, is how inexpensive it is, how great it tastes, and how nutritious it is. When I was a Hare Krishna monk (circa 1982) and started feeding the homeless plant-based meals in New York City, we made this. With some greens and bread, it provided all the nutrition anyone needed for their day. It's all in the spicing, which is abundant as f*ck. So do yoga mantras over it while you cook in order to keep that PMA (positive mental attitude).

Serves 6

For the Chapatis:

3 cups whole-wheat flour

1½ teaspoons sea salt

½ cup melted vegan butter, plus more for serving

1⅓ cups lukewarm water

For the Stew:

2 tablespoons coconut oil

2 tablespoons organic vegan butter (I like Miyoko's), divided

2 fresh chilis, seeded and minced

3 teaspoons cumin seeds

2 teaspoons grated fresh ginger

2 teaspoons ground coriander

2 teaspoons ground turmeric

4 cups cubed and peeled eggplant

3 cups cauliflower florets

8 tomatoes, chopped

4 cups stemmed and chopped spinach

2 cups cooked (or canned and rinsed) chickpeas

3 teaspoons Himalayan pink salt

For the Rice:

1 teaspoon coconut oil

½ teaspoon vegan butter

1 teaspoon ground turmeric

3 cups white basmati rice

½ cup whole cashews

1½ teaspoons sea salt

Make the chapatis: In a large bowl, combine the flour and salt. Slowly add the butter and water as you stir with a wooden spoon. When you have a soft, moist dough, transfer it to a clean, dry surface. Knead the dough with your hands for 8 to 10 minutes. Cover the dough with a clean, damp cloth and let it rest for 2 hours.

When ready to cook your meal, separate the dough into pieces the size of a golf ball and form them into balls. You should have about 20 of them.

Flour a clean, flat surface and roll out the balls until they're flat and about ¼-inch thick. Heat a medium skillet over medium heat. Place a chapati in the pan and cook it for 30 seconds. Use tongs to flip it and cook for another 30 seconds. Flip it one more time and cook until the edges of the chapati start turning up. Over the open flame of another burner, use the tongs to transfer the chapati directly over the flame, putting the side down that was previously facing up. It should immediately puff up and fill with air. After a few seconds, flip and let it continue to puff. Remove and douse with a little extra butter if you want. Repeat with the remaining chapatis.

Make the stew: In a large saucepan over medium heat, heat the oil and 1 tablespoon of the butter. When melted, toss in your chilies, cumin seeds, ginger, coriander, and turmeric and toast for 30 seconds, or until fragrant.

Add the eggplant and cook until it begins to get soft and browned. Stir in the cauliflower and cook until slightly tender, about 5 minutes. Add the tomatoes and spinach, and stir to combine.

Pour in the chickpeas, salt, and ¾ cup water. Reduce the flame to medium-low, cover, and simmer for 10 minutes. Stir in the remaining tablespoon of butter. Continue cooking, stirring occasionally so it doesn't stick, until the water cooks out. You're done when your stew is nice and thick.

Make the rice: In a medium pot over medium heat, combine the oil and butter. Add the turmeric, followed by the rice. Stir to combine and cook for 3 minutes, making sure the rice doesn't burn.

Add the cashews and salt along with 6 cups of water. Bring to a boil, stir, and reduce the heat to low. Cover the pot and cook for 15 to 20 minutes, until there is very little water left at the bottom of the pot, practically none. Remove the pot from the heat and set aside, still covered. The heat will evaporate the rest of the water, leaving your rice fluffy.

Nutritional Totals per Serving:
Calories: 725   Fat: 33.7 g
Protein: 19.7 g   Fiber: 16.8 g
Carbohydrates: 95 g

Legendary Tuscan Potato Soup

Contributed by **Robert Cheeke**, *bodybuilder*

This is one of the all-time great soups that my wife has been making for years. When we have guests over, this is always a crowd-pleaser, for vegans and nonvegans alike. Though we typically make this Italian soup for dinner and serve it with ciabatta bread and a side salad, since it's usually just the two of us, we end up enjoying this amazing soup for lunch over the next few days. Therefore, we actually consume it as a midday meal more often than as a dinner entrée. Soups are always versatile and can be enjoyed for lunch any day of the week, any time of year, and this is no exception. But it's particularly nice during winter, served hot with chunks of potatoes in it.

This particular soup is packed with flavor, largely because of the plant-based Italian sausages. The recipe makes a huge batch, which you will appreciate because you can reheat it and enjoy it for days to come.

Serves 8

1 package of Field Roast brand Italian sausages (4 sausage links)
1 large onion, diced
4 garlic cloves, minced
8 cups vegetable broth
4 large russet potatoes, diced
½ cup plant-based heavy cream (such as Silk, Ripple, or Califia Farms)
2 teaspoons liquid smoke (optional)
1 bunch of curly kale, leaves stripped from the stems and chopped
Kosher salt and freshly ground black pepper to taste

Chop the sausages into small bite-sized pieces. In a large pot over medium heat, lightly brown the sausage and transfer it to a bowl.

In the same pot (which should have some fat residue from the sausage) over medium heat, cook the onions until they begin to brown, about 6 minutes. Add the garlic and cook just until fragrant, about 1 minute. Stir in the broth and potatoes. Bring the pot to a boil, reduce to a simmer, and cook until the potatoes are fork-tender, about 20 minutes.

Add the cream, along with the liquid smoke if using. Add the sausage back to the pot, along with the kale. Cook until the kale turns vibrant green, about 2 minutes. Stir, taste, and adjust the seasoning with salt and pepper if desired.

Serve on its own or with bread such as ciabatta, French, or sourdough. Or, of course, a green salad.

Nutritional Totals per Serving:
Calories: 341   Fat: 10.7 g
Protein: 18 g   Fiber: 5.7 g
Carbohydrates: 44.5 g

DINNER

Mediterranean GoodBowl

Contributed by **Dotsie Bausch**, *cyclist*
Used with permission by chef Jason Wrobel

This bowl is layered with so many flavors and textures, you could easily eat this every night of the week and not get bored. It's loaded with za'atar-spiced rice pilaf, fresh arugula salad, gem-colored steamed beets, creamy cucumber tzatziki, and crunchy chickpeas.

Serves 2

For the Roasted Chickpeas:

  1½ **cups store-bought preroasted chickpeas (such as Biena brand)**

For the Tzatziki Sauce with Cucumbers:

  ½ **cup unsweetened plain nondairy yogurt (soy, almond, or coconut)**

  ½ **large English cucumber or 2 Persian cucumbers, finely chopped**

  ½ **teaspoon apple cider vinegar or lemon juice**

  1 **tablespoon chopped fresh dill or 2 teaspoons dried dill**

  ¼ **teaspoon sea salt**

For the Rice Pilaf:

  1 **tablespoon low-sodium vegetable broth, nondairy butter, or olive oil**

  2 **tablespoons minced onion**

  1 **small clove of garlic, minced**

  2 **cups store-bought precooked frozen or shelf-stable white basmati or brown rice (such as Trader Joe's or Seeds of Change brand)**

  ⅛ **teaspoon ground turmeric**

  ⅛ **teaspoon ground cumin**

  ¼ **teaspoon smoked paprika**

¼ cup finely chopped fresh parsley

Sea salt and freshly ground black pepper, to taste

For the Arugula Salad:

2 cups wild or baby arugula

½ cup diced tomato

½ cup sliced cucumber

1 tablespoon extra-virgin olive oil

1½ tablespoons fresh lemon juice

1 tablespoon za'atar spice mix or ground sumac

Sea salt and freshly ground black pepper to taste

For Assembly:

⅓ cup sliced red onion

⅓ cup sliced cooked beets

¼ cup black or kalamata olives, pitted

⅓ cup crumbled nondairy feta cheese (such as Violife brand),
    optional

2 tablespoons store-bought hummus or baba ganoush, optional

2 tablespoons raw, unroasted pine nuts or almonds from bulk
    section or a bag, toasted in a dry pan until fragrant

½ cup store-bought roasted chickpeas

Make the tzatziki: Combine all the ingredients in a medium bowl, stir until well combined, cover, and refrigerate until ready to use. This will keep in the fridge for up to 3 days.

Make the rice pilaf: In a small skillet, warm the vegetable broth over low heat. Add the onions and sauté until translucent, about 5 minutes. Add the garlic and sauté for another minute, until fragrant. Add the cooked rice, turmeric, cumin, and paprika. Stir to combine and heat through, about 5 minutes. Stir in the parsley and season to taste with salt and pepper. Remove from the heat and set aside.

Make the salad: In a medium bowl, combine the arugula, tomato, and cucumber. Drizzle with the olive oil and lemon juice and sprinkle with za'atar, salt, and pepper.

Assemble: In a medium serving bowl, make a bed of arugula salad. Add a few scoops of rice pilaf and a dollop of tzatziki sauce. Top with the red onion, cooked beets, olives, dairy-free feta (if using), hummus (if using), toasted pine nuts, and a few tablespoons of the roasted chickpeas.

Nutritional Totals per Serving:
Calories: 372
Protein: 12.6 g
Carbohydrates: 64.5 g

Fat: 7.8 g
Fiber: 9.8 g

Curried Chickpeas

Contributed by **Robert Cheeke**, *bodybuilder*

One of the most protein-dense legumes out there is the mighty chickpea. They're even shaped like little shredded biceps! Chickpeas are a great post-workout food because they help with muscle repair and growth. And legumes in general are an outstanding foundation for a meal, especially once you've added in some herbs and spices. These curried chickpeas are great over rice, which together with the chickpeas contribute plenty of replenishing carbohydrates, proteins, fats, and fiber. Add a side salad of leafy greens for added nutrition and drizzle a citrus dressing to help the absorption of iron, and you've got a powerhouse meal. Don't shy away from making it spicy—the added heat will encourage you to hydrate more!

Serves 4

1 yellow onion, chopped

2 garlic cloves, minced

1 (13.6-ounce) can lite coconut milk

4 cups (or two 15.5-ounce cans, rinsed) garbanzo beans (chickpeas)

1 (14.5-ounce) can diced tomatoes (preferably fire-roasted)

2 cups diced Yukon gold potatoes, boiled until tender

1 tablespoon tomato paste

1 tablespoon curry powder

1 tablespoon garam masala

½ teaspoon crushed red pepper flakes, plus more to taste

2 cups spinach

Brown rice or whole-wheat pita for serving

In a large pan over medium-high heat, add 1 tablespoon of water and sauté the onions and garlic until tender, about 3 minutes. Add more water to the pan if necessary to prevent burning. Add the tomato paste, curry powder, garam masala, and red pepper flakes and mix well. Add remaining ingredients, except for the spinach. Cook until the mixture is heated through and the flavors have melded, stirring occasionally, about 10 minutes. Add the spinach and cook for another 5 to 10 minutes, until the spinach is wilted and the flavors have come together. Adjust the seasoning to taste, adding more crushed red pepper flakes if desired.

Serve over brown rice or whole-wheat pita.

> Nutritional Totals per Serving
> (excluding rice or whole-wheat pita):
> Calories: 489   Fat: 21 g
> Protein: 16.3 g   Fiber: 16.6g
> Carbohydrates: 65.3 g

E2 Black Beans and Rice

Contributed by **Rip Esselstyn,** *swimmer and firefighter*
From his book The Engine 2 Cookbook

This staple dinner dish is as basic as they come and, oh, so good. Just like my morning bowl of cereal, I've been eating this meal for more than three decades. This is also a great meal to serve when you're having extra guests over for dinner.

Serve with healthy chips or warm corn tortillas.

Serves 4

2 (15.5-ounce) cans black beans, rinsed and drained

1 to 1½ cups vegetable stock or water

2 cups cooked brown rice

1 tablespoon Bragg Liquid Aminos

1 teaspoon chili powder

2 to 3 tomatoes, chopped

1 bunch green onions, chopped (white and green parts)

1 (8-ounce) can water chestnuts, drained

1 cup corn, fresh, frozen, or canned

2 red, yellow, or green bell peppers, seeded and chopped

1 bunch cilantro, rinsed and chopped

1 avocado, sliced

Store-bought salsa or tamari to taste

In a medium pot, heat the beans with the stock or water, liquid aminos, and chili powder.

To serve, place several big spoonfuls of the brown rice onto large plates and ladle the beans on top. Add generous handfuls of chopped vegetables, cilantro, and avocado on top of the beans. Add salsa or tamari to taste.

Nutritional Totals per Serving:

Calories: 474	Fat: 8.3 g
Protein: 18.8 g	Fiber: 24.7 g
Carbohydrates: 85.6 g	

Curried Lentil Stew

Contributed by **Mary Schneider,** *marathoner*

From her book Green Body Cookbook

This is probably my favorite soup because it has potent anti-inflammatory properties. The curries in this dish are what give it superpowers, as the mix of spices work together to promote good digestion and a healthy metabolism, relieve pain and inflammation, boost the immune system, and improve bone health. This soup is also full of nutrients from the vegetables and protein from the lentils.

I like to prep a batch of this soup in advance and heat it up for lunch during the week. You can also serve it over a bowl of rice to make a heartier dinner meal.

Serves 2

    4 cups vegetable broth or water (vegetable broth is preferred for
       depth of flavor)

    3 large carrots, chopped

    2 large stalks of celery, chopped

    1 large yellow onion, chopped

    2 teaspoons diced garlic (about 2 cloves)

    ¼ teaspoon red pepper flakes or ¼ teaspoon cayenne pepper for
       heat (optional)

    1 (15-ounce) can full-fat coconut milk

    1 (15-ounce) can diced tomatoes

    1 cup uncooked lentils

    2 tablespoons curry powder

    1 teaspoon sea salt

    ¼ tsp ground turmeric

    ¼ teaspoon freshly ground black pepper

    1 dried bay leaf

    2 overflowing cups of spinach, chopped

    Brown rice for serving (optional)

Heat a large pot over medium heat. Add 1 to 2 tablespoons of the vegetable broth or water and sauté the carrots, celery, and onion until just tender, 5 to 7 minutes. Add the garlic and red pepper or cayenne, if using, and sauté for another 2 to 3 minutes, until the vegetables have softened further.

Stir in the remaining broth or water, coconut milk, diced tomatoes, lentils, curry, salt, turmeric, pepper, and bay leaf. Bring the soup to a boil, cover, and reduce the heat to a simmer. Cook for 30 minutes.

Remove the bay leaf and discard. Add the spinach and stir until it wilts. If you prefer a thinner soup, adjust the consistency by adding ⅓ cup of water at a time. Serve as is or over a bowl of brown rice.

Nutritional Totals per Serving (excluding brown rice):

Calories: 832	Fat: 34.6 g
Protein: 32.3 g	Fiber: 27.6 g
Carbohydrates: 110.2 g	

Spaghetti Squash with Tempeh Bolognese Sauce

Contributed by **Mary Schneider,** *marathoner*

From her book Green Body Cookbook

I love this recipe because it is more nutrient dense than your typical pasta dish. Pasta is a minimally processed food, whereas spaghetti squash—whose texture mimics pasta—is not processed at all. Plus, it contains so many vitamins and minerals, including B vitamins, folate, potassium, omega-3s and omega 6s, calcium, iron, phosphorus, and zinc. And it's naturally gluten free! You can certainly sub in your favorite boxed pasta, which is what I do when I'm pressed for time and still want a healthy homemade meal.

This recipe is great any time, but I like to use it as a recovery meal after a hard workout to rebuild muscle and thereby boost recovery. If you are a strength athlete and looking to build muscle, it is an especially helpful dish to incorporate because it is high in protein. An 8-ounce package of tempeh has 2 servings, with 20 grams of protein per serving!

Serves 2

- **1 medium spaghetti squash**
- **1 teaspoon sea salt, divided**
- **1 teaspoon garlic powder, divided**
- **½ teaspoon freshly ground black pepper**
- **1 (25-ounce) jar of store-bought marinara sauce of choice (or more if you like it saucy!)**
- **1 teaspoon diced garlic (about 1 clove)**
- **½ teaspoon red pepper flakes**
- **1 (8-ounce) package of tempeh, diced**
- **½ teaspoon paprika**
- **½ teaspoon dried basil**
- **½ teaspoon dried oregano**
- **1 (8-ounce) package of cremini mushrooms (or sub the same serving size of another vegetable of choice, such as squash or zucchini), sliced**
- **Nutritional yeast for serving (optional)**

Preheat the oven to 400°F. Line a large baking sheet with foil and set aside. (This will help with cleanup!)

Cut the spaghetti squash in half lengthwise, scoop out the seeds, and discard. Sprinkle the flesh of the squash with ½ teaspoon of the salt, ½ teaspoon of the garlic powder, and the pepper. Place the squash cut-side down on a baking sheet and bake for 40 minutes.

Meanwhile, heat a large saucepan over medium heat. Add 2 tablespoons of the marinara sauce, just enough to lightly coat the bottom of the pan. Once the sauce begins to bubble, add the garlic and red pepper flakes. Stir and let the sauce infuse for 1 minute.

Add the tempeh and 1 more tablespoon of the sauce, enough so that the tempeh is lightly coated. Stir in the paprika, basil, oregano, and remaining ½ teaspoon of salt and garlic powder and cook, stirring continuously, for 3 to 5 minutes, until the tempeh heats through. If the tempeh begins to stick, stir in another tablespoon or two of marinara.

Push the tempeh mixture to one side of the pan. On the other side, add 2 more tablespoons of sauce and the sliced mushrooms. Stir to combine and sauté for 3 to 5 minutes, until the mushrooms (or vegetable of your choice) are tender. Stir the tempeh periodically during this time so it doesn't stick.

Stir together the mushrooms and tempeh and add the remaining marinara sauce. Reduce the heat to low, just to keep the sauce warm and to help meld the flavors. Stir occasionally until the squash is ready.

When the spaghetti squash is cooked, carefully use a spatula to flip the squash cut-side up. Be mindful that this will release hot steam from beneath the squash. Allow the squash to cool for several minutes, then use a fork to shred the flesh.

Add the "spaghetti" to a large bowl and top with the tempeh Bolognese. If desired, sprinkle with nutritional yeast.

Nutritional Totals per Serving:

Calories: 578	Fat: 21 g
Protein: 35.2 g	Fiber: 18 g
Carbohydrates: 78.4 g	

Sloppy Vegan Chili

Contributed by **Natalie Matthews**, *bikini competitor and fitness model*

Part sloppy joe, part chili, what's not to love? Serve it on some cornbread, make a sloppy sandwich, or serve it up with chips and vegan queso. Don't forget the napkins!

Serves 10

- ½ cup water (4 ounces)
- ¼ cup minced onion
- 3 garlic cloves, minced
- 2 (15.5-ounce) cans of black beans, rinsed
- 1 cup textured vegetable protein (TVP)
- 1 cup tomato sauce
- ½ cup tomato paste
- 2 tablespoons coconut sugar
- 2 tablespoons mustard (any kind will work)
- 1½ tablespoons white vinegar
- 2 teaspoons chili powder
- 2 teaspoons cumin
- 2 teaspoons dried or fresh oregano
- 1 teaspoon salt
- 4 cups vegetable broth or water

In a large pot over medium heat, add the ½ cup of water and the onion. Cook until the onion becomes translucent, about 5 minutes. Add the garlic and cook until it turns golden, stirring constantly to prevent burning, about 3 more minutes.

Stir in the beans, TVP, tomato sauce, tomato paste, coconut sugar, mustard, vinegar, chili powder, cumin, oregano, and salt. Add the vegetable broth or water and stir until well combined. Bring to a boil, cover, and reduce to a simmer. Cook for 20 minutes, remove from the heat, and serve.

Nutritional Totals per Serving:

Calories: 155	Fat: 1 g
Protein: 11 g	Fiber: 9 g
Carbohydrates: 27 g	

Black Bean Veggie Burger Patties

Contributed by **Brendan Brazier**, *ultramarathoner*

From his book Thrive Energy Cookbook

Here's a classic protein-rich black bean burger staple. It's delicious paired with vegan cheddar cheese, such as Mind-Blowing (Nut-Free) Vegan Cheese Sauce on page 326, and layered on a bun with all your favorite veggie toppings, crumbled over grains, or just eaten on its own. Keep a batch of these in the fridge so that a tasty burger is never more than a few minutes away.

Makes 10 patties

- 2 cups cooked (or rinsed canned) black beans
- 1 cup rolled oats
- ⅔ cup cooked whole-grain brown rice
- ⅓ cup nutritional yeast
- ¼ cup shredded Daiya or your favorite cheddar-style dairy-free cheese
- 1 large onion, grated (or chopped in a food processor)
- 1 large handful of fresh cilantro leaves, chopped
- 2 tablespoons ground coriander
- 1 tablespoon paprika
- 1 tablespoon grainy mustard
- 2 tablespoons tamari sauce
- 1 teaspoon sea salt, plus more to taste
- 1 to 2 cups fresh breadcrumbs from sprouted bread (I like Silver Hills Chia Bread for a gluten-free option)
- Coconut oil for frying

In a medium bowl, combine the black beans, oats, rice, nutritional yeast, and cheese. Mix thoroughly with your hands.

In a blender, combine the onion, cilantro, coriander, paprika, mustard, and tamari. Blend just until mixed.

Add the onion mixture to the bean mixture; add salt and mix well. Adjust the seasoning with more salt, if desired. Add the breadcrumbs and mix with your hands until the mixture is firm to the touch and no longer sticky. You will find that the breadcrumbs and oats absorb the moisture and it will become harder to mix.

Form the mixture into 10 patties, ¾-inch thick. Heat a skillet over medium heat. Add a little coconut oil and fry the patties until lightly brown, about 1 minute per side.

Store in a covered container in the fridge for up to 5 days.

Nutritional Totals per Serving:
Calories: 226
Protein: 10.1 g
Carbohydrates: 39 g
Fat: 3.6 g
Fiber: 8.9 g

Garden "Meatballs"

Contributed by **Breana Wigley**, *bikini competitor*

These lentil-based "meatballs" are packed with flavor and take minutes to make. Grab your favorite legume or bean and enjoy them with your favorite pasta. This is a great recipe to make in an air fryer if you have one. Otherwise, they're just as delicious baked in the oven.

Serves 2 (makes 8 meatballs)

For the Meatballs:

2 cups vegetable broth or water

Sea salt, to taste

1 cup lentils

¼ cup diced carrots

¼ cup peas

¼ cup chopped mushrooms

¼ cup chopped onions

2 tablespoons tomato paste

2 tablespoons vital wheat gluten, breadcrumbs, or chickpea flour for a gluten-free option

1 tablespoon vegan Worcestershire sauce or Dale's liquid marinade

½ teaspoon extra-virgin olive oil

For the Sauce:

1 jar store-bought marinara sauce

1 tablespoon nutritional yeast

½ tablespoon garlic powder

½ tablespoon onion powder

½ tablespoon dried oregano

1 teaspoon cane sugar (optional)

For Assembly:

1 package of your favorite noodles

Make the meatballs: Preheat the oven to 375°F, if making the meatballs in the oven. In a medium pot, bring the broth or water to a boil. Add a pinch of salt and the lentils. Cook according to the package instructions until the lentils are tender, 20 to 25 minutes. Drain and set aside.

In another small pot, bring 2 cups of water to a boil. Add a pinch of salt and add the carrots and boil for 2-3 minutes. Add the peas and boil until just tender, about 1 minute. Drain and set aside.

In a food processor, combine the cooked lentils, carrots, and peas with the mushrooms, onions, tomato paste, wheat gluten (or alternative), and vegan Worcestershire sauce. Pulse until the mixture is just combined. Don't overmix or it will get mushy; three to four pulses will do the trick.

Form the mixture into 8 meatballs. They should be roughly 1- to 1½-tablespoons-sized.

If making the meatballs in an air fryer, line the air fryer with foil and coat it with the oil. Air fry on 375°F for 12 to 13 minutes, checking after 10 minutes. The meatballs should be golden brown and cooked through.

Otherwise, line a baking sheet with foil and coat it with the oil. Bake for 20 minutes, until the meatballs are golden brown and cooked through.

Allow the meatballs to cool slightly before removing them from the foil; otherwise, they may stick.

Make the sauce: In a medium pot over medium-low heat, combine the marinara sauce with the nutritional yeast, garlic powder, onion powder, oregano, and sugar, if using. Simmer for 5 to 7 minutes, stirring frequently. When the flavors have melded, add the meatballs, coating them in the sauce. Serve over pasta.

Nutritional Totals per Serving:
Calories: 588
Protein: 36.2 g
Carbohydrates: 102.4 g
Fat: 7.1 g
Fiber: 17.7 g

Asian Noodle Bowl

Contributed by **Sonya Looney,** *mountain biker*

This is one of my favorite bowls because it comes together quickly, is loaded with a variety of vegetables, and is super satisfying. I highly recommend doubling or tripling the peanut sauce and storing it in the fridge for future ready-in-a-minute meals.

Serves 2

For the Peanut Sauce:

4 tablespoons peanut butter

2 tablespoons tamari or soy sauce

Juice of 1 lime

2 teaspoons chili garlic sauce

For the Noodles:

1 (8-ounce) package smoked tofu, sliced

1 (9-ounce) package buckwheat soba noodles (or any whole grain, if you want to avoid noodles)

1 cup shiitake mushrooms, sliced

½ cup bean sprouts

½ cup shredded carrots (you can buy them shredded to save a step)

½ red or orange bell pepper, seeded and sliced

Black sesame seeds, for serving

Make the peanut sauce: Combine all the ingredients in a blender with 2 tablespoons of water and blend until smooth. Set aside.

Make the noodles: In a large nonstick pan over medium-low heat, dry-fry the smoked tofu until warmed through, about 3 minutes. Remove the tofu from the pan and set aside. Add 1 tablespoon of water to the pan and add the mushrooms. Sauté until tender, about 5 minutes.

Cook the soba noodles according to the package instructions. Add them to the bottom of your bowl and top with the mushrooms and tofu. Add the peanut sauce, toss to coat, and top with the sprouts, carrots, peppers, and sesame seeds.

Nutritional Totals per Serving:
Calories: 500
Protein: 32.4 g
Carbohydrates: 51 g

Fat: 23.7 g
Fiber: 12.2 g

Vegan Mac & Cheese
with Carrot-Potato Cheese Sauce

Contributed by **Julia Murray,** *former Olympic skier,*
plant-based nutritionist

You won't miss butter, cheese, and cream thanks to this reinvention of a comfort food classic. Not only are you taking out foods that aren't doing your health any favors; you're also adding high-nutrient ingredients such as carrots, potatoes, and nutritional yeast. Nutritional yeast has a nutty, cheeselike flavor; is loaded with minerals, vitamins, and antioxidants; and is particularly good at repairing cell damage and decreasing inflammation.

Serves 4

For the Carrot-Potato Cheese Sauce:

3 medium russet potatoes, peeled and chopped

4 large carrots, chopped

1 garlic clove

1 teaspoon onion powder

¼ cup miso paste

⅛ cup Dijon mustard

¾ cup nutritional yeast

Juice of 1 lemon

1 teaspoon apple cider vinegar

¾ cup unsweetened, unflavored soy milk

Sea salt and freshly ground black pepper, to taste

For the Pasta:

1 large head of broccoli, chopped into florets (save stalks for your
next hummus plate as dippers!)

1 (16-ounce) package of pasta of choice

1 teaspoon avocado oil or other high-heat oil of choice

1 package vegan sausage (I use Field Roast brand)

Smoky Vegan Parmesan (page 325) or store-bought vegan
parmesan for serving

Make the Carrot-Potato Cheese Sauce: In a steamer or a large pot with a
couple inches of water on the bottom, steam the potatoes and carrots until
you can easily pierce them with a fork, 10 to 15 minutes.

Transfer them to a blender and combine with the remaining ingredients.
Blend until smooth. You may need to use the tamper to get it going, but it'll
get silky after a couple minutes.

In a steamer or large pot with a couple of inches of water at the bottom,
steam the broccoli until tender, about 5 minutes. Set aside.

Cook the pasta for 1 minute less than the package instructions.

Meanwhile, heat the oil in a large pan over medium heat. Add the sausage
and cook, flipping every minute or so until evenly browned and warmed
through, about 5 minutes. Set aside.

Strain the pasta, then add it to the pan with the sausage. Toss in the
broccoli and smother with the cheese sauce. Mix until everything is well
coated and creamy, sprinkle with vegan parm, and serve.

Nutritional Totals per Serving (including cheese sauce):
Calories: 960   Fat: 13.9 g
Protein: 57.6 g   Fiber: 37.5 g
Carbohydrates: 167.9 g

3-Bean Tempeh Chili

Contributed by **Robert Cheeke**, *bodybuilder*

This chili is delicious, filling, and quick and easy to make, and it hits the mark for low calories and high nutrient density. It makes a big batch and tastes even better the next day, so it's perfect for cooking over the weekend and eating throughout the week. You could also transfer it to smaller containers and store it in the freezer until you're ready to defrost and reheat. It never gets old because you can load it up with your favorite toppings. Enjoy it after a workout or for lunch or dinner.

Serves 4

2 cloves garlic, minced

½ onion, diced

3 stalks celery, diced

3 carrots, diced

½ green bell pepper, seeded and diced

1 (8-ounce) package tempeh, crumbled

1 tablespoon ground cumin

½ tablespoon chili powder (use less if you prefer less heat)

1½ cups cooked (or one 15.5-ounce can, drained and rinsed)
   black beans

1½ cups cooked (or one 15.5-ounce can, drained and rinsed)
   pinto beans

1½ cups cooked (or one 15.5-ounce can, drained and rinsed)
   red kidney beans

1 (14.5-ounce) can diced tomatoes (preferably fire roasted)

1 (4.5-ounce) can roasted green chilies

1 cup frozen or fresh corn

Sliced avocado for serving (optional)

Sliced tomato for serving (optional)

Shredded romaine lettuce for serving (optional)

Sliced black olives for serving (optional)

Crushed red pepper flakes to taste (optional)

Bread or crackers for serving (optional)

In a large pot over medium heat, add 2 tablespoons water and sauté the garlic, onion, celery, carrots, and pepper for 5 minutes, or until the vegetables have started to soften. Add the crumbled tempeh, cumin, and chili powder and continue to cook for a few more minutes as the flavors come together, adding water as needed to prevent burning. Add the remaining ingredients plus 1 cup of water, reduce the heat to low, and simmer until heated through and thickened slightly, about 20 minutes.

Serve with your toppings of choice and, if desired, a side of bread or crackers.

Nutritional Totals per Serving (excluding optional toppings):
Calories: 465
Protein: 32.2 g
Carbohydrates: 71.3 g
Fat: 8.7 g
Fiber: 23.9 g

Raise-the-Roof Sweet Potato–Vegetable Lasagna

Contributed by **Rip Esselstyn**, *swimmer and firefighter*
From his book The Engine 2 Cookbook

I prepared this lasagna for my first cooking demonstration at the new Whole Foods Market Culinary Center in Austin, Texas. Tim Lafuente, an award-winning chef who is also an Austin firefighter, asked me to join him at this event, where he made an angel hair pasta with chicken, bacon, butter, and oil. Firefighters are competitive, so the demonstration quickly turned into a contest. No one was declared the winner, but I walked away with my head high because the lasagna was a smashing success: another triumph for plant-happy cuisine!

This lasagna is so good that my wife and I chose this to be the main dish at our wedding reception.

Serves 10

1 onion, chopped
1 small head of garlic, all cloves chopped or pressed
8 ounces mushrooms, sliced

1 head of broccoli, chopped

2 carrots, chopped

2 red bell peppers, seeded and chopped

1 (15.5-ounce) can of corn, rinsed and drained

1 (16-ounce) package firm tofu

½ teaspoon cayenne pepper

1 teaspoon chopped fresh oregano

1 teaspoon chopped fresh basil

1 teaspoon chopped fresh rosemary

2 (24-ounce) jars store-bought pasta sauce

2 (16-ounce) boxes whole-grain lasagna noodles

16 ounces frozen spinach, thawed and drained

2 sweet potatoes, cooked and mashed

6 Roma tomatoes, sliced thin

1 cup raw cashews, ground

Preheat the oven to 400°F. In a wok or nonstick pan over high heat, add a tablespoon of water and sauté the onion and garlic until tender, 3 minutes. Add the mushrooms and cook until they become limp and give up their liquid, about 5 minutes. Transfer the mushroom mixture to a large bowl with a slotted spoon. Reserve the mushroom liquid in the pan.

Add the broccoli and carrots to the pan and cook for 5 minutes, until just tender but not mushy. Transfer to the bowl with the mushrooms. Sauté the peppers and corn until just soft, about 3 minutes, and add them to the vegetable bowl.

Drain the tofu by wrapping it in paper towels. Carefully crumble it into the bowl with the vegetables. Add the spices and toss to combine.

Cover the bottom of a 9-by-13-inch casserole dish with a layer of sauce. Add a layer of noodles and then cover the noodles with more sauce. (The noodles will cook in the sauce as the lasagna bakes, saving you time and hassle.) Evenly spread the vegetable mixture over the sauced noodles. Cover with another layer of noodles and another dressing of sauce. Spread the spinach over the second layer of sauced noodles. Cover the spinach with the mashed sweet potatoes, followed by another layer of sauce, a final layer of noodles, and one last layer of sauce. Arrange the sliced tomatoes over the top of the lasagna, cover the pan with foil, and bake for 45 minutes. Remove the foil, sprinkle the top of the lasagna with the cashews, and bake for another 15 minutes. Let the lasagna rest at room temperature for 15 minutes before serving.

Nutritional Totals per Serving:

Calories: 612

Fat: 14.5 g

Protein: 29.5 g

Fiber: 18.3 g

Carbohydrates: 101.9 g

Taco Bake

Contributed by **Breana Wigley**, *bikini competitor*

This simple Taco Tuesday-inspired dish is great for feeding a family, entertaining guests, or just making batch meals for yourself. You can spice things up by serving this over tortilla chips or multigrain tortillas or go with fresh, crisp greens.

And you don't have to wait until Tuesday to make it; any day is a great day for a taco bake.

Note: If you don't have instant rice, you can use another variety. Just bake for 45 minutes, or until the rice is tender.

Serves 6

2 tablespoons vegetable oil of choice (I like grapeseed oil), divided

8 to 10 ounces protein of choice (tofu, seitan, tempeh)

1 packet of taco seasoning

2 cups seeded and sliced bell pepper (I like a mix of red and green)

1 yellow onion, sliced

1 cup instant rice

2 cups vegetable broth

1 to 2 (15.5-ounce) cans black beans (low-sodium), drained and rinsed

1 cup frozen corn kernels

1 (10-ounce) can RO-TEL brand fire-roasted tomatoes

2 cups fresh spinach

2 tablespoons shredded dairy-free cheese

Chopped red onion for serving

1 ripe avocado, mashed, for serving

Chopped fresh cilantro for serving

Preheat the oven to 400°F. Heat 1 tablespoon of the oil in a large skillet over medium heat. Add your protein of choice and season with a generous pinch of the taco seasoning. Cook for 7 to 8 minutes or until the protein is cooked through. Transfer to a small bowl and set aside.

Add 3 tablespoons of water to the skillet over medium-high heat. Add the bell peppers and onions and season with a pinch of the taco blend. Cook until the peppers are tender and the onions are slightly translucent, 5 to 7 minutes. Remove the pan from the heat and set aside.

Lightly oil a medium casserole dish with the remaining oil. (You may not need an entire tablespoon.) Spread the rice evenly over the bottom of the dish and pour over the veggie broth. Next, create a layer of the beans and sprinkle them with the remaining taco seasoning. Add a layer of the cooked protein, followed by the corn, fire-roasted tomatoes, spinach, pepper and onion mixture, and, finally, the shredded cheese. Do not stir to combine! You want your taco bake to have beautiful layers of all the ingredients.

Tightly cover the dish with foil and bake for 30 to 35 minutes, until the rice is tender and has absorbed all the liquid. Remove the foil and bake for an additional 10 to 15 minutes, or until the cheese is bubbly and slightly browned.

Top with red onion, mashed avocado, and a sprinkle of cilantro.

Nutritional Totals per Serving:

Calories: 287	Fat: 8.1 g
Protein: 14.5 g	Fiber: 12.3 g
Carbohydrates: 42.7 g	

DESSERT

Healthy Fudge Bars

Contributed by **Laura Kline**, *duathlete*

Dessert?? Yes, I do sometimes enjoy a sweet treat when I'm in peak training. For when the craving strikes, I keep these date-based fudge bars on hand.

Serves 8

1 cup pitted dates

½ cup almonds

¼ cup walnuts

½ cup unsweetened cocoa powder, divided

2 ripe bananas

¼ cup almond butter

¼ cup agave nectar

Soak the dates in warm water for 30 minutes, then drain.

In the bowl of a food processor, combine the dates, almonds, walnuts, and ¼ cup of the cocoa. Blend until the mixture is well combined. Press the mixture into the bottom of a 9-by-5-inch or 8-by-8-inch baking pan and set aside.

Wipe out the bowl of the food processor and combine the bananas, almond butter, agave, and remaining ¼ cup cocoa powder. Blend until the mixture is well combined. Spread it evenly over the date mixture and freeze for at least 30 minutes before cutting into 8 equal bars. These should be stored in the freezer—just pop one out and let it thaw when you want one!

Nutritional Totals per Serving:

Calories: 232. 8   Fat: 11.6 g

Protein: 5.8 g   Fiber: 6.8 g

Carbohydrates: 34 g

Raw Frozen Banana Truffles

Contributed by **Matt Frazier**, *ultramarathoner*

These truffles, created by my sister, Christine, are what I like to call "sneaky healthy." With very little added sugar plus some healthy fat from tahini, you get a sweet, satisfying ice cream-like bite. It also doesn't hurt that bananas help store glycogen in your muscles and use it for fuel.

Makes about 14 1-inch truffles

- **4 very ripe frozen bananas, chopped**
- **2 tablespoons tahini**
- **4 teaspoons maple syrup**
- **2 teaspoons alcohol-free vanilla extract**
- **½ teaspoon sea salt**
- **⅓ cup cocoa powder**
- **½ cup shredded unsweetened coconut, finely chopped**
- **½ cup walnuts, finely chopped**

In a stand mixer fitted with the paddle attachment or a blender, combine the bananas, tahini, maple syrup, vanilla, and salt. Mix until smooth and creamy. Taste and adjust the sweetness with more agave if desired.

Pour the mixture into three pint-sized containers and freeze until solid, 4 hours up to overnight.

When ready to make your truffles, spread the cocoa, coconut, and walnuts over individual plates. Remove one container of the banana mixture from the freezer. Using a melon baller or mini ice cream scoop, create a bite-size truffle from the frozen banana mixture. Roll the truffle in one of the toppings to coat. Repeat with the remaining truffles—working as quickly as possible—then return the coated truffles to the container and freeze once again. Repeat the process with the second and third containers of the banana mixture.

Freeze the truffles until firm, about 1 hour, before serving. Or store them in the freezer for up to 2 weeks.

Nutritional Totals per Serving (based on 14 servings):

Calories: 99

Fat: 6.1 g

Protein: 2 g

Fiber: 2.6 g

Carbohydrates: 11.4 g

Avocado Mousse

Contributed by **James Newbury**, *CrossFit athlete*

This sweet treat takes minutes to throw together and delivers the kind of creamy, chocolaty decadence that you need every once in a while, not to mention healthy fats from the avocado and calcium, iron, magnesium, and antioxidants from the cacao.

Serves 1

- **1 avocado**
- **1 tablespoon raw cacao**
- **1 tablespoon pure maple syrup**
- **1 pinch of sea salt**
- **Dash of almond milk**

Blend everything together in a food processor or blender until smooth. Eat immediately or chill in the fridge for a more fudgelike consistency.

Nutritional Totals per Serving:
Calories: 378   Fat: 28.1 g
Protein: 4 g   Fiber: 11 g
Carbohydrates: 32.5 g

Sweet Potato Brownies

Contributed by **Meagan Duhamel**, *figure skater*

This recipe's secret weapon: sweet potatoes! High in vitamins A, B_5, B_6, and C; potassium; and fiber, sweet potatoes are incredibly versatile. Here is a yummy and chocolaty brownie recipe chock-full of sweet potato nutrients.

Makes 16 brownies

- **1 cup coconut sugar**
- **¾ cup mashed sweet potatoes**
- **½ cup nut butter (I like peanut butter)**
- **½ cup cacao powder**
- **⅓ cup all-purpose flour (I use Bob's Red Mill gluten-free blend)**

1 teaspoon baking powder

1 teaspoon vanilla extract

½ cup chocolate chips or chunks

Preheat the oven to 350°F. In a large bowl, combine the sugar, sweet potatoes, nut butter, cacao, flour, baking powder, and vanilla. Mix well. Fold in the chocolate chips.

Pour the batter into a 9-by-9-inch baking dish and bake for 40 minutes, until the edges are crisp and the center is gooey but cooked through. Let the brownies cool for 15 minutes before slicing into 16 equal bars.

Nutritional Totals per Serving:

Calories: 183   Fat: 6.7 g

Protein: 4.9 g   Fiber: 4.1 g

Carbohydrates: 29 g

Protein Pudding

Contributed by **Vanessa Espinoza**, *powerlifter*

Once again, here's more proof that you don't have to go without when you're eating a plant-based diet. Not only can you satisfy your sweet tooth; you can also satisfy your daily macro needs.

If you don't have a high-speed blender, you will need to soak the cashews overnight, and this pudding is best served chilled after a few hours—so it does require a little advance planning. But otherwise, it's very easy to make.

Serves 4

1 cup cashews

1 package silken tofu

2 scoops chocolate protein powder (I like TRU plant-based protein powder)

2 tablespoons pure maple syrup

2 tablespoons cocoa powder

1 teaspoon vanilla extract

In a blender, add 1 cup of water with all the ingredients. Blend until smooth.

Nutritional Totals per Serving:

Calories: 345	Fat: 18 g
Protein: 26.8 g	Fiber: 2.2 g
Carbohydrates: 21.3 g	

Banana Bread

Contributed by **Christine Vardaros**, *cyclist*

Banana bread is one of my favorite treats to make. As a vegan for more than twenty years, I don't feel I'm ever missing out on anything, as I focus on lots of variety with my meals. But since I typically eat for athletic performance, focusing primarily on healthy, whole-plant foods, banana bread is a guilty pleasure of mine, especially after a grueling race or when I have a day off from training. To make it even more decadent, you can sprinkle it with a crumble topping before it bakes—though it's just as delicious without it. I hope you love it as much as I do!

Makes 1 loaf

Serves 6

For the Crumble Topping (optional):
- **2 tablespoons all-purpose flour**
- **½ teaspoon cinnamon**
- **¼ teaspoon nutmeg**
- **1 tablespoon margarine, coarsely chopped**

For the Banana Bread:
- **¼ cup soy milk**
- **1 teaspoon apple cider vinegar**
- **1 cup all-purpose flour**
- **1 cup whole-wheat flour**
- **½ cup granulated sugar**
- **½ cup brown sugar**

½ teaspoon baking soda

1 teaspoon cinnamon

½ teaspoon nutmeg

½ teaspoon sea salt

3 ripe bananas, mashed

½ cup margarine, softened, plus more for greasing the pan

1 teaspoon vanilla extract

Make the crumble topping: In a small bowl, combine the flour, cinnamon, nutmeg, and margarine. Stir until the mixture takes on a crumbly consistency.

Make the banana bread: Preheat the oven to 350°F. Grease a loaf pan with margarine or line it with parchment paper. Set aside.

In a small bowl, combine the soy milk and apple cider vinegar. Set aside.

In a large bowl, combine the flours, sugars, baking soda, cinnamon, nutmeg, and salt. Mix well. Fold in the soy milk and vinegar, mashed bananas, softened margarine, and vanilla. Mix until well combined.

Pour the batter into the prepared loaf pan. If adding the topping, evenly crumble it over the batter. Bake for 1 hour to 1 hour and 15 minutes, until a toothpick or sharp knife inserted into the center comes out clean.

Nutritional Totals per Serving
(without optional crumble topping):

Calories: 382	Fat: 16 g
Protein: 5.9 g	Fiber: 4.6 g
Carbohydrates: 56.4 g	

Coconut Caramel Cookies

Contributed by **Christine Vardaros**, *cyclist*

This is my go-to recipe when I need to get into a happy zone. Whether it is the day after a race when I didn't perform well, or a day after I rocked a training or a race, this cookie never, ever fails to lift my spirits. And the best thing about it is that it is (almost) guilt free!

Note: You could also dip the bottom of each cookie in chocolate for an extra chocolate kick. Just increase the melted chocolate to ⅓ cup and the coconut oil to ¾ teaspoon. Dip the base of each cookie in the chocolate first, then lay them on the tray and drizzle the remaining chocolate over the top.

Serves 4

½ teaspoon coconut oil, plus more for greasing

1 cup shredded unsweetened coconut

1 cup dates

¼ cup dark chocolate chips or bar

Preheat the oven to 375°F. Lightly grease a baking sheet or large plate with the coconut oil and set aside.

Spread the coconut over a clean, dry baking sheet and toast it in the oven until golden brown, about 3 minutes. Keep a close eye on it so as not to burn it.

In a blender, combine the toasted coconut with the dates and blend until the mixture comes together. Form the mixture into 2-inch balls and arrange them on the prepared baking sheet or plate. Flatten them slightly with your thumb. Freeze for 20 minutes.

Melt the chocolate (30 seconds in the microwave does the trick). Stir in the coconut oil. Drizzle the mixture over the cookies, then return the cookies to the freezer until the chocolate is set, at least 10 minutes.

Nutritional Totals per Serving:

Calories: 267	Fat: 19.5 g
Protein: 2.9 g	Fiber: 5.3 g
Carbohydrates: 23.6 g	

CONDIMENTS, DIPS, AND DRESSINGS

Cucumber Avocado Dressing

Contributed by **Brendan Brazier**, *ultramarathoner*

From his book Thrive Energy Cookbook

A clever and tasty way to pack more vegetables into your salad.

Makes 8 ¼-cup servings

- 2 medium English cucumbers, peeled and coarsely chopped
- 1 ripe avocado, peeled and coarsely hopped
- 2 large handfuls fresh cilantro leaves
- 2 medium garlic cloves, peeled
- ½ cup fresh lime juice
- ¼ cup plus 2 tablespoons grapeseed oil
- ¼ cup plus 2 tablespoons filtered water
- 1½ tablespoons sea salt, plus more to taste
- ¼ teaspoon freshly ground black pepper

In a blender, combine all the ingredients. Blend on high speed until smooth and creamy. Season with salt to taste. Keep in a sealed container in the fridge for up to 1 week.

Nutritional Totals per Serving:

Calories: 132	Fat: 12.9 g
Protein: 0.8 g	Fiber: 1.9 g
Carbohydrates: 5 g	

Shiitake Bacon

Contributed by **Matt Frazier**, *ultramarathoner*

Sometimes you just need a little something chewy, salty, and smoky. Make a batch of these crispy mushroom bits and you'll have the perfect finishing touch for stir-fries, grain bowls, salads, soups, and tofu scrambles.

Makes about 1 cup

8 ounces shiitake mushrooms, thinly sliced

1 tablespoon extra-virgin olive oil

½ teaspoon sea salt

⅛ teaspoon freshly ground black pepper

Pinch of sweet smoked paprika

Preheat the oven to 350°F. On a baking sheet, toss the mushrooms with the olive oil, salt, pepper, and paprika. Bake for 25 minutes, or until crispy on the outside and still barely chewy on the inside.

Nutritional Totals per Serving (1 cup):
Calories: 197   Fat: 14.6 g
Protein: 5.1 g   Fiber: 5.7 g
Carbohydrates: 15.6 g

Smoky Vegan Parmesan

Contributed by **Julia Murray,** *former Olympic skier, plant-based nutritionist*

Any of your savory dishes will benefit from a sprinkle of this better-than-the-real-thing "cheese." Cashews provide you with 100 percent of your copper needs (crucial for metabolizing iron and fueling energy production in the body); paprika (which is ground-up red pepper) is packed with antioxidants and anti-inflammatory properties, and sunflower seeds are another amazing source of copper, in addition to vitamin E and vitamin B_1, which helps break down fats and protein and improves cardiovascular function.

Makes 4 ¼-cup servings

¾ cup raw cashews

1 tablespoon sunflower seeds

¼ cup nutritional yeast

1 teaspoon garlic powder

¼ teaspoon smoked paprika

¾ teaspoon sea salt

In a mini food processor or a blender or spice grinder, blend the ingredients until the mixture resembles a parmesan-like consistency. It should take about 30 seconds. Store in a covered container in the fridge for up to 3 weeks.

Nutritional Totals per Serving:

Calories: 204   Fat: 12.4 g

Protein: 12.6 g   Fiber: 4.6 g

Carbohydrates: 13.7 g

Mind-Blowing (Nut-Free) Vegan Cheese Sauce

Contributed by **Julia Murray,** *former Olympic skier,*
plant-based nutritionist

This is an all-purpose sauce that not only scratches the itch when you want something gooey and cheesy but also delivers tons of nutrition thanks to cauliflower, carrots, onions, and garlic. Mix it into pasta, drizzle it over vegetables, serve it as a dip, or just eat it by the spoonful.

Makes 4 ¾-cup servings

1 medium head cauliflower, roughly chopped

6 medium carrots, chopped

½ large sweet onion, diced (or 1 tablespoon onion powder)

2 garlic cloves (or 1 tablespoon garlic powder)

¾ cup nutritional yeast

1 tablespoon Dijon mustard

1 tablespoon miso paste

¼ teaspoon ground turmeric

⅛ teaspoon smoked paprika (optional, but it lends a nice
   smoky flavor)

1 cup unsweetened almond milk (or any other plain plant-based
   milk)

Use a steamer or a large pot with an inch of water in the bottom to steam the cauliflower and carrots until tender, about 10 minutes.

Meanwhile, in a large pan over medium heat, add a tablespoon of water and sauté the onion and garlic until tender and turning golden brown, about 7 minutes. (Skip this step if using onion and garlic powder.) Add more water to the pan as needed if the vegetables begin to stick. Once the vegetables have browned, add 1 to 2 tablespoons water to the pan while scraping up any brown bits from the bottom with your wooden spoon or spatula.

Combine the onion and garlic mixture, cauliflower, and carrots in a blender with the remaining ingredients. Blend until smooth. If serving as a dip, transfer the sauce to an oven-safe dish and broil on high for 3 minutes, until golden and bubbly.

Nutritional Totals per Serving:

Calories: 264

Fat: 3.5 g

Protein: 27.5 g

Fiber: 16.6 g

Carbohydrates: 35.6 g

Edamame-Spinach Hummus

Contributed by **Natalie Matthews**, *bikini competitor and fitness model*

It's not shocking news that hummus is a healthy snack, but this recipe takes it to the next level and is packed with more nutrients than any hummus you could buy at the store. It's is a great way to sneak in some extra greens and has added protein from the edamame. Eat this with raw vegetables or spread on a sandwich.

Makes 6 servings

1 cup shelled edamame

1 cup fresh spinach

3 tablespoons fresh lemon juice

2 tablespoons tahini

1 tablespoon nutritional yeast

1 teaspoon agave nectar

½ teaspoon onion powder

½ teaspoon garlic powder
¼ teaspoon sea salt

Combine all the ingredients in a food processor or blender. Blend thoroughly on high until smooth. Store in a covered container in the refrigerator for up to 1 week.

Nutritional Totals per Serving:

Calories: 76	Fat: 3.7 g
Protein: 5.1 g	Fiber: 2 g
Carbohydrates: 6.5 g	

ACKNOWLEDGMENTS

Matt Frazier would like to thank:

Erin, Holden, and Ellarie Frazier, the three vegan athletes who inspire me the most. Everything I do is for you guys, first.

Robert Cheeke, my friend and coauthor, a true godfather of this movement, and the first vegan athlete who moved me to want to do it too. What an honor it is to have my name on the same book as yours.

Dr. Michael Greger, whose support of this project, my previous work, and most important, the plant-based movement, means so much.

All of the vegan athletes featured in this book, whose willingness to stand apart from the crowd I admire deeply. Thank you for sharing your stories, and for inspiring the next generation of plant-based athletes.

Matt Tullman, my friend and business partner. I'm endlessly grateful for the wisdom, drive, trust, and enormous vision you bring to our partnership—and for all the work you've done to build this incredible group of people we get to call our team.

Our teams at No Meat Athlete, Complement, 80/20 Plants, and Plant Bites: Doug Hay, Esther Jaffa, Jerry Sever, Andrew Carter, Michael Palm, Chris Lambrou, Julia Murray, Matt Jager, Izzy Fischer, Alyssa Hodenfield, Mckenna Walker, and Emilia Guidobono. I'm continually made proud by the magic you do every day, and especially by how deeply each of you cares about this mission and our work.

Our broader community of partners in these brands: Dr. Joel Kahn, Ocean Robbins, T. K. Pillan, Marco Antonio Regil, and Brian and Andrea Borg.

Seth Godin and Brian Clark, my earliest mentors in writing and marketing, without whom nothing would look or feel the same.

Sydney Rogers at HarperOne, Rachel Holtzman, and Janis Donnaud, the true professionals who have helped to shape this project into what it is—something larger and more beautiful than we ever envisioned.

Finally, every individual who's a part of the No Meat Athlete community. It's such a privilege to be able to do this work for you, and I'm so grateful for your eagerness to engage with it and share it—and, most of all, for your drive to make this world better.

Robert Cheeke would like to thank:

Karen Oxley, my beautiful wife and partner for more than ten years. Karen, thank you for supporting me through a full decade of writing self-published books, which led to this book that we're so proud of. The expression rings true, I couldn't have done it without you. I love you, and I thank you for your thoughtfulness, your patience, and your belief that this was possible.

Benny and Ellie, our rescued Chihuahuas who spent countless hours sleeping by my feet while I worked on this book for years, keeping me company during long days and late nights.

Matt Frazier, my friend and coauthor, who has taught me so much about priorities and what is truly important in life. Matt, we did it. Thank you for your commitment to excellence in this pursuit, and for your passion for this movement. You are an inspiration to many.

Dr. Michael Greger, because his work has had such an important impact on our lives, and he has played a critical role in how Matt and I approach plant-based nutrition. What an honor it is to have your support, Dr. Greger. We are grateful and honored to have your endorsement for such a meaningful project.

My mother, Edna, and my father, Peter, who encouraged me to follow my dreams to create truly meaningful work. And to my sister, Tanya, who inspired me to become vegan more than a quarter century ago. It is because of my greatest influences that this book became a reality.

My teachers, Carol Young, Lillian Smith, Eric Dazey, Tony Vandermeer, and Maynard Freemole, for embracing my dream of becoming a writer, helping me believe as far back as third grade, that I would someday be in this position, writing an impactful book that will make a difference in the lives of thousands of individuals.

My childhood friend, Jordan Baskerville, who not only introduced me to the sport of bodybuilding, making my role in the plant-based athlete community relevant, but who has also supported my writing career from day one, challenging me to create my best work.

Charles Chang, Shawn Kowalewski, Satish Karandikar, Shaleen Shah, Chris Chamberlin, and Susan Peters, for giving me the opportunity to pursue my passion for writing, while I worked full-time for entities such as Vega and Vegan Strong.

Brian Wendel for giving me an opportunity to work for Forks Over Knives, which changed the way I approached plant-based nutrition, and for introducing me to Janis Donnaud, which ultimately led to this book becoming a reality.

Janis Donnaud, Rachel Holtzman, Sydney Rogers and the Harper-One team for taking a chance on this book, for guiding us through the publishing process, and for truly believing this book could become a big success. We are grateful for your vision, your wisdom, and your guidance, and we are so proud of what we created together.

Dotsie Bausch for introducing me to amazing plant-based athletes I had the honor of interviewing for the book, and Rip Esselstyn for helping me discover incredible plant-based athletes who had been flying under the radar.

Linda Plowright, MD, Christine Kestner, MS, T. Colin Campbell, PhD, Caldwell B. Esselstyn Jr., MD, and Michael Klaper, MD, the experts who were the first to support this book, and whose work has been such an inspiration to me over the years.

Sheryl and Bob Greenberg for their generous support of my writing career over the years, which has meant so much to me.

The nearly 100 plant-based athletes we interviewed for this book, for paving the way to a more compassionate future for all of us, through your example of what it means to be a successful plant-based athlete.

Kai Wu and Matt Sedlacek for their mentorship, their vision, and for injecting their creative spark into www.veganbodybuilding.com, shaping it into what it is today.

Lastly, my Vegan Bodybuilding & Fitness community, many of whom have been with me for nearly twenty years. Thank you for your years of support, encouragement, friendship, and dedication to the plant-based athlete lifestyle. This book is the result of all of your support over the years, and I thank you.

NOTES

Chapter 1: Becoming a Plant-Based Athlete

1   Sean Coughlan, "Gladiators Were 'Mostly Vegetarian,'" BBC News, October 22, 2014, https://www.bbc.com/news/education-29723384#:~:text=Roman%20gladiators%20had%20a%20diet,the%20arena%20fighters%20were%20buried.&text=They%20found%20the%20gladiator%20diet,drink%20made%20from%20plant%20ashes.

Chapter 2: Understanding the Power Behind the Food: Macronutrients, Micronutrients, and Calorie Density

1   G. H. Boutros et al., "Is a Vegan Diet Detrimental to Endurance and Muscle Strength?," *European Journal of Clinical Nutrition* (April 24, 2020), https://doi.org/10.1038/s41430-020-0639-y.
2   K. Wirnitzer et al., "Health Status of Female and Male Vegetarian and Vegan Endurance Runners Compared to Omnivores—Results from the NURMI Study (Step 2)," *Nutrients* 11, no. 1 (January 2019): 29, https://dx.doi.org/10.3390%2Fnu11010029.
3   N. D. Barnard et al., "Plant-Based Diets for Cardiovascular Safety and Performance in Endurance Sports," *Nutrients* 11, no. 1 (January 2019): 130, https://dx.doi.org/10.3390%2Fnu11010130.
4   "Macronutrients: The Importance of Carbohydrate, Protein, and Fat," McKinley Health Center, Univ. of Illinois at Urbana-Champaign, February 4, 2014, https://mckinley.illinois.edu/sites/default/files/docs/macronutrients.pdf.

Chapter 3: It's Time to Have the Protein Talk

1   K. M. Mangano et al., "Dietary Protein Is Associated with Musculoskeletal Health Independently of Dietary Pattern: The Framingham Third Generation Study," *American Journal of Clinical Nutrition* 105, no. 3 (March 2017): 714–722, https://doi.org/10.3945/ajcn.116.136762.

2 S. Mettler, C. Mannhart, and P. C. Colombani, "Development and Validation of a Food Pyramid for Swiss Athletes," *International Journal of Sport Nutrition and Exercise Metabolism* 19, no. 5 (October 2009): 504–518, https://doi.org /10.1123/ijsnem.19.5.504.

3 W. Chai et al., "Dietary Red and Processed Meat Intake and Markers of Adiposity and Inflammation: The Multiethnic Cohort Study," *Journal of the American College of Nutrition* 36, no. 5 (2017): 378–385, https://dx.doi.org/10 .1080%2F07315724.2017.1318317.

4 GBD 2017 Causes of Death Collaborators, "Global, Regional, and National Age-Sex-Specific Mortality for 282 Causes of Death in 195 Countries and Territories, 1980–2017: A Systematic Analysis for the Global Burden of Disease Study 2017," *Lancet* 392, no. 10159 (November 10, 2018): 1736–1788, https://doi.org/10.1016/S0140-6736(18)32203-7.

5 Loma Linda University Adventist Health Sciences Center, "New Study Associates Intake of Dairy Milk with Greater Risk of Breast Cancer: Evidence Suggests Consistently Drinking as Little as One Cup per Day May Increase Rate of Breast Cancer up to 50%," *ScienceDaily*, February 25, 2020, https:// www.sciencedaily.com/releases/202%2/200225101323.htm.

6 S.-W. Park et al., "A Milk Protein, Casein, as a Proliferation Promoting Factor in Prostate Cancer Cells," *World Journal of Men's Health* 32, no. 2 (August 2014): 76–82, https://dx.doi.org/10.5534%2Fwjmh.2014.32.2.76.

7 A. Thompson, "From Fish to Humans, a Microplastic Invasion May Be Taking a Toll," *Scientific American*, September 4, 2018, https://www.scientific american.com/article/from-fish-to-humans-a-microplastic-invasion-may -be-taking-a-toll/.

8 J. K. Nelson, "Expert Answers: Fish and Polychlorinated Biphenyls," FAQ-20348595, Healthy Lifestyle, Nutrition and Healthy Eating, Mayo Clinic, https://www.mayoclinic.org/healthy-lifestyle/nutrition-and-healthy-eating /expert-answers/fish-and-pbcs/faq-20348595#:~:text=Farmed%20salmon%20 that%20are%20fed,lakes%2C%20streams%20and%20drinking%20water.

9 "Thirsty Food: Fueling Agriculture to Fuel Humans," *National Geographic*, accessed June 2020, https://www.nationalgeographic.com/environment /freshwater/food/.

10 N. Babault, "Pea Proteins Oral Supplementation Promotes Muscle Thickness Gains During Resistance Training: A Double-Blind, Randomized, Placebo-Controlled Clinical Trial vs. Whey Protein," *Journal of the International Society of Sports Nutrition* 12, no. 3 (2015), https://dx.doi.org/10.1186%2Fs 12970-014-0064-5.

11 J. M. Joy et al., "The Effects of 8 Weeks of Whey or Rice Protein Supplementation on Body Composition and Exercise Performance," *Nutrition Journal* 12, no. 86 (2013), https://dx.doi.org/10.1186%2F1475-2891-12-86.

12 National Research Council, *Recommended Dietary Allowances*, 10th ed. (Washington, DC: National Academies Press, 1989).

13 D. T. Thomas, K. A. Erdman, and L. M. Burke, "Position of the Academy of

Nutrition and Dietetics, Dietitians of Canada, and the American College of Sports Medicine: Nutrition and Athletic Performance," *Journal of the Academy of Nutrition and Dietetics* 116, no. 3 (March 1, 2016): 501–528 , https://doi .org/10.1016/j.jand.2015.12.006.

14 "High-Protein Plant-Based Diet Versus a Protein-Matched Omnivorous Diet to Support Resistance Training Adaptations: A Comparison Between Habitual Vegans and Omnivores," https://link.springer.com/article/10.1007/s40279 -021-01434-9.

15 "Soy," NutritionFacts.org, accessed June 2020, https://nutritionfacts.org /topics/soy/.

16 G. Paul and G. J. Mendelson, "Evidence Supports the Use of Soy Protein to Promote Cardiometabolic Health and Muscle Development," *Journal of the American College of Nutrition* 34, no. sup1 (2015): 56–59, https://doi.org /10.108%7315724.2015.1080531.

Chapter 5: Fat: It's Not All Bad

1   G. Zong et al., "Monounsaturated Fats from Plant and Animal Sources in Relation to Risk of Coronary Heart Disease Among US Men and Women," *American Journal of Clinical Nutrition* 107, no. 3 (March 2018): 445–453, https://doi.org/10.1093/ajcn/nqx004.

Chapter 6: Supplements: Should I or Shouldn't I?

1   A. S. Prasad, "Zinc Is an Antioxidant and Anti-inflammatory Agent: Its Role in Human Health," *Frontiers in Nutrition* 1 (September 1, 2014), https://dx .doi.org/10.3389%2Ffnut.2014.00014.

2   M. Foster et al., "Effect of Vegetarian Diets on Zinc Status: A Systemic Review and Meta-analysis of Studies in Humans," *Journal of the Science of Food and Agriculture* 93, no. 10 (August 15, 2013): 2362–2371, https://doi.org/10.1002 /jsfa.6179.

3   M. Ruscigno, "What Every Vegetarian Needs to Know About Iron," No Meat Athlete, accessed June 2020, https://www.nomeatathlete.com/iron-for -vegetarians/.

4   S. J. Bailey et al., "Dietary Nitrate Supplementation Reduces the O_2 Cost of Low-Intensity Exercise and Enhances Tolerance to High-Intensity Exercise in Humans," *Journal of Applied Physiology* 107, no. 4 (October 2009): 1144–1155, https://doi.org/10.1152/japplphysiol.00722.2009.

5   J. L. Viana et al., "Evidence for Anti-inflammatory Effects of Exercise in CKD," *Journal of the American Society of Nephrology* 25, no. 9 (September 2014): 2121–2130, https://doi.org/10.1681/ASN.2013070702.

6   K. C. Carpenter et al., "Baker's Yeast ß-Glucan Supplementation Increases Monocytes and Cytokines Post-Exercise: Implications for Infection Risk?," *British Journal of Nutrition* 109, no. 3 (February 14, 2013): 478–486, https:// doi.org/10.1017/S0007114512001407.

7   S. Talbott and J. Talbott, "Effect of Beta 1, 3/1, 6 Glucan on Upper Respiratory

Tract Infection Symptoms and Mood State in Marathon Athletes," *Journal of Sports Science and Medicine* 8, no. 4 (December 1, 2009): 509–515.

8   T. C. Campbell, "Casein Is a Carcinogen," T. Colin Campbell Center for Nutrition Studies, December 4, 2014, updated January 4, 2019, https://nutritionstudies.org/provocations-casein-carcinogen-really/.

9   S.-W. Park et al., "A Milk Protein, Casein, as a Proliferation Promoting Factor in Prostate Cancer Cells," *World Journal of Men's Health* 32, no. 2 (2014): 76–82, https://dx.doi.org/10.5534%2Fwjmh.2014.32.2.76, https://www.ncbi.nlm.nih.gov/pmc/articles/PMC4166373/.

10 W. Lu et al., "Dairy Products Intake and Cancer Mortality Risk: A Meta-analysis of 11 Population-Based Cohort Studies," *Nutrition Journal* 15, no. 91 (2016), https://dx.doi.org/10.1186%2Fs12937-016-0210-9.

11 See https://www.health.harvard.edu/heart-health/brewing-evidence-for-teas-heart-benefit. See also D. M. Main, "Citrus Juice, Vitamin C Give Staying Power to Green Tea Antioxidants," Purdue University, November 13, 2007, https://www.purdue.edu/uns/x/2007b/071113FerruzziTea.html.

Chapter 8: Recover Better, Train More

1   "Foods That Fight Inflammation," Harvard Health Publishing, June 2014, updated August 29, 2020, https://www.health.harvard.edu/staying-healthy/foods-that-fight-inflammation.

2   G. Howatson et al., "Influence of Tart Cherry Juice on Indices of Recovery Following Marathon Running," *Scandinavian Journal of Medicine and Science in Sports* 20, no. 6 (December 2010): 843–852, https://doi.org/10.1111/j.1600-0838.2009.01005.x.

3   P. G. Bell et al., "Montmorency Cherries Reduce the Oxidative Stress and Inflammatory Responses to Repeated Days High-Intensity Stochastic Cycling," *Nutrients* 6, no. 2 (2014): 829–843, https://doi.org/10.3390/nu6020829.

4   Bell et al., "Montmorency Cherries"; J. L. Bowtell et al., "Montmorency Cherry Juice Reduces Muscle Damage Caused by Intensive Strength Exercise," *Medicine and Science in Sports and Exercise* 43, no. 8 (August 2011): 1544–1551, https://doi.org/10.1249/mss.0b013e31820e5adc.

5   Z. Yu et al., "Associations Between Nut Consumption and Inflammatory Biomarkers," *American Journal of Clinical Nutrition* 104, no. 3 (September 2016): 722–728, https://dx.doi.org/10.3945%2Fajcn.116.134205.

ABOUT THE AUTHORS

Matt Frazier is a vegan ultramarathoner and entrepreneur, best known as the founder of the No Meat Athlete movement. Matt's books have sold over 100,000 copies in five languages, and he and his work have been featured in books by Rich Roll, Seth Godin, and Kathy Freston; print magazines such as *Runner's World*, *Trail Runner*, *Outside*, *Health*, and *VegNews*, and other media including CNN, *Sports Illustrated*, *People*, *Huffington Post*, *Forbes*, *Business Insider*, and WebMD. Matt is the cofounder of Complement, 80/20 Plants, and Plant Bites, three brands that share a mission to grow the plant-based movement and help vegans thrive. He lives in Asheville, North Carolina, with his wife, two children, and rescued dog.

Robert Cheeke grew up on a farm in Corvallis, Oregon, where he adopted a vegan lifestyle in 1995 at age fifteen, weighing just 120 pounds. Today he is the author of the books *Vegan Bodybuilding & Fitness*, *Shred It!*, and *Plant-Based Muscle*. He is often referred to as the Godfather of Vegan Bodybuilding, having grown the industry from its infancy in 2002 to where it is today. As a two-time natural bodybuilding champion, Robert is one of *VegNews* magazine's Most Influential Vegan Athletes.

He tours the world sharing his story of transformation from a skinny farm kid to a champion vegan bodybuilder. Robert is the founder and president of Vegan Bodybuilding & Fitness and maintains the popular website VeganBodybuilding.com. He is a regular contributor to No Meat Athlete, Forks Over Knives, and Vegan Strong; is a multisport athlete and an entrepreneur; and has followed a plant-based diet for more than twenty-five years. Robert lives in Colorado with his wife and their two rescued Chihuahuas.

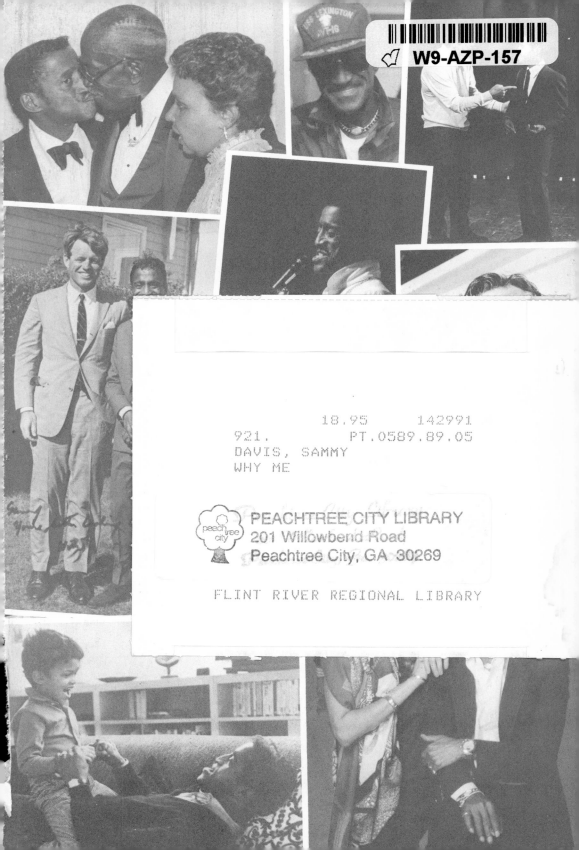

Why Me?

Also by Sammy Davis, Jr.,
and Jane and Burt Boyar

Yes I Can

Why Me?

The Sammy Davis, Jr.
Story

Sammy Davis, Jr.
and
Jane and Burt Boyar

Farrar, Straus and Giroux
New York

The authors would like to thank Jenny Plath,
their editor, for her taste and talent and for her
hard work, which have made this a better book.

Copyright © 1989 by Sammy Davis, Jr., and Boyar Investments Ltd.
All rights reserved
Published simultaneously in Canada by Collins Publishers, Toronto
Printed in the United States of America
Designed by Susan Hood
First edition, 1989
Second printing, 1989

Library of Congress Cataloging-in-Publication Data
Davis, Sammy.
  Why me?
  1. Davis, Sammy. 2. Entertainers—United
States—Biography. I. Boyar, Jane. II. Boyar, Burt.
III. Title.
PN2287.D322A3 1989   792.7′092′4 [B]   88-36327

Every reasonable effort has been made to trace the ownership
of copyrighted material included in this volume. Any errors are
inadvertent and will be corrected in subsequent printings.

Grateful acknowledgment is made to the following for permis-
sion to reprint their copyrighted material: lyrics from "The
Candy Man," written by Leslie Bricusse and Anthony Newley
© 1970/1979 Taradam Music, Inc., from the motion picture
Willy Wonka and the Chocolate Factory; from "Five Minutes
More," words by Sammy Cahn and music by Jule Styne © 1946
Morley Music Co., copyright renewed and assigned to Morley
Music Co. and Cahn Music Company; from "Paper Doll," writ-
ten by Johnny Black © Edward B. Marks Music Company; "Say
It Loud—I'm Black and I'm Proud," by James Brown and
Alfred James Ellis © 1968 by Unichappell Music, Inc. All rights
reserved. Used by permission. Drawing by Charles E. Martin
© 1965 by the New Yorker Magazine, Inc. Photo of Tracey and
Guy Garner's wedding from the July 21, 1986 (Vol. 70, No. 18),
issue of Jet magazine.

For my father

A star. What is a star? In the same way that live performance is an impermanent art, a star is an impermanent illusion who lives only in the memory of those who have seen him and then dies with them. He is carried on people's shoulders and he falls on his face, all within a minute. He is an insecure egocentric, a tyrant and a teddy bear. Is the mike right? The music good? Hey, what are those musicians doing reaching for cups of water while I'm singing? A star is the fool who'll try anything in public and the genius when it works. A star has a thick skin that you can pierce with a frown. Draw me happy, draw me sad. He has been gifted with talent, with the ability to see deeper, hear wider, laugh harder. Also to cry more easily because he bruises more easily. And he was given the hunger, the need to excel. He is amazed by his fame, thrilled by applause, made incredulous by the money. And a thousand times he has wanted to ask, "Dear God, I don't deserve all this. Why *me*?"

Why Me?

1

THE FEAR OF losing success begins when you become entrenched with it. In my case it became an obsession. When I came out of the Army, desperate to become a star, if the devil had been waiting for me I think I would have made the deal.

It didn't happen that way. There was no devil involved, at least not the one with the pitchfork and the tail, but the manic pursuit of success cost me everything I could love: my wife, my three children, some friends I would have liked to grow old with. And it cost me two or three fortunes which I might still have if during those desperate years I hadn't been so single-sighted that a million dollars was just three words.

Yet there was never a reasonable alternative. I've heard people say, "When you finally reach the top you find that everything you wanted was there at the bottom." That is not how it was for me.

My home has always been show business. That's where I've lived since the age of three. I've slept in hotels and rooming houses, in cars, on trains and buses, in our dressing rooms, with my father and a man I called my uncle, Will Mastin; and, when we were out of work, with my grandmother, Rosa B. Davis, whom I called Mamma, at her place in Harlem. But home was where the lights were, the people out front, the laughter and applause, the acts that I watched from the wings all day long—Butterbeans and Susie, the Eight Black Dots, and Pot, Pan and Skillet. And the Green Rooms where between shows I played pinochle with my father and listened to the show talk. I had traveled ten states and played over fifty cities by the time I was four. We carried our roots with us: our same boxes of makeup, our same clothes hanging on iron-pipe racks with our shoes under them. Only the details changed, like the faces on the men sitting inside the stage doors.

We'd arrive in a town, check into our rooming house, and ask, "Where's the restaurant?" There was always one good restaurant and they served soul food, though Will and my father would only let me eat chicken. The other acts would be there and from town to town there was a continuing camaraderie.

As far as I knew, everybody liked us. The audience was throwing money at me when I was six. We were judged on how good our act was. If we were the best on the bill, we got the first dressing room and our names went up out front. If there was a better act than ours, then we took second, or third, on the dressing room and the billing.

I was seven and we were in New York when Will started taking me with him and my father to the booking offices. We dressed in our best clothes and went downtown. While we were with one of the bookers Will said, "I want you to listen carefully to everything that's said, Sammy. There's two words in show business, 'show' and 'business,' and one's important as the other. The dancing and knowing how to please the audience is the 'show' and getting the dates and the money is the 'business.' I know you like to dance and sing and be on the stage in front of the people but if you don't get money for it, then you ain't doing nothing but having a good time for yourself. You have to know how to make deals, which to take and which to let go by."

The man behind the desk, Bert Jonas, said to me, "You're learning the business from the right man. Follow his ways. His handshake is all the contract anybody needs."

I couldn't read much but I knew my name when I saw it and the first time I'd ever seen it on the front of a theater Will read the sign out loud: "Will Mastin's Gang Featuring Little Sammy." I asked, "What's 'featuring' mean?" My father said, "That means you're something worth seeing. Ain't many eight-year-olds got their name out front like this."

Will said, "From now on we're a trio and we'll split our money three ways. You're an equal partner now, Sammy, and we're counting on you. Your daddy and me will open strong to form the

impression. Then you've got to go out there and keep 'em going."
He put his arm around my shoulder. "Do your best, Mose Gastin,
but don't ever worry, 'cause whatever you do your daddy and me'll
come on and it'll be okay." Why he called me Mose Gastin or
where he got that name I don't know.

The three of us shook hands and went inside to dress for our
first show.

My father rubbed his chin thoughtfully. "I'd say I'm kinda in
the mood for the glen plaid with the pearl-gray shirts." He'd chosen
our best clothes for our first look around Joplin, Missouri. Will and
I nodded. My clothes were exact miniatures of theirs, with breast-
pocket handkerchief, vest, gold watch and chain, spats, and a cane.
My father set the pearl stickpin into my necktie and we went
downstairs to the bulletin board, where there was always the name
of a nearby restaurant that had good food.

Will nudged my father and me. "Look who's here." Vern and
Kissel, a good act, and friends of ours, were on their way to eat
too, so we all went together. "How you been making out against
the talkies?" "Great. We just played some time for Dudley in
Detroit." We walked down the street, happy to be working, talking
show talk, laughing all the way to the restaurant. It was a big square
room with a completely round counter. "Sammy's a full partner
now and pullin' his weight. Wait'll you see him doin' my African
Zulu Charleston Prance."

The counterman smiled. "Evening, folks. You niggers'll have to
sit on the other side."

The countertop was painted white halfway around and brown on
the other half. He was pointing to the brown section.

Vern said, "But we're together."

"Sorry, bub. Black 'n' white don't sit together in here even if
you're brothers." He grinned. "Although 'tain't likely."

Vern was on his feet. "Let's get out of here."

The muscle in Will's cheek was moving up and down. "No point
in spoiling your meal. If we leave here you won't have time to find
someplace else."

The counterman shrugged. "Fact is, it's no different elsewhere
in these parts, so you might as well make do."

My father took my hand, and he, Will, and I sat on the brown
side. Vern and Kissel moved to the seats next to us on the white

side where the line ended. Nobody said much anymore. We finished eating quickly and went back to the theater.

Vern and Kissel were talking to the stage manager, angrily pointing down the street. My father and Will stood with me on the stairs waiting for them. The stage manager strode over to the bulletin board and tore the restaurant's sign down. "I'm sorry about this, Mr. Mastin, Mr. Davis . . . ."

My father said, "I'd as soon not discuss it now." He moved his eyes toward me. Will took my hand. "C'mon, Sammy, we'll get ready for the show." My father called out, "I'll be right up, Poppa." That's what he'd called me ever since I can remember.

Will didn't say a word as we got undressed.

"Massey?"

"Yes, Sammy?"

"What's goin' on?"

Again the muscles of his face tightened and started moving. "Nothing for you to be worrying yourself over."

"I'm not worryin'. I'm just wonderin' what happened. We were havin' fun and then everybody got mad and now downstairs they're talkin' about it . . ."

"Talk-*ing*, Sammy. Say the word the way it's supposed to be said. Don't be lazy."

"What's a nigger?"

Will walked over to his makeup chair and sat down. "That's just a nasty word some people use about us."

"About show people?"

"No. It's a word about colored people. People like us whose skin is brown."

"What's it mean, Massey?"

He faced me. "It doesn't mean anything except to say they don't like us."

"But Vern and Kissel like us, don't they?"

"Yes. But show people are different. Most of 'em don't care about anything except how good is your act. It's others, some of the people outside—someday you'll understand . . ."

My father walked in. "That man was just jealous of us 'cause we're in show business and he's gotta be pushin' beans all his damned life. Don't you even give it a thought, Poppa."

But Vern and Kissel were in show business and he hadn't called them niggers. The way Will and my father were so angry I knew the word must have meant just us and it must have been terrible. The closest I could come is that somehow it meant we were different from other people in a way that was bad. But that didn't make any sense. I wasn't different from anybody else.

"Betcha I can make you laugh, Poppa."

My father was crouched in front of me making his poker face. I fought it, as I always did, but within a minute I was rolling on the floor, laughing.

2

A PFC WAS sitting on the steps of a barracks, sewing an emblem onto a shirt. I walked over to him. "Excuse me, buddy. I'm a little lost. Can you tell me where 202 is?"

He jerked his head, indicating around the corner. "And I'm not your buddy, you black bastard!" He turned back to his sewing.

The corporal standing outside 202 checked my name against a list on a clipboard. "Yeah—well, you better wait over there till we figure out what to do with you."

It was 1942. I was at the Infantry's Basic Training Center at Fort Francis E. Warren in Cheyenne, Wyoming. I sat on the steps where he'd pointed. Other guys were showing up and he checked them off against his list and told them, "Go inside and take the first bunk you see." I looked away for a moment and heard him saying, "Sit over there with Davis."

A tall, powerfully built guy dropped his gear alongside mine. "My name's Edward Robbins." We shook hands and he sat down next to me. One by one, men were arriving and being sent inside but no one else was told to wait with us. Finally, it was clear that we were the only ones being held outside while all the white guys were going right in.

The corporal went inside. We were sitting in front of a screen door, so I could hear every word he was saying. "Look, we got a problem. Those niggers out there are assigned to this company. I'm gonna stick 'em down at that end. You two guys move your gear so I can give 'em those last two bunks."

Another voice said, "Hey, that's right next to me. I ain't sleepin' near no dinge."

"Look, soldier, let's get something straight right off. I'm in charge of this barracks and . . ."

"I ain't arguin' you're in charge. I'm only sayin' I didn't join no nigger army."

Edward and I looked straight ahead.

"What about the can? Y'mean we gotta use the same toilets as them?"

"That's right, soldier. They use the same latrine we all use. Now look, we ain't got no goddamned choice. They used to keep 'em all together, but now for some goddamned reason somebody decided to make us the first integrated outfit in the Army and they sent 'em here. We just gotta put up with 'em . . ."

It was impossible to believe they were talking about me.

"Yeah, but I still ain't sleepin' next to no nigger."

"What the hell's the Army need 'em for? They'll steal ya blind while ya sleep and they're all yeller bellies . . ."

"Awright, knock it off. I don't want 'em any more than you do, but we're stuck with 'em. That's orders."

There was the sound of iron beds sliding across the wooden floor. The corporal beckoned from the doorway. "Okay, c'mon in," he snapped, "on the double." We picked up our gear and followed him through the door. I felt like a disease he was bringing in.

There were rows of cots on both sides with an aisle down the center. The guys were standing in groups. They'd stopped talking. I looked straight ahead. I could feel them staring as we followed the corporal down the aisle. He pointed to the last two cots on one side. "These are yours. Now, we don't want no trouble with you. Keep your noses clean, do as you're told, and we'll get along." He walked away.

I looked around the barracks. The bed nearest ours was empty. All the cots were about two feet apart from each other except ours, which were separated from the rest by about six feet—like we were on an island.

A few of the men sort of smiled and half waved hello. Some wouldn't look over at us. The nearest, a tall, husky guy who must have been a laborer or an athlete, kept his back turned.

A sergeant came in and from the center of the barracks announced, "I'm Sergeant Williams. I'm in charge of this company and I . . ." His glance fell on the space between the beds. He turned to the corporal. "What the hell is that?"

The corporal explained how he'd handled things. Sergeant Williams listened, then spoke sharply. "There is only one way we do things here and that's the Army way! There will be exactly three feet of space, to the inch, between every bed in this barracks. You have sixty seconds to replace the beds as you found them. *Move!*"

He came over to me. "What's your name, soldier?"

"Sammy Davis, Jr."

"Did you arrive at this barracks first or tenth or last or what?"

"About in the middle."

"Did you choose this bunk?"

"Well, no. I was told . . ."

He looked around. By this time the barracks had been rearranged. "All right, Davis. Move your gear one bunk over." He turned to Edward. "You do the same."

He addressed us all. "No man here is better than the next man unless he's got the rank to prove it."

I sat on the end of my bunk, the shock gone, anger growing inside of me until my legs were shaking. I couldn't give them the satisfaction of seeing how they'd gotten to me. I saw one of the other guys polishing his boots. That was a good idea. The boots were a brand-new, almost yellow leather, and we'd been told to darken them with polish. I took off my watch and laid it safely on the bed. It had been a present from my father and Will, a gold chronograph, the kind the Air Force pilots were using. I'd been dying to own one. It cost them $150, so the rent didn't get paid, but Will said, "We always had the reputation as the best-dressed act in show business. Can't let 'em think different about us in the Army."

I opened my shoeshine kit, took out the polish and brush, and began rubbing the polish into the leather, doing the same spot over and over, working so hard that I could blank out everything else from my mind. Suddenly another pair of boots landed at my feet. "Here, boy, you can do mine too."

I looked up. It was the guy who had the bed next to me, and he'd already turned away. I grabbed for the boots, to throw them at his head—but I didn't want to make trouble. I put them down beside his bed.

"Hey, boy, don't get me wrong. I expected t'give you a tip. Maybe two bits for a good job."

"I'm no bootblack. And I'm no boy either."

"Whoa now, don't get uppity, boy." He shrugged and walked over to Edward. "Here y'are, boy. You can do 'em."

"Yes, suh! Glad t'do 'em, suh."

"Well, that's more like it. And you don't have to call me sir. Just call me Mr. Jennings. Y'see, in the Army you only call the officers sir."

"Yes, suh, Mr. Jennings. And my name is Edward. Anything you needs . . ."

I wanted to vomit. I was alone in that barracks.

Jennings was talking to a couple of the other guys. "This may work out okay. One of 'em's not a half-bad nigger." He came by Edward's bunk with three more pairs of boots. Edward's face fell for a second but he brightened up right away. "Yes, suh, you just leave 'em here and I'll take care of 'em."

"You oughta thank me for settin' up this nice little business for you."

"I *do* thank you." He smiled broadly. "Oh, yes, suh. I thanks you kindly."

Edward was avoiding my eyes. Eventually he looked up and moved his head just the slightest bit. For a split second he opened up to me and I saw the humiliation he was enduring. I hoped he'd look up again so I could let him know I was sorry I'd judged him. Perhaps this was how he had to live, but I wasn't going to take it from anybody. I wasn't going to let anybody goad me into fights and get myself into trouble either. I was going to mind my own business and have a clean record.

Jennings flopped onto his bunk. He sat up, reached over, and took my watch off my bed. "Say, this ain't a half-bad watch." He looked at me suspiciously.

"Put it back."

"Hold on, now. My, but you're an uppity one." He stood up. "Hey, Phillips . . . catch!" He tossed the watch across the barracks. I ran to get it back, but just as I reached Phillips he lobbed it over my head to another guy, who threw it back to Jennings. I ran after it, knowing how ridiculous I looked getting there just as Jennings threw it over my head again, that I shouldn't chase after it, that I was only encouraging them, but I was afraid they'd drop it and I couldn't stop myself.

"Atten-*shun!!!*" Every head in the barracks snapped toward the doorway. Sergeant Williams walked straight to Jennings. "What've you got there?"

Jennings showed him my watch.

"Whose is it?"

Jennings shrugged.

"It's mine."

Sergeant Williams brought it to me. Jennings grinned. "Hell, Sarge, we were just kiddin' around."

"You're a wise guy, Jennings. In the Army we respect another man's property. You just drew KP for a week." He left the barracks.

Jennings looked at me with more hatred than I had ever seen on a man's face. "I'll fix you for this, black boy."

Hours after lights-out I lay awake. How many white people had felt like this about me? I couldn't remember any. Had I been too stupid to see it? I thought of the people we'd known—agents, managers, the acts we'd worked with—those people had all been friends. I know they were. There were so many things I had to remember: the dressing rooms—had we been stuck at the ends of corridors off by ourselves? Or with the other colored acts? No. Dressing rooms were assigned according to our spot on the bill. And the places we stayed? They *were* almost always colored hotels and rooming houses, but I'd never thought of them like that. They were just *our* rooming houses. But did we *have* to go to them? Didn't we just go to them because they knew us and because they were the cheapest? Or wasn't that the reason? Sure, there were people who hadn't liked us, but it had always been: "Don't pay attention, Poppa, he's just jealous 'cause we got a better act." Or: "They don't like us 'cause we're in show business." And I'd never questioned it. I remembered several times Will telling me, "Someday you'll understand." But I didn't understand and I couldn't believe I ever would.

MOST OF the men in our barracks gave me no problems, either because they didn't care or because after a day of Basic they were too tired to worry what the hell I was. But there were about a dozen I had to look out for. They clustered around Jennings and their unity alone was enough to intimidate anybody who might have wanted to show friendliness toward me. When that group wasn't around, the others would be pleasant, but as soon as one of them showed up, it was as if nobody knew me. The sneers, the loud whispers, the hate-filled looks were bad enough, but I didn't want it to get worse. I tried to keep peace with Jennings without Tomming him as Edward was doing. I hoped that if I was good at my job he'd respect me, but when I was good on the rifle range he hated me all the more. If I was bad he laughed at me. I found myself walking on eggs to stay out of his way, casually but deliberately standing on a different chow line, always finding a place at one of the tables far away from him in the mess hall.

I was fastening the strap on my watch before evening mess and it slipped off my wrist and fell to the floor next to Jennings's bed. Before I could reach it he stood up and ground it into the floor with the heel of his boot. I heard the crack. He lifted his foot, smiling coyly. "Oh! What *have* I gone and done? Sure was foolish of you to leave your watch on the floor. Too bad, boy. Tough luck."

The glass was crushed and the gold was twisted. The winding stem and the hands were broken off and mangled. I put the pieces on the bed and looked at them, foolishly trying to put them together again.

"Awwww, don't carry on, boy. You can always steal another one."

I looked at him. "What've you got against me?"

"Hell, I ain't got nothin' against you, boy. I like you fine."

I knew I should swing at him or something, but I was so weakened from the hurt of it that I couldn't get up the anger. I wrapped the pieces in some paper and put it in my pocket. Maybe it could still be fixed.

Overnight the world looked different, it wasn't one color anymore. I could see the protection I'd gotten all my life from my father and Will. I appreciated their loving hope that I'd never need to know about prejudice and hate, but they were wrong. It was as if I'd walked through a swinging door for eighteen years, a door which they had always secretly held open. But they weren't there to hold it now, and when it finally hit me it was worse than if I'd learned about it gradually and knew how to move with it.

SERGEANT Williams walked out of the mess hall with me. "I was looking over the service records and I see that you were in show business. We have shows at the service club every Friday. If you'd care to help out I'm sure it would be appreciated, and perhaps you might enjoy doing it."

After the show, I was standing backstage with one of the musicians, a guy from another company, and I suggested we go out front and have a Coke. He said, "Maybe we'd better go over to the colored service club. We don't want trouble."

"Trouble? I just entertained them for an hour. They cheered me. Hey, look, God knows I don't want trouble, but there's gotta be a point where you draw the line. Now, I don't know about you, but I'm thirsty and I'm going in for a Coke."

A few of the guys who'd seen the show saw us walking in and made room for us at their table. Jennings was seated with four of his buddies. They looked over at me and smiled or smirked, I couldn't be sure which. I sat with a group from our barracks and it was the best hour I'd spent in the Army. I luxuriated in it. I had earned their respect; they were offering their friendship and I was grabbing for it.

After an hour or so I said good night and headed for the door. As I passed Jennings's table he stood up. "Hey, Davis, c'mon over here and let's get acquainted." He was smiling, holding out his hand. It would have been satisfying to brush him off, but if he was trying to be friendly it seemed better to accept it and keep the peace. "I was going to the barracks . . ."

"Hell, you got time for one little drink with us." He pulled out a chair for me. "Man, where'd you learn to dance like that? I swear I never saw a man's feet move so fast. By the way, notice I ain't callin' you boy."

"Have a beer, Davis." One of the guys pushed a bottle toward me. "Here y'are," Jennings said.

"If you don't mind, I'd rather have a Coke."

"Hey, old buddy, you're in the Army. It's time you got over that kid stuff. Try it. You're gonna like it."

The others were watching me. One of them grinned. "Yeah, you gotta learn to drink if you're gonna be a soldier."

Jennings said, "Listen, you're gonna insult me in a minute. Any man who won't drink with me . . ."

"Okay, I'll try it."

"That's better. Now I'll tell you how to drink beer. It can't be sipped like whiskey or Coke. To really get the taste of beer you've gotta take a good long slug."

The others nodded and raised their bottles. Jennings said, "Here's to you." I picked up my bottle to return their toast. I had it halfway to my mouth when I realized it wasn't cold. It was warm. As it came close to my nose I got a good whiff of it. It wasn't beer.

"Hell, don't smell it, man. Drink it!"

I took another smell and all at once I understood the smiles, the handshakes, the friendliness from Jennings. Somebody had taken the bottle empty into the men's room and came back with it filled.

Jennings was saying, "Come on, drink up, boy . . ."

I put the bottle on the table. The faces in front of me zoomed in like a movie close-up and I could see every bead of perspiration, every blink of their eyes. The noise in the room was growing loud then low, loud then low. Suddenly I snapped out of it. "Drink it yourself, you dirty louse."

Jennings laughed. "He even curses like a Coke drinker." I tried to stand up but my chair wouldn't move. He had his foot behind a leg of it, trapping me. The hate was back in his face. "You wanta live with us and you wanta eat with us and now you came in here to drink with us. I thought you loved us so much you'd wanta . . ."

I felt a warm wetness creeping over the side of my shirt and pants. While he'd been talking he had turned the bottle upside down and let it run out on me. I stared at the dark stain spreading over the khaki cloth, cringing from it, trying to lean away from my wet shirt and wet pants. My pocket was too soaked to put my hand in for my handkerchief.

Jennings jumped up, pointing to me, jeering loudly, "Silly niggers can't even control themselves. This little fella got so excited sittin' with white men—look what he did to himself."

I was out of the chair and on top of him. I had my hands on his throat with every intention of killing him. I loved seeing the sneer replaced by shock as I squeezed tighter and tighter, my thumbs against his windpipe. He was gasping for breath. In a desperate effort he swung around fast, lifting me off the floor. My own weight dragged me off him and I flew through the air and crashed into one of the tables. Within seconds the area was cleared as though we were in a ring together.

Until this moment it hadn't been a fight, it had been an attack by 115 pounds of rage propelled by blind impulse. I hadn't known it was going to happen any more than Jennings had. The weeks of taking it, of looking for peace, of avoiding trouble, had passed, and it just happened, like a pitcher overflows when you put too much into it.

But we both knew it was going to be different now: he was a foot taller than me and half again my weight, or more, and without the advantage of surprise I was like a toy to him. He was taking his time, grinning to his friends, caressing the knuckles of one hand with the palm of the other. He raised his fists and began circling, licking his lips, anticipating the pleasure he was going to take out of me.

I flew into him with every bit of strength I had. His fist smashed into my face. Then I just stood there watching his other fist come at me, helpless to make myself move out of the way. I felt my nose crumble as if he'd hit an apple with a sledge-hammer. The blood spurted out and I smelled a dry horrible dusty smell.

"Get up, you yellow-livered black bastard, you stinking coon nigger . . ." I hadn't realized I was on the floor. I got to my feet and stumbled toward him. He hit me in the stomach and I collapsed. I was gasping for breath but no air was coming in and I was suffocating. Then suddenly I could taste air, and the figures in front of my eyes straightened out and became people again. I got up and went for him. He was methodically hitting me over and over again, landing four to every one of my punches, but they weren't hurting me anymore, they were just dull thuds against my body. Then his fist was beating down on the top of my head like a club. Someone shouted, "Don't hit 'im on the head, Jen. Y'can't hurt a nigger 'cept below the forehead." He kept pounding me and I grabbed his shirt with one hand to keep myself from falling so I could hit him in the face with my other hand. I had to stay on my feet and keep hitting him, nothing else mattered, and I was glad to trade being hit ten times for the joy of feeling my fist smash into his face just once. I hung on and kept hitting him and hitting and hitting . . .

A guy named O'Brien, from my barracks, was holding a wet

cloth against my face. "You'll be okay," he said. "The bleeding's stopped."

We were outside. I was propped up against the side of the PX. Another guy was there. Miller. He smiled. "You might feel better to know that you got in your licks. You closed one of his eyes and you broke his nose. He's wearing it around his left ear." I started to laugh but a shock of pain seared my lips. My head was pounding like it was still being hit.

They walked me to the barracks. Sergeant Williams was waiting in the doorway. He shook his head in disgust. "Very smart! Well, get over to the infirmary with Jennings." He walked into his bedroom.

I had sent Jennings to the infirmary. What beautiful news. Gorgeous! Miller and O'Brien were waiting to take me there. I shook my head and thanked them. I wasn't going to give Jennings the satisfaction of seeing me in the infirmary, not if my nose fell off entirely.

I got into bed. The bruises were murder. Still, the worst pain wasn't so bad that I wouldn't do it again. Jennings had beaten me unconscious and hurt me more than I'd hurt him, but I had won. He was saying, "God made me better than you," but he lost the argument the minute he had to use his fists to prove it. All he'd proven is that he was physically stronger than me, but that's not what we were fighting over.

I'd never been so tired in my life, but I couldn't sleep. I hated myself for those weeks of tiptoeing around trying to avoid trouble. I'd been insane to imagine there was anything I could do to make a Jennings like me. I hadn't begun to understand the scope of their hatred. I was haunted by that voice yelling, "Y'can't hurt a nigger 'cept below the forehead." My God, if they can believe that, then they don't even know what I am. I'm a whole other brand of being to them.

There was so much to think about. How long would I have gone on not knowing the world was made up of haters, guys in the middle, Uncle Toms . . . I couldn't believe I was going to spend the rest of my life fighting with people who hate me when they don't even know me.

WE WERE loaded with Southerners and Southwesterners who got their kicks out of needling me, and Jennings and his guys never let up. I must have had a knock-down-drag-out fight every two days. I had scabs on my knuckles for the first three months in the Army. My nose was broken again and getting flatter all the time. I fought clean, dirty, any way I could win. They were the ones who started the fights, and I didn't owe them any Marquis of Queensberry rules. It always started the same way: a wise guy look, a sneer—once they knew how I'd react, they were constantly maneuvering me into fights. To them it was sport, entertainment, but for me the satisfaction which I had first derived diminished each time, until it was just a chore I had to perform. Somebody would say something and my reaction would be: oh, hell, here we go again. But I had to answer them. Invariably, I'd walk away angrier than when the fight had started. Why should I have to keep getting my face smashed? Why did I have to prove what no white man had to prove?

I kept in touch with my father and Will by phone. "We're makin' ends meet, Poppa. They ain't what you'd call huggin' and kissin' but we're gettin' by till the day you come home. So do your job in the Army and then get back as fast as you can." I never bothered to tell them what my job in the Army was exactly.

THE GUY in front of me finished with the washbasin, and as I moved forward, a big Southerner, Harcourt, grabbed me by the T-shirt and yanked me back so hard that I stumbled clear across the room, hit the wall, and fell down.

"What's *that* for?"

He drawled, "Where I come from niggers stand in the back of the line."

I got up, gripped my bag of toilet articles, and with all the strength I had, hit him in the mouth with it. The force and shock knocked him down. I stood over him, fists ready. But he made no attempt to get up. Blood was trickling out of his mouth. He wiped it away with his towel, then looked at me. "But you're still a nigger."

Sergeant Williams was standing in the doorway. He motioned for me to follow him to his room and closed the door. "Sit down, Davis." He offered me a cigarette and I took it. "That's not the way to do it, son. You can't beat people into liking you."

The moment I heard, "You're still a nigger," I'd known that.

"You've punched your way across the camp. Have you stopped the insults? After you beat them up, did they respect you?"

"When a guy insults me, what should I do, Sergeant? Curtsy and tell him thanks?"

"You've got to fight a different way, a way where you can win something lasting. You can't hope to change a man's ideas except with a better idea. You've got to fight with your brain, Sammy, not with your fists."

It seemed as though I passed Harcourt a hundred times a day, and I was haunted by that voice: "You're still a nigger." He never said another word to me, but his eyes were saying it in the way they passed over me—as though I wasn't there.

We finished Basic and took our physicals for overseas duty. I was rejected because of an athletic heart. I didn't qualify for any of the Army's specialist schools where I might have bettered myself. My lack of education closed everything to me. They didn't know what to do with me, so somebody sent down an order, "Put him through Basic again," probably hoping that by the time I came out I'd be somebody else's problem. When I came out I was sent back in again, like a shirt that hadn't been done right. Four times. I was disgusted with myself. Outside a club or a theater I was totally unequipped for the world, just another uneducated laborer.

I was on latrine duty and I passed Sergeant Williams's room. The door was open and he was on his bed, reading. He must have had a hundred books in there. "These all your books, Sergeant?"

"Yes. Would you like to read one?"

I wanted to, but I'd never read a book and I was afraid of picking something ridiculous and making a fool of myself.

He sat up. "You'll get a lot more out of them than you do from those comic books you read." He chose a book and gave it to me. "Start with this one. You may not enjoy it right away but stick with it."

It was *The Picture of Dorian Gray* by Oscar Wilde. After taps, I went into the latrine, where the lights stayed on, and sat on the floor reading until after midnight. The next day I bought a pocket dictionary at the PX and started the book from the beginning again, doing my reading in isolated places so people wouldn't see me looking up words.

When I'd finished it I gave it back to Sergeant Williams and we talked about it. He handed me more and we had discussions as I finished them. He took a book from his shelves. *The Complete Works of Shakespeare.* "Now you're going too far. I mean, I never spent a day in school in my life."

His voice had a slight edge to it. "I never said you should be ashamed of no schooling. But it's not something to be proud of either."

He gave me Carl Sandburg's books about Lincoln, books by Dickens, Poe, Mark Twain, and a history of the United States. I read *Cyrano de Bergerac*, entranced by the flair of the man; by the majesty of speeches I read aloud in a whisper, playing the role, dueling in dance steps around the latrine; imagining myself that homely, sensitive man, richly costumed in knee breeches, plumed hat, a handkerchief tucked into my sleeve, a sword in my hand. I feasted on the glory of the moment when, making good his threat, he drove the actor from the stage, and as the audience shouted for their money back, tossed them his last bag of gold and admitted to Le Bret, "Foolish? Of course. But such a magnificent gesture." And it was. Glorious! I put my hand in my pocket, and clutching a fistful of silver, I slipped out into the night, sword in hand, to drive the actor from the stage. Then, as fops and peasants alike shouted for their money back, I bowed and hurled my handful of coins into the air. They landed clanging against the side of the barracks. A light went on. A voice yelled, "Corporal of the guard!" I ran like hell.

The more education Sergeant Williams gave me, through his books and our discussions, the greater a hunger I developed for it. When I ran through his books I found others at the post library and then reread the ones he had.

As I got offstage at the service club, a fellow standing in the wings came over to me. "That was one hell of a show you just did. Will you have a drink with me? My name is George M. Cohan, Jr."

We sat together and he said, "You've heard about the show every camp's going to be doing for the intercamp competition? Well, with all the stuff you know and with my dad's special material, which I know backwards, I'll bet we could get that assignment. All the guys trying for it will just be using stuff out of the Special Services books. But with us writing our own, something fresh, we couldn't miss."

20

We auditioned for the general and then we were invited to describe the show we'd do. While we talked a WAC captain, his adjutant, found enough stumbling blocks to build a wall around the entire camp and she said she'd let us know in about a week.

Outside, George said, "Well, she's the power as far as our show's concerned. We've got to butter her up."

We thought up excuses to go to her office and always brought bunches of flowers that we'd picked. The captain seemed to be swinging over to our side, so we redoubled our efforts.

I stopped off to leave some new material we'd worked out. She asked, "You were a professional entertainer, Davis?"

"Yes, Captain. Since I was three."

"Tell me something about it." She leaned back, listening, waving away clerks who tried to speak to her. Her interest triggered a stream of show talk and "the old days" poured out of me. She smiled. "When I first heard your ideas they seemed so professional that frankly I doubted you'd be able to execute them. But now that I understand your background, and from what I know of George, I'm convinced you and he are more than up to the job. I'd like you two to work out a budget for props and costumes as soon as you can." She walked me to the door, shook hands with me, and smiled. "I probably shouldn't say this but you boys have quite an edge over the others. We'll have the official word by Friday."

Leaving, I felt like doing a Fred Astaire number, tap-dancing across the tops of the row of desks leading to the front door. I was a specialist. Show business had given me something to offer the Army.

As I started toward my barracks, a couple of headquarters clerks called out to me. One of them, a PFC with a heavy Southern drawl, smiled. "The captain told us to take you to meet her at Building 2134."

I grinned. "Her wish is my command." Maybe she wanted me to look at props and scenery they'd used in other shows. We walked about half a mile, to a semi-deserted part of the camp, to barracks that weren't in use. I followed the PFC into 2134. One of the men closed the door behind us. They shoved me into the latrine. Four others were in there, obviously waiting for us.

"Sorry, nigger, but your lady love won't be here."

"What is this?"

"Nothin' but a little meeting some of us in the office thought we oughta have with you." They took hold of my arms. The PFC spit in my face. I tried to reach up to wipe it away but I couldn't move my arms. "Oh, I'm sorry. Here, I'll wipe it for you." He slapped me across the face, then backhanded me.

The seven of them crowded around me. The PFC was breathing heavily and a vein in his forehead was pulsing quickly. "We've been watching you makin' eyes at the captain for a week now, and we decided we oughta have a little talk with you."

"Making eyes? Wait a minute . . ."

He hit me again. "Niggers don't talk 'less they're spoken to." He punched me in the stomach and I collapsed, hanging by the arms from the two guys who were holding me. "Now, like I was sayin', we just get so sick seein' you playin' up to her, and bringin' her flowers, and tryin' to make time—not to say the captain would give an ape-face like you the time of day, but we figured we should smarten you up some so you won't be makin' such a fool of yourself.

"Now, what you gotta learn is that black is black and it don't matter how white it looks or feels, it's still black, and we're gonna show you a little experiment to prove it so's you won't think we're tryin' to fool you none."

One of the others was stirring a can of white paint. Two of them ripped my shirt open and tore it off me. The PFC had a small artist's paintbrush, which he dipped into the paint. They held me in front of a mirror. Across my chest he wrote, "I'm a nigger!" Then he wrote something on my back. When he was finished with that he took a larger brush and began to cover my arms and hands with white paint, going back and forth over the hair on my arms until every strand was plastered down.

"Now," he said, "we're gonna let this paint dry so we can finish our lesson. So while we're waiting, you c'n give us a little dance."

They let go of my arms. My legs felt like cardboard buckling under me. Two of them were blocking the door and the other five were surrounding me.

"Come on, Sambo, give us a little dance!"

I stood motionless, dazed. The PFC said, "Guess he don't understand English." They held me again while he picked up the brush and wrote on my forehead, grinning, taking great pleasure in his work, doing it slowly, carefully. When he finished they dragged me back to the mirror. He'd written "Coon" in white paint that was starting to drip into my eyebrows.

"Now listen," he said, "you gotta understand me. When I tell you we wanta see you dance for us, then you gotta believe we wanta see you dance. Now, we're trying to be gentlemen about this. We figure you don't teach a hound nothin' by whipping him, so we're trying to be humane and psychological with you, but if we're takin' all this trouble on your education, then you gotta show a little appreciation and keep us entertained durin' all the time we're givin' up for you. So, come on, Sambo, you be a good little coon and give us a dance."

They let go of my arms again. The PFC punched me in the stomach. "Dance, Sambo." When I got my wind back I started tapping my feet, incredulous, numbed.

"That's better, Sambo. A little faster . . ."

I danced faster, stumbling over my own legs.

"Faster, Sambo, faster . . ."

As I got near the PFC, he hit me in the stomach again. "Didn't you hear me say faster, Sambo?" They made me keep dancing until I couldn't raise my feet off the ground.

"Okay, that's enough of that. You're not that good." He turned to the others. "I really thought we were gonna have us a treat, didn't you?" They all nodded and acted disappointed. "Well, I guess we can't be mad 'cause you don't dance good. Anyway, we gotta get back to your education."

I could feel the paint tightening on my skin.

"Now, we figure you've got the idea you're the same as white 'cause you're in a uniform like us and 'cause you dance at the shows and you go in and sit down with white men and because you think you got manners like a white man with the flowers you give our women. So we gotta explain to you how you're not white and you ain't never gonna be white no matter how hard you try. No matter what you do or think, you can't change what you are, and what you are is black and you better get it outta your head to mess around with white women.

"Now, look at your arm. Looks white, don't it? Well, it ain't. Watch and see." He poured turpentine on a rag and began wiping my arm in one spot. When my skin showed through the paint, he grinned. "There. Y'see? Just as black 'n' ugly as ever!"

He rubbed some turpentine on his own arm. "See the difference? No matter how hard I keep rubbin', it's still white. So, like I said, white is white and black is black." He poured the rest of the turpentine down the drain.

"Okay, you ugly little nigger bastard. We're lettin' you off easy this time. I mean, we coulda been nasty and painted all the rest of you, but we figured you're a smart nigger and you'll get the idea fast, so because we're peace-lovin' fellas we don't wanta hurt you none, so we didn't do that. Now we're gonna be leaving you here, but remember that we did you this favor, see? And if you should decide to tell anybody anything about our little lesson, well, we'd just have to admit we caught you makin' passes at the captain and that sure wouldn't do neither of you no good, and then besides that we'd have to find you again and give you another lesson, 'cept we'd have to try harder to make you understand, like maybe open up your skin a trifle and show you it's black under there too. So just take our little lesson in the spirit we meant and we're willin' to let bygones be bygones and you'll stay away from the captain, right? Okay, Sambo, we'll be goin' now . . ."

Then I was alone. I looked at myself in one of the mirrors. I wanted to crawl into the walls and die. I sat down on the floor and cried.

I looked at the part of my arm they had cleaned with turpentine. I rubbed the skin and watched it change color under the pressure, then darken as the blood flowed through again. How could the color of skin matter so much? It was just skin. What *is* skin? Why is one kind better than another? Why did they think mine made me inferior?

I stayed there for an hour, maybe two hours. I lost track of time, trying to understand it. Why should they want to do this to me? I'd have given my life to hear my father say, "Hell, Poppa, they're just jealous of our act." I wanted to believe anything but that people could hate me this much.

As the paint hardened it drew on my skin. It was starting to pull the hairs on my arms and it itched terribly. I tried to wipe some of it off with toilet paper, but it tore and stuck to the paint and only made it worse. I had to get back to the barracks. I dreaded being seen. Some of the guys would laugh and some would feel sorry for me and one would be as bad as the other. But I wanted

Sergeant Williams to see me. I wanted to hear him tell me again, "You've got to fight with your brain."

It was already dark. Most of the camp was in the mess halls, so it was easy to hide behind buildings back to the barracks. It was empty. I got my towel and after-shave lotion and went into the latrine. I poured half a bottle on the towel and rubbed until it hurt, but it didn't help at all. There were voices outside, Sergeant Williams and some of the guys. I hid in the shower, praying they wouldn't come in. When I heard the other guys' steps going toward their bunks I ducked into Sergeant Williams's room.

He closed the door. "Who did it?" I shook my head. "Don't be a fool. You don't have to fear them. They'll be court-martialed and sent to the stockade for years . . ."

I wasn't afraid. I just wanted it to be over. If they were arrested there'd be a trial and everybody in camp would know about it. I just wanted to forget that it ever happened.

There was no pity in his face—just sadness. Not only for me but for the depth of what he could read into what had happened. He left the room, cautiously, so nobody would see me, and sent to the motor pool for turpentine. Then he locked the door, soaked his towel, and began wiping the paint off my skin. For the next hour and a half he didn't say one word. I sat there naked to the waist until he was finished. Then he gave me soap and a brush and sent me to the shower room.

Bits of paint clung to my pores. I stood under the hot water rubbing until rashes of blood trickled to the surface, brushing until I'd scraped the last speck of white out of my skin.

I got into bed. *Nobody, nobody in this world is ever going to do this to me again. I'll die first.*

THE BAND was playing the overture. George made room for me to peek through the curtain. Among all the faces, I saw Harcourt from my barracks. How can you run out and smile at people who despise you? How can you entertain people who don't like you?

I did my opening number, forcing myself to concentrate on the one thing I was out there to do: entertain the audience.

As I was taking my bow, enjoying the applause, I glanced at Harcourt. He wasn't applauding. Our eyes met and I caught something in his face that I'd never seen there before. It wasn't warmth or respect—he was trying to show no recognition at all. At that moment I knew that because of what I could do on a stage he could never again think, "But you're still a nigger." Somehow I'd gotten to him. He'd found something of me in six minutes of my performance which he hadn't seen in the barracks in all those months.

My talent was the weapon, the power, the way for me to fight. It was the only way I might hope to affect a man's thinking. The same man who had caused the question had provided the answer. The man who had shown me that my fists could never be enough was showing me how to fight with whatever intelligence and talent God had given me.

We played the show for a week and when I was on that stage it was as though the spotlight erased all color and I was just another guy. I could feel it in the way they looked at me, not in anything new that appeared in their faces, but in something old that was missing. While I was performing they forgot what I was and there were times when even I could forget it. Sometimes offstage I passed a guy I didn't know and he said, "Good show last night." It was as though my talent was giving me a pass from their prejudice. I didn't hope for camaraderie. All I wanted was to walk into a room without hearing the conversation slow down, and it was happening. I was developing an identity around camp and it was buying me a little chunk of peace.

I was transferred into Special Services and for eight months I did shows in camps across the country, gorging myself on the joy of being liked. I dug down deeper every day, looking for new material, inventing it, stealing it, switching it—any way that I could find new things to make my shows better—and I lived twenty-four hours a day for that hour or two at night when I could stand on that stage, facing the audience, knowing I was dancing down the barriers between us.

I WALKED around the camp remembering my first months in Cheyenne. Now that I was leaving the Army I had a detached feeling about it, as though it had happened to someone else. But it was me all right, and I wasn't about to let myself forget it. I'd gone into the Army like a kid going to a birthday party, and I'd seen it. They'd taught me well all that my father and Will had so lovingly kept from me.

I'd learned a lot in the Army and I knew that above all things in the world I had to become so big, so strong, so important that those people and their hatred could never touch me. My talent was the only thing that made me a little different from everybody else, and it was all that I could hope would shield me *because* I was different.

I'd weighed it all, over and over again: What have I got? No looks, no money, no education. Just talent. Where do I want to go? I want to be treated well. I want people to like me and be decent to me. How do I get there? There's only one way I can do it with what I have to work with. I've got to be a star! I have to be a star like another man has to breathe.

3

WE WERE OUT of work, living in two-dollar hotel rooms in Los Angeles. It was a Saturday night in 1945 and I turned on the radio to hear "Your Hit Parade." The music came pouring out playing the Axel Stordahl arrangement, opening a path for Frank Sinatra's voice to come through singing, "I'm going to buy a paper doll that I can call my own . . ."

When the chorus started doing a Lucky Strike Extra, I said, "Dad, you wanta hear something unbelievable?" I switched from station to station and the same voice came out, ". . . five minutes more, only five minutes more in your arms . . ."

He was "Frankie," "the Voice," and "the Bow Tie."

"Poppa? You eatin' yourself up over how he's doin'?"

"Oh, come on, Dad. He's too big to envy. But I can't help thinking we were on the same bill with him when nobody knew him either. *Now* look where he is, and we haven't budged." I turned it off. "I'm going down there to see him next week."

"Hell, he ain't about to remember you, and you ain't gonna get nowheres near him anyway."

"I know, but I want to watch him work."

I walked across Hollywood to NBC. After the show I hurried around the corner to the stage door. There must have been five hundred kids ahead of me, waiting for a look at him. When he appeared, the crowd surged forward like one massive body. Girls were screaming, fainting, pushing, waving pencils and papers in the air. I stood on tiptoe trying to see him. He was so sure of himself, completely in control. He concentrated on one person at a time, signing, smiling. He got to me and took my paper. He used a gold pen to sign his name. He looked at me. "Don't I know you?"

"Well, we were on the bill with you and Tommy Dorsey in Detroit about five years ago."

"What's your name?"

"Sammy Davis, Jr."

"Didn't you work with your old man and another guy? Yeah, sure. I hate Sammy. I'll call you Sam. Why don't you come back next week and see the show? I'll leave a ticket for you . . ." The kids were pressing toward him, shoving papers in his face for autographs. He touched me on the arm. "See ya next week, Sam."

The following week I was looking for a box office when an NBC guard walked over to me. "Hey, you! End of the line."

"But Frank Sinatra left a ticket for me." As I said it I was struck by how ridiculous it sounded.

The guard was giving me a "Yeah, sure" look, but he took me to the Guest Relations desk. There was nothing for me. I was almost out the door when a page came running up and asked my name. "Then this must be for you." It had my name on it. "Sam." He ushered me to a seat in the front row and after the show he came back. "Mr. Sinatra wants you to come to his dressing room."

Important-looking people were coming in. "Beautiful show, Francis." ". . . that last song, Frank." ". . . great voice, baby, great!"

He had the aura of a king about him. And that's how people were treating him. He didn't say anything to me and I was beginning to wonder if he remembered who I was and that he'd sent for me, but as he was leaving he turned to me. "Hey, Sam. Maybe next week you'll come around and watch rehearsal." He put his arm around my shoulder and we walked out the stage door together and into the mob of screaming kids. He was reaching for his gold pen to sign autographs. He smiled at me and spoke over the uproar around us. "So long, Sam. Keep in touch."

MY FATHER came into the dressing room and flopped onto a chair. "Nothin'. Guess we'll have to sleep in here."

Will asked, "You mean there's nothing in the whole city of Spokane?"

"There ain't that many colored rooming houses to start with."

"What about a hotel?"

"Ain't a single colored hotel around."

Colored rooming houses? Colored hotels? Colored, colored, colored! And the way they were accepting it, so matter-of-factly. "Whaddya mean *colored* rooming house? Why must it always be colored rooming houses and colored hotels . . ."

"Now, Poppa, you know better'n this."

"I do like hell! Why do we have to live *colored* lives? Y'mean we have to let people say, 'You're colored, so you've gotta sleep in your dressing room'? Where, Dad? Where do we sleep? On the goddamned floor?"

"Now, Poppa, that's how it is and there ain't no use fightin' it. That's how people are."

"Nobody has to tell me about people. I found out how they are. And it ain't 'cause they're jealous we're in show business." He backed up hurt. I was sorry, but the heat was pouring out of my body. "I'll get us a room. In the whitest goddamned hotel in town."

Dressed in my best clothes, as I spun through the revolving door I glanced at the clean lobby, the uniformed bellboys, and the elevators. I sauntered up to the front desk. "I'd like three single rooms for the next ten days. We're appearing in the show downtown."

"I'm terribly sorry, sir, but we're entirely filled." *He's turning me down.* I hadn't really believed he would. "Swamped. Truly swamped. Busiest we've seen it in . . ."

The revolving door seemed so much heavier as I pushed my way to the outside.

"Nervy nigger wanted a room. Some crust." A bellboy was telling the story to the doorman. "Go on," he said, "go back where you belong." He was looking at me with the contempt you have for something you dispose of with a DDT spray gun. All the strength in the world was in my body as I hurtled toward that face and hit it.

I was sitting on the ground smelling the same awful, dry, dusty smell that I had when Jennings first broke my nose.

My father and Will were waiting for me outside the stage door. I should have been embarrassed returning like this after all my big talk, but all I could think was that my nose was broken and I had to keep the blood from staining my best shirt. There was nothing to say. We made beds on the floor out of canvas tarps, used our overcoats for blankets, and I made a pillow out of a rolled-up pair of pants. All I'd accomplished was to get my damned nose broken, so that for at least two weeks I'd be limited in what I could do onstage. I'd slid back and tried to hit an idea with my fists. I couldn't afford that mistake again.

In the morning Will was reading *Variety*. " 'Bill Robinson's salary at the Palace is five thousand dollars per week.' " He kept rereading it. "No colored act in the world is ever going to get more than five thousand a week."

I said, "Massey, I'd like to put in impressions of Jimmy Cagney and Durante and Edward G. Robinson."

He put down the paper. "Sammy, what's the matter with you? You wanta do impressions of *white people?*"

"Why not?"

"You just can't. They'll think you're making fun of 'em. No colored performer ever did white people in front of white people."

"But I did them in the Army and they went over great."

"That's a whole other story. Those soldiers are hungry for shows. Plus the fact of getting 'em free. You just stick with Satchmo and B and Stepin Fetchit. I've watched what'll go over and what won't for nearly forty years and you can't get away with something like that."

"Massey, you're the boss of the act, but it seems to me that all that should matter is if they're good or not."

He was shaking his head sadly. "Sammy, what's right and what's wrong don't always have say over what is."

In Seattle, Will told us, "We're booked as the opening act at El Rancho Vegas in Las Vegas, Nevada, for five hundred dollars a week."

The trade papers were bursting with news about Las Vegas. El Rancho and the Last Frontier were the first luxury hotels and there was talk about more new hotels being planned.

My father was heating coffee on the hot plate. "The word is they're payin' acts twice as much as anywheres else. Free suites and food tabs."

Will said, "They're out to make it the number one show town. *Variety* says the whole business is watching what's happening in Vegas."

I walked over to Will. "I'm going to do those impressions."

He stared out of his bedroom window. I knew by his long silence that he wasn't going to fight me. "Sammy, I don't think you can get away with it. Still, you're a third of the Trio and you've seen a lot of show business, so I won't stop you. I'm just going to hope you're right."

THE BAND was the biggest we'd ever worked with; the floor of the stage was springy; the lighting was the most modern I'd ever seen. After rehearsal we asked about our rooms. The manager said, "We can't let you have rooms here. You'll have to find a place on the other side of town."

The hotels we passed in downtown Las Vegas looked awful compared to El Rancho but even they were out of bounds to us. In Reno we could stay at the Mapes. But Vegas was a different Nevada for us. The cab continued to Westside. "There's a woman name of Cartwright takes in you people." It was Tobacco Road. A child, naked, was standing in front of a shack made of wooden crates and cardboard.

I glanced at my father. *Look where they put us!*

The driver sounded almost embarrassed. "Guess ya can't say a lot for housing out here. Not much cause for your kind t'come to Vegas. Just a handful of porters and dishwashers they use over on the Strip."

Who else would live here?

The cab stopped in front of one of the few decent houses. My father followed me into my room. "Not half bad." I started unpacking. He sat down and I could feel him watching me. I threw a shirt into a drawer and slammed it closed. "All right, Dad, for God's sake, what is it?"

"*That's* what it is. Exactly what you're doin', eatin' yourself up, grindin' your teeth. Y'can't let it get t'you, Poppa. I know how you feels. But the fact is, when it comes time to lay your head down at night, what's the difference if it's here or in a room at El Rancho?"

"Dad, I don't give a damn about their lousy rooms, I really don't. Right now, the only thing in this world that I want is their stage!"

As I danced, I did Satchmo. I shuffled across the stage like Stepin Fetchit. Then I spun around and came back doing the Jimmy Cagney walk to the center of the stage and faced my father and

Will, doing Cagney's legs-apart stance, the face, and then "All right
. . . you dirty rats!" The audience roared.

In the wings Will smiled warmly. "I'm glad I was wrong,
Sammy." My father laughed and picked me up. "Poppa, you was
great!" He put me down. "Whaddya say we get dressed after the
next show and go look around the casino? I got fifty dollars that's
bustin' t'grow into a hundred."

We walked out the stage door. The casino was blazing with light.
The door opened for some people and there was an outpouring of
hilarity: slot machines clanging, dealers droning, a woman shriek-
ing with joy—and behind it all the liveliest, gayest music I'd ever
heard. As I held the door open for my father, my eyes moved in
all directions—to slot machines, dice tables, waiters rushing around
with drinks, a man carrying a tray of silver dollars.

I saw a hand on my father's shoulder. A deputy sheriff was
holding him, shaking his head.

We rode to Mrs. Cartwright's in silence. As we passed under
the viaduct, leaving the million-watt excitement of the Strip, we
disappeared into a darkness broken only by the headlights of our
cab. There were no streetlights, the shacks did not have electricity.
Then, in the distance, there was a little patch of light and my father
said, "That must be the Cotton Club and the El Morocco. Hey,
driver, how 'bout dropping us there."

Every colored act in town was at the El Morocco, among them
Paul White and Elroy Peace. Billy Eckstine, who was headlining
on the Strip, picked me up and hugged me, "Hey, you longhead
motherfucker," and my father pounded his back. "Listen, B., just
tell me if the crap table is straight."

B. put me down. "What's the difference? You can play for two
bits."

We got hysterical over that and in a few minutes we were playing
with rolls of quarters. Will didn't gamble but he stood there watching and smiling. My father had gorgeous girls on both sides of him
and he let go of them only long enough to place his bets and pull
in his winnings. A cocktail waitress with *legggggggs* asked him what
he wanted to drink. "Bring me a coupla skullbusters, darlin'. And
a Coke for my son here." He gave me a shot on the arm. "Ain't
this place fantastic, Poppa?"

It really was. I looked around me, enjoying the show business camaraderie, the music, the beautiful chicks, and I was thinking that maybe I could get one to have a Coke with and talk to, when I had the sudden realization that we were all colored people and we were all there because that was the only place they *allowed* us to be. This was *our* corner of the world. Even Billy Eckstine, a *headliner*, couldn't go into a casino on the Strip.

I told my father, "Catch y'later, Dad," and he called out "Have fun, Poppa, while Daddy Sam makes ten the hard way." I got a cab and went downtown where there was a movie theater, where for a few hours I could lose myself in other people's lives.

A hand gripped my arm like a circle of steel, yanking me out of my seat, half dragging me out to the lobby. "What're you, boy? A wise guy?" He was wearing a sheriff's star and a big Western hat. His hand slapped across my face.

"What'd I do?"

"Don't bull me, boy. You know the law."

When I explained that I'd just gotten to town he pointed to a sign. "Coloreds sit in the last three rows. You're in Nevada now. Mind our rules and you'll be treated square. Go on back and enjoy the movie, boy."

I went back to Mrs. Cartwright's and tried reading but I couldn't keep my mind on the book. I stared out the window at the glow of the lights from the Strip in the distance until it faded into the morning sun. The next night as eight o'clock drew near I was vibrating with energy and I couldn't wait to get on the stage. I worked with the strength of ten men.

We did our shows and went out to get a cab to Mrs. Cartwright's. I looked away from the lights of the casino but I couldn't avoid hearing the sounds. Night after night I had to pass that door to get a cab. Once, between shows, I stood around the corner where nobody could see me, and listened to the bursts of gaiety that escaped as people went in and came out. I sat on the ground for an hour, listening and wondering what it must be like to be able to just walk in anywhere.

My FATHER looked into my room. "Hey, Poppa, come out and wrap yourself around some of the best barbecue you'll ever taste. Then we could look in on the bar. They got a Keno game going and we c'n double our money." He was selling me, as he had been every day for a week.

"Thanks, Dad. You go ahead."

"Hell, son, come on and get some laughs outta life."

"I'm happy, Dad."

"No you ain't."

"The hell I'm not."

"The hell you is. You sit here all day listenin' to them records when already you sound more like them people than they do. Then you're blowin' the horn . . ."

"And I'm getting pretty good. Here, listen . . ."

"I know." He tapped on the wall, causing a hollow knocking sound, and smiled. "This ain't exactly made outta three-foot-thick cement." He sat down on the bed. "Poppa, you do impressions, you dance, you play drums and trumpet, but you don't know doodly squat about livin'. You're not havin' your fun."

"I will, Dad. Bet your life on it. I will!"

He stood up, frustrated. "Okay, son, I don't know how to help you. So just tell me . . ."

I watched him walking down the street toward the commercial section of Westside. There were a few decent places over there but the idea that I was being told, "That's your side of town, stay there," made it impossible for me to go near them.

He looked back and waved, offering me a chance to change my mind. I waved back and he turned and kept walking. I picked up the trumpet and started playing.

MAMA's kitchen in Harlem was the warmest room, but even so, my father and I wore overcoats and had the oven on low. The refrigerator, unplugged to save electricity, was open, scrubbed clean, and empty except for some ads my father had clipped from magazines: pictures of roast beef, eggs, butter, sausages, and a bottle of milk.

Every morning we'd go downtown to a booking office. When a call came in for an opening dance act we'd sit there hoping it was we who had the best connection. We weren't an attraction that drew people to a theater, we were just a tool to open another man's show fast and lively, interchangeable with countless others just as fast and just as lively. We were one of a million like us in a world that was buying tickets to see one of a kind.

Lucky Millander's band was doing the stage show at the Strand. A colored comedy act was going on as I sat down. They were funny and I was laughing, but I wasn't enjoying myself. Something was bothering me. I listened to them saying, "Ladies and gen'men, we's gwine git our laigs movin' heah." They were talking "colored" as Negro acts always did. I'd heard it a thousand times before, but for the first time it jarred me. I watched them doing all the colored clichés, realizing that we were doing exactly the same thing. We'd always done them. It was the way people expected Negro acts to be, so that's the way we were. But why can't we say "gentlemen"? Why must it be "gen'men"? Must we downgrade ourselves? Must we be caricatures of cotton-field slaves? Can't we entertain and still keep our dignity? We were contributing a means for mockery by characterizing all Negroes as shuffling illiterates who carried razors, shot craps, lied, and ate nothing but watermelon and fried chicken.

I went from theater to theater, wherever there were colored acts. They were all "yassuhing" all over the stages. Does the public really want this? If the joke is funny, won't they still laugh if we call them "gentlemen"?

Then I saw the trap of it: they were making no personal contact with the audiences. None! And how could they even *hope* to with their real personalities buried beneath ten feet of "yassuh, gen'-men"? Negro performers worked in a cubicle. They'd run on, sing twelve songs, dance, and do jokes—but not to the people. The jokes weren't done like Milton Berle was doing them, to the audience, they were done between the men onstage, as if they didn't have the right to communicate with the people out front. It was the reverse of the way Mickey Rooney and Frank Sinatra played. We'd been on the bill with them and they both worked directly to the people, talking to them, kidding them, communicating with them, making them care about them. Touching their emotions.

By a lifetime of habit, by *tradition*, I too had been cementing myself inside a wall of anonymity. It didn't matter how many instruments I learned to play, how many impressions I learned to do, or how much I perfected them—we were still doing a flash act. That was how we set ourselves up, so that was how the audience would see us.

I strode the floor of Will's hotel room explaining everything I'd seen, everything I felt and wanted to do. He was gazing past me. "Okay, Sammy. The only thing is, I've been doing an act one way all my life, and making a living. Only a fool would throw away what he lived on for forty years. But I won't stop you from trying new things if you believe in them. Maybe you're right that we've been sneaking in the impressions instead of framing them to get the most out of them. Take a straight eight minutes in the middle of the act and use it however you want. But your father and me'll do what we know and always did."

We were up north playing Portland when Will received a telegram: OPEN CAPITOL THEATER NEW YORK NEXT MONTH, FRANK SINATRA SHOW. THREE WEEKS, TWELVE FIFTY PER. We passed that telegram back and forth like three drunks working out of the same bottle.

My father was gazing at it. "Ain't lookin' no gift horse in the mouth, but damned if I can figure how come us." Will shrugged. "Frank Sinatra always has a colored act on the bill with him." "Yeah, Will, but why *us?* I mean, with all the powerhouse acts around like Moke and Poke, Stump and Stumpy, the Nicholas Brothers, the Berry Brothers . . ." "We're as powerhouse as the next and I guess Harry Rogers did a good job of agenting."

We had three weeks to get ready. I could feel myself on the stage with our new act, smooth, organized, everything displayed to give it the best possible chance to go over—and at the Capitol Theater with Frank Sinatra where the *world* would have a chance to see us!

Alan Zee, the general manager of the Capitol, came over to us at rehearsal. "You ran too long. Drop the impressions, all we want is the flash dancing. Just give me six minutes."

I ran after him. "Is there any chance of taking a little time out of Lorraine and Rognan?"

He kept walking. "Just cut your act. Don't worry about anybody else's."

On opening day I was putting on my makeup when a man came in. "Mr. Sinatra would like you to come by his dressing room."

Frank Sinatra came out of the second room of a suite. "Hi ya, Sam. Good to see you. How's your family?" We walked toward the wings. "Glad we're working together."

The orchestra played the first bars of "Night and Day," the pit rose with Skitch Henderson conducting, the curtains opened, and

Frank Sinatra was onstage. He sang two numbers, then said, "We've got three cats here who really swing and they're all too much, but keep your eye on the cat in the middle because he's my man! Here they are, the Will Mastin Trio and Sammy Davis, Jr."

Frank took me completely under his wing. He had our names up out front, he was wonderful to my family, and he had me to his dressing room between almost every show. If I was there at dinnertime he'd take me out to eat with him.

I was standing in the wings watching him work, as I did at every show. Sidney Piermont, the head of Loew's booking, was standing beside me. "Your trio is doing a fine job."

"Thank you very much. And for this chance, sir."

"Don't thank me. You were booked strictly because of Frank. I suggested the Berry Brothers, but he said, 'No, there's a kid who comes to my radio show, he works with his family, his name is Sam something. Use him.' I tried to figure out who he meant. 'You don't mean Will Mastin's kid?' Frank said, 'Yeah, that's them.' I said, 'They're unknowns. Why gamble on them?' Frank insisted. 'All right, Frank. How much do you want to give them?' 'Make it twelve fifty.' Well, that was ridiculous. 'We can get the Nicholas Brothers for that kind of money. And they've even got a movie going for them.' He said, 'Twelve fifty. That's it. I don't want the Nicholas Brothers. I want Sam and his family.' "

Frank had never even hinted at it. Just "Glad we're working together."

He invited the cast to a Thanksgiving dinner the day before closing. He had a basement rehearsal hall converted into a party room and his mother sent over pots and pots of homemade Italian food. We were eating our heads off when somebody yelled, "Hey, Sammy, do the thing for Frank like you did for us."

I'd been playing around with an impression of him. Watching him all the time I was able to catch the physical things he does, his hands, his mouth, and his shoulders, as well as the voice.

"Let's see it, Sam." He had no idea what it was and I was afraid he'd be offended. But I did it and he laughed. "Beautiful, beautiful. It's a scream." In his dressing room he asked, "Why don't you sing?"

"Well, I sing when I do impressions. But for straight singing I don't have a style of my own."

"Let me hear the impressions." I did a few and he began nodding his head. "Put those in the act. And you should sing straight. You've got the voice, work on it, develop a style. And do as many of those impressions as you can. Do them all." He frowned. "You should have been doing them here. You wasted three weeks of important exposure."

There was no point in explaining they'd been cut.

After the closing show, as members of the company came to his dressing room to say goodbye, I stood off to the side thinking how a star of Frank's stature had taken the time and thought to help me.

When the last person had gone we shook hands. "So long, Sam." He looked me in the eye. "Anything I can ever do for you—you've got yourself a friend for life." I nodded the best thank-you I could and went to the door. He called out, "Hey, Charley." He was smiling. "Take care of yourself, Charley. And remember—if anybody hits you, let me know."

4

I SPENT twenty minutes making a perfect knot on a ten-dollar tie I'd bought at Saks Fifth Avenue that afternoon.

My father asked, "What're you doin' tonight?"

"Nothing much . . ." I played it cool. "Just going over to the Copa to catch Frank Sinatra."

His forehead wrinkled. "Listen, Poppa . . ."

"It's okay, Dad. I'm going with Buddy Rich. He's a hip guy, right? He must know it's okay or he wouldn't have invited me."

Although the subway downtown was half empty I stood all the way so I wouldn't wrinkle my suit. Over the grinding of the wheels I heard myself whistling in the past with my father as we walked downtown from Harlem, whistling to keep warm in the cold so we could stand in the doorway of the building at 15 East Sixtieth Street and look across the street at the Copacabana and watch the people arriving, the doorman helping them out of their limousines and cabs, tipping his hat, holding the door open for them until they disappeared inside, laughing, beautiful, rich, going to see Joe E. Lewis, Tony Martin, Jimmy Durante, Martin and Lewis . . . the best performers in the business. That's where they played. The Copa. We'd wait two hours for the audience to come out, just to see their faces after they'd seen the show, and hopefully to get a look at one of the headliners.

I was in front of the Copa entrance at a quarter to eleven. Buddy and his friends pulled up in a cab. As we got to the steps the doorman stopped us. "Only people with reservations." He rushed in front of us. "Hey, didn't you hear me?"

"I'm Buddy Rich and I have a reservation."

He shook his head. "You better wait here while I check." He was back in a few minutes. "They don't know anything about a reservation for you." He gave me a meaningful look, then turned to Buddy. "Maybe if you go away and come back in a little while they'll be able to find it."

Buddy's arm was cocked to swing. "Are you saying that if we come back without our friend we'll get a table? 'Cause if you're saying it I want to hear it."

The doorman's face reddened. "I didn't say that. Now, look, don't make trouble . . ."

I pulled Buddy away. "Come on, let's go." We walked up the street. I couldn't face him. "Look, this is ridiculous. You guys go in. Why should you miss Frank's show?"

"If you say that again I'm going to belt you." We walked in silence toward Fifth Avenue. As we reached the corner I looked back at the awning that said "Copacabana." I felt Buddy's hand on my shoulder. "You'll dance on their tables someday."

My father was waiting up in the kitchen. "How'd it go?"

"They didn't let us in. Good night, Dad."

I went into the bedroom and began undressing. It was hot but I closed the window to keep out the smell of garbage which people threw out their windows and which piled up in the courtyard. I heard his steps coming into the room. "Look, Poppa, they never did want us in them places and they never will and it kills me seein' you gettin' yourself hurt over somethin' you oughta know by now."

"Any word from Will, yet?"

"Yeah, we're set to play the Flamingo in Vegas. Will signed 'cause they upped us to $750 plus pickin' up our fare out. I know you get mad havin' to stay over in Westside, but we can't afford to turn down that kinda money, Poppa."

"Dad, I'll play the Governor's Mansion in Alabama if it'll help us to get off the ground a little faster! *Anything* to change the way we've gotta live. I've gotta get away from it! I've *got to!*"

He was looking at my hand, at the necktie I hadn't realized I'd been holding in my fist, crumpling it into a wrinkled mess. He shook his head slowly, sadly. "Sammy . . . you ain't gonna get away from it till you die."

BUDDY SAID, "I talked to Frank last night. He wants you to call him." I looked up from my coffee. He nodded. "Certainly I told him." He pointed to the phone booth. "Eldorado 5-3100."

"You are coming to the club tonight, Charley. I made the reservation and you're walking in there alone."

"Look, Frank, I'd rather not. I appreciate . . ."

"We don't discuss it. Just be there." His voice softened. "When something is wrong it's not going to get right unless you fix it. I know it's lousy, Charley, but you've got to do it."

Buddy told me, "Frank had a confrontation with the maître d', he told him, 'You keep that fucking table open for him. I don't care if he never shows up.' "

I walked slowly toward the Copa. Even if it goes smoothly, if I get in and get a table—at best, forcing my way in where I'm not wanted is even more degrading than being turned away. But I could never face Frank if I backed out. He was in a decline and he needed the Copa more than they needed him. Despite that he was fighting for me.

I walked up the three front steps. The doorman stood at the curb, watching. I pulled open the door and walked in, braced to be facing people, but I found myself alone in a vestibule. I paused, then pushed open the next door. People were standing around a bar to the right of me. I couldn't see anything but a mirror on the left, so I turned right. A captain smiled too brightly. "Good evening, sir. A drink at the bar?"

"No, thank you. I have a reservation for the show."

"The show is downstairs." He smiled indulgently, pointing to the left.

There were two groups of people ahead of me downstairs. The headwaiter asked their names, checked them off on a list, and sent them to their tables. I stepped forward but before I could give my name he snapped his fingers and a captain appeared, telling me, "Right this way, sir." He left me at a table. I was so far back that I could see what was happening in the kitchen better than what was going on onstage.

The stares, like jabs against my skin, were coming from every direction. I sipped the Coke I'd ordered. I lit a cigarette, and took a long drag, holding the cigarette at the tips of my fingers, trying to do all the suave Cary Grant moves I'd just seen in *Mr. Lucky*. Two guys were coming across the room straight toward me. A hand moved forward. "Sam? We're friends of Frank. He said you wouldn't mind if we sat at your table." Frank had wanted me to walk in by myself, leaning on nobody, but he had sent them to sit with me so I wouldn't feel like I was alone on an island.

Up in his dressing room Frank put an arm around my shoulder. "You did something good, Charley."

The subway lurched from side to side and I swayed with it. For the first time I could remember, I enjoyed that ride uptown and I nestled into the restful, anonymous cheapness of it. Usually I saw just the seamy side of Harlem and resented being glued to the second-bestness of everything, but now I welcomed the peace it offered. I knew that I was thinking wrong, and I tried to bring myself out of it. *I've been to the Copa*. I kept repeating it till I heard it roaring back at me in time with the wheels: "I've been to the Copa . . . been to the Copa . . . been to the Copa . . ." but all I felt was like I'd bought a brand-new Cadillac convertible— for a hundred thousand dollars.

At breakfast I lit a cigarette and dropped the Copacabana match-book on the table. My father grabbed it. "Hey! How'd you get these? Were you inside?" I nodded. "Damn!" He laughed, giddily. "What's it like?"

"It's unbelievable! You go downstairs and a guy in a black coat is waiting with the reservations list. He turns you over to a guy in a red coat who takes you to your table. Then a guy in a blue coat takes your order and a waiter in a white jacket brings it to you. And when you're finished along comes a maroon jacket who takes away the dishes . . ." He was hanging on every word.

IN VEGAS, for twenty minutes, twice a night, our skin had no color. Then, the second we stepped off the stage, we were colored again. I went on every night, turning myself inside out for the audience. They were paying more attention and giving us more respect than ever before, and after every performance I was so exhilarated by our acceptance onstage that I expected one of the owners to say, "You were great. To hell with the rules. Come on in and have a drink, enjoy yourselves." But it never happened. The other acts could gamble or sit in the lounge and have a drink, but we had to leave through the kitchen with the garbage. I was dying to grab a look into the casino, just to see what it was like, but I was damned if I'd let anyone see me with my nose against the candy-store window. Yet I couldn't help imagining what it must be like to be acceptable, to be able to walk into any casino in town. I kept seeing the warmth on the faces of the people we'd played to that night. How could they like me onstage—and then this?

My father spent his time around the Westside bars and the El Morocco playing two-bit craps and blackjack. I'd have loved to be a part of all that fun and the show business camaraderie but I couldn't stand being told that that was the only place I could be. So I went to my room trying to ignore the taunting light from the Strip until finally the irresistible blaze of it drew me to the window. It was only three in the morning, which was like noon in Las Vegas. I felt as wide awake as the rest of the town, which was rocking with excitement. I pictured myself in the midst of it all, the music, the gaiety, the money piled high on tables, the women in beautiful dresses and diamonds, gambling away fortunes and laughing.

It took a physical effort to tear myself away from the window. I forced it all out of my mind and kept telling myself: Someday . . . Listening to records and reading until I was tired enough to fall asleep, always wondering when "someday" would be.

WE WERE booked into Ciro's in Hollywood. The sign out front said "JANIS PAIGE," then underneath in smaller letters: "The Will Mastin Trio."

There is never a night that a supporting act opens anywhere when he, she, or they don't think, "This is the night. This is the time we hit that stage and the audience won't let us off. They'll stand up and cheer and no act will be able to follow us. Then, tomorrow night, *we'll* be the star attraction, the headliners, and we'll close the show. And from then on we'll be stars." It happens only once in ten thousand openings, to only one out of thousands of performers—and it happened to us.

It was Academy Awards night, there was going to be only one show, at midnight, and every celebrity in Hollywood was there to see Janis Paige. The band hit the first notes of "Dancing Shoes."

My father and Will moved into our opening number. Eight bars later I joined them and we might have been barefoot on hot sand, our feet weren't on the stage as much as they were in the air. We'd started probably faster than any act this crowd had ever seen and we kept increasing the pace, trying as we never had before. We finished the opening number and we didn't wait to enjoy the applause before we were off and dancing again, first Will, then my dad, and then me. Our frenzy of movement got to the audience from the moment we started until soon it was like they were out of breath trying to keep up with us. The applause was great when my father and Will finished their numbers and stepped back. I took the mike and did Sinatra and they screamed. I went through the rest of the singers, Billy Eckstine, Mel Tormé, Nat "King" Cole, Vaughn Monroe, the Ink Spots, Frankie Laine, and by the time I finished Satchmo they were pounding the tables so hard I could see the silverware jumping up and down. I switched into the movie stars: Bogart, Cagney, Garfield, Edward G. Robinson, Lionel Barrymore, George Sanders, James Mason, Ronald Colman—suddenly I felt the whole room shifting toward me. From one second to another they'd become involved with me. They were reacting to everything, leaning in, catching every inflection, every little move and gesture. I was touching them. It was the most glorious moment I'd ever known. I was really honest to God touching them.

We swung into our dances again, never letting them catch up with us or grow tired of anything, switching, changing pace, and when we'd finished, after being on for forty minutes, the audience wouldn't let us off. It was as though they knew something big was happening to us and they wanted to be a part of it. They kept applauding, and began beating on the tables with knives and forks and their fists, screaming for us to come back. We'd been ordered not to take more than two bows, that it was in Janis Paige's contract. My father and Will stood in the wings, hesitating. I looked at them. "To hell with her contract. I ain't gonna miss this for *nobody!!!*" We went out twice more. They kept shouting for an encore. I'd already done every impression I'd ever tried. But we had to do something, so, seeing Jerry Lewis sitting in the audience, I did Jerry Lewis, which I'd never done before. The sight of a colored Jerry Lewis was the absolute topper. He screamed. Everyone did.

It was *over*. When I heard that scream I knew there was nothing we could do to top that!

Janis Paige couldn't even get their attention. There was a post-pandemonium atmosphere out there and she was only one girl coming on to sing after three strong, hungry men had just given the show of their lives.

Dean Martin and Jerry Lewis came backstage. Jerry had made notes of things that would help me. Dean said, "You're going all the way, pally." Bogart came back, and a dozen other major stars we'd never met but who wanted to be generous. Unfortunately, Frank was in Europe.

We waited up until eight o'clock and the three of us went out and brought the morning newspapers back to Will's room. I read Herb Stein's review in the Hollywood *Reporter*: "Once in a long time an artist hits town and sends the place on its ear. Such a one is young Sammy Davis, Jr., of the Will Mastin Trio at Ciro's." Paul Coates's column in the *Mirror*: "The surprise sensation of the show was the Will Mastin Trio, a father-uncle-son combination that is the greatest act Hollywood has seen in some months." And *Daily Variety*: ". . . a riotous group of Negro song and dance men whose enthusiasm, brightness, and obvious love for show business combine to form an infectious charm which wins the audience in a flash . . . walloping success . . ."

Will was reading the Los Angeles *Times*. "Listen to what Walter Ames says: 'The Will Mastin Trio, featuring dynamic Sammy Davis, Jr., are such show-stoppers at Ciro's that star Janis Paige has relinquished the closing spot to them.' "

Only a few weeks before, we had been in Vegas feeling abused, hurt, and angry. At that time I could have made a list of every bug-infested mattress we'd slept on for ten thousand nights; I knew every heartache, frustration, and pain, every brush-off which had tormented us for twenty-three years. They had scarred deep, and forgetting them seemed as impossible as undoing them. But as we sat in Will's room reading those reviews the novocaine of success had already begun numbing our memories, making the past indistinct until miraculously there were no yesterdays.

Abe Lastfogel, head of the William Morris Agency, came backstage and we signed to be represented by the Morris office. He invited me to play golf and have lunch with him at the Hillcrest

Country Club. I hadn't exactly had the time to take up the sport but I was happy to walk around the course with him. He was "putting his arms around me." Why? With all the major stars he could be with, why did he reach out to pull me up?

In the clubhouse he said, "That's Jolson sitting over there. After lunch I'll take you over and introduce you. You should begin to meet these people. They are soon going to be your peers."

Groucho Marx was there, George Burns, Jack Benny, Al Jolson, all sitting at a round table with Harry Axt, Jolson's piano player. Mr. Lastfogel introduced me to everybody. Jack Benny said, "I saw him the other night. You're wonderful, son. I'm going to keep you in mind for something."

"Thank you, Mr. Benny."

He turned to the others, "This is the kid that Cantor had on."

I stood there with Mr. Lastfogel looking at the greats. Groucho Marx said, "This kid's the greatest entertainer. And this goes for you, Jolson. He does everything, sings better than you did . . ." Jolson just smiled and waved. "Nice to see you."

During the next few weeks Mr. Lastfogel took me there several times and we always said hello to them. You would stand at that table. They would never ask you to sit down. They didn't ask Abe Lastfogel to sit down. There was no "Bring another chair over." It was not something that occurred to them. They were the kings and other people stood around and paid homage. You were in awe. Business people, old-timers, new celebrities milled around the table, but nobody sat down; there was no intrusion. There was an unwritten law: "Respect this . . ." You were glad you could approach.

The Morris office booked us on the bill with Georgia Gibbs and Jackie Miles at Bill Miller's Riviera just across the river from New York. After that the Beachcomber in Miami Beach and then the Copacabana in New York.

Milton Berle, the King of Television, came to see our act at the Riviera, then he came backstage and told us all the things a performer dreams of hearing. Afterward, he took me aside. "That joke about the swimming pool is cute but you might find it works better if you frame it differently." He told me how the same joke would work better, and why. I was impressed with how right he was. It was no mistake that he was the most important comedian of our time. And I was touched that he would take the trouble to reach back and try to pull me up with him.

As he was leaving he said, "After your second show c'mon over to Lindy's and have a sandwich with me." Milton Berle's nightly table at Lindy's was a Broadway institution. I was dying to go, to sit there with him, with the top comedy writers and the major Broadway characters. But the last time a friend had invited me to have a sandwich at Lindy's the doorman hadn't let me in.

I felt ice in my stomach as the cab pulled up in front of Lindy's. I gave the driver a five for luck. It was after closing time and the revolving door was locked. I could see Berle inside at the head of a round table, a large cigar in his hand, holding court. I saw the doorman inside. I tapped on the glass door with my ring. He waved me away. Simultaneously Milton Berle saw me and snapped his fingers, pointing toward me, and the door opened.

The people at his table were all pros on close terms with lots of stars, and they knew I was just a "kid who's moving up," but they treated me almost as if I was already there. I accepted the hug they were giving me. I could still feel the nights when I hadn't known how to try any harder, how to make myself dance better, to be funnier—but that was behind me, I had their attention, everything was working and the ghettos of my life were shrinking.

As we left there an hour later Berle's Cadillac limousine was at the curb. "Can I drop you at your hotel?"

I thanked him but I'd been on exactly long enough. The world was beautiful and I felt like walking in it.

I headed downtown, crossed Fifty-first Street, and as I passed the Capitol Theater, I thought of Frank. I looked across the street and, incredibly, there he was. I started to run after him, call out to him, but I stopped, my arm in the air. He was slowly walking down Broadway with no hat on and his collar up—and not a soul was paying attention to him. This was the man who only a few years ago had tied up traffic all over Times Square. Now the same man was walking down the street and nobody noticed. God, how could it happen?

I couldn't take my eyes off him, walking the streets, alone, an ordinary Joe who'd been a giant. He was fighting to make it back up again. By himself. The "friends" were gone. He was walking slowly. A hundred people passed him in those few minutes, dozens who must have been fans who'd screamed for him only a few years before, but now nobody cared. I was dying to run over to him, but I felt it would be an intrusion, that he wouldn't want me to see him this way.

And then I thought: My God, if it can happen to him, then how easily it could happen to me. This fragile acceptance could be shattered by a wrong move, or by complacence. The doors could start closing again.

I didn't want to walk anymore.

I took a cab to our hotel. I had to get better, I had to think of everything I could do to keep our momentum going. I couldn't shake the image of Frank Sinatra walking by himself on Broadway. He'd been so big, so entrenched. How could it happen?

5

THERE WAS A sign on the wall of the railroad station: "WELCOME TO MIAMI." Inside were the waiting rooms: "WHITE," "COLORED."

The Lord Calvert was a first-rate hotel in the heart of the Negro section of Miami. Niggy Stein, one of the bosses of the Beachcomber, checked my room. "Everything okay?"

"Yeah, sure, it's fine. Everything's crazy."

He pointed out the window to a new Corvette. "That's yours while you're here. Only white cabs can cross the bridge from Miami onto the Beach and they aren't allowed to ride colored guys." He was telling it to me fast, like a man jumping into cold water. "Here, I got you these cards from the Police Department. There's a curfew on the Beach for all colored people and they can arrest you unless you show 'em this, which explains you're working there."

"But there's a desegregation law!"

He looked at me simpatico. "Not if they won't enforce it."

The headliners at the Beachcomber were Sophie Tucker and Harry Richman. He MC'd the shows, and when I met him backstage on opening night, he said, "I hear you do a great job with 'Birth of the Blues.' Give 'em hell, cousin, that song was good to me."

Arthur Silber, Jr., who was traveling with me, came into the dressing room holding a newspaper. "There's a guy peddling this in front of the club." The headline was "NIGGER ON THE BEACH," and the story was entitled "Stamp Out Sammy Davis, Jr." It said,

50

"The black people are an un-American disease which threatens to spread all over the Beach . . ."

The chorus kids and the crew were giving me sympathy looks, like "How can he possibly do a show now?" But there was no choice. I could let it bury me or turn the hurt and anger into energy to propel me.

I did three encores. Arthur was in the dressing room when we got off. "Well, the guy is gone. But who do you think chased him? Only Milton Berle. I'm outside when Berle gets out of a car and hears the guy shouting, 'Nigger on the Beach.' He smashes him in the mouth, a shot that knocks him right off his feet. The papers go flying in the air and Berle is kicking them into a mudhole."

Niggy came back after the second show. "Whaddya say we bum around, have some laughs?" I knew he was trying to make me feel that I didn't have to run back to the hotel. He took me to a few jazz spots where I was tuned in half to the music and half to the people around us. Nobody said anything. But they didn't have to, the pressure was there.

I woke up at around two in the afternoon. The pool area was jumping: Nat Cole and Sugar Ray Robinson were there, and the ball clubs were in town for winter training, so the Campanellas and Jackie Robinson were there. I was enjoying the crowd of chicks around me until one of them sighed, wistfully, "Gee, I sure wish I could see your show." I was embarrassed to be playing a club that wouldn't let me in either if I weren't starring there.

I made a date with her for that night and we hit the best colored clubs, had laughs, champagne, and everywhere we went the MC introduced me from the stage. I got back to the room around six in the morning, tired but unable to sleep any better than the night before. I'd had a million laughs but no fun. It should have been, and it would have been, if it wasn't being forced down my throat, if I weren't being told this is your side of town, stay here.

WILL CLOSED the dressing-room door. "Eddie wants us back next season. He's offering . . ."

"The next time *I'm* playing Miami Beach is never! Not till they let colored people come in as customers. I don't care how much the money is."

He was smiling. "I already told him no." He waved away my

apology. "I'm only telling you so you can enjoy that we're in a position to choose. And you'll be glad to hear that I turned down another Vegas deal. They're up to $7,500 but they still won't give us rooms in the hotel."

"They must be crazy wanting us that badly but expecting us to live in a slum."

"You won't believe the nerve they got. They know we won't go live in Westside no more, so they came up with a compromise, a new thing some of the colored acts have been taking: three first-class trailers parked on the hotel grounds."

I SAT AT a table on the upper level of the Copacabana. Morty Stevens, who'd been in the band at the Riviera and was now traveling with us as our conductor, was running through our opening number with the band. They were playing it loud and flashy, as it was supposed to be. I listened to music I had heard a thousand times but suddenly I disliked what it was saying.

I walked over to Morty. "Baby, can I talk to you for a moment?" He gave the guys a break and we sat down at a table. "Morty, I want to change the opening number."

"Not for tomorrow night?"

"I'm sorry. I don't care if I have to pay ten guys to stay up all night copying new music—I can't use that number."

"But what's wrong?"

"I don't want to come running onto the stage tomorrow night the way we always have—panting and puffing like 'Is this good enough, folks?' I want to do something that no Negro dance act has ever done before. From now on I'm going to *walk* onto the stage." I hoped I wouldn't have to explain: "With dignity. I'm a headliner. I want to walk on like a gentleman."

He was looking past me, thinking. "There's a number from *Street Scene*. It's soft, New Yorky . . ." He hummed it.

"That's perfect. Start with twelve bars of what you were just rehearsing, to get their attention, then drop into *Street Scene* and I'll walk on."

My father and I left our hotel on West Forty-fourth Street at six-thirty that evening and I told the cabdriver, "The Copacabana." As we turned off Madison Avenue into Sixtieth Street, I said, "Driver, stop on the other side of the street." My dad and I got out of the taxi and walked over to our old doorway. He could appreciate the corny "show business" mood of the moment. Ten years had passed. My father was staring across the street and back through the years as I was. I remembered the doorman's face when he was chasing me away. I remembered Buddy saying "You'll dance on their tables someday."

The time I was onstage might have been a minute or an hour or my lifetime, it was as unreal, as immeasurable as a dream which covers a year but takes only seconds to happen. There were no tomorrows, no yesterdays. I was welded to the emotions of the audience. Suddenly the bond between us was snapped by a tentative crackling of applause, answered by a sharp burst from across the room. Another picked it up and it began gaining urgency like something wild breaking loose, rolling toward me with such force that I couldn't hear the music playing or the words I was singing— only that monumental roar growing and growing and wrapping itself around me.

My head fell to my chest. My arms hung limp at my sides. When I could look up I saw a wall of people rising all around us; table by table they were getting to their feet, standing and applauding us. I was unable to feel my feet on the floor or the fingers I knew I was digging into my palms, or hear anything except one vast, magnificent roar that went on and on. I looked at my father and Will and the tears were pouring from their eyes as they were from mine. After more than twenty years of performing together this was the climax, the ultimate payoff. I lost count of the bows we took and the encores we did before I was stumbling offstage, exhausted, stunned, crying for joy.

THE REAL estate broker drove me straight up to Central Avenue, which leads to Watts. An hour away from all the action, Sunset Strip, the Mocambo, Ciro's, Chasen's.

"Nothing up in the hills, in the Hollywood section?"

"Well—you see—uh . . . Mr. Davis, try to understand. If you were buying it would be a lot simpler. But renting presents certain additional problems . . ."

Obviously I wasn't big enough yet. "Will you take me back to the Sunset Colonial, please?"

"But don't you want to see any of these?"

I shook my head. I was never again going to live in a ghetto. Not if the walls around it were made of solid gold.

Mama had come out to California to live with me. She had a spacious, comfortable house, but I had told her we'd get a house with a pool and palm trees and she wouldn't have to suffer through any more cold New York winters. I took a cab to the house she was sharing with my father and his girlfriend Peewee. "I'm sorry, Mama. You'll have to stay here with Dad and Peewee for a while until I can work this out somehow."

My father spoke softly. "Sammy, they ain't about to let you have a house up there in the hills. Why tear yourself apart over it? You can't change these things."

We were booked as summer replacements for Eddie Cantor's Colgate TV shows. I'd started recording for Decca and "Hey There" was starting to appear on the record charts. It's not just moths that are attracted to flame and heat, so are chicks, and I was swinging like my father always had, taking them out two at a time. For the quiet nights Tony Curtis, Janet Leigh, and Jeff Chandler were buddies I could be with endlessly, and my friendship with Frank was precious to me. I could relax with him more than I had in the early days, but I was still "the kid" to him and he was still "Sinatra" to me. He took me up to the Bogarts' and those were beautiful evenings. With Bogart there was no "he's a this" or "he's a that." Bogart could have been color blind. He got to know a man before he decided if he liked him or not.

The summer was over and I was packing when the phone rang. It was Will. "Sammy, I'm at the Morris office and something just came up. How fast can you get down here?"

The receptionist led me to the room where he and my father were waiting with one of the agents from the nightclub department. "We're playing Vegas," Will said. "We'll be working the Old Frontier and we'll be *living* at the Old Frontier! In the best suites they got! And free of charge besides. Plus food and drink and $7,500 a week."

The Morris guy said, "They're asking for November, which means you play Detroit, Chicago, Atlantic City, Buffalo, Syracuse, Boston, and then into Vegas. That's twelve straight weeks with no day off except for travel . . ."

I wasn't looking for days off. If Vegas could open up to us like that, then it was just a matter of time until the whole country would open up, and I couldn't wait to hit the road and sing and dance my head off toward that moment.

AFTER THE late show in Vegas one of the boy dancers came into the dressing room. "No party tonight?"

"Sorry, baby. Gotta run into L.A. I'm doing the sound track for *Six Bridges to Cross*."

He looked at my rack of clothes and stroked the sleeve of a gray silk. "Crazy-looking threads."

I lifted the suit off the rack. "Wear it in good health."

"Hey, no—I didn't mean . . ."

"No big deal, baby. I'd like you to have it."

I heard him down the hall. "You won't believe what Sammy Davis just did. I was standing in his dressing room looking at this suit . . ."

I felt like Frank had always looked—like a star, to my fingertips.

As I stepped out of the dressing room, someone grabbed my arm. "How's it goin', chicky?" It was Jess Rand, my press agent. He walked outside with me.

"We're doing all the business in town and it's been the ball of all time. Listen, here's the scam. I'm driving to L.A., I'll be back tomorrow, sixish, we'll grab some steam, then it's a little din-din and you can catch the show." I tapped him on the arm. "Meanwhile, grab a chick, have some booze, sign my name, and I'll see you tomorrow."

I took the long way around to my room, through the casino, just for the sheer joy of walking through it. The deputy sheriff standing inside the doorway gave me a big "Hi ya, Sammy." I waved back and kept moving through all the action. Some guys at a dice table made room for me. "C'mon in, Sammy, we've got a hot shooter."

I loved the way the crowds opened up for me and I circled the room twice getting loaded on the atmosphere they'd kept us away from the other times we'd played Vegas, and now the joy of it swept through me every time I walked through that door. Two of the chorus chicks standing at the roulette table waved and made room for me between them. I had no desire to gamble, but people were gathering around to watch my action. I dropped five one-hundred-dollar bills on the table. "On the red, please." An excited murmuring rose around me. "Sammydavis . . . Sammydavis . . . Sammydavis . . ." The chicks were digging the big-time move. The dealer spun the wheel. I shook my fist at him. "If you yell black at me there's gonna be a race riot." It got a laugh and the ball clicked into the red six. The dealer matched my money with a stack of chips and pushed it all back to me. I slid one pile to each of the girls, and playing it Cary Grant on the Riviera with a bow and "Thank you for bringing me luck, ladies," I turned and rode away on their gasps.

It was as though a genie had materialized out of show business and said, "You're a star and anything you want is yours, now you're as good as anybody," and he'd handed us a solid-gold key to every door that had ever been slammed in our faces.

I sat on an easy chair in my living room, absorbing the acceptance, enjoying the luxury of the suite and the picture of myself in the middle of it. I took out a pair of Levi's and a sweater to wear in the car and I called room service for a hamburger. I'd just finished showering when there was a knock on the door. One of the chorus chicks was standing there smiling.

"Hey, this hotel has crazy room service."

She didn't understand the joke but she laughed anyway. When you're making it you get laughs with "Good morning."

I told her, "Darling, I sent Charley around to say there'd be no party tonight. I have to go into L.A."

"I know." She stepped in. "But I thought maybe you'd like some company while you're getting dressed." The doors weren't only opening, they were swinging!

THE GRINDING, steel-twisting, glass-shattering noise screamed all around me. I had no control. I was just there, totally consumed by it, unable to believe I was really in an automobile crash. I saw the impact spin the other car completely around and hurl it out of sight, then my forehead slammed into my steering wheel.

As I felt pain and saw my hand moving, I was stunned by the knowledge that I was still alive.

Cars were stopping, people were running out of a diner and gas station. Someone said, "It's Sammy Davis." I started up the road to see what had happened to the people in the other car. "They're all right, but we'd better get you to a hospital." He pointed to my face and closed his eyes.

I reached up. As I ran my hand over my cheek I felt my eye hanging there by a string. Frantically I tried to stuff it back in, like if I could do that it would stay there and nobody would know, it would be as though nothing had happened. The ground went out from under me and I was on my knees. "Don't let me go blind. Please, God, don't take it all away . . ."

People were picking me up and carrying me and putting me somewhere but I couldn't see, I couldn't move. I was half awake, half asleep, hanging somewhere between the past and the future. But there was no future anymore. All the beautiful things, all the plans, the laughs—they were lying out there, smashed just like the car. The doors were going to close again. The people who'd been nice when I was somebody would turn away from me. None of them were going to say "Hi ya, Sam" anymore.

I heard a siren. There was movement under me and I knew I was in an ambulance. Can it really happen this way? Twenty-six years of working, and taking it, and reaching—was all that for nothing? Can you finally get it and blow it so fast? Was that little touch all there was for me? For my whole life? I'm never going to be a star?

They're going to hate me again.

"NURSE? What's that smell? Flowers?" The doctor had removed my damaged eye. My head was completely bandaged.

"It's all the flowers in San Bernardino. We can't bring any more into the room or you'll suffocate. But there's a line of baskets all the way down the hall. You've also gotten over five hundred telegrams."

"I don't even know five hundred people. You don't have to do cheer-up bits with me."

She took my hand and ran it against a stack of envelopes that must have been a foot high. "We've got eight bundles like this one."

"There's gotta be a mistake. Will you read me the names on the flowers?"

"Betty and Charles Schuyler . . ."

"Darling, I don't know anyone by that name."

"The card says, 'Though we have never met you, our prayers are with you. Have courage. Betty and Charles Schuyler.'"

What a beautiful thing! Total strangers to go to the trouble and expense of sending me flowers. She went through the other cards and the telegrams, reading off names of governors, mayors, movie and TV producers, bit players, stars, headwaiters, and vaudeville performers I hadn't seen or heard of in years. But mostly they were from total strangers.

I heard someone coming in. "Well, chicky, this was a great little publicity stunt you dreamed up." I recognized Jess's voice. "You've won the hearts of a grateful Hollywood for knocking Eddie and Debbie off the front pages. Even Korea couldn't do *that*."

"Baby, slow up a minute. Are you saying I've been on the front pages?"

"Don't they read newspapers around here?"

"Jess, there's been a few other things going on. Like, for openers, I lost an eye."

"I'm hip. Well, you've made page one clear across the country for two days running. Pictures, stories, the whole bit. The wire services haven't been off my phone since it happened."

"Jess, if this is your idea of a gag . . ."

"Chicky, it's emmis! You're the hottest thing in the business. The coverage has been fantastic: 'Can the little man with the big talent survive this blow to his career?' . . . 'Just as the dreams of a lifetime were being fulfilled . . .'"

I listened to Walter Winchell's Sunday night radio program. "This is your New York correspondent winding up another edition with a word of advice to young Sammy Davis, Jr., in a hospital somewhere in San Bernardino, California. Sammy: if you can hear me . . . remember . . . no champ ever lost a fight by being knocked down. Only by *staying* down."

THE NURSE was taking away the breakfast tray when I heard my father and Will burst in. "Poppa, what would you like to have more than anything in the world?"

"Oh, come on, Dad."

"No kiddin'!"

"I'd like to have my goddamned career back."

Will said, "Sammy, this is a telegram from the New Frontier in Las Vegas. It says: 'Firm offer for Will Mastin Trio Featuring Sammy Davis, Jr. *Twenty five thousand per week*, first available date, please advise.'"

I COULD hear the excitement in the halls. Nurses were running from room to room gasping, "He's here, in the hospital! Frank Sinatra!" They were going out of their minds, dropping thermometers and grabbing for lipsticks. He had won an Oscar for *From Here to Eternity* and he was back on top.

Frank was standing in the doorway, smiling. "Hi ya, Charley." He came in, flipped his hat onto a chair, and looked at me carefully. "You're going to be all right." The nurse was rooted to the floor, staring at him, so flustered that she didn't think to give him a chair. He smiled at her. "Hi ya, honey." She nodded like a drunk, with the grin and the glazed eyes.

He pulled up a chair and straddled it, arms resting against its back. "Well, what's happening with the eye?"

"I'll have to wear a patch until the socket heals, then I get a new eye. Plastic." I took a cigarette out of a pack and held up my lighter, but the flame missed the end of the cigarette. When I finally got it lit Frank smiled, "You're full of little party tricks, Charley."

"Stick around. For an encore I light my nose."

"How long do the docs figure for you to straighten out?"

"They say maybe three months, but they're not sure."

"You still got the place in the Sunset Colonial?" I nodded. "Well, we've got to get you out of there. You should have a house."

"I tried to get one, but . . ."

"You'll have a house in the hills where you can get some quiet and still not be in the Yukon." He looked at my father. "I'll be in touch with you on it." He turned back to me. "We'll get you something small, a rental until you know exactly what you want. You should have a couple of guys living with you until you're on your feet. Meanwhile, come out to the Springs and spend a couple of weeks with me. Have you decided where you want to open?"

"Well, that Vegas money looks awfully good, but I've got a funny kind of a feeling about our first date. Herman Hover can only give us five thousand and though I hate to go for the short money, well, I've been thinking maybe we should go back to Ciro's, where it all began for us."

"You're definitely right. The important thing is to start strong, and in L.A. you'll be home where you know you have friends around you. The Vegas money'll still be there. Meanwhile, Charley, get your health back, rest, don't rush."

"I wish it was that simple. Let's say it takes three months. By then, all this fantastic publicity won't mean beans—I'll have blown all this momentum. On the other hand, obviously I can't come back too early, coming on like I'm stumbling around for sympathy."

"You wait till you're ready! Don't worry about the momentum. They'll wait for you. The day you go back to work you'll be as hot as you are today."

"I wish I could believe that."

He raised an eyebrow. "You want to talk about comebacks?"

He picked up his hat. "I'll see you at the Springs." He put his hand on my shoulder. "Relax. You're going to be bigger than ever, Charley. Bigger than ever."

6

WHEN WE OPENED at Ciro's we got front-page coverage and there were lines outside the club for every performance. And after the shows I was at Frank's house or the Bogarts' or Judy Garland's.

It was almost light as I started up the hill to my house, and when I got there it was all I could do to find a parking spot. The place was swinging with young actors and performers from all over town. Some of them were drinking, listening to music, some were half asleep—but they were all waiting for me. "I'm awfully sorry. I got hung up." They waved away my apologies like they understood. Dave Landfield, a young actor whom I'd asked to move in with me, was careening around the room doing charming bits with the best-looking starlets in town.

I went downstairs to see Mama in her living room on the first floor. "You okay, Mama? Is there too much noise upstairs?"

"I'm fine, Sammy. I'm glad to hear all that happiness."

Dave grabbed me by the arm. "Hey, you had a call from Judy Kanter. She wants to throw a party for you Wednesday night."

"Crazy, but she'll have to make it Thursday, between five and eight."

"Sam! Her father's president of Paramount. Don't get her angry. They could make me a star."

"Sorry, old buddy, but I happen to be very big on Wednesday. I've already got two parties in my honor."

He was looking at me wistfully. "It must be fantastic to make it like this."

"Yeah, I've got to admit it. The world is my oyster, and I'm the little black pearl."

He stood there, smiling at me, transplanting himself into my life, enjoying a glimpse of what he wanted so badly.

"Listen, Dave, I've got a wild idea. Come on the road with me as a sort of secretary-buddy. You'll make some money, be around the business, maybe you'll meet somebody who'll do you some good—I'll help you with anyone I can. And we'll have a million laughs besides."

"You just hired a secretary-buddy."

I gave him a shot on the arm. "The first thing you do is take care of our rooms in Chicago. It's your hometown. Get us the best two-bedroom suite in the best hotel there."

"Hey, that runs into money."

"Dave, you're working for a star! And if we ain't goin' first cabin, then the boat ain't leavin' the dock."

THE ROOM clerk shuffled through a stack of reservations, glancing at them in a way that you knew he knew he wasn't going to find what he was looking for. He smiled weakly. "I'm terribly sorry, Mr. Davis, but there's no reservation for you. And we're entirely filled up!"

Dave didn't catch on. "I wired you two weeks ago."

"Well, uh . . . we tried to notify you—but we didn't have the address."

Morty glared at him. "Why didn't you try sending it to Sammy Davis, Jr., U.S.A.?"

Dave called another hotel. I sat in the cab between him and Morty while the doorman put our bags into the trunk. I'd thought this was all behind me. I really had. There was a sharp crack. The sunglasses I'd been holding had snapped in my hand.

"Take it easy, Sam."

I looked at the cracked lenses and the trickle of blood coming out of my palm. "I *am* taking it easy." I rubbed the skin over my knuckles, watching the color lighten under the pressure of my thumb and then come back to normal. Morty sat next to me, silent. I stared up at the ceiling of the cab. I'm a star! This isn't supposed to happen anymore.

OUR LIMOUSINE moved through the downtown Las Vegas traffic, past the Golden Nugget, Horseshoe Club, Jackpot, and onto Highway 91. Dave was Charley Tourist: "Hey, is this the Strip?"

"Yeah, baby. This is it."

"Wow! Wild! What's it like in those places?"

I didn't answer, not wanting to deflate him or embarrass myself by explaining that I'd never been to any of them, that I had the run of the hotel where I was working but I was not welcome at the others.

I stopped off at my father's room. "Any word from Mama?"

"They called from a gas station. Oughta be here by six."

"Great. I'll arrange a table for the dinner show."

"Poppa? You sure maybe you're not pushin' the horse a little faster'n he can run? Colored people sittin' out front in Vegas?" He was shaking his head. "I just hope you ain't stickin' your neck out too far."

"I'm not sticking my neck out. But I ain't pullin' it in like a goddamned turtle either. My grandmother is going to sit and watch me perform or there ain't nobody gonna sit and watch me perform."

I picked up the phone and asked to be connected with the Copa Room. "Hello, this is Sammy Davis, Jr. . . . Fine, thanks. I'd like a table for six, for my family, at the ringside, for the dinner show tonight."

"Well? What'd they say, Poppa?"

"They said, 'Yes, sir, I'll hold a center ringside. And have a great opening, Mr. Davis.'"

MY LIVING room was jammed. I sat down next to Mama and put my arm around her. "Did you have a good time tonight?"

"Just seeing what people think of you and how they're treating you is a good time for me, Sammy. I'd better be getting my sleep, though." I walked her to the door.

There were about a dozen people left when Dave said, "Hey, whaddya say we start at one end of town and hit every place along the way?" His face was still reflecting the excitement of the evening. "I hear there's a wild lounge act at the Desert Inn . . ."

The wave of ice passed across my stomach. "Baby, we're comfortable, it's late, we've got everything we want."

"It's only four o'clock. Come on, let's celebrate."

"I don't know about those places, Dave." I had to explain. "Baby, this is Vegas. It's one thing for me here where I'm working, but I'm not so sure about those other hotels. Now, do you want to see a lounge act or a lynching?"

Somebody else said, "Don't you know how big you are? They'll roll out a red carpet anywhere you go."

Dave shrugged. "He's out of his mind." He picked up the phone. "Years ago it was one thing . . . Hello, may I have the Desert Inn, please?"

I got busy putting my records into their cardboard covers. Conversation had stopped. Dave crossed one leg over the other and blew smoke rings at the ceiling. "Connect me with the lounge, please, darling . . . Hello, I'd like to reserve a table for about twenty minutes from now for Sammy Davis, Jr., and a party of . . ." There was a burst of red across his cheeks. He lowered the phone back on the hook. "Sam . . . I'm sorry." There were murmurs of "Well, if that's how they are, then who the hell needs them . . ." "They're a hundred years behind the times . . ." Everyone was embarrassed for me. The evening was lying on the floor dead.

I stood up. "Morty, do me a favor. Have room service bring over twenty steak sandwiches, and a case of their best champagne, quick style. And swing by the casino and tell Sonny and the kids it's a party. Invite everybody you see that we dig."

I turned on the hi-fi set loud. Within ten minutes the crowd of chorus kids was drowning it out, and the room came alive like somebody'd plugged us in.

Dave came over to where I was standing. "You okay?"

"Thanks, baby. I'm fine." I had the feeling of having waited all my life to own a raincoat and when finally I got one it wasn't working, the water was coming through.

I asked Jack Entratter, the president of the Sands, "Can I do a third show next Saturday? I'd like to invite all the performers on the Strip."

Al Freeman, the Sands' publicist, saw the potential for goodwill and word of mouth. For me it was a fast introduction to everyone in town and I knew that after they'd seen me perform most of them would like me.

And I began running movies after the shows, on the second floor, in the Emerald Room. I had two features flown in from L.A. every night and I invited the line of "Texas Copa Girls," our opening act, everyone in the show. I put in a standing order for a steam table with Chinese food, a table of sandwiches, and a bartender. Nothing started until around 3 a.m. because the "Texas Copa Girls" were required to spend one full hour at the bar after the last show in case a high roller wanted a companion. It was standard for show girls at all the Strip hotels. They were not there just because they were gorgeous and kicked high.

My father came in one night. "Sammy, can I talk to you a minute?" Outside in the hall for privacy, he gave me a newspaper clipping. The headline was "Is Sammy Ashamed He's a Negro?"

Sammy Davis, Jr., who recently sparkled like a 14-carat-gold star on the stage of the Fairmont, was a rare pleasure to us as a reviewer and as a Negro. But, unfortunately, persistent reports of his offstage performances leave much to be desired. His all-night, all-white, orgy-style parties are the talk of Las Vegas, where he is currently appearing. We are sorry to be the ones to remind Mr. Davis of his obligation to the Negro community, but even sorrier for the necessity to do so.

"I don't get it, Dad. Why should they want to write lousy stuff like this about me?"

"Poppa . . . well, right in that room there, just look who you got around you. Ain't nothin' but ofays."

"Dad! Where in the goddamned hell am I going to find colored people in Las Vegas? Should I go over to Westside and find cats I don't know? To dress up the room?"

"Well, maybe you could cut down on the parties some."

"What else am I supposed to do? I drain myself dry on that stage every night, don't I have the right to unwind? Okay, I can't do it like everybody else; I can't do drop-ins at the Desert Inn, and 'Hey, let's catch the new lounge act at El Rancho.' I'm not complaining, but I'm on an island here at the Sands. I shouldn't have to draw pictures for you why I bring people over." He didn't fight me and my anger turned to a rotten, hollow feeling. "They don't mention that because of me colored people sat out front in a Las Vegas hotel for the first time in history. Just that I have parties."

I stared at the clipping. "I swear to God I'd have thought they'd be happy every time one of us breaks out and lives good."

The stage managers of other hotels began calling: "What's the picture tonight?" and they'd post it on their backstage bulletin boards and soon I had all the performers in Las Vegas. Guys would come up to me. "Jeez, Sammy, we can't get laid. All the chicks in town are up there in your fuckin' place watchin' the fuckin' movie. Y'gotta stop this."

Okay, I'd brought the mountain to Mohammed, I'd made my own world and it wasn't bad. But I didn't want my own world. I wanted to live in the same world as everyone else.

I had to get bigger, that's all. I had to get bigger.

LENNY HIRSHON, my agent at the William Morris office, was not very interested in my problem. "Sammy, if you were white you'd have been in pictures a year ago."

"Hold it, Lenny. I've *got to have* the importance of motion pictures. I've got to expand, break out of being a singer-dancer-comic, and you've got to help me."

"Well, it's not easy. There just aren't parts for Negroes. Plus, they couldn't begin to meet your price."

"What's my price?" I leaned across his desk. "My price to make a movie is fifty dollars! You hear what I'm saying? *Fifty dollars!* And I'll take a cut if necessary."

His phone rang and he grabbed for it, extending the other hand to me. "Sammy, I'll bring it up at the next meeting."

I went down the hall to the television department.

"Sammy, the truth is we just haven't been able to find a dramatic role for you. But you can have all the variety shows you want. At top money."

"Fine. But I need dramatic television too."

"Well, for a star of your importance we have to find the right vehicle."

"Don't give me the vehicle jazz. I'm not asking for Rolls-Royce parts. Find me a little used Chevy. It could be one scene if it's the right one. Let *me* be the one to say, 'No, it's too small.' "

"Sammy, what're you knocking yourself out for? Why risk bombing in dramatic television? You're a first-rate Sammy Davis, Jr.; why be a second-rate Sidney Poitier?" I held on, telling myself,

Don't make an enemy, you need him, you need him. "You're a great entertainer, but that doesn't mean you're an actor. Maybe if you took some drama lessons, like the Actors Studio, something that'd give us a little background to work with."

I stood up and ground a cigarette into his ashtray. "You want some background? How's twenty-four years in the business? How's *eight hundred thousand dollars* a year, of which you guys get ten percent? How's the fact that I'm a star that you don't have to lift a finger to get booked in clubs, all you have to do is answer phone calls. Please, let's stop kidding each other. The problem is racial."

"Well, it *is* awfully touchy. We all know that on certain networks Negroes are banned except if they appear as servants."

"Look, we both know they aren't running around town hoping to find colored actors. But I'm a name. Maybe I can draw a rating, right? The door isn't locked. It's just closed and there must be a way to get it opened."

I left there knowing they would continue taking the easy way out, avoiding the extra work of selling me, taking the attitude: "Who needs problems?"

A month later we were playing Vegas and Jule Styne came into the dressing room, shy, yet bristling with energy. I'd met him at Frank's house. He and Sammy Cahn had written a lot of Frank's hit songs. "Sammy, I saw your show. Fantastic! You're a great talent but you'll suffocate that talent in saloons. You've got to expand, you need dimension . . ." His enthusiasm was dizzying. "The place for you is Broadway."

I was staring at him like he was Charley Messiah. "Jule, keep talking. But keep your distance or you may get a kiss on the lips."

"You should star in a musical. You can sing and dance and do everything you do in clubs. I'll produce it and we'll get some good writers to do a modern musical comedy. You can't possibly miss. And the prestige would be enormous for you."

When he left I found myself smiling at the walls: if television and movies don't want me, to hell with them—there's *nothing* that can match Broadway for stature and dignity.

7

I RECEIVED a telegram: WELCOME TO NEW YORK. PLEASE DROP
IN AND VISIT US. ED WYNNE, THE HARWYN. I had just opened in
Mr. Wonderful. I called Jule's co-producer, George Gilbert. "What
kind of a place is the Harwyn?"

"East Side supper-clubbish. It's the hot place. Whatever *that*
means."

I read him the telegram. "That's damned nice of them."

"Well, really! You *are* the star of a Broadway show."

"Baby, I admit that I'm one of the great stars of our time. I even
admit that I'm adorable, but I'm not exactly in demand around the
chic supper clubs." In fact, the only restaurant I went to in New
York was Danny's Hideaway, because Danny had reached out to
me and I knew I was safe there. As I spoke, the tone of George's
voice caught up with me and I realized that he'd understood; I
could picture him smiling, but he was considerably playing it cool.
"The least we can do is accept the man's invitation, right? Let's
make up a party of six and do it tonight, baby."

"Sure, *baby.*"

When I saw the Harwyn's doorman from down the street I felt
the usual ice in the stomach. But when our cab stopped he opened
the door. "Nice to see you, Mr. Davis." He moved quickly to
open the front door for me. I let George and the others go in first,
aware that I was letting them run interference for me.

A tall, good-looking man extended his hand. "Sammy, my name
is Ed Wynne. Thank you for coming in."

The dance band started playing "Mr. Wonderful"; people all over the room were smiling and waving at me; Ed led us to a prominent table, removed the "Reserved" sign, and introduced our table captain. "Mac here will see that you have everything you want." A waiter brought over a bucket with champagne bottles in it. "Compliments of Mr. Wynne."

My stomach and the skin around my jaw were loosening up. I leaned back against the soft banquette and smiled at the group. "That's how it is when you're with a star, folks. It's a definite first cabin all the way."

When we were leaving, Ed walked me to the door. "Thanks for coming in, Sammy. Now come back soon. Please. Think of this as your home."

We left the others and George and I walked toward Park Avenue. When we were far enough away from the club I grabbed his arm and hung on it like a half-hysterical nitwit. "Do you want to know about a small Negro lad from Harlem who just saw his first chic supper club and the owner told him, 'This is your home'?" I did a few Bill Robinson steps up the stoop of a private house.

George shrugged. "Now really. What's the big deal?" But his face was bursting with concealed pleasure for me and I danced back down the steps and gave him a shot on the arm.

"Ow."

"I'm a star and it's in my contract that I can hit my producer any time I feel like it."

I WAS invited to Sunday dinner at D.D. and Johnny Ryan's apartment. I'd been surprised to see his name, John Barry Ryan III, in Cholly Knickerbocker's column, and learn that a guy who worked as my stage manager and dressed like he couldn't afford to get his name in the telephone book was Charley Social Register. He'd said it would be an informal dinner. To me that would mean Levi's and hamburgers, but with them it might be a sit-down dinner with only three forks instead of five.

On Friday afternoon I left my apartment at the Gorham, a West Fifty-fifth Street hotel. I walked a few blocks to Tiffany, glanced at the window display—a golf club poised in midair, ready to swing at a large diamond resting on a tee—and pushed the revolving door slowly, trying to get my bearings before I was inside. A store detective smiled. "Hello, Mr. Davis." The showcases sparkled as though every time a customer touched one a hand came out and polished it.

As I stepped off the elevator into the silver department a saleswoman approached me. "Mr. Davis, so nice to have you in the store. May I help you?"

"Thank you. I'm interested in two things." I selected a water pitcher to bring Johnny and D.D.

"You said there was something else?"

"Yes . . . it's a favor I'd like to ask of you. Just between us, I don't know the first thing about the different kinds of silverware and I want to learn. I thought about looking it up in Emily Post but then I figured she probably learned it *here*."

She lowered her voice. "You wouldn't believe how many people don't know an oyster fork from a bouillon spoon. It will be my privilege to show you."

On Sunday I took the package from Tiffany out of the closet. A few dozen roses would be more appropriate for one dinner, but Johnny and D.D. had been great to me when we were on the road with the show and I wanted to give them something nice. I could always play it as though it was in return for the books on fine art they'd given me. I dressed in a gray tweed suit, an eggshell shirt, and a black knitted tie, put on a vicuña polo coat, and left the apartment.

A strong gust of wind from the East River almost knocked the box out of my hand as I stepped out of the cab in front of River House. I gripped the box securely against me and walked toward the building. At the front entrance a doorman stuck his head out and pointed to the left. "Delivery entrance is up the street." He closed the door.

My phone was ringing as I got home. I didn't answer it. I put the Tiffany box in the closet. I made myself a drink and looked out the window at New York. God, it was cold out there. So warm and so cold.

On Monday evening Johnny Ryan came to my dressing room. "Sam? You weren't sick last night? We called . . ."

I turned around. "I'm sorry about dinner, baby, but something came up."

"Oh . . . okay."

I went after him and stopped him in the hall. "Look, John . . . I'm sorry. I didn't forget. I just couldn't make it."

He was confused and hurt. "Sammy . . . D.D. spent the whole day cooking a turkey for you. Couldn't you at least have called?"

"I'm sorry, John. I couldn't. I really couldn't."

His eyes became veiled, as if a stone wall had risen between us. "All right, Sam. We'll do it some other time." He turned and I stood there watching him walk away from me.

JUST ON the rumor that Frank was going to play the Copa the two-week engagement was sold out. On opening night there was a famous face at every table, from DiMaggio to Dietrich. I got Julie Podell to give me the impossible, a ringside table for ten for every night. A few days after the opening Humphrey Bogart died and I got a call from Julie. "Frank can't go on tonight. I've got Jerry Lewis for the first show. I need you for the second." When I came off Julie was beaming at me like an angel. He held my face in his hands with more affection than I'd ever seen from him. "You did me a big favor, buddy. How many people can fill in for Frank? We'd have had to close down." He gave me a fistful of hundred-dollar bills. "And the tabs you been signing every night, they're on me. The joint is yours."

I went into the lounge with some buddies. Bruno, the maître d', grabbed my hand with both of his. "It was wonderful, Sammy. Thanks." Every captain and waiter at the Copa went out of his way to smile at me.

Frank was back the next night and I was at ringside again—but center-center ringside—with buckets of champagne and bottles of scotch on the table, preordered by Julie Podell.

As I cut into my steak a voice behind me snarled, ". . . little nigger in front of me." I continued cutting my food and without raising my head shot a glance around my table. The voice continued: "Waiter, let's have the captain over here." Then he was saying, "You got any authority around this place?"

"Is something wrong, sir?"

"Damned right. I want a table without such a lousy view." A woman was trying to quiet him down. George took a shot of scotch and closed his eyes as it seared through his chest. The captain must have signaled up above, because I heard Bruno asking, "Can I help you, sir?" I kept cutting away at my steak. "Maybe you can do better than your flunky here. You look like a man who knows right from wrong." The voice softened, becoming fraternal, conspiratorial. "It's obviously some kind of a mistake. I come in here thinking I'm spending my money in a first-class place, so you can understand my surprise when I find my wife and I seated behind that little jigaboo. Now I'm sure that you . . ." The words ended in a gasp. George was staring past me, his face chalked by shock. I turned. The table was empty. Bruno and the captain had the man under each arm and were already halfway out of the room with him. A woman was hurrying after them.

People around us were whispering, looking toward me, speculating on what happened. My group was limp, doing self-conscious smiles, not knowing if they should look at me or away from me, and I felt the sympathetic stares burning into me like I was caught in the headlights of a dozen converging cars.

A hand was on my shoulder. Julie Podell was looking at me simpatico. "The bum is out on the street where he belongs." My guests were getting their wind back, talking, but their voices were like a record being played at the wrong speed. "I'm sorry, Michael, what did you say, baby?" He blushed. "It wasn't worth repeating. Just something insipid, like 'Keep a stiff upper lip, things'll get better someday.' "

"Baby, if you'll excuse a little well-earned bitterness: colored people don't really have big lips, we just look this way from *keeping* them stiff for so long."

The lights dimmed and Joey Bishop was opening the show. I put a smile on my face because people would be watching me. Joey looked at me with feigned curiosity. "Don't I know you from somewhere, sir?" The crowd laughed, and I played the scene of enjoying myself, stamping my feet hilariously.

As Frank sang I thought: *If I can make myself remember the first time I ever came in here, if I can appreciate how far I've come . . . I'm a star. So much has changed.* But nothing had changed. Not really. And I remembered my father's voice despairing: "You ain't gonna get away from it till you die."

As soon as I could I made a break for it. My new car was in front of the door, a Cadillac Brougham, the best, most expensive American car built. I got into it and started driving uptown. Maybe in Harlem I'd be able to breathe, to get a reprieve from the grasping for quicksilver acceptance, from the constant looking over my shoulder, the listening, waiting. I had to break the spasm of suspense. I tore my collar open and kept pushing uptown, stopping at lights, not aware that the car had lost its motion until they changed and I was surging forward again, straining to get there. I passed 110th Street—I was beginning to feel better, looser. Turning west on 125th, I drove slowly over to Seventh Avenue, parked, and let a crowd form around me. They were shoving to get near me, excited, calling down the street to their friends. But they didn't give a damn that I was Sammy, that I was home, standing on the corner. I was just another celebrity, that's all they saw—that and my car and my clothes. I pushed my way through them and got back into my car . . . drove uptown toward Mama's old place, speeding, suddenly afraid it might have been torn down.

I put my hand on the banister, trying to feel as I had when Mama had been in the kitchen and I could race up the stairs and inside for dinner. The rich warm smells of the food she was cooking, the home smells, used to be all the good things in the world to me. I looked around me at the walls, the stairs, the banister—not really surprised at finding it no different, but not the same. I thought of going upstairs and standing in front of our door. Somebody'd come by and say, "Aren't you Sammy Davis, Jr.?" and I'd nod. "I used to live here." They'd ask me in and I'd sit in the easy chair next to the window and the whole family would come in and watch me. "That's Sammy Davis, Jr., he used to live here, right here in this room." They'd be poor like we were, and when I left I'd find the landlord and pay up their rent for a year. But I knew that I was only romancing my unhappiness, playing a corny scene from any one of a thousand old movies—that I didn't even feel like I was home.

AFTER THE show I sat behind my bar autographing pictures, occasionally glancing up to see how the "family"—George, Chita Rivera, who was in the show with me, and Michael Wettach, our assistant stage manager—were doing. The bell rang and Michael opened the door for Jane and Burt Boyar. He was a columnist and we'd become very close. I waved. "So the wandering journalists have returned home after another glittering night of gathering tomorrow's news today, eh?"

Jane slipped off her shoes and walked over to glance at herself in the mirror. George asked, "And where were Mr. and Mrs. Manhattan *this* evening?"

"The usual." Burt's voice came from the closet. "There was an opening at the Plaza . . . we looked into Morocco . . ."

"Don't knock it," George grumbled. "These four walls!"

I listened to them, realizing that it had been weeks since we'd been anywhere. It was always the show, then benefits, then straight back to the apartment, to the island I'd created, to the few people I'd allowed to live on it with me—avoiding aggravation. But by doing so I was giving sanction to the idea that the world was white and I shouldn't try to live in it. It was frightening. I was the guy who comes home from the office and goes for a dip in the ocean, closing his eyes, luxuriating in feeling the tensions and pressures easing—unaware that he's drifting from shore.

"Burt."

"Yes, Sam?"

"What's it like at El Morocco?"

"I guess it's about the best place of its kind in town, probably the world. Sophisticated-type crowd, glamorous . . ."

"But you're never going to take me there, right?"

"Just say when."

"It's only one o'clock. Let's go tonight."

Chita jumped up. "You really mean it, Sammy?"

"How long will it take you to go home and change your clothes?"

She rushed for her coat. "I'll be back in less than half an hour." Michael was already out the door and ringing for the elevator.

I told Burt, "You'd better make a reservation. Tell them I'm in your party."

He dialed a number. I got a camera and started taking shots of the lighted buildings, appreciating the tripod which kept the camera steady, concentrating on the methodical clicks of the shutter that cracked across the room until they were drowned out by the sound of Burt's voice, angry, vibrating with emotion. I glanced around and saw the skin pulled tight around his jaw, the muscle in his cheek throbbing; Jane started going through her purse, George picked up a photography magazine which he'd already looked through earlier in the evening. I heard the phone being set slowly on the receiver.

"They don't want me, right?"

His face was drained of color, chalky. I walked over to him and gently pinched his cheeks. "Baby, it's okay to be white but you're overdoing it." I sat behind my bar. "Well, I went for broke and I got it." I looked at Burt. "Let's hear it, don't leave me in the dark. Oops. What do I mean by *that?*"

He was shaking his head slowly. "It was unbelievable . . . he started to say they didn't have any tables but he knew I'd know that's ridiculous at this hour. Then he said he wanted to speak to John Perona—the owner. He came back in a minute and asked me what you looked like."

"What I look like?"

"He said, 'He's very black, isn't he?' "

"You're kidding!"

"I wish to God I was. Then he started copping out by saying, 'I mean, he's not light-skinned. I mean, it's awfully dark, isn't it?' Then he had a new idea. He said you've been in *Confidential* and the scandal magazines and that's the reason they don't want you— because they don't want to encourage people like that. . . . Sam, I should have mentioned a dozen of their steady customers who've been in those magazines, to say nothing of Bob Harrison, who publishes *Confidential*, but I was so dazed I . . . I just hung up."

"Did they actually say, 'No, he can't come here'?"

"No. They know that's against the law. They just said you're not welcome and that you won't be treated nicely if you appear there."

I ground my fist into my hand, drawing my fingers tightly over the knuckles, watching my skin changing color under the pressure, overwhelmed for the millionth time by the great goddamned difference people saw in it, embarrassed by my incredibly naïve optimism that had again, inexcusably, suckered me into hoping that this time it would be different.

"Sam?"

Burt's face was racked by the pain of someone who'd always known fire was hot but now the first searing touch of it had shown him how hot it really was. He smiled grimly. "As I hung up—the dance band was playing 'Mr. Wonderful.' "

When they'd gone home I sat at my bar. There was a puddle of water from a Coke bottle and, dipping my finger into it, I wrote my name on the varnished wood top. I stared at the autograph I'd given away so many thousands of times. I was a star. On Broadway!

When you star on Broadway you're supposed to be accepted. This wasn't supposed to happen anymore.

I saw a fly come into my living room and in trying to get out he landed on the window. He could see through the glass to where he wanted to go, and he kept trying to get there, but not understanding what it was that was stopping him, he kept trying and trying and finally, exhausted, he fell, trapped by the glass, and died.

8

As soon as I got out to the Coast I went to the Morris office. I'd heard about this new guy, Sy Marsh, who was head of the television department and also the liaison with Universal, the largest studio in the world. I didn't call for an appointment. I didn't want to give him time to figure out how to tell me, "It's a problem."

His secretary phoned inside: "Sammy Davis, Jr., is here . . ." The door of his office burst open and this young guy rushed out and grabbed my hand. "Come in, come in, I'm thrilled to death. You're my idol as an entertainer." He was in his early thirties and as we rapped I found out he was a kid from Brooklyn who'd tried to be a performer before he'd become an agent.

"Sy, I want to get into dramatic television. Now, I know there's a problem, I'm a Negro, and there aren't parts written for us except as servants, but I think that there's a place for me somewhere, that I can act . . ."

He said, "It's outrageous. A great talent like yours. It's insulting. Of course you're an actor. When you do impersonations, what is that, chopped liver? It's acting." He shrugged. "I guess the reason has been that the sponsors aren't going to stick their necks out and take a chance on jarring customers in the Southern markets."

"Baby, have you any idea how jarring it must be for about five million colored kids who sit in front of their TV sets hour after hour and they almost never see anybody who looks like them? It's like they and their families and their friends just plain don't exist."

"Terrible. It's wrong." He was thoughtful for a moment. "Universal does the *GE Theater*. The producer is Harry Tugend . . . let's give him a shot." In a minute he was saying, "Harry, listen, you and I have an opportunity to break through an important barrier. Sammy Davis, Jr., is a great name, he's hot as a pistol, he's starred on Broadway, whenever he appears on variety shows he draws tremendous ratings across the country, North and South, and he should be starring on dramatic television. He's performing right now at the Moulin Rouge over on Sunset. I would like you to be my guest and I think you will see a quality outside of singing and dancing. You'll see sensitivity, dramatic ability . . ."

I had put them at center ringside. I did Cyrano de Bergerac, a scene from *The Caine Mutiny*, Olivier doing *Hamlet*, things I never did normally, plus all the standards: Bogart, Cagney, Ronald Colman, Frank, Jerry, and as I worked I could lip-read Harry Tugend saying "Great! Fantastic!" and it was the fuel that drove me higher and higher.

We had supper at the Villa Capri and Harry said, "I have a property that was done on Broadway, a playlet called *Auf Wiedersehen*. It's a heartrending thing . . ."

The script was marvelous, we cleared the dates, I got lucky and acted over my head, and everybody on the set was crying. On the last day of shooting, Ronald Reagan, the host on *GE Theater*, said to Sy, "It's going to be a wonderful episode. When I introduce it what do you think would be appropriate for me to say about Sammy?"

Sy suggested, "This is the first time that a transition is being made by a Negro entertainer to a leading dramatic role, so the emphasis should be that the world's greatest entertainer has come to GE to star in a dramatic show."

Later, he came into my dressing room. "Well, sweetheart, you've made television history. When they write books about the tube they've got to write that Sammy Davis, Jr., was the first Negro actor to star in episodic television. And the doors are going to open for a lot of other Negro actors. You'll have opened those doors for others to follow."

I could imagine the pleasure of turning on the television set and seeing young Negro actors and actresses playing doctors and lawyers, cops and robbers, good guys and bad guys . . . it didn't matter what as long as they broke out of it being just maids and butlers.

I PARKED my motorcycle in the driveway of the Beverly Wilshire Hotel and went to the penthouse suite. I'd met Elvis Presley on the set of his third picture, *Loving You*. Both of us were rebels in our own ways and we'd gravitated toward each other. We both had motorcycles. I had a cut-down Harley and we ran together whenever we were in the same town. Up in his living room he was at the piano. Nicky Blair, Nick Adams, Natalie Wood, Dennis Hopper, and some kids not in the business were there.

Elvis started doing Ray Charles. He was a marvelous impressionist. I could do Ray but not with the piano. Elvis did the best white Ray Charles I've ever heard. I said, "Okay, pal of mine, I've got one for you. Dr. Jekyll and Mr. Hyde." Elvis went over to a couch and the kids who'd been standing around him at the piano all took their places to watch me.

I was wearing my hair very long and I roughed it up and strung it out like the mad Mr. Hyde. I took out my bridge, I did the crazy eyes, and, bent over, I did the heavy breathing, the whole transition that Fredric March did. I leaped onto the couch next to Elvis, screaming, "I'm free . . . I'm free . . ." He cringed. "Don't touch me." He was really upset, so I came out of the character. He was still half nervous. "Put your teeth back and comb your hair." Then, when I looked like me again, he relaxed. "You've gotta put that in the act."

A few nights later I was in my dressing room at the Mou getting ready for the second show when I was told, "Elvis is at center ringside." I went over to Big John Hopkins, my road manager. "Elvis is here and I'm gonna do something. Be in the wings to catch me 'cause I'm gonna come off flying in the air."

I did the whole show, did the impression of Elvis with the white shoes and the guitar. Then I said, "This is for my man." I did about two minutes of Jekyll and Hyde dialogue, ending in screaming, "I'm free, freeeee . . . ," and I ran and leaped high into the wings and John caught me. Blackout.

The people were still yelling when I came back onstage. Elvis stood up at ringside and we shook hands.

A few days later when I arrived to hang out with him at the Beverly Wilshire, he took me aside. "Stanley Kramer has a script he's going to make. The two leads are chain-gang prisoners who escape but they're chained to each other. One is colored, the other is a white Southerner, and they hate each other's guts, but they have to tolerate each other because they're chained together and being hunted down. By the end of the film they develop a deep respect for each other. The title is *The Defiant Ones*. He's been thinking about me for the white guy but he didn't have any ideas about the colored guy till he saw you at the Mou a few nights ago. He saw us shaking hands and he liked our chemistry . . ." He was looking at me hopefully. "Whaddya think? Would you be interested?"

"*Interested?????* I'm dying to do something like that."

"Oh Lord, me too. I'm up to here in these beach-and-bikini pictures." I knew that Elvis's idols were dramatic actors like Marlon Brando, Rod Steiger, and Jimmy Dean. He said, "I'd really like to act, do something serious. Mr. Kramer's sending me a script. Why don't you tell the Morris office you're interested and have them get him to send one to you?"

After all the begging and cajoling to get my agents to find a movie for me it had happened because of a handshake in a nightclub at a moment when Stanley Kramer happened to be there with his mind on a script starring a white and a Negro. But was that all coincidence? Or hadn't God put all those circumstances together?

The hundred pages of everything I wanted in the world arrived within twenty-four hours and after my late show Elvis and I read the script out loud. It was real heavyweight drama. Dynamite. Our chemistry on the screen and in the press would be sensational.

Elvis was elated. "I'm gonna be an actor! Hey, do you think the kids'll be interested in me without the guitar and the tight pants and the pompadour?" His high level of animation lowered. "Course, I'll have to talk to Colonel. He's really got the say about what I do." Colonel Parker was not in Beverly Hills with Elvis. "He'll be here in five days," Elvis said. "I'm not going to tell him about this on the phone. I do better with him face to face."

"You think he'll go for it?"

"The only thing I can guess against it is he may not see as much money in it with Stanley Kramer as when we do the teenage pictures, plus which they sell records."

"Will he see the value of a change of style, I mean the dramatic thing to prolong the career?"

"I sure think so. Colonel's smart. He's never made a bad decision. And the great plus is that he likes you. He respects you. We're a sure thing. Let's read it again."

I called the motion picture department at the Morris office and told them, "When you get down to negotiating the contract, I don't care about the money. Or billing. I just want a chance . . ."

"Well, I don't know, Sam. Big as Elvis is in his business, you're the world's greatest entertainer, you've starred on Broadway . . ."

I started sweating. "Look, I'm still the new boy in town for pictures. Don't do a Bud Abbott with me. Let me pay the two dollars. Please! I'll happily take second to Elvis. Just don't lose it for me!!"

Tony Curtis came backstage on closing night. "Come on to the house. We're having some people over." I knew almost everybody there and Janet was introducing me to the few I hadn't met before.

Kim Novak held out her hand and smiled. "I'm awfully glad to meet you. I admire your work tremendously."

The next afternoon Arthur Silber came into the Playhouse of the house I'd bought for Mama and myself on Evanview Drive in the Hollywood Hills. He sat down at the end of the bar. I was listening to one of the new sides I'd just made for Decca. He said, "I never thought you'd hold out on me like this."

I put the next side onto the turntable. "Like what?"

His grin broadened into a misterioso smile. "You know what I mean. Come on, you don't have to do bits with *me*. It's all over town."

"*What's* all over town?"

"You and Kim Novak. Didn't you see the papers today?"

"Certainly I saw them but they didn't say nothing about me and no Kim Novak."

He showed me one of the columns. "Kim Novak's new interest will make her studio bosses turn lavender . . ." I'd skimmed past it earlier, never imagining it meant me. I started to tell him that we'd hardly spoken twenty words to each other, but as I looked up and saw the admiration in his face I smiled and shrugged noncommittally.

When he left I got her telephone number. "Kim, this is Sammy Davis, Jr."

"Hi. How are you?"

"I'm feeling horrible over a rumor going around."

"I heard it."

"I'm calling to say I'm sorry as hell and I hope you know I didn't have anything to do with it."

"Of course I know that."

"We can handle it any way you think best. I realize the position you're in with the studio."

"The studio doesn't own me! Listen, I'm cooking some dinner. It's not much, but would you like to join me?"

I called Arthur and told him to come back, and I was dressed in Levi's and a leather jacket when he got to the house. "Now, here's the scam: I'm going to Kim's house for dinner." I caught his smile of satisfaction. "Obviously I can't leave my car parked in her driveway. I need you to drop me off in yours." Half a block from her house I said, "I'll get out here. Now check your watch with mine. At exactly ten o'clock, to the second, I want you pulling up. I'll be running out of there on schedule and I don't wanta have to stand around on the street and get picked off by no photographers or neighbors. And have the car door open for me." I pulled up my collar, slipped out of the car, and ran the last half block, ducking behind trees and slinking across her lawn. As I touched the bell the door opened. I slipped inside and she closed it.

She'd made spaghetti and meatballs and as we were eating I thought: *Wouldn't the papers give their eyeteeth for an eight-by-ten glossy of me having dinner with Kim Novak?*

She smiled conspiratorially. "An hour after I spoke with you the studio called. They wanted to know if we'd ever met."

"What'd you tell them?"

She seemed pleased with herself. "The truth. I said, 'Yes, I met him at a party. He's such a delightful man.' "

I laughed. "Then what?"

"Then there was what the scripts call a moment of stunned silence while the studio gathers itself together and, in a voice tensely casual, asks, 'Is that the only time you've seen him?' I told them we hadn't met since then." The amusement left her face. "Oh, how I loathe people interfering in my life. Do you know what I mean?"

"Sort of."

She smiled, simpatico. "Well . . . at least you don't have an entire studio checking every move you make. I mean, they must really believe they *own* me."

"I guess it gets to be a drag sometimes but let's be honest, it's not *all* bad."

"You're not much fun, are you?" Then, looking at me, dramatically, she said, "You're a wall of wet paint."

"And all the signs say 'Don't touch.'" She nodded, pleased. I'd known it the moment she'd invited me to dinner. Through me she was rebelling against the people who made rules for her. And wasn't I doing the same thing? We'd spent a few hours in each other's company at a party, and when we'd said good night there'd been no slipping of private phone numbers, no thought of getting together again. I was impressed with the glamour of a movie star and she was impressed by my talent. But when it was forbidden, we became conspirators, drawn together by the single thing we had in common: defiance. I'd sensed it on the phone and in the way she'd been waiting behind the door, playing the scene like it was a B movie, and I was aware that I too had done everything but wear a cloak and mustache.

At exactly three seconds before ten I opened the door and dashed to the street. Arthur had timed it on the button; his car door swung open as I reached the curb and before he'd come to a full stop I was inside and we zoomed away like he was driving a getaway car.

I still had a few days free in L.A. before I opened in Las Vegas and during every free minute we had Elvis and I read our scenes. Colonel Parker arrived in town on a Friday. Elvis said, "He's in his room sleeping. I'll get him at breakfast."

When I woke up there was a message for me to call Elvis. He said, "Can I come over and see you? Or can you come over here?" The second I walked in I knew it was bad news. "Colonel's against it."

I sat down. "Did he say why?"

"Like what I guessed, about how it wouldn't be something that would sell records, and we probably can't get the kind of a deal from Kramer for me as an actor as we get when I do the fuckin' musicals."

I saw tears in his eyes and tried to comfort him. "Hey, you'll get your chance. There'll be another . . ."

He started sobbing. "It's not that. It's that you're my friend and

I'm bullshitting you. I'm sorry, Sam. The real reason is because he says that all those people out there who buy my albums, among them are lots who won't want to see me chained to a colored guy and end up liking him."

The elevator at the Beverly Wilshire seemed like it would never get there. Why did God make me with brown skin if He didn't like brown skin? Would God make people to have them tortured for life by frustration? I caught myself. Bullshit! It's not God, it's people. I tried to keep from wallowing in depression by looking at "the doughnut instead of the hole," a slogan I'd seen when I was a kid on a sign outside the Mayflower doughnut shop on Broadway and Forty-fifth Street. Okay, so I don't make a picture with Elvis. But I'm still big in clubs, I've still got *GE Theater*.

My dresser had tired of traveling and I'd hired a new man named Murphy Bennett. I was packing to leave for Vegas and then the East. In the bedroom he gazed at the camera cases, pipe racks, guns and holsters, tape recorders, Gucci leather carrying cases for books, and clothes piled high on the bed and every chair. I enjoyed the way he was looking at everything Alice in Wonderland style. I said, "After a while you'll get bored with packing and unpacking everything for just a few days or a week or two that we stay in a town. But when you get sick of it, try to remember that packing and unpacking is your job. And it might help if you understand that I *need* all those shirts and suits and hats and all the canes and shoes because I have to *look* like a star even when I'm crossing a hotel lobby or sitting in a plane. That's part of *my* job. Yes, I enjoy the clothes, but basically they're props. I get written about and talked about for what I do offstage as much as for what I do onstage.

"Also, I'm not like the business cat who makes a quick trip and he carries a two-suiter and suffers the inconvenience till he gets home. The road *is* my home. I'm out there forty-eight weeks a year. So I try to make life pleasant by carrying familiar things, some ashtrays and lighters I bought, cigarette boxes friends have given me, a few pictures. They make all those hotel rooms a little more personal. Y'dig? And for the dressing room, which is my entertainment center, I carry that box of framed pictures of friends and family. When you set up the dressing room the hotel will always put in a full bar, but make sure we have a couple of bottles of Lafite-Rothschild, some Puilly-Fuissé, and some Dom Pérignon or any other premium champagne."

He took out a pencil and paper. "Would you mind spelling those wines for me?"

"Spell 'em? Get outta here! I just learned how to say 'em!"

I called Sy Marsh to say goodbye and he said, "Sweetheart, I'll be in touch with you as soon as I get an air date."

"When do you think that will be?"

"I always get a date a few weeks after it's been shot."

" 'Cause I'm going to take full-page ads in the trades to say 'Thank you' to GE."

"Beautiful. The whole industry sees those ads. We're on our way, sweetheart."

ALL I could see were the red lights at the tip of the wing and I had the feeling that it would be so peaceful to sit out there, my legs hanging over the edge, riding through space, the clean, fresh air bathing away all the pressures.

"Look at this." Arthur was pointing to an item in one of the papers we'd picked up at the airport. ". . . Guess which sepia entertainer's attentions are being whispered as the Kiss of Death to guess which blond movie star's career? . . ."

I opened a scandal magazine and skimmed "The Real Story Between KIM and HIM," a rehash of all the rumors and gossip items. The real story I saw was the insult to me and to all Negroes. Didn't it occur to the people who wrote those things how it might feel to hear "A woman's career can be ruined just by association with you"? Didn't they understand that's what they were saying? Didn't they care? Worse—they didn't think. They couldn't feel anything that might *make* them think because their sensitivities were covered by a thick callus that it had taken centuries of stupidity to develop.

I rested against the seat. The stewardess came by. "Would you like a pillow, Mr. Davis?" Her eyes flicked to the magazine, and she maintained her smile, making a businesslike attempt to camouflage the condemnation in her eyes. As she moved down the aisle Arthur leaned over to me, reading aloud. " 'Advice to Sammy Davis, Jr., before it's too late. Sammy, I consider myself your friend, so I'm speaking up to beg you to show some sense. Don't damage a promising career, and probably your own too. Wouldn't it be more fitting for a man of your prominence to be a credit to his people, instead of one whose life is scandal, scandal, scandal?

Think it over, Sammy, you're too smart for this.' " Arthur asked, "What are you going to do? Y'going to keep seeing her?"

"Why the hell not?" I turned to him. "Do you know how sick I am of being watched and judged and criticized? Do you realize that even the goddamned stewardess is ready to cast her vote how I oughta live?"

He looked around frantically, afraid somebody was listening, and he spoke softly, pacifying. "I only meant maybe you're letting yourself in for more trouble than it's worth."

"You can't drop it, right, Arthur?"

"But do you really think it's smart to keep it going?"

"No, but I'm going to."

"But with the whole world saying the same thing . . ."

I looked away from him. "If I'd listened to what the whole world says I'd be in Harlem shining shoes."

ON OPENING night in Vegas I had a respite from all the innuendo, the unsolicited advice. The show caught fire and the audience and I were tucked away in a vacuum, just me and those people whom I didn't know by name, yet who were the best friends I had. Obviously they'd heard all the bad talk and they didn't seem to care, so I wanted to tell them some of the good. "For years now I've been dying to do some dramatic acting on television but those doors have always been closed to colored people . . . but I've got good news. I was just in L.A., where I had the privilege of playing the lead in an upcoming episode on *GE Theater* . . ." A man at ringside began applauding. "Thank you. I love you. Obviously you're friends or you wouldn't be here. Which is why I wanted to share my news with you, because if not for you I wouldn't be standing here, and consequently I wouldn't be starring on any *GE Theater*. So thank you. And keep an eye out for the show. I'd love for you to watch it. And if you happen to be in the market for a new iron or an icebox, there is one manufacturer I would like to recommend . . ."

I called Sy. "When's it going on, baby? I've been telling all my audiences to watch for it."

"That's great, sweetheart. Keep it up. I haven't been given an air date, but if I don't hear from them in another week I'll call Harry."

I looked through the papers. "Sammy Davis, Jr., has been warned by top Chicago gangsters that if he ever sees that blonde movie star again both of his legs will be broken and torn off at the knee." . . . "The boss of a certain moom pitcha company has a photo of SD, Jr., on his office walls. Flings darts at it."

It had to mean Harry Cohn, the head of Columbia, Kim's studio. He was known to be well connected and the suggestion was that he had a contract out on me. I called a number in Chicago and asked for "Dr. Goldberg," the name Sam Giancana used when he called me, like if we were in the same town and he wanted me to go out with him and Phyllis McGuire, whom he was dating.

"Who's calling him?"

"Sammy Davis, Jr."

"Where are you? He'll call you back."

Within five minutes Murphy asked, "Do you know a Dr. Goldberg?" Murphy was still new.

"I'll take it, babe." When we'd done the pleasantries I asked, "Sam, am I in trouble with your guys?"

"No. And if you were, you know I'd handle it for you."

"Thank you. I knew that. I just wanted to be sure."

I RENTED a beach house at Malibu so Kim and I could meet secretly and Arthur was driving me there for the sixth night in a row. As we neared the beach I said, "Baby, it's still light out, so pull over and let me get in the back. I'd better stay flat on the floor and under a blanket, 'cause the way the rumors are flying, them cats on the papers may have movie cameras set up all along this road."

The floor smelled lousy. There was a clump of dirt a few inches from my head. From one second to the next the game ended and it was as though I was standing back, seeing myself on the floor of a car, hiding, like a criminal. So I could say, "I showed them." What was I showing them? I wasn't making my own rules. I was sneaking around theirs, doing everything I'd thought I'd always refused to do. They were saying, "You're not good enough to be seen with a white woman." And I was hiding on the floor of a car, confirming it.

Arthur whispered, "We're almost there." He looked in the rear-view mirror and saw me sitting up in the back seat. "You crazy? I said we're almost there."

"Turn around. Don't go to the house."

"You spot somebody?"

"Just turn around. Keep driving—anyplace." I rested against the back of the seat.

As we passed through a bad neighborhood we stopped for a light and a bum with a week's growth of beard and filthy, torn clothes staggered up to the car. He looked at me and then asked Arthur, "Buddy, can y'give a guy a little help?"

I started to reach for some money but I stopped. Why should I? Underneath all that filth his skin is white: he'd been given a pass through the world and he'd blown it. I stared at the wasted life holding out his hand and I had a weird, ridiculous picture of Kim arriving at a movie premiere, escorted by this old rummy in the same clothes and no shave and everybody smiling and applauding as they walked in. An eccentric, they'd think. He could be a pimp or a dope peddler but still he'd be okay. There's nothing he could ever do to get himself as low as me.

"C'mon, buddy, be a pal," he whined at Arthur. "Whaddya say, just a few cents?" I took a hundred-dollar bill out of my pocket, folded it, and rolled down the window. He turned, stared at me, then took the money. "Thanks a lot, mac. Damn white of ya." He stuffed it into his pocket and stumbled away. He probably thought it was a single. He'd put it on a bar and get change for a dollar. He would never know what he had in his pocket.

I OPENED at Lake Tahoe. What you hope for when you die is that it will be as good as it was when you were a headliner at Harrah's Club. Bill Harrah paid top dollar and all the vigorish, a casino word for extras. Bill's attitude was: "These are unusual people who have a certain lifestyle in Beverly Hills or Bel Air or wherever. I want them to come onstage and give the best show they're capable of, and not be distracted because their room, the food, or the service isn't what they're accustomed to. With all the perks we can think of, if it costs another $5,000 a week to have that quality performance, it's worth it."

Bill provided a four-bedroom house on the lake with twenty-four-hour domestic service, a staff which ironed, sewed, cooked anything you liked, and had the hotel kitchen as a backup for anything else you wanted. The house had a pool and as many Rolls-Royces as you could use.

When I got past the opening I called Sy. I still hadn't got an air date on *GE Theater* and I asked if something might have gone wrong.

"Sweetheart, what could be wrong? It's in the can. Ready to go. Network scheduling is complicated, it's a chess game. I'll let you know the second I hear."

I watched *GE Theater* every week. Two months had gone by when I saw that they were putting on a show that Bob Culp had made. I remembered him telling me he was doing it, and it had been shot *after* ours. I called Sy and pointed it out. "Plus, there isn't that much left of this season."

"You're right," Sy said, "this is not normal. The second we hang up I'm going out to Universal and demand that they give me an air date. I'll get back to you in a few hours."

When I got back to the house after the second show, Sy was calling. "Sam . . ." Something was wrong, he never called me by my name. "Listen, I'm here in Tahoe. In the hotel lobby . . ."

I was waiting at the door and gave it the Jack Benny reading: "Well . . . so you got on the wrong freeway and you figured as long as you were in the neighborhood . . ." I led him into the living room. He tried to grin but he couldn't make it. He was hurting, and I knew it was for me, for something he had to tell me. "Look, Sy, I'm hip you didn't fly to Tahoe to give me good news. It's bad, right?"

"I couldn't give it to you on the phone. I'm sick about this, but I can't lie to you, and there's no way to soften this: GE wants to kill the show."

"Kill it?"

"Yeah. Dump it. Take their losses rather than show it."

"But why? Everybody loves it."

"I'll tell it to you like it happened. I went out to speak to Alan Miller, president of Universal, and I demanded that he give me an air date. He said, 'Sy, sit down and let's talk. We're going to have to kill that show. Here's the problem. General Electric's advertising agency sends representatives out here to review the film, they see a colored man in a starring role, they have sixty-three percent of all GE products sold below the Mason-Dixon line, they say they will be ostracized by their white customers and dealers: "So, there's no way we can use that show." '

"I was devastated. I said, 'Alan, this news will wreck Sammy.

He's been counting on this. He's been telling his audiences, plugging GE, he did a great job acting.' Alan said, 'It's not my decision, Sy. On a personal level I agree with you. But the sponsor is the boss. I'm sorry, Sy, but GE paid for the show, and it's GE's right to bury it.' I told him, 'This is going to kill Sammy. It's wrong. It's not justified. If this show is not aired I'll go to the press. I'll ruin General Electric.' And I left.

"As soon as I got to my office my secretary told me that Abe Lastfogel wanted to see me the minute I came in. He'd had a call from Alan Miller telling him that I'd threatened him. He said, 'Sy, I hardly have to explain to you that we work all year round with Universal. Now, do you want to weaken our relationship there over this one incident?'

"I said, 'No, sir, I do not want to weaken us with Universal. But I tell you, Mr. Lastfogel, this is unfair and I cannot allow it to happen.' He looked at me very coldly. 'Are you willing to jeopardize your job?' It was such a shock, I got so scared that I asked, 'Do you mean that my job is on the line if I pursue this?' I got so mad that I said, 'If that's the case, then, yes, sir, I'll be willing to lose my job.' "

I couldn't stand it. "Sy, I'm sorry . . ."

"Wait, sweetheart, let me finish. Mr. Lastfogel looked at me for a hell of a long time, then he goes from beady-eyed to I see a smile coming on his face. He says, 'Well . . . let's see what we can do,' and he phones Alan Miller. 'Alan, it seems that Sy Marsh is a motivated young man. I've threatened him with his job but he will not back down. If I fire him, then he'll have nothing to lose and he'll blow this out of proportion to the point that everybody will suffer. I think you should speak to the sponsor.' And that's where it stands, sweetheart. They have to make a decision to use the show or I take it to the press."

I didn't know what to say to him, what words to express how I felt about putting his job in jeopardy, and at the very least causing him to lose a major connection with Universal.

When he'd left I stared out at the lake. I could understand Tom Parker, a Southerner, fearing that Elvis would be hurt by association with me. Elvis could go on making beach-and-bikini pictures forever at a million apiece. Don't jeopardize *that*. But I could not get it through my mind that the opposition to my skin was so great that a commercial sponsor preferred to take $50,000 worth of really good film and throw it away.

A few days later, in New York, at the Copa, I'd just come offstage when Sy called. "You won't believe what I'm going to tell you."

"They're really going to burn it."

"Worse. They're going to use it to open next season. But that's not good like it sounds. It's a more sophisticated way of burying you. *GE Theater*'s in a bind against Dinah Shore, who, I don't have to tell you, is the hottest show on the air, and she is going to open the season with Rock Hudson, who has never made an appearance on variety television. Every TV set in America will be tuned to them. GE is slotting you against *that* in order to get the least exposure for your show."

"They figure nobody'll notice I've been on."

"They've won. We can't raise a fuss in the press, or sue. They'd say, 'But what's wrong? We're putting Sammy on to open our season.'"

I had an hour and a half before the second show. If I stayed in the dressing room I'd have to entertain visitors. I told Murphy, "I'll be back in an hour," and I slipped out onto Sixtieth Street and walked toward the anonymous darkness of Madison. I didn't look across at our old doorway as I did every time I went in or out of the Copa. I didn't feel corny. Corny is pleasant, romantic. I felt terrible. Apart from my own loss, my dreams of glory of being a trailblazer for my people were hanging in shreds on the fucking Mason-Dixon line.

As I tried to lose myself in the night, for all the money in the world, if it were a matter of life and death, I could not begin to feel like anybody should hate me. Why? For God's sake, why? I thought that there was no way I could stand on the stage of the Copa and tell jokes, and try to be adorable, and amuse people. But then I thought: *No! I'm an entertainer, a professional, and fuck 'em if they don't like the fact that my skin is brown, fuck anyone who doesn't like my skin, let 'em stay home, but I'll be there singing and dancing.* And then, in my mind, I saw their faces, those eyes that stare across the tables with love, those people who applaud until their hands hurt. Are they the ones who won't buy a GE toaster if they see me on a TV program?

It made no sense. Nothing did. Except to do my job. Without

that I had no hope at all. I walked back to the Copa, willing myself to remember how things had changed there. I had reason to be an optimist. Maybe they would change elsewhere. Maybe I could help change them.

SY CALLED me in Miami, at the Eden Roc, the morning after my *GE Theater* was aired. "Sweetheart, the local ratings are in and in New York, Chicago, Philly, and L.A. you outdrew Dinah."

When the full ratings picture was in, we were only a half point behind Dinah. GE waited for the mail pull at the studio. The letters said, "It's about time you featured a Negro . . ." There was some hate mail, but proportionately little. GE told Sy they wanted to buy me for one show a year. And then I got nominated for an Emmy.

WILL MASTIN came over to my house in Hollywood. "Sammy, I'm quitting the act. I had another examination and the doctors say I can't keep it up. Truth is, they told me I should stay home and rest, but I'll keep traveling with the act as manager."

I would finally be on the stage by myself, putting an end to years of "What're those two guys still doing on that stage? It's embarrassing." That was industry talk, performers, agents, press. Then my father had retired during *Mr. Wonderful* and it was even more ludicrous with just Will standing behind me, but I certainly wasn't going to put him off the stage. If it was embarrassing to anybody, it was to Will, not to me. The public loved the fact that the kid was loyal.

I'd expected that when Will retired we'd open an office in L.A. or New York and save the $20,000 a year in travel expense for him and his dresser. "Massey, maybe you should listen to what the doctors say. If they think you should stay home . . ."

"No. Doctors don't know everything about a man. If I had to stay away from show business, I'd have nothing to live for." And though he stepped down and began traveling only as manager, he carried with him all of his costumes and makeup and set them up in a dressing room at every club I played.

9

ON OPENING NIGHT in Vegas, a friend of mine—a very well-connected friend of mine—was waiting in the dressing room. He said, "We gotta talk." I took him into my makeup room and closed the door. "Sam, you've got a problem with the guys."

"No, babe, it's okay. Thanks, I appreciate it, but I talked to Sam in Chicago and that was just phony shit in the columns. Anyway, that relationship is over."

He was shaking his head. "I'm not talking Chicago. I'm talking L.A. West Coast. Harry Cohn's mad. There's a contract out. To break your legs. But these guys have a habit of crushing kneecaps with a sledgehammer so they never mend. Be careful, Sam, they enjoy hurting people and they could decide they should balance off your eyes too." I sat down, unable to stand up. When this man spoke it was fact. "Now, we can protect you while you're here in Vegas, you know that. Nobody's coming in. You're safe when you work here, Chicago, Miami, New York—we'll be there, we can protect you. But don't you go back home unless you straighten out with Cohn."

"How do I do that?"

"I don't know. That's between you and him. But, talkin' as a friend, if I was you I'd think of something."

My father had come in from L.A. for the weekend and I knew by the way he closed the dressing-room door that it wasn't going to be "Great show, son." He handed me a newspaper clipping.

"Poppa, I've gotta show you what they're writin' about you in our papers. Mama saw this one and it made her feel real bad."

Sammy Davis, Jr., once a pride to all Negroes, has become a never-ending source of embarrassment. The legend of Mr. Davis's amours trips gaily from one bedroom to another, leering out at us from the covers of endless scandal magazines, dragging us all through the mud along with him. Perhaps Errol Flynn can prosper from this kind of publicity but on one of us it doesn't look good. Mr. Davis has never been particularly race conscious but his current scandal displays him as inexcusably *unconscious* of his responsibility as a Negro. Look in the mirror, Sammy. You're still one of us.

I dropped the paper. "I don't need a mirror to remind me. *Nobody* in this whole goddamned world'll let me forget it."

Will had come in with him. Now he glared at me. "All my life I did a clean act, but the way you're rolling around in the mud there'll come a day when people are going to stop bringin' their families in to see us." He walked out of the room.

"Poppa, I . . ." There was a long silence. Then: "Hey, whaddya say we go get us a little somethin' to eat? Maybe some Chinese food, just you and me?"

"I'm not exactly hungry, Dad."

"Well . . . I guess I'll stop by the casino."

When I'd dressed and gone out he was standing at a crap table. His face brightened. "Glad t'see you, son."

"You're sure it's okay for me to be in here now? You don't worry the papers'll call me Uncle Tom or nigger rich?"

"Sammy . . ."

"Catch y'later, Dad." I wandered over to the cashier's window. "Baby, let me have five thousand." I sat down at a blackjack table and put five hundred dollars on the line. At least fifty people were gathered around me, groaning as I went down hand after hand. "Baby, you'd better get another five thousand for me." I signed the slip and kept playing. It all seemed so silly: I sign my name, a man gives me a stack of chips, I put them on a table, and another guy takes them away. "You'd better get me another five, baby."

A cocktail waitress came by. "Coke, Sammy?"

"That's last year's publicity, darling. It's Jack Daniel's now." I walked over to the crap table and tapped my father on the shoulder. He turned around and smiled. "I thought you'd like to know, Dad. I just lost thirty-nine thousand dollars!" I waited for him to be shocked or get angry but he just looked sad and I wanted to kill myself. I touched his arm and walked away.

I did my second show, got boozed up in the lounge, and stumbled into my car half stoned. When I didn't feel like driving anymore, I looked around. I was in front of the Silver Slipper.

Pounding the bar top, I called out, "Innkeeper! Wine for my horses and nothing for my men!" Oh, fine. Lines from the act.

The bartender grinned. "What'll it be, Sammy."

"A little Daniel's, old buddy, a little double Daniel's for old Sam t'make up for lost time." The show had ended and the girls were coming out front. *Hmmmmmmmm, which wench will ye have, m'lord?* . . . One of them was walking toward me. The body looked familiar . . . but I couldn't place the face.

"Hello, Sammy."

I tried to focus on her but she kept moving. I was bobbing my head back and forth trying to get in rhythm with her. "Don't I know you? . . . I *know* I know you . . . oh, for God's sake, hello, Loray, what're *you* doing here?"

"I'm working here. I hope you didn't drive over in the shape you're in."

"Nobody was driving, Officer, we were all in the back seat singing. How've you been, Loray honey?"

"Fine, Sammy. How about you?"

"Swingin'. Crazy! Dontcha read the papers?" She nodded. "I'm a big star, huh? Have a drink, Loray! Whaddya drink?"

"I'll have a glass of champagne."

"That's right. Now I 'member. Barkeep! Champagne for the lady, and more red-eye for old Sam." I grinned. "Hey, where've you been, Loray?"

"I played some places in South America . . ."

"Rio or Mississippi?" Oh God. "C'mon, y'wanta gamble?"

"No, Sammy. I don't think you should gamble either."

"Hey! Hol' everything. No one tells *me* when to gamble." I took out a roll of bills. "Y'see this? Thousands!" I gave her a handful and steered her over to the crap tables. "Let's *be* somebody." I got on a winning streak right away but I couldn't get interested. "C'mon, Loray, this is a bore."

She gasped. "You're crazy. You're *hot*."

"I'm hot and hot-blooded." I stuffed the hundred-dollar chips I'd won into my pockets. "Goddamned tight pants bulge." I took out a handful and gave them to her. "Buy a hat." She was startled. "Tut-tut, wench. A mere farthing. I've a thousand acres of the finest cattle land, as far as the eye can see . . ." We went back to the bar. "Y'know, you're a beautiful girl, Loray. You're one swingin' chick, y'know that? How come we stopped going around together?"

"That's something you know better than me, Sammy. You just disappeared."

"We had a good little thing goin' for us. Nothing fantastic—but it was kinda nice, right?" Oops! It came back to me. She couldn't play it: catch-you-next-time-around. I'd smelled a cottage small by a waterfall, so I'd left town without even calling her. *Maybe that was stupid . . . maybe a wife's what I'd needed all the time, maybe that's what I need now. If I had a wife, I'd belong. The papers would get off my back. Harry Cohn would be happy. She's beautiful. Better-looking than ever. Hey, this is a beautiful chick, Charley. She understands the business, she's a lady.* "Y'know, Loray, if I had any sense I'd marry you. Never been more serious in my life. Y'think I tell that to everyone I meet? I don't have to do this jazz to get a chick. I've got 'em comin' out of my ears. Just 'cause I made a mistake once doesn't mean I have to keep making the same one all my life, does it? Does it?"

"I don't mean to be ungracious but you're drunk, Sammy."

"Sure I am, but I know what I'm doing. Whaddya think I came in here for in the first place? Hey, have another drink, Loray. What're y'drinkin'?"

"Still champagne."

"Waiter, some champagne for the lady and booze for Sam. Cert'n'y, Loray honey. Whaddya think? They don't have booze at the Sands? I didn't exactly have to come here to buy a drink, y'know."

"Please, maybe this is laughs for you . . ."

"Hey, cool it! Did I ever ask you to marry me before?"

"No, but—"

"Answer the question. Did I ever ask me to marry you before?"

She smiled. I knew I'd screwed up the words.

"Okay. I accept your proposal."

"You do? Hey, that's pretty crazy." I leaned back to focus on her. *This is a natural. Just what I need. A nice girl to come home to, someone I can be proud to introduce as my wife; I'll come across to the public as Charley Straight. They'll drop the "wild kid" jazz in the papers. And the Negro press'll go out of their minds; they'll eat it up like a hundred yards of chitlins. There'll be hugging and kissing and front pages with come-home-son-all-is-forgiven.* And Harry Cohn would be solved! What could make him happier than I'm married and out of circulation? One great move would solve all my problems.

I stood up. "C'mon. We'll announce it." As I led her to the bandstand, the whole idea kept getting better all the time. *Here goes Charley Single.* "Scuse me, guys. Got a li'l announcement to make." The room quieted down immediately. "Ladies and gentlemen, your 'tention, please . . ."

The club's press agent pushed his way through the crowd around us. "Will you wait here till I get a photographer? Please? Just a few minutes?" I nodded and as he turned to dash away I nudged him. "Congratulations, baby."

People were offering us drinks. *This is beautiful, everybody loves it.* "A li'l booze f'r th' happy couple! How often's a guy get married? What're y'drinking, Loray honey?"

ARTHUR was standing close to my head. "Sammy? You up?" What the hell's he whispering for? If I'm awake, why doesn't he just talk? But if I'm sleeping, then leave me alone. "Sammy, your father's on the phone. He wants to know about your engagement to Loray White."

Oh God. I started to sit up but I grabbed my head and fell back onto the pillow. "I'll call him back. And, Arthur, gimme a Coke, with a lot of ice." I rested, trying to piece the evening together. "How'd my father hear about it?"

"On the radio. And it's in all the papers today. Front page here in Vegas. When'd you start seeing Loray again?"

"Baby, cool the questions. I've got to think."

"Whaddya mean? Isn't it true?"

"Arthur, I got drunk and my whiskey asked her to marry me."

"But you haven't seen her in years. Not that she isn't a hell of a nice girl . . ."

"Arthur, she's a lovely girl. So is Eleanor Roosevelt, but I'm not in love with *her* either."

"Then you're not going to marry her?"

"What do *you* think? You know Loray and I were all over two years ago. Do you really think I'm about to *marry* her now?" My head killed me when I yelled.

"Loray's smart. Probably wondering if you still mean it."

"She knows I was gassed . . ." I felt hopeful.

He gave me a stack of phone messages. "All the L.A. papers have been calling. There's a guy outside now from one of the wire services. The Negro press has been on the phone every ten minutes. *Jet, The Courier,* some woman in New York—someone Cunningham."

"*Evelyn* Cunningham?"

"Yeah, that's her. She's all excited . . ."

The toughest columnist in the Negro press. Even if Loray lets me off the hook they'll wrap this around my ears: "He was just using her for publicity." "He doesn't want her because she isn't white." Before they're finished there won't be a colored cat in the country who'll talk to me.

I picked up the phone to call Billy Rowe, who was handling the New York press for me. He could fend her off. But the other phone rang and I heard Arthur saying, "Yes, he is, Mrs. Cunningham."

I hissed, "I'm still sleeping."

He covered the mouthpiece. "But I said you're awake."

I shook my fist at him and took the phone. "Hello, Mrs. Cunningham, so nice to hear from you."

"Hello, Sammy. I believe congratulations are in order."

She said it tentatively, a test question. "Thank you, Mrs. Cunningham. Very kind of you."

"Then it's true?" I could feel the phone warming up. "You and Loray White *are* engaged?"

The nails were in the coffin. "Yes, ma'am. We became betrothed, as they say, last night."

"Well, this is wonderful." It was as though she was thinking: are we wrong about him? "When will you be married?"

"We haven't set the date. Soon, though, I hope."

"Will Loray keep her career? Or will she travel with you?"

"Well . . . if she wants to keep up her career, I certainly won't object—she's talented, you know."

"Perhaps she'll want to do an act with you?"

Another partner. "Well, that's certainly an interesting idea. Of course, nobody could ever replace my father and my uncle." Bullshit, bullshit, bullshit.

"Sammy, I think this is wonderful. I'm very happy for you. Sometimes a man needs some responsibility."

Arthur was gaping at me as I hung up. I glared viciously. "And thank *you*, Arthur. One of the great, *stupid* moves of our times."

The phone was ringing. "Go ahead, baby, you can't bury me any deeper."

He whispered, "Dr. Goldberg." I grabbed the phone.

"Sammy, listen, when we talked I didn't know you had a problem in L.A. I'm calling you now because I was just talking to an associate in L.A. and he said, 'You're a friend of Sammy's, so you can tell him that Mr. Cohn says that'll be fine.' You can relax, kid, the pressure's off."

I told Arthur, "Call Loray and ask her to come over this afternoon at five."

He hung up. "She'll be here. What're you gonna do?"

I couldn't breathe without causing waves of nausea. "I'll explain the whole thing and ask her to go along with me. We'll get married, we'll make it look good for a while, and then we'll get divorced."

"You think she'll go along with it? You didn't treat her so well that she'll be looking to do you favors. And once a chick becomes Mrs. Sammy Davis, Jr., she's not going to let go so easily."

"Arthur, may I assume this is *all* the good news you have for me today?"

"What I mean is, maybe it's not worth it. You've been in trouble with the press before."

"Of course it's not worth it. But this time I can't afford trouble."

"Why now more than ever?"

"Baby, just know this: if I back out now, I'm dead."

Will arrived. "This true, Mose Gastin?" He hadn't called me that in years. He looked confused, which, all things considered, was as good a way to look as any other. I nodded. "Do you love this girl?" He searched my face. "You get her in trouble?"

"Not the kind you're thinking of. Massey, I got drunk and I asked her to marry me. Publicly."

"Well then, you gotta come out and say it was all a mistake."

"Sure, I'll take full-page ads in *The Defender, The Amsterdam*

News, and *The Courier*: 'Sorry, folks, it was all a mistake. Old Sam got loaded. Heh, heh, heh.' Massey, I've thought it over. There's no other way to handle it." I walked into the bathroom but he followed me in with Arthur behind him.

"Sammy, nothing's as bad as to marry someone you don't love." He was speaking gingerly—like I was an inmate at a mental institution.

Arthur nodded. "I agree with Will, Sammy."

I glared at him. "*Do* you, Doctor?" He backed up. "Now look, you guys, it's my life. I did it and I'll straighten it out."

LORAY SAT stiffly erect on the couch, expecting me to tell her, "It's all a mistake." I said, "Loray . . . I need your help."

"You don't have to marry me, Sammy."

When I'd finished explaining what I had in mind, she just stared at me, then she stood up. "Fine."

"Great. I can't thank you enough. I'll call you as soon as I need you."

My father tried to talk me out of it; everyone knew what was best for me. I made arrangements for the ceremony. The sooner, the better.

On the night of the wedding I did only one show at the Sands. Loray was at ringside. I introduced her and did all the shtick the audience expects from a guy who gets married. I had a few shots of bourbon with some of the people who'd come to the dressing room, but I couldn't keep up the front any longer. I sent them ahead to the party with Loray. I don't know why they thought I wanted to be alone, but they winked and grinned and left. I locked the door. I couldn't have taken it to see them nudging each other: "Look, he's so happy, he's crying."

I read a few of the telegrams that were coming in from all over the country, from people wishing something good for me. How cheap could I get? Abusing their warmth and affection, letting them put themselves in unflattering positions like this.

From the day of the wedding everybody in the business, the press, all the "smart money" knew it was a phony. They didn't know why or how, so they grabbed for the most obvious reasons and the papers broke loose like I was World War III: "A blonde movie star just lost 20 lbs. No diet. Simply begged the love of her life to marry another to save her career and now she misses him. Boo-hoos herself to sleep every nite." . . . "The facts: Mrs. Sammy Davis, Jr., has a six-month contract with her husband. The deal: a flat $10,000 and no options." . . . "Insiders say Harry Cohn paid $50,000 to guess which song-and-dance man, to take the heat off Columbia's top box-office property."

Almost everything I read was wrong except for the single truth, that nobody was fooled by it. They sensed the hoax. Yet somehow they stayed with me. As I moved across the country the crowds grew bigger than ever. I was *hot*. They had overlooked an interracial scandal and an obviously phony marriage.

As I looked out at them and felt their warmth coming at me, I thought that not only had God given me the talent to entertain them but He had opened a door between me and them so that they felt something for me like you feel for a friend when he screws up and you wish he hadn't but he's still your friend. Why had I been given this pass? I couldn't understand why He would have such patience with me, nor did I question it, I just felt grateful that God still had his arms around me.

I tried to express my feelings with humor. "Ladies and gentlemen, I've always believed that up in heaven all the angels are sitting around God while He puts everything together. I've always had this mental picture of Him looking down at earth and saying, 'Look at that baby down there, cute . . . He's going to be called Harry Belafonte. Make him six foot two, handsome, talented, a good businessman . . . and give him some shirts that don't have buttons in the front. . . .

" 'Let's see who else we've got . . . Sidney Poitier. Hey, I like the sound of that name. Let him be the first colored guy to win the Academy Award. He should be a brilliant actor, sensitive . . . Good, marvelous. Next.

" 'Sammy Davis, Jr. Hmmmmm. Hey, Tom, come over here a minute. I know you've got Shortness. Gimme some for that kid Sammy. Yeah, fine. And, Charley, over by the cloud, what're you going to do with that Accident you've got laying around over there? Yeah, with Losing an Eye. Give it to me for Sammy. Let's see now. Eddie, you've got three Broken Noses, yeah, that's fine for him. Also, we'll make him Jewish.'

"Then God calls out to another of his angels, 'Johnny, you've got All the Talent in the World, we'll give him that too and on top of that he should enjoy what he does . . .' Then God calls to another angel, 'Let him have a Lot of Friends . . . and make them the kind of people who'll stay with him when he messes up, that hang in with him anyway . . .' "

I bowed to them. "Thank you . . . and good night."

10

I WAS HAVING lunch at the Fox commissary when a tall girl with long blond hair walked in and sat down at a table by herself. Her hair was very straight and I dug the dramatic way it framed her face, which was unbelievably beautiful. I clenched my teeth and nudged Barbara Luna, a friend of mine who was working on a remake of *The Blue Angel*.

She followed my gaze across the room. "That's May Britt."

"Now, that's a girl. Yeah. I mean that's a *girl*."

"Forget it."

"I saw her in *The Young Lions* and she was wild-looking, but in person she's unbelievable."

"Forget it. I see her on the set every day. She's a nice girl but she doesn't do anything but work. She goes nowhere with nobody!"

A few nights later I was in my Jag, heading down Santa Monica. I stopped at a light. May Britt was walking across the street. There was no missing the style of her hair. She was wearing a bluish-gray skirt, a button-down-collar man's shirt, and a jacket. She stood very straight and walked with a driving energy. There was an older woman with her, probably her mother.

There was a knocking on the roof of my car. A cop was leaning in my window. "Shall we dance, Sammy?" The light had changed and cars behind me were honking. "Excuse me, Officer." I grinned like an idiot and drove off.

I mentioned her name to some friends and I got "Forget it. The best have tried but she's not interested in dating, parties, nothing!

She's strictly work. She's getting a divorce from some kid who's got millions and she won't take a nickel from him."

I got back to the Coast again about three weeks later and had some kids over. Rudy Duff, a man I'd hired to drive for Mama, was making drinks and running the movies. I sat down next to Barbara Luna and told her I wanted to meet May Britt. "I'll make up a party for Dinah Washington's closing at the Cloisters."

"I'll give you her phone number and you can invite her."

"No good. With this girl, if I call her cold it's a definite turndown. You've got to call her for me."

Barbara called me the next day. "Well, I spoke to her."

"She can't make it, right?"

"She said, 'If he wants to talk to me, why doesn't he call me himself?' "

"Whaddya mean?" I knew exactly what she meant.

SOMEONE answered briskly, "Tell me." Tell me? What the hell is *that*? Again the voice said, "Tell me."

How Swedish can you get? "May I speak with Miss Britt, please?"

"Who's calling?"

From her voice *alone* I wished I had on a heavy sweater. "This is Sammy Davis, Jr."

"Oh, hello there." Some of the chill disappeared. She was still a little crisp, but she didn't sound angry that I'd called.

I gave her the Orson Welles voice, resonant, full of timbre: "Miss Britt, you don't know me . . ."

"I know that." Oh, swell. I needed this. She said, "But I've seen you perform. At the Moulin Rouge. I thought your show was marvelous."

Hey, she didn't have to say that. "Miss Britt, I'm having a little party—I mean a large party, at the Cloisters, Thursday night, and I wondered if I might have the pleasure of your company." I rushed in with a little protection. "Barbara Luna will be there."

"I'd like that but my mother is visiting me from Sweden."

"Please bring her along."

"Thank you. That will be fine."

The show was about to start when I saw her walking in with George Englund, who'd produced *Odds Against Tomorrow*. I nudged Barbara. "Your friend sure has a strange-looking mother." I walked over to greet them.

She smiled. "My mother was tired. Do you know Mr. Englund? I hope you don't mind my asking him."

I walked them to the table. "Do you care for champagne?"

"I hate it."

"Oh. Well, how about some vodka? Scotch? Bourbon?"

"I don't drink. I'll have a plain tonic, thank you."

"Schweppes or Wildroot?" She looked blankly at me, not understanding what in the hell I was talking about. *Very smart, Charley.* "Well, enjoy yourselves . . . catch you later."

After the show I danced with Dinah and Barbara but I kept watching May and Englund. If she were dancing I could cut in but I wasn't about to risk walking over there and getting "I'm sorry. I don't dance." When the party was breaking up I went over. "Everybody's coming to the house for a nightcap. Would you like to join us?"

"Nope."

"Well, don't let anybody tell you you're not direct."

She shook my hand. "Thank you for inviting me."

I waited a few days and called her. "I'm having some friends up to the house tonight—running a few movies—would you like to come by?"

She was wearing slacks. I could have spent the whole night just watching her move. She walked like an athlete. But oh, was she a *girl* athlete! I wondered how old she was. Twenty-three maybe. She was so definite, so sure of everything. It was such a youthful, attractive thing. She said, "You know what I hate?"

"What's that?"

"I don't mean to embarrass you."

"Go right ahead. Please."

"You called me May."

"Oh. Well, I beg your pardon. I'll call you Miss Britt and you can call me Kato." Oh God. Green Hornet bits!

She gave me the blank look of all time. "All I mean is that it's spelled M-a-y but it's pronounced 'My' not 'May.' My real name is Maybritt Wilkens."

"I'm sorry, I didn't know."

"I hope you don't mind my telling you."

"No. I'm glad you did. I really am . . ." We got hung up on it and started laughing. When the evening was over I offered to drive her home. I had someone follow us in my car while I drove May's

Thunderbird toward the beach. She sat next to me, silent except to give me directions through Malibu Colony to a large estate on which she rented the guesthouse.

I wanted to kiss her good night but I felt it couldn't be like with other chicks, with grabbing and squeezing and what-could-I-lose? Do I ask, "May I have a kiss?" like Andy Hardy? She stopped at her door. I held out my hand. "Thank you very much for coming tonight. I'm going to Las Vegas tomorrow. May I call you?"

"I'd like that very much." She smiled and cocked her head and the moonlight shining on her face lit it so beautifully that I felt a weakness pass over me. She had freckles and her skin and her hair looked more lovely than anything I'd ever seen or imagined. I felt a glow within me like nothing I'd ever experienced. The moment was something apart from all moments through all the years of my life. She lowered her eyes, turned, and went inside.

11

THE MARQUEE in front of the Sands was a classic:

FRANK SINATRA
DEAN MARTIN
SAMMY DAVIS, JR.
PETER LAWFORD
JOEY BISHOP

A few months earlier, when we'd made plans to shoot *Ocean's Eleven* and play the hotel simultaneously, the newspapers had been filled with stories about Eisenhower, De Gaulle, and Khrushchev planning a Summit Conference, and Frank had joked, "We'll have our own little Summit meeting." One of the papers printed it, others picked it up, and it stuck.

We'd get offstage at one-thirty, quarter to two, and booze in the lounge until it was light out. We'd been in Vegas for a week and still plane-, train-, and busloads of people were pouring into town, sleeping in lobbies, cars, anywhere, hoping to get rooms.

Senator John F. Kennedy, campaigning for the presidency, was in Vegas for a meeting with the Nevada delegates at the Convention Center. Frank had been getting the theatrical community behind Kennedy and the five of us had begun doing rallies and campaigning for him.

There was only one star dressing room at the Sands, so for the fun of it all five of us used it. As we were getting ready for a second show, Frank told us, "JFK is going to be out front."

We always had celebrities in the audience. All five of us were onstage and we'd introduce them round-robin, each of us taking one, always saving the biggest for last, as is normal. That night Frank stepped back to where we had a bar on the stage and as I was pouring a drink he said, "Smokey, you introduce the President."

Frank threw that to me. Instead of taking the glory for himself and doing a number with it—which I would have done if I'd been that close to the man—he gave it to me. He was still pushing me up front, still had his arm around me.

Later the senator and his party came upstairs and had drinks with us. Everybody was calling him "Number One." After a while one of his aides told him they should leave so he could get some sleep because the plane was leaving in six hours. He was enjoying himself. "Don't worry about me, I'll sleep on the plane."

Peter took me aside and whispered, "If you want to see what a million dollars in cash looks like, go into the next room; there's a brown leather satchel in the closet; open it. It's a gift from the hotel owners for Jack's campaign."

I never went near it. I was also told there were four wild girls scheduled to entertain him and I didn't want to hear about that either and I got out of there. Some things you don't want to know. Like when gangsters are talking and you're sitting there, you don't want to know these things. I'd be sitting in the booth with Julie Podell at the Copa and he'd have some very heavyweight visitors, like Frank Costello. I'd stand up. "Excuse me, gentlemen . . ." "No, sit down, kid, you can listen," and they'd shrug at each other. "Who the fuck is *he* going to tell? Siddown, Sam."

With the President you'd hear rumors, you had your suspicions, but you'd rather not know. I'd be with Peter and he'd drop a few words, or I'd go out to Santa Monica to Peter and Pat's house and there'd be three or four chicks running around. Well, you don't have to be a Dunninger to figure out why they're there. The President was due to arrive. Did I see them humping? No, I did not. Did I see them kissing on the lips? No, I did not. But I also know they ain't there to play shuffleboard.

When we'd settled into our shooting schedule, I called May.

"Tell me." I smiled at the already familiar greeting. She said, "I hear it's fantastic there."

"How'd you like to come down for the weekend and see for yourself?"

"But I hear it's impossible to get a hotel room?"

I played it like the King of France wandering through Paris in disguise—the classic scene in which the loyal subject whose wife is wrongfully imprisoned asks hopefully, "Can you possibly get my case to the attention of His Majesty?" and the King chuckles behind his disguise: "I believe I can manage it." I was so delighted with myself it was practically incest.

As she came through the gate she smiled and her face was like sunshine. She put out her hand. "Hello there."

"Hello there yourself." I took the makeup bag she was carrying. A lady was standing behind her and there was a definite family resemblance.

"I'd like you to meet my mother, Mrs. Wilkens."

I did one of the great recoveries of my life with an eighteenth-century bow. "I'm so glad you could come, Mrs. Wilkens." My nose should have grown twelve inches.

"My mother is going back to Sweden next week and I thought she'd enjoy seeing Las Vegas before she leaves."

I introduced May from the stage with the other celebrities. I met them in the lounge after the second show and we had a bite to eat with Frank and the guys. I didn't have any scenes the next afternoon, so I took them sightseeing. As we drove back across the desert from Lake Mead, May said, "My mother's a little tired. We'll have dinner in our room so she can go to sleep early. Can I come to your second show by myself?"

"Of course. I've got a permanent table. There'll be some of my friends there, so you won't have to sit alone."

As soon as I got off I sent Murphy out front to escort her backstage. "Hello there. I liked your show." Murphy did a sneaky-foot out the door and we were alone. She was wearing a bright yellow dress. She had a sunburn, which highlighted her freckles, and her hair was hanging long and golden over her shoulders.

"Would you like something to drink?"

"No. Thank you very much. But you have one if you like."

"No, thanks. I don't feel like one either."

"The club was really packed."

"Yeah . . . things sure are swinging." I was desperate to make conversation, but I'd never really *talked* to a girl before. It was always laughs, jokes, and pow! into bed or not. She walked over to the TV set and stood there, her eyes glued to it. I stared at it too.

It was impossible to believe. Here's a girl I could get drunk just from looking at, she's just seen me do the show of my life, she's in my dressing room, the door is closed—and we're standing like idiots watching a twenty-year-old movie.

She glanced up as she sensed me staring at her. The haughty look she'd had in *The Blue Angel* and when we'd met was gone. Her cheeks were flushed, and she seemed self-conscious. I walked the two steps over to her, put my hands on her shoulders, and kissed her.

She was a little tall. I asked, "Would you mind taking off your shoes?" She laughed and kicked them off. I kissed her again. Suddenly it was easy to talk. I remembered the closed door and opened it and as I turned I caught a look of satisfaction on her face.

I HUNG UP the phone before she answered. I looked out at my pool. There wasn't a ripple in the water. Everything was quiet and orderly. I could have affairs with a thousand chicks and walk away but every time I even thought about May I felt myself getting drawn in deeper. It defied all logic. Where could it go? I'd have to be a lunatic to leave myself that wide open. I bummed around with the buddies, sticking out each night until I was tired enough to fall asleep. I was in the middle of planning how to kill another evening when I pulled myself up short. *I'm out of my mind. Here I've got the first free time I can remember in years—two weeks, and I'm wasting it. I've been making too much out of this. If I'm careful, why can't I keep it free and winging with May? Nobody forces anyone to get involved.*

From the moment she said "Tell me" I was happy. I invited people over to the Playhouse; showed movies; chartered a boat, and we cruised for a week and had wonderful dinners. I loved talking to her, listening to her, looking at her, photographing her.

The Kennedy campaign was picking up momentum. My role was "Let Sam take care of all the ethnic people—he's Jewish and colored and his mother's Puerto Rican—and we'll take care of all the brown shoes," and wherever I was playing, a campaign official would give me a list of rallies and cocktail parties at which I could sing a song or just mix and shake hands and add to the excitement that was building around the figure of JFK. The campaign was tightly organized. We'd spread out and I'd do rallies in L.A., San Diego, and up the coast to San Francisco, then we'd meet back at Frank's. "How'd it go? What happened?" Or out at Peter and Pat's in Santa Monica. "How was it today? Any problems?"

At the Beverly Hilton, in the Presidential Suite there were meetings going on in five different rooms. John came out of one room as I arrived and it was "Hi, Sam . . ." with two jokes and he was off into another room, another meeting. There were always groups huddling, planning activities, and it was exciting to be there, everybody knew you and you knew everybody and you were all giving yourselves to something in which you deeply believed. It was like belonging to a club.

If Frank was doing a fund-raiser for Kennedy he'd call me, "Are you available?" and I would go there and do it. Rarely did we see Bobby Kennedy. Bobby was not as enamored of the group, or of show business, as John was. I saw Bobby mostly when I was in Boston playing Blinstrub's. Occasionally I'd be playing New York at the Copa, or Chicago at the Chez, and I'd come into the club and there was a message, "Bobby Kennedy called you." He was courteous, appreciative, but all business, and I had the feeling that though he recognized our value at rallies he also saw a negative that our flashy show business association brought to the campaign.

It was mid-March and May's birthday was on the twenty-second. We were shooting interiors for *Ocean's Eleven* and this was the only day I had free to buy her a present. I knew it was going to be a piece of jewelry but I wanted plenty of time to select just the right thing. I'd invited her over for dinner on the twenty-second, only the two of us: a little candlelight, a great bottle of wine, and I would hand it to her when her birthday cake was served.

The photographer who was doing my darkroom work dropped off an envelope of eleven-by-fourteens I'd had made up of May. I spread them on the floor. From every possible angle she was beautiful. I picked up the nearest one and as I held it I was struck by the contrast of my thumb against her arm. I put the picture down and went into the bedroom. I forced myself to look in the mirror at my broken face, my bad eye, the scar across my nose . . . I thought of her beauty, of the desirable men she could have. Still, she wasn't telling me to go away, she was seeing me every day. *Sure, Charley, she needs you! You want to fool yourself that you're Charley Dapper, Charley Star? Well, you go right ahead, keep forgetting you're colored and you're short and you're ugly—until you get reminded. Better still, throw yourself in front of a truck! It's quicker and it'll hurt less.*

I couldn't cancel our date for her birthday, not without giving a good reason. I'd go through with it, playing everything down, and let it taper off. On the twenty-second when we broke for lunch I called my housekeeper, Etheline, and told her to pick up a birthday cake. There was no point in being rude. We finished shooting early and I headed home. I felt rotten having no present for her. She had no family over here . . . what the hell, maybe I'd get her something silly, something that doesn't mean anything. I drove to Beverly Hills and browsed through the Toy Menagerie, looking at joke-type presents, like a giant stuffed giraffe. But I didn't want to give her a giant stuffed giraffe.

I walked a few blocks to Sy Sandler's and gazed at the beautiful rings and clips and pins in the window. I'd never wanted anything like I wanted to give her one of them. But she was no "chick" who'd accept an expensive gift from a guy she wasn't serious about. She'd hand it back and feel bad about embarrassing me. I stared into the window. What could I lose? Who was I kidding? I was in so deep that I couldn't walk away from her anymore. She'd have to send me away.

I RAISED the lid of the box and set it down on the coffee table in front of her. It contained a simple diamond cocktail ring, one that couldn't possibly be mistaken for an engagement ring. "Okay. You can open your eyes now." She looked at it. She didn't speak or move. I shrugged. "Not everybody likes jewelry, so I won't be offended . . ."

She lifted the ring out of the box and put it on her finger. Her voice was a whisper. "Thank you."

MAY WAS at the Sherry Netherland in New York to shoot *Murder, Inc.* I knew I couldn't give my name to the telephone operator. Maybe because it was Sunday I thought of the characters in "Peanuts," the comic strip we both liked, and when the hotel operator asked, I said, "Tell her it's Charlie Brown calling Peanuts."

May was laughing as the connection was made. "Tell me, Sharlie Brown, are you somebody I just left a few hours ago?" I kidded her about the way her accent slid over the "Ch" sound, softening it to "Sh," and, maybe to take the emphasis off the fact that I had to use a code name, I laughed a little harder than it was worth.

On Monday I browsed around a flower shop. I enjoyed choosing what I thought she'd like, and it occurred to me that in the last ten years I'd probably sent out thirty thousand dollars' worth of flowers, but this was the first time I'd ever been in a florist's shop.

We spoke on the phone as often every day as we could. I had scenes to shoot all week and at night I went to sleep early. On Sunday I called to say good morning and we spoke until afternoon. Neither of us had anything to do all day but there were three thousand miles between us.

I bumped around the house trying to get involved in books, television, records. It was incredible that with all the things I'd done, all the people I knew, one girl with a funny Swedish accent, who answered the telephone "Tell me," could fill my life—or leave it so empty. I knew that if I had a brain in my head I'd have the place swarming with chicks. But I had no eyes for all the chicks in Hollywood. There was no suddenly saying, "This is the woman I love," yet it was impossible to imagine the day I'd ever stop seeing her, and I knew that compared to what was coming, I'd never had a problem in my life.

What do I do when she becomes aware of how much I love her and she says, "I'm sorry. I like you, maybe even love you, but I . . . well, I never dreamed you were thinking of marriage."

How can I hope for anything else? Let's say she loves me. It's one thing to have quiet dinners together, go on private boats, come to Las Vegas with her mother. But marrying me brings it out in the open. She thinks she doesn't care about her career, but how will she feel when they take it away from her? How can I expect her to face the world and her family and say, "This is my husband. He's a little dark, folks . . ."

Night after night I placed my calls to her, like an alcoholic watching the bartender pour his drink, then, finally, relaxing as the warmth of her voice spread through my being, suspending my fears. Then, as the phone touched the receiver, the fears and the doubts gripped me again and I lay stretched out on the bed, hating myself for breathing life into a relationship which I'd known was condemned before it was born.

We'd been on the phone for almost an hour, we'd counted the days she'd been gone, and I said, sort of wistfully, "Wouldn't it be great to be married?" The instant I heard my own words slip out I hurried to make a joke of it. "Listen, at these prices on the phone, two could live cheaper than one."

She said, "It sure *would* be great, wouldn't it?"

I was unable to continue speaking. I told her I'd call back and we hung up. I sat on the edge of the bed, my hand still on the phone, hearing her answer over and over again. But she was in New York and I was in California and she couldn't see my skin through the phone. Had she considered that after marriage comes children? And with us they might be colored? Was she prepared for that? I let go of the phone, trying to break contact, forcing myself to face some reality. Did she know what she was saying? Had she thought seriously about it before? Or had she answered too quickly?

I walked around the room thanking God she hadn't said no, but knowing I couldn't let us go blundering happily on until a month or who knows when from now when we'd talk about children and she'd say, "I guess I didn't really give it enough thought." I owed it to her and I owed to it myself, now, to be sure she understood what she was doing.

I called her back and after we'd talked for a while I said, "You know how I love kids. Won't it be great when we're married and have lots of little brown babies?"

"I'd love to. Lots of them. Sammy? . . . Sammy, don't *you* want little brown babies?"

The tears were running down my face. I don't know exactly what I'd feared—a deathly silence, or words that would cut me in half. I'd dreaded being one inch from heaven when the gate swings closed. But then to have all the fears disappear like a horrible dream from which you've just awakened and the sun is shining and it's a beautiful day and you know that it always will be a beautiful day—the relief was paralyzing. A few hours earlier I hadn't even known that I was going to propose to her, yet if she had turned me down, if she hadn't wanted my little brown babies, I knew then, as sure as I stand on God's earth, I would have hung up the phone and blown my brains out.

12

"WHAT'S THE MATTER, SAMMY? CAN'T YOU FIND A COLORED GIRL?" . . . "GO BACK TO THE CONGO, YOU KOSHER COON." Neo-Nazi storm troopers, wearing swastika armbands, were picketing me in the middle of Washington, D.C. It was September 1960. We were engaged to be married in October and I'd just arrived in Washington to play the Lotus Club. They had a small black dog walking with them, and they had attached a sign to his back: "I'M BLACK TOO, SAMMY, BUT I'M NOT A JEW."

I could only stare at them, thinking: *This is happening. It's really happening. Thank you, God, for not letting May be here.*

MURPHY tried to slip the hate mail past me, but I needed to know what people were thinking. "Dear Nigger Bastard, I see Frank Sinatra is going to be best man at your abortion. Well, it's good to know the kind of people supporting Kennedy before it's too late. [signed] An ex-Kennedy vote."

Murphy looked pained. "Sammy, why do you bother to read those lousy things? I'll take care of the mail for you."

"Baby, if you thought it would hurt me, you wouldn't tell me, right?"

"They don't mean anything. They don't even sign their names."

"They don't have to sign their names when they vote. Do me a favor. Find an out-of-town-news stand and get me some papers from the South and the Southwest." The first mention I saw was: "Show business and politics have merged more heavily in this election than ever before. Notable among the vote swayers is Frank Sinatra. The crooner, a close friend of JFK, will take time off from politics to serve in the coveted capacity of best man at the wedding of Negro entertainer Sammy Davis, Jr.—another Kennedy booster—to blonde movie star May Britt."

The already stale news that Frank would be my best man continued making the front pages and too often, by "coincidence," right next to it were stories about Frank campaigning for Kennedy.

I too was devoting all spare time to campaigning, in Los Angeles, in Watts, in some twenty large cities. I went with Ethel Kennedy, or Bobby, and on some occasions with John. The Broadway and Hollywood columns were alive with jokes and political humor: "If Kennedy's elected his problem is: should he appoint Sammy Davis, Jr., Ambassador to Israel or the Congo?" . . . "Public opinion experts say that when Frank Sinatra appears at pal Sammy Davis, Jr.'s interracial marriage it will cost Kennedy as many votes, maybe more, as the crooner has been able to swing via his successful JFK rallies."

I hadn't been in Vegas twenty minutes when I got word that the bookmakers were offering three to one that Frank wouldn't show at my wedding. Frank, Dean, and Peter had come down for the weekend and I was in the steam room with Frank. He asked, "How's she standing up under all the garbage?"

"So far so good. But the momentum keeps growing. At least if I could be with her—but I figure the less we're seen together until the wedding, the less they'll have to work with."

When I spoke with May between shows she said, "Frank called me a little while ago. Just to say hello and find out how I am."

I saw him the next afternoon as he and the guys were leaving. "I talked to May last night, Frank. Thanks."

"See you at the wedding, Charley. I'll leave Hawaii on the fourteenth and be back a day early to make sure I won't run into weather."

When I got to the dressing room I looked through the mail. Somebody had sent me a clipping, a two-panel cartoon. The first panel was a picture of me dressed like a butler, grinning and serving a platter of fried chicken and watermelon to John F. Kennedy. In the second panel I was sitting at the table eating it with him. The caption was: "Will it still be the *White* House?"

After the shows, I put a "Don't Disturb" sign on the door of my suite and sat in the living room by myself. Fair or not, my wedding was giving the Nixon people the opportunity to ridicule Kennedy and hurt him at the polls. I could imagine the pressure Frank must be under: eighty guys telling him, "Don't be a fool. You've worked hard for Kennedy, now do you want to louse him up?" And it was understandable. If he stood up for me at a controversial interracial marriage only a few weeks before the election there would be votes he'd lose for Kennedy. And the innuendo and publicity so far was only a hint of what would happen after he appeared at the wedding and they had a piece of hard news to work with.

How can I call myself his friend when I'm keeping him in this kind of a bind? If he's holding out for me like this, how can I not be equally his friend and take him off the spot?

But aside from the fact that I couldn't imagine being married without him present at my wedding, at this point if Frank did not appear it would backfire. They'd make it look as if Kennedy's staff had suggested it. Maybe he'd regain the bigot vote but he'd lose some of the liberals and a lot of the Negro vote.

There was only one way to take the pressure off everyone concerned. Postpone the wedding. I knew he was at the Springs with Peter.

"Hi ya, Charley, what's new?"

"Frank, we're going to have to put the wedding off a couple of weeks. You wouldn't believe the problems a poor soul has trying to get married: there's a hitch getting the Escoffier Room for the reception, the rabbi can't make it 'cause he's already booked for a bar mitzvah. Anyway, I don't know when it'll be but I'll give you plenty of notice."

"You're lying, Charley."

I hesitated, but it was pointless. "Look, it's best that we postpone till after the election."

There was silence at the other end of the line. Then: "You don't have to do that."

"I want to. All the talk . . ."

"Screw the talk."

"I know, but it's better this way."

When finally he spoke again, his voice was almost a whisper. "I'll be there whenever it is. You know that, don't you?"

118

"I know that, Frank."

"I'd never ask you to do a thing like this. Not your wedding. I'd never ask that."

"That's why it's up to me to be saying it."

"You're a better man than I am, Charley. I don't know if I could do this for you, or for anyone . . ."

"You've been doing it, haven't you?"

I heard him put down the phone and then Peter was on the line. There were no jokes. None of the usual insults we do with each other. He said, "Frank can't talk anymore." If he got that choked up now, if he could break down in the middle of a phone call, then the pressure must have been greater than I'd imagined.

"Charley?"

"Yes, Peter?"

"Charley, I . . . it's beautiful of you."

I stared at May's picture on my night table. What could I say to her? "We're postponing our marriage because it's so repulsive to some people that they won't want to vote for Kennedy." How does a man explain this to the one person above all others from whom he wants respect and admiration?

I got into my car and drove aimlessly around downtown Vegas, racked by the picture of her excitement of the past few weeks, rushing around and getting the house ready, waiting for her parents to arrive from Sweden, sending out invitations, fitting her dress . . . the sooner I faced it, the faster it would be behind us. I went into a drugstore and sat down in a phone booth. Her excitement soared through the phone. "Sharley Brown, our first presents arrived. Six of them. One is from George and Gracie Burns, the others have the names inside. I can't wait till you get back so we can open them together."

"May, I have something important to tell you, but before I do I want you to know that this is the first and only thing that concerns us both that I'll ever do without consulting you." As I explained it, I knew by her silence that she was hurt and saddened. "Darling, it boils down to this: during a period of over twenty years Frank has been aces high, aces up—everything a guy could be to me. Now he needs something from me, so there can be no evaluating, no hesitating, no limit. It's got to be to the end of the earth and back for him if he needs it."

"I understand," she said, "and I agree with you. There was nothing else to do."

Rogers and Cowan, who were handling my public relations, sent an announcement to the press: The Sammy Davis, Jr.–May Britt wedding has been postponed due to a legal technicality in Miss Britt's Mexican divorce from her previous husband.

That was the lie and that's how we told it.

THERE WERE bomb threats on my opening at the Huntington Hartford Theater in Los Angeles: "We've got guns and we've got hand grenades and we're coming to blow up the place." "Is that black bastard still going to open there? There's a bomb in the theater right now." The stage manager had called the police and they were searching the building. Another call came in: "We'll fix him and we'll get his nigger-loving girlfriend too."

I called May. "You should know this from me before you hear it on the news. We've had some threats and I don't want you here tonight."

"What kind of threats?"

"Just idiots. But I'm not about to take chances."

"Are you going to do the show?"

"Yes."

"Then I'll be there."

"May, it's out of the question."

"Don't argue with me, Sammy. Nobody is going to frighten me away from you."

I called the sheriff of Los Angeles County and hired ten off-duty detectives to be sitting in front of and behind her seat.

Murphy brought me a folded sheet of paper. "Somebody slipped this under the stage door." A bullet was drawn in the center of the paper. Below, it said, "I'm going to shoot you dead during your show. Guess when?"

Cranks, sadists, idiots. Certainly. Yet among the empty threats could be the one that might materialize. How do you anticipate the workings of a man's mind when he himself isn't in control of it?

May came into the dressing room. Her face was drawn tight. "Sammy, do you think you should go on? Shouldn't you put the opening off for a few days so the police will have time to be sure?"

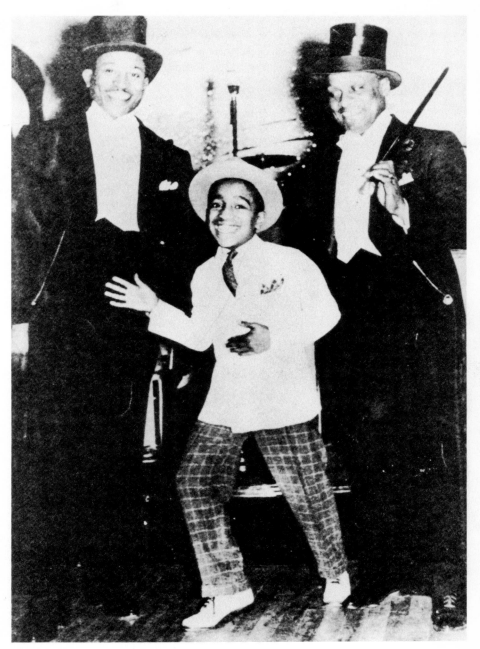

Age nine, with Sam Sr. and Will Mastin

When I was nine I told my father, "I can outdance you."
"Oh yeah? What makes you think that?" he asked.
" 'Cause you taught me everything I know."
"Yeah, but I didn't teach you everything *I* know."

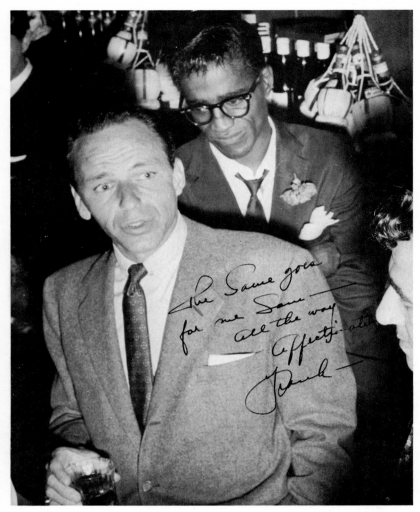

"The same goes for me Sam—all the way. Affectionately, Frank."

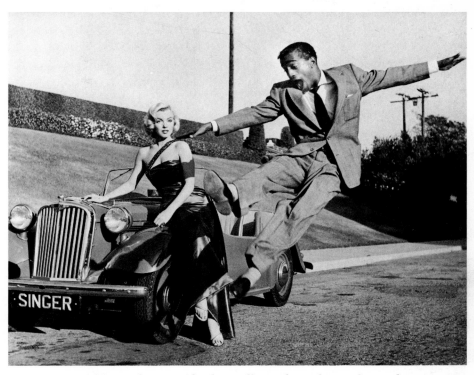

An innocent publicity shot outside the Hollywood Bowl. Marilyn and I were rumored to be "an item." We were friends. Nothing more. To me, Marilyn was one of the sweetest creatures that ever lived.

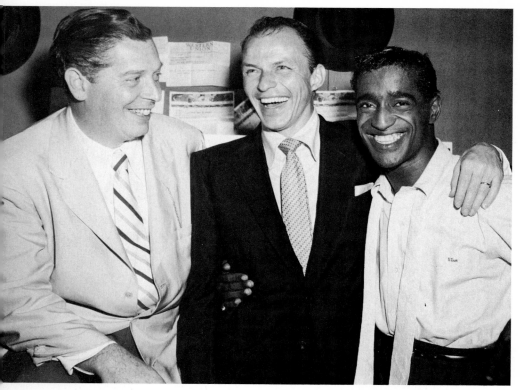

Milton Berle is always funny. "Sammy, you look great. You've taken off height."

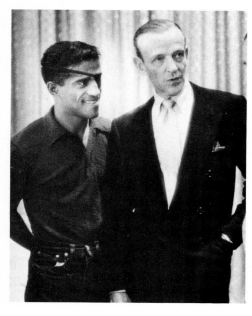

Fred Astaire always greeted me, "Hello, tap dancer." I appreciated it, but I always replied, "Not around you, I ain't. Around you I'm a singer."

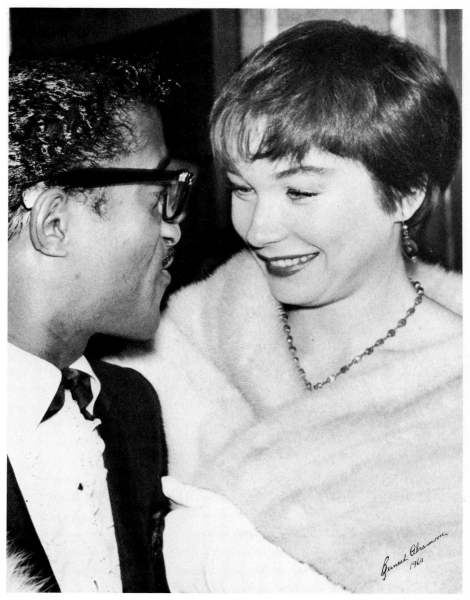

One of the two Shirleys in my life. I love them both. In each case, there has never been anything but work and deep friendship. We are closer, more indivisible, than lovers. When you lose a lover it's like getting a bad haircut. It grows back in time. But if you ever lose a friend as special as either of my Shirleys, it's like a finger got cut off.

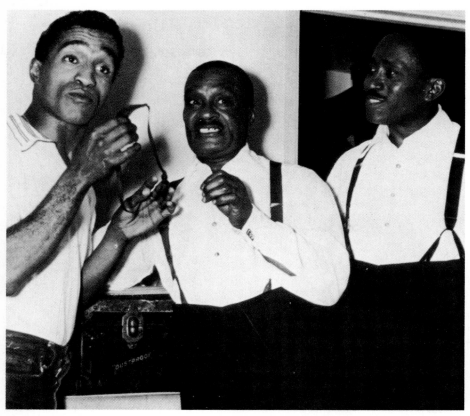

With Will Mastin and Sam Sr., on eve of first performance without eyepatch, 1955

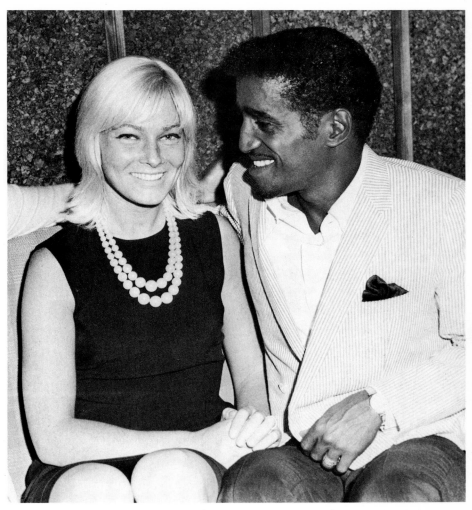

May is the finest mother I have ever heard of. Singlehandedly, she raised our children into young people who make me proud. Once, when she was going with somebody special, I urged her to marry him. "I couldn't," she replied. "It wouldn't be fair. If ever there was a problem between him and the kids, I'd be on the side of the kids, even if I knew they were wrong."

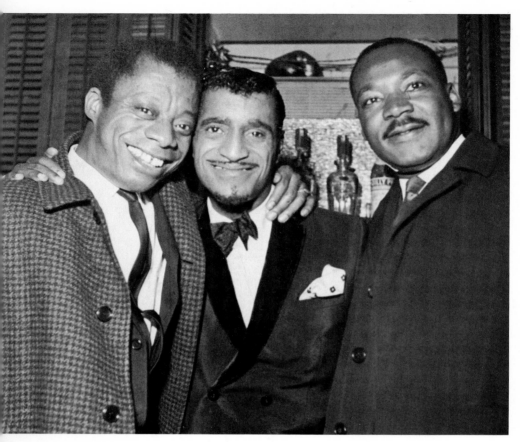

With James Baldwin and Martin Luther King, Jr.

"We ain't what we oughta be,
we ain't what we wanta be,
we ain't what we gonna be,
but thank God we ain't what we was."

—Martin Luther King, Jr.

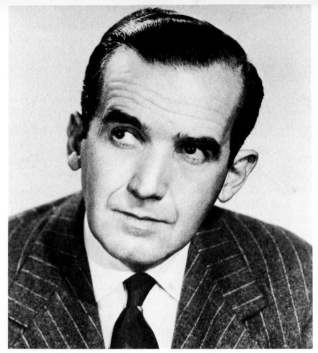

Though I was constantly on the road I bought a house in the Hollywood Hills and brought my grandmother from Harlem to live in it with me. Ed Murrow visited us in our new home on *Person to Person*, the most prestigious show of its time. I was happy that the viewers would see that I'd accomplished something. But, the joke went, "It's the damnedest thing. I see the maid going in and out all the time, but the people who live there never leave the house."

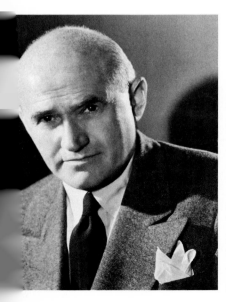

During the filming of *Porgy and Bess*, I told Mr. Goldwyn I couldn't work on Yom Kippur. He couldn't believe it. Suspending production for one day would cost him $25,000. I said, "Sir, I'm sorry for the problems I'm causing you, but I go to temple a lot less than I would like because when I do, people still look at me as if they think it's a publicity stunt. However, I must draw the line at working on Yom Kippur."

He took off his glasses. "Sammy, you're a little so-and-so, but go with your yarmulke and your tallis— we'll work it out somehow." He sighed, like now he'd seen everything, and as I left his office he was behind his desk talking to the four walls.

"Directors I can fight. Fires on the set I can fight. Writers, even actors I can fight. But a Jewish colored fellow? This, I can't fight!"

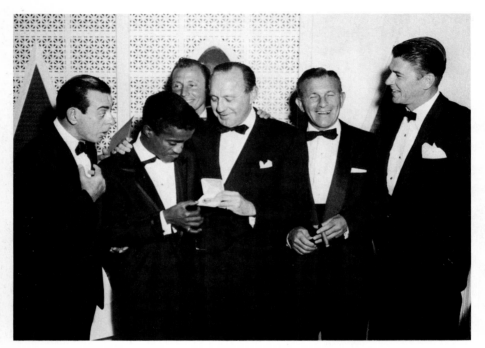

Getting an award from the Beverly Hills Friars Club. L–R: Eddie Cantor, (uniden-tified,) Jack Benny, George Burns, and a man we used to call Ron

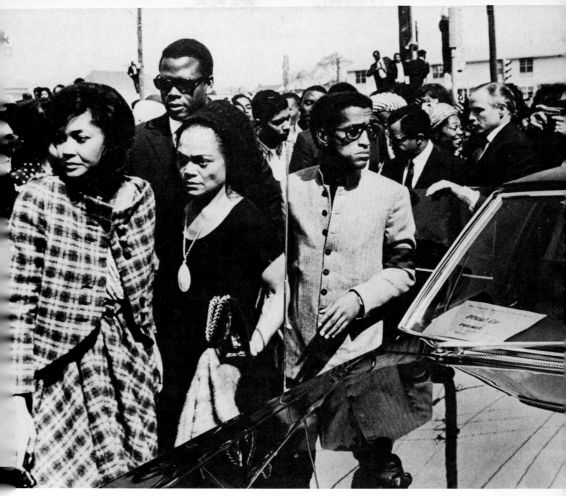

At Martin Luther King, Jr.'s funeral. L–R: Nancy Wilson, Eartha Kitt, Sidney Poitier, Berry Gordy, Marlon Brando

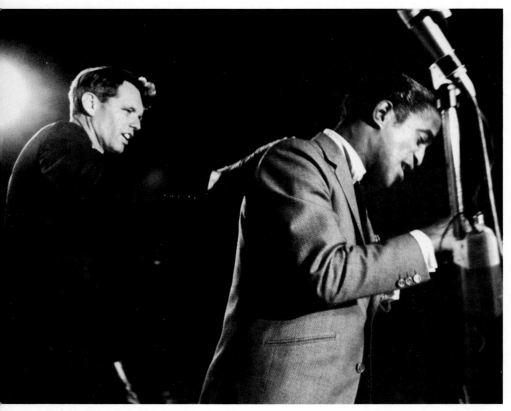

I believed in Bobby. Campaigning for him, introducing him at rallies, was an attempt to give back something to this country that has given me so much.

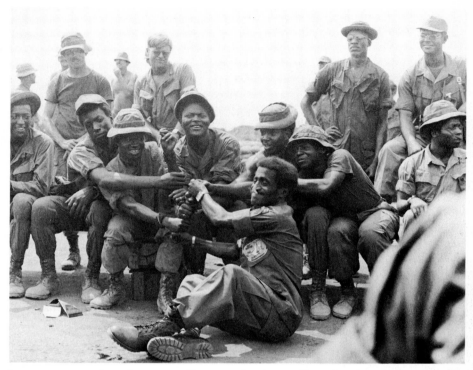

I was so opposed to the war in Vietnam that I initially refused President Nixon's urgings for me to go there. It finally occurred to me that none of our kids wanted to be there, either. It was the most rewarding experience of my life.

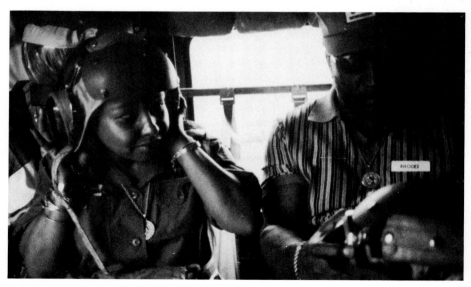

Shirley and George Rhodes in a helicopter in Vietnam

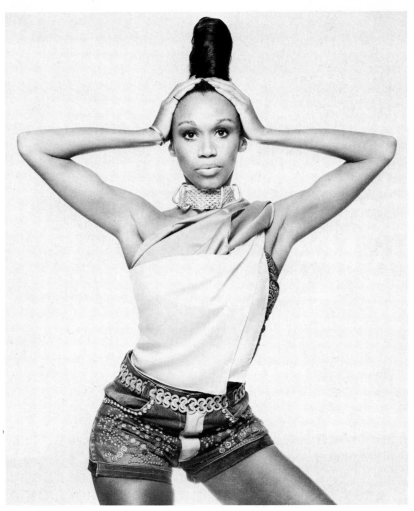

Altovise in 1973. When Jock Mahoney (Tarzan) first saw Altovise, she was stepping out of the water in Hawaii, wearing a bikini. He said, "Sam . . . this time I think you've overmarried."

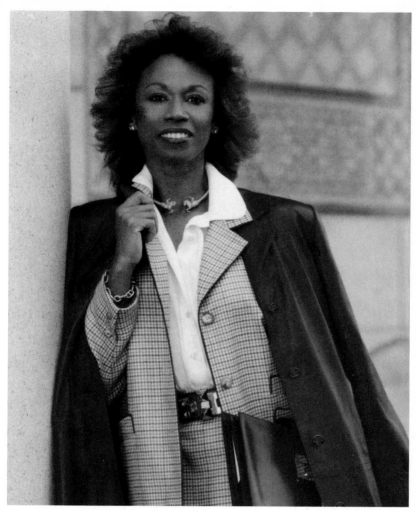

Altovise in 1983. She was the first black woman invited to become a member of SHARE and she became its chairman.

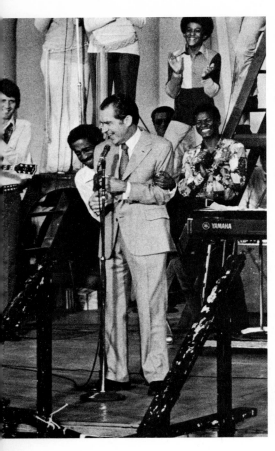

President Nixon sent me an inscribed copy of this photograph and a letter wryly observing that, as it had received "such wide coverage in the press [I was all but lynched by blacks and whites], I thought you might like to have a copy as a memento."

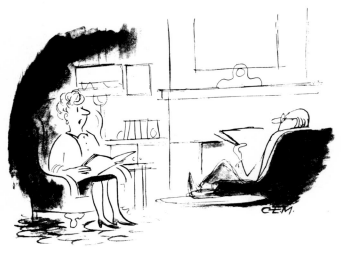

"Is it all right not to like Sammy Davis, Jr.?"

The civil rights movement wasn't easy for anybody

I put my hands on her shoulders. "Darling, know now: I'm not doing hero bits with reckless and dramatic and the-show-must-go-on. But I can't let myself be chased off the stage by anyone who makes a threat or I'm going to spend the rest of my life running from shadows." I walked to the wings. Policemen were stationed all over the backstage area. I looked through the curtain, scanning the audience. How do you entertain them while wondering if a bomb will explode? How do you do two hours of singing, dancing, and jokes, distracted by the thought that at any moment a lunatic might shoot you?

ON THE DAY of our wedding people were leaning out their windows all the way up the hill with telescopic lenses trained on my house, crowded onto the porches of the houses above us as if they'd bought tickets for a ball game. Reporters and newsreel men clustered in front of the door. Photographers were perched in trees to get a free line of sight to the doorway.

Frank was completely in character, a cigarette in one hand, a glass in the other, intense, yet with a casual air in the way he punctuated his sentences with the familiar Sinatra hand gesture. I thought, it's easy enough for others who sit in a relatively obscure corner of fame to say, "It's only right for him to be there, he's your friend, isn't he? He *should* be there!" But it's not that simple. With all his independence, still he knows where it comes from, and how quickly a career can go down the drain on the whim of the public. For him to state, "This is my friend and in your ear if you don't like it," means putting in jeopardy everything he'd worked for, lost and regained, and must fight to hold on to. It was not a minor thing for Frank to be my best man, nor for Peter and Pat, the President's sister and brother-in-law, to be in the wedding party.

I took my place in the living room under the canopy of flowers. Frank was at my side. Peter was next to him. Mama and my mother and father and Will were gathered around us.

May appeared from the next room with her father, walking toward me. She was every fine and lovely, precious thing that God ever put into a woman. Her father kissed her and smiled at me as I stepped forward. She put her arm in mine and the rabbi began the ceremony.

"Almighty God, supremely blessed, supreme in might and glory, guide this groom and bride. Sammy and May, you are standing in front of me to join your lives even as your hands are joined together, and custom dictates that I, as your rabbi, give you some advice. Your marriage is something more than just two people in love, and it is most certainly that or I have never seen two people in love in twenty years of the ministry. But as you come together as man and wife something more is involved. You are people without prejudice. You represent the value of the society that many of us dream about but, I suspect, hesitate to enter. As such, because you are normal in an abnormal society—society will treat you as sick. To be healthy among the sick is to be treated as sick as if the others were healthy . . ."

THE DAY after our wedding the manager of the Geary Theater in San Francisco called me at home. "Mr. Davis, we've had a number of bomb threats and threats against your life."

May was still resting. She'd been up late packing for San Francisco, our first trip together and what we had planned would be the honeymoon we lost when we postponed the wedding.

Obviously there could be no more hoping that the commotion at the Hartford was merely a flurry before the wedding. This was the tip-off that they'd be waiting for me all across the country. I couldn't bring May with me into the unknown. I had to keep her here, at home, where I could have her protected.

I opened the bedroom door. May sat up. "Good morning, Sharley Brown." Her suitcases were packed, her travel outfit was ready and hanging on the closet door.

I sat on the bed. "Darling . . ." She stopped smiling, sensing something serious. I forced the words out. "I'm sorry but you can't come to San Francisco." May listened without interrupting as I explained what was going on. "We can say it's wrong, it's lousy, but that's not going to change it. In the days of King Arthur, or the days of the Romans, they'd have a trial by ordeal: they'd say, 'We'll put him in with a hungry lion,' and if he survived he was set free. It's going to be something like that with us. The first year will be the tough one. If we can survive that, then I think we'll have it made."

"Do you really think it will take a whole year before they'll leave us alone?"

"I don't know. But I do know that I have to protect what I hold dear. We'll have to adopt a routine, a security procedure that we'll follow until the pressure is off. You won't arrive in any city with me. I'll go ahead and get a feeling of what's up. If it looks safe after a few days, then I'll be on the phone telling you to grab the first plane."

She got out of bed and casually closed the closet door so that I wouldn't be reminded that her travel outfit was hanging there ready, and she sat down beside me.

"Meanwhile I've hired someone who'll move in and stay here while I'm gone. Naturally, Rudy'll be here too, but it won't hurt to have another man in the house."

"A guard?"

"He's a private detective."

"Do you think . . . do I really need that?"

"No. Nor do I expect the house to burn down but I carry fire insurance against the remote chance that it might." I stood up. "May? Thank you for not making a fuss over something I can't change." I took her hand in mine. "I want you to know how sorry I am about all this and how much I appreciate you."

Embarrassed, she smiled. "Do you think I'm marvelous?" I gave her a look. Then it was time to say goodbye and she walked with me toward the front door. "Sammy . . ." Her face was losing the façade of cheerfulness. "I'm afraid I'm not going to be so marvelous . . ." Her voice was starting to quaver. I held her in my arms, stroking her head while she got it out of her system. "A fine Joan of Arc I turned out to be." Her ears became red and suddenly, abruptly, she pulled herself together and strode briskly across the living room. "Okay, that's enough of that." She faced me. "I'm sorry. That's the last time I'll ever do this to you. I promise. I won't make it harder for you than it already is."

THE THREATS and hate mail continued heavily in San Francisco. I told May not to come. "Maybe Reno."

I called her from Reno. "I'm sorry but you can't come here . . ."

And then a few weeks after that I told her, "I'm sorry but you can't come to Chicago . . ."

And then I told her, "I'm sorry but you can't come to Philadelphia . . ."

She didn't fight it. She didn't complain. She hurt in private, trying not to make it harder on me. May was young and beautiful, we were legally married, but she was caught in the prison of my skin.

THE APPLAUSE increased, kept growing louder, but I could only think of it as an ideal shield for the sound of a gunshot. Despite the plainclothesmen spread all over the Latin Casino in Camden, New Jersey, despite every possible precaution, I found myself unable to devote myself fully to each song, each dance: I was looking for hints of trouble, studying hazy faces as far as I could see into the lights. As I did the impressions, my mind's ear wasn't tuned entirely to Cagney or Robinson, and as I sang, only half of me was absorbed in the words of the song while the other half was praying that somebody hadn't left a window or a door unlocked at the house. I was afraid. Somewhere out there, in this audience or the next, was the guy who'd make trouble. Or, worse still, was he in Hollywood creeping up to the house planning some horrible revenge against May?

Suddenly I wasn't so sure where I could best protect her. Even with a professional security man there was always the human factor. Maybe it would be safer to have her where I could be on top of her security. And I wanted to see my wife. So far, more than ninety percent of our marriage had taken place on the phone. I took a chance and brought her to New York.

Earl Wilson reported, "The Sammy Davis, Jr.'s are expecting. If it's a boy they'll name him Mark Sidney, or Tracey if it's a girl." Hundreds of letters arrived at the Copa: "God will strike you down for what you are doing. You have sinned against God's will." "What about the children?"

Would it be better if I'd married a Negro woman? Would they treat my child any better? Erect fewer barriers? No. My baby would have it tough no matter what, until *no* baby would have it tough no matter what.

MAY PULLED back the curtains excitedly. "Look. It must have snowed all night." I put my arm around her and we stood at the window of our suite in the Sherry Netherland admiring the beauty of Fifth Avenue. "Sammy, can we go walking in the snow?"

"Darling, may I tell you something?

"Sure."

"That's the *worst idea I ever heard!* A woman takes a singer who dances—a dancing singer—and wants to turn him into a ski instructor? First of all, have you any idea what happens when a small colored fella like me goes walking around in snowdrifts? Right away people point and yell, 'Hey, look, it's a penguin, it's a penguin.'"

I stood at the window watching the snowflakes swirling through the trees in Central Park, wishing I could take her out and we could run around like a couple of nitwits. I had bought her a mink coat at Maximilian. Knowing I couldn't afford it she'd insisted I return it, but I wouldn't. It was for self. It was a way of compensating, a way of saying, "It ain't *all* bad. You're locked out of this, you're locked out of that, you've lost your contract at Fox, they don't want you anymore, you're a nigger lover, but it ain't *all* bad. Look—I can give you this." I yearned to take her out in it—window-shopping along Fifth Avenue and maybe going into some of the stores and buying things together. We'd had dozens of nice invitations but I didn't accept. Even the idea of taking her to Danny's or the Harwyn, where it was as safe as any public place could be— still, the hotel and dressing room were safer. Nobody could insult her there or do icy stares from across the room.

May was putting on her boots. "I'm going for a walk around the block. I've got to get some air."

"Why don't you wear your mink coat?"

She was surprised. "I'm saving it to wear for the first time with my husband."

I wiped the frost off a window and watched her as she turned the corner at Fifty-ninth Street. Paul Newer, my bodyguard, was a few yards behind her. It had been more than ten days of confinement to the club and the hotel. There'd been some questions like "How come we don't go to Danny's?" and "What's the Harwyn like?" and I'd covered with trumped-up reasons why we had to be at the hotel: an interview, business meetings, exhaustion—always something, but I was afraid that she was beginning to suspect that we were in hiding. I couldn't let her think that. It would be too denigrating, too depressing, even for May.

The frost was re-forming on the glass, blurring the outside, reducing the world to the rooms of our suite.

She stamped the last of the snow off her boots, her face pink from the cold, smiling as though she'd opened a safety valve and all the tension had been released. I helped her off with her coat. "How was it?"

"*Beautiful.* There's hardly anybody on the streets and the snow is so fresh . . ." She saw the hot chocolate I'd ordered for her. "Heyyyy . . . I was just thinking I could use something like that to hit the spot."

"I got four tickets for *Camelot* for the matinee tomorrow."

She beamed at me, savoring the moment. "You mean my husband and I are really honest-to-God saying to heck with meetings and stuff and going to a matinee?"

"And I've asked Jane and Burt to come with us." Apart from being friends whom I know she liked, having another couple with us, a white couple, would dilute the impact of just the two of us together.

I woke up afraid. I felt it physically, like whirring motors in my stomach, down my legs, and an ache in my heart for her when she finds out she's not a beautiful girl going out to a matinee with her husband, but a "nigger lover." It was out of the question to risk it. I knew I couldn't protect her forever but I had to wait until I could be sure that she was emotionally prepared for whatever we might run into, until I was certain that we had enough background together so that the threads of our marriage could absorb the shock of the kind of abuse that was waiting for us outside.

She was moving around quietly, believing I was still asleep. She'd washed her hair and had a towel around her neck. I didn't move. I heard her open the bedroom door, then close it softly. Her mink coat was hanging outside the closet door. Under it was an orange dress and pink beads. Her boots were on the floor directly under the coat. It was one o'clock. It seemed like a long time before I heard the door opening.

"Sammy? It's one-thirty."

". . . five minutes, darling, just five more minutes . . ." I heard the phone ring in the other room.

"Sammy, that was Jane and Burt. The traffic is heavy and we should be waiting downstairs or we'll miss the overture."

I rolled over, keeping my eyes closed. "Five more minutes . . ."

"But, Sammy, if you don't get up now we'll miss the show." I could smell her perfume. I didn't want to look at her and see her all dressed and ready with her makeup on. "Well, if you're this tired you'd better sleep for another hour or two. We can see the show some other time." I was aching to tell her, "Darling, I don't want to sleep away our day. I love you and I want to see you happy. I don't want to keep your beauty locked in a closet. I'd give anything to be able to take you to the show as we've planned, to take you anywhere, but I don't dare." I stayed in bed long after she'd left the room, certain I'd done the best thing, yet what was it costing? Disappointment by disappointment, would it become so unpleasant for her that eventually, layer by layer, it would wear away the love?

I stood in the doorway of the living room, wearing a robe and pajamas. May got up and hugged me. I held her tight. Jane and Burt were sitting on the couch. "I'm sorry, guys. I just couldn't have gotten out of bed if my life depended on it."

Burt shrugged. "We've already seen it."

"Look, I've been doing two shows a night and three on weekends and I plain ran out of strength."

May poured a cup of coffee for me and looked at Jane and Burt. "Coffee?"

Jane smiled pointedly. "No, thanks. We're already awake."

"Hey," May said, "he's my husband and if I'm not angry at him, then you guys have no right to be."

They didn't care about the show. They were annoyed and puzzled by the way I was treating May. There was no way they could understand without my telling them and it was better that they didn't understand and couldn't pity her. I played it Charley Cheerful. "I've got a swingin' idea for dinner tonight. Instead of ordinary room service we'll have a dinner party. The guys'll wear black tie and the girls long dresses. We'll order caviar, lobster cocktails, steaks or maybe some duck. Then for dessert we can have a soufflé, cordials with our coffee—we'll do it banquet style for two hours and we'll keep a waiter and a captain here to serve the whole meal . . ."

Jane and Burt left to get dressed and sent flowers. I'd ordered a magnum of champagne and poured drinks for the four of us. The evening went off with the luxury I'd planned, but all I'd accomplished was to raise the level of the prison.

THE MAIL brought our invitation to John F. Kennedy's inauguration, in a large flat envelope with a piece of cardboard to keep it from bending. I showed it to May. "How's this for a sense of history? For knowing that everyone who receives one of these is going to want to frame it."

Looking at my name on the invitation, I thought, *It really can happen in America. Despite all the obstacles, still in 1960 an uneducated kid from Harlem could work hard and be invited to the White House.* I felt May watching me and I was embarrassed to be so proud of receiving the invitation. I copped out, "These are not exactly being sent out to every cat on the corner."

She squeaked out, "I'm very impressed . . ." Tears were streaming down her face, which had a huge sunshine smile on it.

"Hey, don't cry."

"I'm not crying . . ."

I mopped up her eyes. "Well, then you've sprung a helluva leak."

"I'm so happy for you, Sharley Brown."

We both sat there in a happy funk, allowing the moment to press back some of the twisted muscles, to knead them soft and back into shape. Then I said, "Tomorrow it's a definite hit Bergdorf Goodman and buy the most elegant, most knock-their-eyes-out gown you can find. That will be for the night of the Inaugural Ball. Frank's putting together the show and I'll be performing. You'll also need something afternoony like a Chanel suit for the swearing-in ceremony."

"Sammy, I thought we were going to be on an economy drive."

"Darling, if when I was a kid in Harlem somebody had told me, 'You'll be performing at the White House,' I'd have saved my money for your dress. However, as I just got this news today . . . Look, don't worry about it, we'll save money later. Which reminds me, I'd better call Sy Devore and get a new tux made."

"But you have fifteen or twenty tuxedos."

"Would I be so crass as to wear a previously worn tux to entertain the President? And after I wear it at the White House it's going into mothballs. I'll have them deliver it to the house and when you fly in to Washington you can bring it with you. I'll be coming in from the Latin in Camden."

On closing night at the Copa, May said, "I'm going to hate going back to the Coast without you."

"Let's be happy that we're getting together in Washington, which is an extra we hadn't expected."

THE PHILADELPHIA *Inquirer* ran a story: "Sammy Davis, Jr., will be among the luminaries attending the presidential inauguration parties. The singer-dancer's performances at the Latin Casino in Camden will be canceled for the night of January 20."

Three days before the inauguration I was in my hotel room when Murphy woke me at eleven in the morning. "Sammy, President Kennedy's secretary is calling . . ."

It was Evelyn Lincoln, JFK's personal secretary, whom I knew from the campaign. "Mr. Davis . . . Sammy . . . the President has asked me to tell you that he does not want you to be present at his inauguration. There is a situation into which he is being forced and to fight it would be counterproductive to the goals he's set. He very much hopes you will understand . . ."

I felt a torrent of words bubbling up in my throat: "No, don't ask me to understand. Don't do this. Don't humiliate me. Don't cut me in half in front of my wife. In front of all the people I've told about it, my family, my friends, my audiences. My God, my wife called her parents in Sweden! If John can do this to me, then tell him I hate him. Please!! I have goals too. I campaigned, I earned better . . ."

But I didn't say any of that. I said, "I understand. Thank you for calling."

And I did understand, that hatred got noticed and had to be neutralized, whereas love could be put on hold. I understood that in politics a thousand votes were exactly one thousand times more valuable than one friend. I sat down on the bed, then, feeling ill, I stretched out flat. I could handle it from the idiot in the street who pickets or calls me a name or writes a letter. But when the President of the United States does it? To someone he knows. Someone he shook hands with and told, "I won't forget your help . . ." My God, if he'll do this to me, then what hope have the millions of invisible people got?

Murphy was looking at me fearfully.

"Cancel our reservations to Washington, Murph. And tell them at the club that I won't be needing that night off."

I had the feeling that Murphy was hurting more for me than I was, and *I* was just short of bleeding. "But, Sammy, you worked hard for him—he told you 'Thanks,' I heard him."

"They don't want me, baby. Now let's not make a three-act play out of it." I lay on my back trying to understand it. The election was over. The votes were in! We'd all worked so hard for Jack to be President . . . and all those moments you're never aware of the difference. I was with May at some occasions. I'd introduced her to them. They had seen me with white women and black women, and there were never any raised eyebrows. They were sophisticates in every sense of the word.

Obviously my presence would be bad for him. I knew that I was expected to understand that. I was supposed to be worldly. To understand. My hurt and embarrassment turned to anger at my friends, at Frank and Peter: why didn't they stand up for me? But I knew they had, to the extent they could.

Murphy opened the door. Peter's calling. I said you were sleeping, I didn't know if you wanted . . ."

"I don't. But I will." I didn't want him to know it got to me. Yet I did. I took the call with our usual kind of insults. "Listen, I don't care if you *are* the President's brother-in-law, I don't want to go to school with you."

"Sam . . . Pierre told me what happened. They talked the President into it. They said, 'Look, this is our first time out. Let's not do anything to fuck up. We've got Southern senators, bigoted congressmen. They see you as too liberal to start with. Peter Lawford's an actor, we've still got residue from 'The Clan's Taking Over the White House.' If we have Sammy here, is he going to bring his wife? We can't ask him not to bring her.' The President said, 'Okay, then dump it. Call Sam. He'll understand.'

"Charley? You'll be interested to know that Bobby argued for you, 'That's bullshit! It's wrong. The man campaigned.' But he was overruled. He got so angry he walked out of the rest of the discussion."

I suppose I was pleased to hear that about Bobby, but it didn't help much. I had the desire to slam the phone so hard it would go through the floor. I hung up. How could I tell May? What could I do to soften it, to make it less embarrassing? To not have her feel sorry for me?

It was noon. Only nine in the morning on the Coast. Too early to call her. Bullshit! I knew very well that she was up. She was accustomed to motion picture hours. I was procrastinating, knowing that she would expect me to be sleeping for the next few hours. I forced myself to pick up the telephone, and I told her.

"Oh, Sammy, they must have broken your heart." She wasn't brushing over the snub, playing it light, like "So what? It's just another party."

I appreciated the honesty but I couldn't return it. "I'm not going to come apart and die. Darling, I'm a controversial figure, I always have been, and they don't need anything to rock the ship of state—oh, he *can* turn a phrase, can't he! Seriously, I am *not* so important, as much as sometimes I would like to think I am, that they're going to have a cabinet meeting over me. At this point in John's career he's wondering about his inaugural address, and whether I'm there or not is, at best, minor. The whole discussion took less time than it's taking us to discuss it."

"Sharley Brown . . . I'm really very sorry. If it weren't for me . . . that people would see us there together, this would never have happened. I don't need to go. He's not *my* President. Maybe Peter could let them know that you'll be coming alone . . ."

I had never craved so much to put my arms around her and tell her the value I put on her, but again, we were three thousand miles apart. "Darling, I wouldn't go without you. Period. But thank you."

"Yes, I realized that as I was saying it. Hey, I've got an idea . . ." Suddenly her voice sounded buoyant. "I'm going to Miami Beach to be with you. I know you'd rather check things out, but, Sharley Brown, there's a time for a husband and wife to be together, and the time is now. I'll bring my new dress and your tux and we'll have our own party . . ."

"Darling . . . Florida is not the place for us."

"I know the South is 'different,' you've told me that and I believe it, but after all, how different can it be? I really want to be with my husband."

A hurt kind of puzzlement was coming across in her voice. I knew that "Darling, it's the South" just didn't mean enough to a girl raised in Sweden. Sure, she'd heard about it in school, about the plantations and then Lincoln freeing the slaves and everybody dancing around singing "Swanee River." But she could have no real understanding of what it meant in 1960 to a Negro, me, who had refused to play to segregated audiences and had succeeded in opening Miami Beach to anyone who wanted to see my show. If they hated me for desegregating audiences, my marriage would outrage them. I feared physical revenge. A gunshot, acid in her face. But I couldn't subject myself to more pity from my wife, or portray my countrymen as so harsh and heartless. I said, "Look, I'll be there for two weeks. Let me get there and check it out," and she accepted that.

The Latin Casino announced that I would not be canceling any performances. Something like "His audiences come first."

Standing in the wings listening to what I used to think of as a glamorous overture, I wondered what the people would be thinking, looking at me onstage in Camden, knowing that the rest of the Rat Pack was in Washington. It hurt like a motherfucker.

I SPOKE to May several times a day from Miami Beach.

"Do you *really* miss me?"

I sat on the bed after we'd hung up, still hearing the flecks of doubt in her voice. When someone doesn't understand the real reasons for something, they begin guessing and they have to come up with the wrong answers: Is he more concerned with his career, afraid a few people might stay away because of me? She could be thinking anything and I realized that in order to spare myself humiliation I was causing her the anguish of doubt.

She answered the phone on the first ring.

"May . . . I want to explain this Miami Beach jazz."

"Well, as long as you mention it, I must say I don't understand, although I sure would like to."

"Okay. Try to understand that we haven't only committed the cardinal sin of the South. Florida has a state *law* against miscegenation—a white person mixing with a colored person. They could put us in jail for a year if they wanted to."

"But we're married . . ."

"Down here I don't have the right to even walk down the street with you despite the fact that we're married."

"I didn't know."

"Darling, I have to have a special police card or if I go out on the streets at night I can be arrested. I need a special police permit so that a taxi driver will take me . . ."

When she spoke there were tears in her voice. "I feel rotten making you tell me that . . . I'm so sorry."

Long after we'd hung up I sat by myself looking, for the millionth time, at my skin. The skin of my hands, my face. Through my living-room window I couldn't help seeing people at the pool, in front of their cabanas, suffering in the sun, trying to darken their skin. What was the great goddamned difference? I was sick of the question. At that moment I wished I could just zip myself out of my skin, out of all this trouble it was causing. I wanted to see my wife and to hold her.

13

A MAN IS NOT complete until he sees a baby he has made, and by the grace of God I stood there looking at mine, seeing her tiny face and hands, her whole delicate self. I watched the nurse taking Tracey away until she was out of sight. I wasn't ready to go downstairs and talk to people. I went into the waiting room and sat down near a window. I prayed that by the time our baby was grown she would live in a world of people who would not care about a layer of skin. But was that possible? Ever? Are people willing to change? Would they ever be willing to understand a child's innocence? I gazed out the window, grateful for the talent I had been given and because of it the thought that perhaps I could have something to do with affecting the world so that someday my children, or maybe only my grandchildren, would be able, finally, to stop fighting.

MARTIN Luther King was in L.A. and he stopped by my house to visit me. When I asked him how his work was going he said, "We're hurtin' for money. We can hardly function."

Like so many others, I had come to look upon him as hope. "How much do you need?"

"A hundred thousand dollars would pay our debts and give us some breathing room."

I didn't have anywhere near that or I'd have given it to him. But I called Frank and Dean and we did a benefit for the Southern Christian Leadership Conference at Carnegie Hall and SCLC got $100,000 to work with.

Backstage, Martin embraced and thanked me. "I'm gonna call on you again."

"If you need me, you've got me. Only I ain't comin' down South. I'll do all the benefits you want—in the North."

"We'll get you down there." Martin was a well-rounded man who loved a good joke, and could laugh at himself. I did my jokes back at him. "You wanta get me down there and get me lynched? You know I'm married to a white woman up here. You must be crazy wantin' me down there." He sat with his hands clasped in front of him, laughing. "Don't worry about it, don't worry. We safe. We in God's hands."

"But suppose He's busy?"

Jesse Jackson was there and he nodded. "You're good for the Doctor. You make him laugh."

I WAS AT home between dates when I got a call from London inviting me to play the Royal Command Performance again. It coincided with my date for a one-man show at the Prince of Wales Theater. I described the elegance of the evening to May: ". . . with the Queen and the royal family and all those cats wearing sashes and medals. Darling, you are going to see a small colored lad perform so good that the Queen's gonna say, 'I ain't leavin' here to go to heaven.' "

"Sammy . . . I'm dying to be with you in London, and to see that performance . . . but I don't see how I can go."

"Why not?"

"I can't leave Tracey."

"We'll bring her with us."

May shook her head. "She can't travel."

I didn't realize how serious she was, so I kidded it. "Darling, it's no problem. There's a new law that until you have a tooth you don't need a passport."

"Seriously, Tracey's too young to travel all the way over there and to live in a hotel."

"Then we can leave her home. We'll get a great nurse. Mama will be here, and my dad can look in every day."

"No. I want her to know the walls of her nursery and to hear my voice and your voice, to never have a moment when suddenly there's a nurse she doesn't recognize. If we give her that kind of security at the beginning, then if she has some rough times later, hopefully she'll have all the feelings of self to help her over them. And it's not just racial. We talked about this before we got married: I want to raise my own child. I'm not going to be one of those Hollywood mothers who stop by the nursery for ten minutes a day. I want our daughter to know us."

"Darling, I agree, but can't Tracey start getting to know us when we come back from London? My life, which I can't change, is traveling. When are we going to see each other?"

"Whenever we can during these early years. Sammy, it's not how I'd choose to be married, but we made a commitment to an unborn child—to give her whatever she needs—so if anyone's got to bend it has to be us." She sat down beside me on the couch in our living room. "Are you angry?"

"Of course not." I took her hand, recognizing that I was just spoiled, always trying to have everything both ways. I'd been looking forward to the trip as a kind of vacation, to have the freedom of being in England with May, to be out of the pressure cooker, and, frankly, to have my wife see me in a more glamorous situation than it had been over here.

May did one of those faces like a light bulb. "Sharley Brown! You'll be gone for Tracey's birthday. She's having a party and a cake. Can you switch your dates around?"

I stood up. "Darling. The one-man show at the Prince of Wales is very important, plus it's worth a lot of money, which we can certainly use, plus the reason why 'the show must go on' is otherwise they'll sue me. And secondly, I cannot dump the Queen of England with 'Sorry, Your Majesty, but my daughter's having a birthday party.' "

"Tracey will be sad that her father isn't with her."

"Darling . . . she's just turning *one*. Lie to her. Tell her I'm there. Tell her I'm hiding, playing spooky games with her."

I STEPPED off the plane and onto the front pages of four London newspapers. Not a little box saying "Sammy Davis is back again," which would have been plenty considering I hadn't done anything yet, but front-page photos with "S.D. Jnr. Is Back," "The Prince of Wails," "Mr. Wonderful," that kind of thing. Of course, I didn't exactly hurt my case by stepping off the plane in a British-cut double-breasted suit, wearing a bowler, and carrying a tightly wrapped umbrella. It was all the sadder that May wasn't with me. After all the downers we'd been through, I wished she could have seen her husband flying.

I called her at twelve every night after the show, catching her at four in the afternoon Los Angeles time. On closing night she said, "Tracey and I have been sitting here eating birthday cake and waiting for you to call. I'll put her on."

"No. Stop! Look, I love our daughter but I am not having a phone conversation with her for at least twelve more years."

"Well, then will you sing 'Happy Birthday' to her?"

"I'm not singing 'Happy Birthday' to a one-year-old. Just tell her Dad says, 'Have a Fabulous First.' Or tell her I'm sending a birthday card."

"Sammy . . . don't you know the words?"

I tried to whisper. "May, listen, I'm calling you from my dressing room. I'm in the back room. Out in the living room is Noël Coward, who's giving a party for me tonight in his town house. And all the muckety-mucks are here with him. Sir Laurence Olivier, Albert Finney, Peter O'Toole, Michael Caine, Stanley Baker, and the cream of the British theater, plus the Duke and Duchess of Kent or York—I can't remember. I've just received a standing ovation with oak-leaf clusters, with the audience singing 'Auld Lang Syne' to *me*. Fifteen hundred people. Now, are you going to make me have them hear me singing into a telephone like a Western Union man?"

"I think it would be sharming. 'The great star is just a loving father at heart.' "

"May, please . . ."

"Tracey and I both have our ears to the phone."

I sang "Happy Birthday" to a one-year-old and her slightly, only slightly, more mature mother.

RUDY DUFF was grilling steaks at the barbecue, Murphy was handling the bar, the sound system was working beautifully, it was a warm night, and six or seven people were in the pool, young actors I admired, Steve McQueen, the Culps, Peter Brown. Clint Eastwood was sitting to the side, looking into the water. I sat down next to him. I knew that *Rawhide* had just been canceled and he was out of work. "Nobody here wants me, Sam. The Westerns are going out. I'm going over to Europe." I tried to comfort him, encourage him. Then I got up and mixed with the others. I saw May sitting by herself away from the crowd and I joined her.

"Sammy, are there always going to be people around?"

"Look, I'm sorry. I made a mistake. Having the buddies around is a lifetime habit. When we were in vaudeville we always hung out with the other acts on the bill. Later, when we were headlining Las Vegas, I enjoyed those parties I gave and the movies I ran every night. The same when I was doing *Mr. Wonderful.* It was always more comfortable to be at home with the buddies and it's become a habit. But, darling, I really want a married life and I'm going to change it. But some of these are real friends. We can't take a broadsword and clean heads, it has to be a gradual process."

"Well, I can wait as long as necessary. I just don't want to feel that whenever we *can* be together I'll be sharing my husband with a pack of people who knew him before I did."

MURPHY KNEW what I'd be taking on the road but I added a few new sweaters and chose the records and the cameras I wanted. Then while he did the packing I made a drink and sat with May. "I've been thinking about our conversation and I'm going to be a better husband. It's only that I don't know how *much* I dare change. If you asked me, 'How do you be a Sammy Davis, Jr.?' I'd have trouble answering. Obviously it starts with being given talent. But there are dozens of better dancers than I am and dozens of better singers—who remain unknown while I've become a star. There are better impressionists than me and I guarantee you that Buddy Rich plays better drums than I do. A painter can mix four colors together and come up with a great blue, that's an exact science. Mine is not. When I walk out onto a stage and say, 'Good evening, ladies and gentlemen,' I know that part of what the people see is the figure of perpetual motion, the little guy with the dazzling energy. They love to say, 'Nobody works as hard as Sammy Davis!' They also see 'the swinger,' 'Sinatra's friend,' 'the colored cat who turned Jewish,' who lost an eye; they see my clothes, they know I spend too much money, I'm always in trouble but somehow I luck out. Yet I wouldn't know how to evaluate each of those elements. If I threw away all my clothes and wore nothing but blue jeans, they wouldn't recognize me. If there was an announcement, 'Hey, he's not a swinger, he's a virgin,' I don't know if they'd believe it or not, or if they'd even care.

"What I do know is that I don't dare lose a single facet of whatever it is that creates 'Sammy Davis, Jr.,' because for me to be 'Sammy Davis, Jr.,' is much more important than it was to you to be 'May Britt' or for Frank to be 'Frank Sinatra.' The color of my skin makes the difference. I couldn't own this house in the Hollywood Hills if I weren't 'Sammy.' Nor do I believe that May Britt would have fallen in love with the Sammy Davis who had to live in Harlem. The only way I can survive in this world is to be 'Sammy Davis, Jr.' I don't say that's right, or wrong, but it's a fact that I live with."

"I sure don't want to change you. I'd just like to see more of you. Especially as Tracey grows up and we have more children, I'd like us to create the atmosphere of a real home. I understand you've got a lot of business guys and friends to see, but in the middle of it all I'd like to sit at a table with just my husband and have dinner with him."

OUR CONVERSATIONS had surprised me. Yet they shouldn't have, because from the beginning she'd been something of a loner. When I'd first seen her in the commissary she'd been sitting by herself, and no one who looks like that had lunch alone except by choice. I liked having the buddies around but I remembered the wistfulness in her voice: "I'd like to sit at a table with just my husband and have dinner with him." I was playing San Francisco and she'd stayed at home with Tracey. I made some arrangements and then called her. "Darling, on Wednesday will you get dressed in something elegant for dinner, something a bit soigné, and be ready at eight sharp?"

"But, Sharley Brown, you have to be in Vegas then."

"You said you'd enjoy a quiet dinner with your husband . . ."

I'd hired a party cook and a waiter, and I'd chartered a plane that would make it possible for me to stop off at home, have dinner, and still get to Vegas when I had to be there.

At eight o'clock, dressed in black tie, I rang the doorbell of my house. May was wearing a powder-blue satin gown, her face radiant, glowing with the happiness I had hoped to create.

Tracey was sleeping. I picked her up, hardly waking her, hugging

139

her gingerly. *Hello, miracle.* I kissed her head and put her back into the crib. "Great kid. No crying, just 'Hi, Dad, how's the show?' and back to sleep."

We sat on a couch while the waiter poured champagne, and we put a nice dent in a tin of fresh beluga caviar.

Candles were burning on the dining table, which was set for just us. "I've been thinking that if God allows us to have more children, that's wonderful, but I'd like to adopt some Negro children too. There are too many colored kids that are orphans, they have nobody that wants them, nobody comes to get them . . ."

"Ohhh, Sharley Brown, I agree with you so much! Maybe we can start with a big brother for Tracey."

I was relieved that she was enthusiastic about adopting Negro children, that some of the wars we had been through had not weakened her, made her lean toward an easier road.

"We'll need more space," I said. "Sy told me that David Selznick's house in Beverly Hills is up for sale. It's got a four-car garage, the bedroom windows work on push buttons, and it's got a projection room with a 35mm setup which I'm dying to have. I hate the rinky-dink thing we've got down in the Playhouse."

"It sounds expensive."

"It *is*, but hey, I make a couple of million dollars a year."

"I know, but hey, we're in debt."

The waiter served the main course. May waited till he was out of the room. "When I asked for a dinner alone with my husband I didn't mean to hire a chef with a waiter, champagne, caviar, and a private airplane."

"Darling, it's just a little parsley, some tissue paper. In a world of meat and potatoes you're allowed to have a little parsley. You don't have to eat it. But it makes life pretty."

"Well, I appreciate what you did this evening, but I've sold stockings and washed dishes. I like luxuries but I can take them or leave them."

" 'Not I,' said the little brown bear. I wanta *take* 'em. All I can get."

She put her hand on mine. "I'm sorry, I didn't mean to hurt your surprise."

Again I was aware of the difference between us. I'd seen her as Mary Movie Star and had assumed that the love for the theatrical, the appreciation for the grand gesture went with it. I was becoming aware that we had different ideas of what a package of happiness looks like. On the way to the airport and on the plane I reflected on how little time we'd spent getting to know each other, never sharing the common everyday things, undoubtedly because we'd never experienced a common everyday life. Our life together had been masked by drama and fear: her courage, guts, love; my protectiveness. Bodyguards, screening the hate mail, hiding, creating fictional worlds to block out the harshness and the embarrassments of the real one.

I was doing turn-away business at the Sands. I did the impression of Louis Armstrong with the trumpet in one hand and the big handkerchief mopping his face in the other. When I was finished and they were applauding, I dropped the handkerchief over my head like a hood. "And there'll be another meetin' tomorrow night."

I could hardly believe the screams of laughter over racial humor from a black man in Vegas in the mid-sixties. Civil rights was moving slowly, we all thought, but I could look back to only 1950 when we'd had to live over in Mrs. Cartwright's house.

Turning to my pianist, George Rhodes, who'd been on the road with me since *Mr. Wonderful*, I said, "George, I know how sensitive you are, but would you mind playing on the *white* keys?"

A redneck stood up and muttered loudly, "I don't have to listen to this shit." I ad-libbed, "Hey, man, th' brothers gonna git you f'that," and he sat down. I was so surprised that I raised a fist and shrugged. "Guess that's what they mean by Black Power." He slunk into his seat. I hadn't intended that, I wasn't up there to scare away my audience, or the high rollers. It had been just a joke line that got away from me, but I couldn't help enjoying the feeling of potency.

It was a strange time, the sixties, a strange feeling suddenly being "black." Yet overnight thirty million "colored people" and "Negroes" had become "blacks." It was difficult to think of myself as a "black" after all the years of hating "black bastard," "black motherfucker." Nobody ever got called "Negro bastard" or "colored motherfucker." It was always "black" and the word was nasty and hard. Only a few months earlier I'd heard someone say, "This black guy . . ." and was offended by it. I berated him: "I've never *seen* a person with black skin. I've seen people with brown skin, tan skin, but never black."

But riding on the mood of social change, James Brown recorded

"Black Is Beautiful," in which the lyrics urged, ". . . say it loud, I'm black and I'm proud . . ." and suddenly we weren't afraid of the word "black" anymore. It was no longer a sneer, but an anthem. ". . . say it loud, I'm black and I'm proud . . ." One song found the pride of a scattered people, one song straightened our backs and raised our heads and drew us together more than we had ever been, uniting us all into blacks.

In the dressing room, Murphy handed me the telephone. "It's Finis. He's in town." Finis Henderson was a Chicago friend from the old days. I said, "Come on over, babe."

"I'm with some of the brothers, over in Westside."

"Bring 'em along. Use my table for the second show."

"I'd love to see your show, ol' buddy . . ." He was backing away from it.

"Hey, don't worry. I'll leave your name and there'll be no problem."

"I know that, Sam, and I appreciate it, but, frankly, it's heavy. Y'know what I mean? I just wanted to say hello, hear your voice. I'll catch you in Chicago or someplace . . ."

I sat behind the bar and made myself a drink. I understood exactly how he felt. Black Power! What a joke! We were still impotent. In my mind's eye I saw my dinner-show audience: there had been no black faces out there. Black people did not come to see me in Las Vegas because if black people didn't arrive at the hotel with the special safe-conduct of "Sammy's guest," they didn't get in. And who wanted *that?* Who wanted to be "allowed in" and then sit there at my ringside table, the only black people in the room, trying to enjoy the show, feeling the stares against the back of your neck? That was fun?

I left the dressing room and walked through the casino. All of the dealers had white hands. I saw cocktail waitresses, change makers, maintenance people. All white. At the front desk of the hotel, nobody, nobody was black.

May was watching television in our suite. A room service table with places for May and Tracey and our new son, Mark, had been pushed near the door. She said, "The children wanted to stay up to kiss you good night but their little eyes were closing, so I put them to bed."

Our suite had three bedrooms, a sauna, a kitchen, and a dining room. The opulence came at me as through a zoom lens. Since 1954 we'd been getting the best suites in the hotels we'd played in Vegas, free, plus all the vig: food, booze, guests; pick up the phone, "Hello, this is Sammy, would you please send up New Jersey?" "On the way, Sam."

I called Jack Entratter and he asked me to come to his apartment. We sat down on a couch. "Jack, I've got to see some of my people sitting out there."

"Sam, you know you can bring anyone you like. Your family is always welcome, your friends . . ."

"I know and I appreciate it but that's not enough. The doors have to open to *everybody*."

He sighed, like Oops! "Sam, we still have the boys from Kansas City; why do we call the line the 'Texas Copa Girls'? Because we get a lot of high rollers from there."

I understood but could not accept the magic wand that okayed anything because "It's business." It wasn't the Texans alone, or the boys from Kansas City. Las Vegas was an inveterate prejudiced city, built by Southerners and Northerners *from* prejudiced cities: Detroit's Purple Gang, the guys from Chicago, Kansas City. But that was a lot of sit-ins and pray-ins ago.

"Jack, keeping black people out is now illegal and it's morally wrong. Plus, it's unkind." He nodded. "Then you'll agree that it has to stop. And we should be the ones to do it. We're the starters, the doers and movers . . . we've got to let black people come see the shows and make them comfortable doing it. And we've got to put black people to work in this town, and where they will be visible. Things are changing, Jack. Even Mississippi is getting ready to change . . ."

"Sammy, antagonizing our high-rolling Southern clientele is not smart business. But lemme talk to the board. I'll try to come up with something to at least get us started."

ETHEL KENNEDY invited me to lunch at Hickory Hill, their home in Virginia. I was performing at the Shoreham Hotel in Washington. It was a small gathering that included Peter and Pat, Pierre Salinger, General Maxwell Taylor, and Art Buchwald. A tray of Bloody Marys in large, stemmed Steuben glasses was passed around as guests arrived.

I was grateful to Bobby for reaching out to me, for as much as saying, "You're welcome in *my* house."

After lunch while Ethel and I watched Bobby and Max Taylor and two others playing tennis, she said, "Sammy, that business about Jack's inauguration, I hope you know we had nothing to do with it. Bobby was outraged by what they did."

"I knew that then. Peter told me. You didn't even have to mention it, but thank you."

Before it was time to leave, Bobby walked me around the house for privacy. "You're not popular with the Klan," he said, "or the White Citizens Council. You're on all of their lists. Whenever you plan to appear in public at anything controversial, anything to do with civil rights, be sure to call me a day or two in advance and at least I can have a couple of men there looking out for you."

SY MARSH called me from California while I was in New York playing the Copa. Ever since *GE Theater* I'd let it be known that I would deal only with Sy. He asked, "Sweetheart, do you remember Clifford Odets's picture *Golden Boy?* A producer named Hillard Elkins wants to make it into a Broadway musical starring you as the fighter. He's got the rights and he's got Odets himself to adapt it for the stage."

In my dressing room Odets said, "I'll write it out of your mouth . . ."

Hilly Elkins was a few years younger than me, he had big, wide-open eyes, and he was all enthusiasm. "One of the major conflicts should be that you're in love with a white girl. I think we can do something important, racially."

For a white man to think that way was remarkable. I had to like him immediately. "And, Hilly, what about a really integrated cast, not just a couple of token black kids in the chorus?"

"Absolutely. Fifty-fifty. Which, by the way, is more than equal. But it's time for the pendulum to swing a little too far the other way."

"And why not a black musical conductor, for the first time? George Rhodes, my pianist, has been conducting for me and writing arrangements. He's a talented, experienced man. He could handle it beautifully."

Hilly agreed with everything. We sat up until dawn talking about

144

it. He said, "I saw you in London about two years ago and I thought of *Golden Boy* and you, and I haven't thought of anything else since. I got Clifford, I've got financing . . ."

"And you've got me."

"NEW YORK?" May was less than receptive to the idea. "But we've just barely moved into this house. I don't know about the schools for Mark in New York . . ."

I'd been premature telling it to her on the telephone. I should have waited until I was home but I'd wanted to share it with her.

"How long do you think we'll have to stay there?"

"Hilly's asking me to commit to three years."

By the time I got out to the Coast, May had sold herself on it. "Boy, Sharley Brown, three years together. I must have been crazy not to see that right away. We're finally going to have a real family life."

While May gave the children dinner in the breakfast nook I shot pictures of them. Tracey was three and Mark was almost six. Then Rudy made some chops for us. I had a week off and didn't have to get into my pants the next night, so I sent down the hill to Will Wright's and we sat on the floor eating ice cream, seeing but not watching television. I could talk about nothing but *Golden Boy*. I said, "And I won't mind the chance to make up for *Mr. Wonderful*, artistically *and* racially."

"Artistically? But I thought it was a big hit. It ran a year."

"On my drawing power as a *nightclub* entertainer, not as a play. Almost the entire second act was my nightclub act. And racially— nothing! But now with *Golden Boy* we have a chance to say something. I think that's important. If I just take the money from clubs and run, if I don't stop and say, 'Hey, I've got an audience that likes me, I've got their attention and I should utilize it,' then I'm a parasite."

HARRY BELAFONTE called me. "Sam, we're planning on you in Washington."

"Of course I'm going to be there. How many people are you expecting to march?"

"If ten thousand show up it will be a success. Twenty thousand would be unbelievable."

Two days before the March on Washington, Bobby Kennedy called me. "Sam, you've been moving up on the White Citizens Council's 'Ten Most Wanted' list. If you're coming to Washington, stay in the mainstream, and when it's over, don't hang around. I'll have some agents identify themselves to you and take you out to the airport and stay with you till your flight . . ."

If Bobby Kennedy ever told you, "Don't worry about your back, I've got it covered," you could walk easy and never worry about anything.

I was playing the Elmwood Casino in Windsor, Ontario. Murphy and I left Windsor at five in the morning and flew out of Detroit to get to Washington by ten in the morning. Already thousands had arrived before us. They were walking toward the Washington Monument and the Lincoln Memorial, clustered in bunches of whites and blacks. Everyone looked tense, apprehensive. Policemen were stationed on street corners, looking hard-nosed and nervous. There had been many threats to disrupt the march. There were no thoughts of assassination yet. But the threats of violence were there. Despite Bobby's help I was frightened. What if it erupts into a riot? In our nation's capital? Yes, it could happen. It was only a few years since I'd been picketed there.

I stood on the steps of the Lincoln Memorial looking toward the Washington Monument, looking over all the heads, into the faces, and then, as if abruptly, the sun burst through the clouds, for no apparent reason, yet all at once people were *smiling* and it was "Hey, man . . ." and you knew there wasn't going to be any trouble, as if a happiness virus had spread among all those men and women. I watched little vignettes of people touching, holding hands; black people who had never touched white people before; a black woman handing a handkerchief to a white boy who was crying from emotion. There were blacks and whites who had never hugged or had a physical line of communication before; white people who had never been next to a poor, humble black woman holding her child. Everybody had love in their hearts and on their faces and it was wonderful, happy-making. The police were relaxed and cordial.

Ten thousand? Twenty thousand? There were three hundred thousand people there and everybody felt the same way. Twenty-four hours before and maybe even twenty-four hours later they might have killed each other, but for that suspended, isolated few hours in time there was more love in that mall than the world has ever known.

The galvanizing of what the civil rights movement was about occurred on that day. It showed that people could live together, black, white, Hispanic, that we could pull together. That massive turnout revealed that the whole country was behind it, not just a hundred thousand blacks and a handful of influential liberals. For me it was the most American day in the history of our country save for perhaps the Battle of Bunker Hill or the signing of the Declaration of Independence. It was on that level.

Civil rights leader A. Philip Randolph introduced Martin Luther King as "the moral leader of our country." And from the Lincoln Memorial, looking out at three hundred thousand Americans, Dr. King began: "I have a dream . . ."

After the march the entertainers met in Harry Belafonte's hotel suite. Harry said, "Call Bobby Kennedy and tell him the artists would like to have a meeting at the White House."

Bobby took my call but he was adamant. "No. The performers can't come up here. Nobody can come up except the civil rights leaders. I'm fighting for my life, Sam, just to get the civil rights leaders in. The President's got a lot of advisers telling him he shouldn't meet with *anybody*, not Dr. King, *nobody*. If the performers come up, then it becomes a spectacle. The press would make it a farce. We don't want any more cartoons."

He was right, of course. We'd served our purpose by getting our pictures in the papers. Now it was up to the legislators and the civil rights leaders.

IN NOVEMBER 1963 we started making *Robin and the Seven Hoods*. Bing Crosby was guest-starring and the studio had said, "Bing will get third billing." Frank said, "No, he won't. Sammy is over the title with us. The billing is: Frank Sinatra, Dean Martin, Sammy Davis, Jr."

"But, Frank . . ."

"That's *it!* Give Bing a separate box."

I was playing the Sands, so I was going to be commuting to L.A. to shoot scenes. I told May, "Come out to the set. Hang out with the guys."

"I'd really rather not."

Something was wrong. "I don't dig."

"Frankly, I can't stand your relationship with Frank, the way he treats you, the jokes, the way you kowtow to him . . ."

"Darling, Frank and I go way back, to when he was 'Sinatra' and I was 'the kid.' Even though we've become best friends, and I'm a star, too, that relationship will never change. Like with Abe Lastfogel. He's my agent, I pay him a fortune in commissions, I could call him 'Abe,' but I don't. He'll always be 'Mr. Lastfogel' to me. And I'll always be 'the kid' to Frank and he'll always be 'Sinatra' to me."

"I don't mind him being 'Sinatra.' But I can't take it when he treats you like 'the kid.' You're a grown man, you're an important star . . ."

I knew that by "kid" she really meant "lackey." And I knew too that I sometimes gave that impression when I was with him. But that was my doing, not his.

My morning plane from Las Vegas was delayed and as I arrived on the set Frank greeted me: "You're fuckin' late. We had to shoot the first scene without you."

"Francis, come on . . . you know I'm workin' your joint."

He grinned. "I told you not to play the fuckin' place. We did the opening scene without you . . . Who needs ya, Smokey?"

I really didn't mind the jokes. But I was just as glad my wife wasn't there.

The shooting continued, a graveyard scene in which the gangsters are burying Edward G. Robinson, and there's a black funeral going on nearby. It was a beautiful, sunshiny day, and a cheerful one despite the fact that we were shooting in a cemetery.

After lunch we had a drink in Frank's trailer, Dean, Frank, Bing Crosby, Joey Bishop. Then I went back to my own trailer to prepare for the next scene. As I walked in Murphy said, "Hey, there's something on the radio about the President . . ." He turned it up louder and we heard "Yes, it is true, the President was shot . . . We don't know if it was a fatal wound. He's been rushed to Park Cities Hospital . . ."

As I went over to see Frank he was stepping out of his trailer and onto the set and I stared after the figure of a man walking in a cemetery. I stood in the doorway watching him grieve for the man who broke his heart when he'd publicly refused to stay in the

148

"Palm Springs White House," a four-bedroom, self-contained home which Frank had built for the Kennedys. I'd seen a sign on the door, "Palm Springs White House," he was that sure that JFK was coming. But Bobby fought John's going there because of Frank's alleged connections in the underworld, and because Sam Giancana had slept in his house. Presidents have a lot of license. The attitude was: "Tell Frank I can't stay there. That's out." And he went up the hill and stayed at Bing Crosby's house. It broke Frank's heart. It became public knowledge. In all the gossip columns.

I have never heard Frank say a bad word about John Kennedy. I've heard "I don't want to discuss that," but I've never heard him do one minute of ". . . that so-and-so . . . I did this . . . and he did that . . ." Two images I remember of Frank, like old photos you carry in a wallet. Frank walking down Broadway in the fifties when nobody recognized him, when he was alone, no hat on, topcoat collar up. And the image of him walking—on that beautiful, sunlit day—in a graveyard.

The following morning a messenger delivered an envelope addressed to "Mr. and Mrs. Sammy Davis, Jr., an invitation to the funeral services for John F. Kennedy, at noon on November 25, 1963." We couldn't go to Washington but we attended a memorial service held in Los Angeles. And I resolved that whenever I had the occasion to be in Washington, I would take flowers to John Kennedy's graveside and pay my respects. He had not been a friend of mine but he had been the President I and my people needed.

14

When Robert Kennedy campaigned for the office of United States senator from New York, happily I was in New York City rehearsing *Golden Boy*. Sarge Shriver got in touch with me. "Bobby says you might be willing to help."

There was no mystery about Bobby. You knew exactly where he stood. He'd shown it as Attorney General when he'd used his power to allow the marches to happen and to protect the demonstrators when he could. It would have been a different civil rights movement without Bobby Kennedy. The voter registration, the lunch-counter sit-ins, the pray-ins were often violent, but he kept it from being the bloodbath it could have been. There is no counting the lives he saved, the bloodshed he avoided.

Bobby was a humanist. He was not a do-gooder, but a good-doer, a knight of old in a button-down-collar shirt, a man who wanted to right wrong. There was no doubt in my mind that I wanted Robert Kennedy as a senator making my country's laws, and then to run for President. Bobby had been the strength in the Kennedy family. John was always "raised eyebrows," thinking about the next advantageous move; the "piano player" who sat out front with the spotlight on him. The other cat who kept time was the drummer, who never got the spotlight, he never took the solos, but he kept time, he kept the beat going. Bobby was the drummer.

Again, I worked the ethnic dates. Sarge called. "Can you get some time off next week, Sam? We're going to the garment district."

We did it a number of times, usually during lunch hour so as not to take people away from work. For an hour or so the police blocked off Seventh Avenue between Thirty-sixth and Thirty-seventh streets, thousands of people came out of the buildings to see Robert Kennedy, and I'd introduce him to "my people." We went to Harlem the same way: 125th Street at the corner of the Teresa Hotel. "I'm here pullin' on your coats to introduce a man who there ain't no questions about, we *know* what he stands for . . ." Harlem loved Bobby. They knew that Bobby Kennedy was special for them.

WE WERE on the road with *Golden Boy* for twenty-two weeks, longer than most plays run on Broadway, because we were afraid to come in. We opened in Philadelphia and got rapped badly. We had four weeks there to fix the show before our next out-of-town tryout in Boston.

Clifford Odets had died before he'd finished modernizing all of *Golden Boy*. Most of it was still yesteryear, so it was pandemonium, with everybody, myself included, writing scenes and dialogue.

May and Tracey and Mark were with me but I could never see them. *Golden Boy* occupied twenty-four hours of every day. We'd do a show at night and the next day we'd be rehearsing new lines right up until curtain time.

May was waiting in the suite when I came in at four in the morning, an ashtray full of cigarette butts and two empty coffeepots on the night table. "I'm sorry," she said. "I hate to complain, but we've been here for three weeks and the children and I haven't had a meal with you. I never see you."

I collapsed onto a chair across from her. "Darling, it's going to get better, as soon as we settle in New York. These are the rough days."

It was a Friday. I got excused from Sunday rehearsal, then I asked May, "What would you say to a family lunch, just the four of us, at Bookbinder's, on Sunday afternoon?"

She had the children dressed and ready before I woke up. I was excited by it myself; a break from the show, from trying to remember new lines, new concepts. I hadn't realized how much I'd needed a few hours with my family.

I sat next to May in the back seat of the limo and the children sat on the jump seats. Tracey was four and Mark was seven. They were adorable and beautifully dressed and they weren't loud or the take-over kind of kids. May hadn't stopped smiling since Friday. She was radiant and I looked from her to the children, and I took May's hand in mine and squeezed it, trying to project: "Thank you for being so patient and so beautiful and so loving, and for bringing up the children so wonderfully, for giving me this miracle . . ."

When we entered the restaurant people smiled and waved, the maître d' led us to the perfect table, and I had the feeling that except for the catastrophic problems with *Golden Boy* life couldn't be more perfect or pleasant.

And then it happened. A voice from a woman at the next table: "Are their kids very dark like him?" She had her back to us, and she must have been hard of hearing, because she thought she was whispering. "I *can't* turn around and look, stupid. Just tell me, are they light or dark?"

I'd really thought people would see us as I did: a wholesome family with two beautiful, well-behaved children having a happy Sunday together.

Tracey and Mark were busy making a log cabin out of breadsticks. May and I looked away from each other, as if by not acknowledging it, it hadn't happened, or it would stop.

"Their hair? Is it straight, like hers, or kinky?"

I didn't eat my lunch because I knew it would get me sick. The children gobbled up lamb chops, potatoes, and string beans while we waited, May helping Tracey cut her meat, and I realized that even though children "gobble up" their food it takes them a long time.

When they were nearly finished I sighed elaborately. "Wow, I can't eat another bite." Quickly May said, "Me either." I said, "I'll ask for the check."

Tracey looked stricken. "Dad, haven't you seen the pie a la mode?" I'd seen waiters go by with it several times. Earlier, I'd planned to have one.

When finally I could ask for the check the owner of the restaurant came by. "You're our guests and we're delighted you came in. Please come back."

My son looked at me with awe. "You don't have to pay, Dad? Wow!" The expression on his face helped, some.

But in the theater that evening, instead of concentrating on my new lines I could still hear that woman's voice, I could hear the jokes people told about us: "What's black and comes in a white box? Sammy Davis, Jr.," and I could only wonder: Is this forever? No matter what I do, will we always be a sideshow event?

IN BOSTON, Elliot Norton, their most astute critic, cut us to shreds. Hilly invited Norton to lunch and picked his brains. He subsequently got William Gibson to rewrite the show, and he replaced our director with Arthur Penn.

Arthur tried to approach me as an actor who had studied acting for twenty years. He'd say, "Prepare."

"Prepare? For what?" I'd put my makeup on and "Let's go. Ready!"

"Okay. As you cannot prepare, then bring to the stage whatever you experienced that day, bring that emotion; up, down, whatever it was. Don't try to act. If you're angry at something and you play angry it will be honest and the audience will see sincerity."

As we ended the first week in New Haven, Hilly said, "We're not ready to go into New York from here. We need more work. I'm booking us into Detroit."

Detroit was in the middle of race riots. There was no way I could bring May and the children there and hope to keep my mind on my work. I told her, "Darling, I've got an idea. Why don't you guys go on into New York a few weeks ahead of me and find an apartment for us?" And she didn't object.

On the first day of rehearsal in Detroit, Arthur Penn watched the second act scene in which Paula Wayne and I discover we're in love and we're supposed to kiss. A white woman and a black man. But with race riots going on all over the city we were afraid to. He said, "I've never seen a love scene in my life in which people don't kiss. Hold hands. Something. There's no declaration of love . . ." He was completely right, of course. If we were a play with a message we'd better deliver it. That evening Paula and I grabbed each other and kissed. Full on the mouth. Embrace. Kiss. In Detroit, Michigan. All of us scared shit.

May called me from New York. "I'm worried about the pollution here. It's terrible for the children's little lungs."

The onstage kiss outraged some people and Hilly got threats.

"We're gonna cut off that whore's tits. And the nigger's balls." Paula had to be given a bodyguard. I already had one.

When I spoke to May she told me, "I've hired a wonderful woman to help me with the children and the apartment. Her name is Lessie Lee Jackson, she has a nursing background, and she can cook great soul food." At almost any other moment in my life that would have tickled me but I couldn't concentrate on it.

We were changing dialogue, putting in hunks at such speed that one night I didn't remember if I was playing a violinist or a piano player. I worked so hard that I had no voice and had to whisper my songs.

Hilly brought in a throat specialist. "You have polyps on your vocal cords. Stop smoking, stop drinking, and above all stop using your voice. Close this show for a month or two and rest, or you may never sing again."

There was no way to close down, not even for three days.

May called daily, wanting to include me as "father" and "husband," to consult, to share the decisions. "I've been looking into schools for Mark and I'm leaning strongly toward Ethical Culture and Dalton. There are others where he might get better athletic programs because they're not in the center of New York; on the other hand . . ." I could not focus on anything except the show and survival.

By the time our scenery arrived at the Majestic Theater in New York, we had a whole new and polished show. On the day of our opening my voice was in shreds. Another throat specialist examined me backstage and it was word for word what we'd already been told. That evening, a little before "half hour," I called a meeting of the cast onstage. "You've all heard what I sound like. They're not going to say they saw 'the colored Caruso' tonight. I've never in my life asked anyone for help on a stage . . . but for this one performance . . . any support you can give me—every song you sing, every dance you do, if you'll just kick it a little harder, sing it a little cleaner—you'll be carrying me and I'll be grateful."

Our opening number exploded on Broadway, stunning the audience so they felt they were in—not just watching—a boxers' gym: fighters working the bags, skipping ropes, sparring, feinting, jabbing to the music; slowly at first, then faster, savagely, a boxers' ballet: jab, feint, cross; jab, feint, cross; every sound, every move sliding click, click, bam, bam; precision, style, pace, all riding on that extra inner strength that starts in the gut and comes through the heart and turns craftsmanship around the corner into art.

The morning papers came in at midnight. ". . . a knockout." ". . . this year's heavyweight champ." "They've broken new ground on Broadway." "Something daring and important is happening at the Majestic . . ." We were a solid hit.

THE APARTMENT May had rented for us was new and large enough, over on Second Avenue in the Eighties. It had a cozy breakfast room and a game room for the children, but now that I had the mentality to see it I did not feel like it belonged to a star. I felt like I was glittering and I wanted the right setting. I told May, "I'm going to find us something that's got a little 'Hey, wow, it's Sammy's place.' " She looked a bit deflated. I asked, "You don't mind, do you, darling? I mean, if we get something better for entertaining?"

She shook her head. "That's fine."

"Something's wrong."

"No. I'm sorry. I hadn't thought about entertaining. What I looked for was a family kind of an apartment."

I rented Serge Rubinstein's town house at 3½ East Ninetieth Street. It had a living room that was made for entertaining and a backyard which would be great for the kids to play in. I bought a navy-blue Cadillac limousine with a bar and a telephone, I got a license plate: SAMMY.

MAY HAD the children in bed around nine and was in my dressing room—blue jeans style—with books and magazines, waiting for me when I came off after the first act. I could only say hello, I had to keep myself in the show, but I loved having her there, sitting around with Murphy and with Shirley Rhodes, George's wife.

After the performance people started coming in, people who'd been out front seeing the show, social and business acquaintances. "Sammy, you were great. Brilliant. Fantastic." I introduced them to May and to Shirley. Others arrived. "Sammy baby, great. Brilliant. Fantastic." May sat through the repetitive chitchat. Shirley slipped out. The chorus kids came by to say good night, gazing at May like fans, doing jokes with me, which I encouraged, for unity.

Then I chased them out. "Okay, kids, go do your hangin' out but get some sleep and go to class tomorrow or you ain't gettin' into gypsy heaven . . ."

Finally, after over an hour, all the visitors had gone. Shirley and George came in from his dressing room. George was not a big talker. "It played well," he said.

Shirley nodded. "It was great, Sammy."

"Oh, yes," May agreed, "brilliant, baby. Fantastic."

I caught them starting to break up and I saw a Wives' Mafia forming but I liked it.

I asked George and Shirley, "You guys feel like a little Sardi's or do y'wanta come home and have some sit-around there?"

George was shaking his head. "Gotta get up in the morning for school." He explained: "Being here in New York I figured I could go to Juilliard and study conducting and theory. Tomorrow's my first class. Nine a.m."

"You gonna study conducting? You already *got* the job!" But I was impressed by a man making top money, whose name was on all the nightclub marquees with me, making the effort to enroll at the Juilliard School of Music and drag himself out of bed to better educate himself. "Damn. Thought you knew 'nuff already! Seems to me the band always ends same time as I do."

He grinned. "Well, you right *there* . . . 'cept one day I'm gonna know how come it works out like that."

I asked Shirley. "What're you going to do while he's in school every day? Y'know, I need an office in New York."

Shirley found us a floor at 120 East Fifty-sixth Street and took over as my secretary and office manager.

LEAVING FOR the theater, I passed the dining room and saw Mark and Tracey seated at the table and May standing at the breakfront lighting a menorah and reciting the Friday evening prayer. Before we had married, she had converted to Judaism as a surprise for me and was conscientiously bringing the children up in our religion.

When she saw me looking into the room she smiled, glancing hopefully at the fourth chair at the head of the table that was set for me. I kissed the kids and left. My mind was on ten different things. I had an idea for the fight scene and I wanted to organize cast parties and competitions. These were good dancers and it was a drag for them to do the same show eight times a week, month after month. Hopefully, if I kept them united during their time off they'd develop an esprit and they wouldn't get bored and leave *Golden Boy* for another, newer musical, which was their habit and the reason they are called gypsies.

As I rode downtown with Joe Grant, the man I'd hired as chauffeur-bodyguard, I looked at my watch. Six-thirty. I had a seven-fifteen radio interview in the dressing room. I felt remiss. I could have sat down with Mark and Tracey and May. Their whole meal wouldn't last more than fifteen minutes. I phoned from the car. "Darling, how about dressing up and meeting me after the show for a little see-and-be-seen."

"Okay."

"Great. Joe'll be there at eleven."

There was a long line at the box office. I sat back in my limo, my thoughts caressing the customers. There are times it's hard to believe you're a hit on Broadway. I mean a no-kidding, real hit on Broadway! Where Jolson was a hit. Where Ziegfeld had those big shows. Get outta here! Maybe it was harder for me to grasp because it was so many millions of miles away from Negro vaudeville and the three-a-day. In those days when we played the "small time," and the Loew's and Keith circuits were the "big time," Broadway just wasn't even dreamed about. We had more hope of going to heaven than to Broadway.

At the theater I asked Hilly, "Do me a favor and make a reservation at '21' for after the show tonight. You and your lady and May and me. And in my name, baby."

As I got into the first scene of the show I knew I shouldn't have started the whole "21" anxiety. It punctured the vacuum I should have been in. I was a second behind the tempo and it took me ten minutes to catch up and get my mind on *Golden Boy* where it belonged.

While I was cleaning off my makeup Hilly came in with May. She looked beautiful in a black Chanel suit with a shocking-pink blouse I'd brought her from Paris. Hilly said, "I told them we'd be there around midnight."

Obviously "21" had accepted the reservation. That was better than I'd done in *Mr. Wonderful* with El Morocco. My thoughts flashed back to that night. Then unaccountably they flashed further back, to a child standing in the wings of a vaudeville theater. I was three or four years old, waiting to go on, and my father was telling me, "Don't put your hand up to your face," because I had blackface on, the burned cork with the big white minstrel lips. That was the modus operandi then, all the comedians had to black up. I had candy-striped overalls and a beige shirt, a little tam on my head, and white gloves and blackface, and my father told me, "Don't put the gloves up to your face, Poppa, 'cause the black'll come off . . ."

As we left the stage door I signed autographs and one of the fans asked, "May I have your autograph, Miss Britt?"

"Thank you, but I've retired. My husband is the star."

I whispered, "Swing with it. I dig the idea that you're an exciting personality, like 'Hey, there's May Britt.' "

Another fan asked her, but she insisted, "No, thank you very much, but my husband is the star in our family."

In the limo going east on Fifty-second Street I felt cold and clammy. Afraid of "21." Why would I believe that my success on Broadway would make any difference in how people felt racially? *Mr. Wonderful* hadn't. Why was I putting myself through this? I was tired of opening doors, weary of being scared. I was too well known, I didn't want to be embarrassed anymore. Yet . . . I wanted to know that I had the freedom of the city.

We were inching up to the entrance of "21." Then we were there. Someone opened our door. I motioned for Hilly to get out first. Ahead of him I could see a glass-covered iron gate, and a short, stocky, ominous-looking man standing behind it. But then I heard "Come in, please, Mr. Davis, Mrs. Davis."

A well-dressed man came over to us, his hand outstretched. "I'm Bob Kriendler. Welcome, Sammy, Mrs. Davis." He led us past a cigar counter and into the bar, then to a table at the left against the wall. I didn't know the room, so I had no way of knowing what it meant. Was it a welcome, or a smoothly handled rejection? A wrong-side-of-the-room?

I glanced around me at the woody, men's club atmosphere and I wondered: if someone really *in*, someone prestigious, a regular customer were to come here, where would they put him? Then I saw we were being seated next to John Lindsay, the mayor of New York. We did our hellos and the jokes, and then he turned back to his party and I sank into the banquette seat.

I ordered Dom Pérignon and a bottle of Napoleon brandy. I needed the jolt of the cognac to turn my stomach back into flesh and muscle from the cast iron it had become as if in defense against a shot to the gut, and to knead the muscles in my shoulders, which were higher than I normally carried them.

I studied the room. I was the only black man in sight. Racial prejudice had obviously not disappeared. But had *I* grown beyond the reach of it? And had I accomplished something beyond the superficiality of having a supper at "21"? Might I have made the color of a man's skin slightly less relevant? Would I come back here another time and find that I'd opened the door for someone else?

Preparing for sleep, I told May, "I'm sorry about dinner tonight. I should have been with you and the kids. I will be next Friday." I was overly rewarded by her pleasure. "And I want you to know that I appreciate that you've been bringing the kids up single-handedly. I'm sorry I'm not exactly an above-the-title father."

She began copping out for me. "It's difficult for you because your work keeps you away . . ."

"I was thinking tonight, when I looked at the table, aside from the fact that *I* should have been there with you, there should have been more kids, the ones we've talked about. Let's get the family going while we're still young. You can keep it swinging until I get done what I have to do and we'll settle into the life we want."

She sat down in the slipper chair across from our bed, and lit a Salem, using it as a prop. "I'll call the adoption agency. But, Sammy? When do you think that will be—settling into the life we want—finding a little time to be a father? You don't want to meet your children when they're all grown up."

"Hey, hold it, I don't deserve that. I'll find time. I'll *make* time. Soon."

"MY GOD, what do you have in here?" May grunted, struggling under the weight of a package about a cubic foot in size, half putting it down, half dropping it at my feet. "It's from Abercrombie and Fitch."

"That's my bowling ball." I lifted it out of the box in its black leather carry bag. "I'm taking the cast bowling tonight after the show. Against the other shows."

"I've never bowled, but I'll try it."

"Darling . . . it's a togetherness thing for the kids and if you're there I can't be all over the place making it into a party."

"Oh. Okay, fine."

"But come to the dressing room during the show, hang out, then take the car home and I'll be along in an hour or two."

"No, that's okay. I'll stay home."

"Don't be silly, come on down."

"Sammy, frankly I'd rather stay home. The dressing-room jazz isn't much fun. It's not like we're together or I get to spend any time with you. In fact, it's boring as hell."

"You're kidding."

"No. I can understand it's fun for you. People come back and tell you how great you were. That's your business. But waiting around all night . . . I'd prefer to wait for you here, or if we're going out meet you there after you've done what you have to do with visitors."

I was astonished. To me the dressing room was the hub, the fun place to be. But from her point of view I suppose it was like watching me onstage without the music or the sound, just seeing me moving around entertaining others.

On Friday as I passed the dining room Tracey climbed off her chair and pulled me by the hand. "Dad, you're having dinner with us tonight."

I stroked her silky hair. I knew I'd promised to take part in the Sabbath dinner. "I'm sorry, Princess of the World." I kissed her and Mark. "Daddy has work to do . . ." and I explained that I had a 6 p.m. photo session with *Life* onstage. "But I'll make it up to you."

May walked me to the door, burning. "You could have told me!"

I hadn't because I didn't want to disappoint her about dinner, and there was always a chance that the photo session would be changed. "Darling, also, they need to bring a photographer over here on Sunday for some family shots." As I said it I guessed maybe that was largely why I'd put off the conversation. I'd known May would hate the idea.

"But the article is about you and *Golden Boy*. The children and I have nothing to do with it. And I don't believe that kids should be brought up seeing their faces in magazines and getting the idea they're something that they're not. Can't *Life* magazine understand that people would like some privacy?"

"I'm thrilled that they can't. We have a good life because people are interested in me. I don't have the moral right to say, 'Sorry, fellas, this is my home, no press,' ignoring the fact that they have a job to do and that by doing their job through the years they've done me a lot of good."

THE *LIFE* piece did us a lot of good at the box office and the lines at *Golden Boy* kept growing. I was nominated for a Tony. This time it was "Welcome to Broadway. You belong." All doors opened to me and I coveted the acceptance, knowing that for me and my wife and my children it was our armor and chain mail.

The Actors' Fund chose *Golden Boy* for a Sunday night benefit. "Sunday?" May stared at the tickets I'd given her for her and Shirley. "This means you work every night this week."

PASSING Saks Fifth Avenue on my way to the matinee, I told my driver to stop. "Pick me up around the corner at the Forty-ninth Street entrance." I took a closer look at the ski outfit I'd seen in the window. What had attracted me was a bright red knitted cap, scarf, and mittens. I went inside and told the saleslady, "Send them to Miss Tracey Davis . . ." I gave her the address and I wrote a card: " 'Cause I love you. Daddy," and had them sent to the house by messenger.

When I got home after midnight May had some of Lessie Lee's soul food keeping warm. I went upstairs to see the kids. It was dark in Tracey's room and as I leaned over her bed to kiss her my hand touched something woolen on her head. She was wearing the cap I'd sent her, and the mittens.

CROSSING New York in my car, I watched Bull Connor and Jim Clark, the sheriff of Selma, Alabama, featured on another bloody news report of police brutality, beatings with rubber hose covered with barbed wire, and stymied voter registration for Selma's black citizens.

Hilly was waiting in my dressing room. "Belafonte called. There's going to be a protest march in Selma. They want all the celebrities possible, to focus the press attention on what's happening there."

"You shouldn't go." The color had drained from May's face.

Gently, I pinched her cheeks. "At this moment you're a little whiter than absolutely necessary."

"It's not funny. I've seen Bull Connor on television. And Jim Clark. They'll kill you if they can. Or hurt you. Sammy, haven't we done enough for integration? My God, even in a war they don't draft married men until it's desperate, and *never* with two children."

I couldn't possibly have expressed how strongly I didn't want to go, how scared I was. I believed she was right. From their point of view, it was bad enough that we were outsiders going into Selma, telling them how to live. But on top of that I was "the nigger who married the white woman."

"Haven't you done enough?"

I had done a lot. I'd been marching since I was seventeen. Long before there was a civil rights movement I was marching through the lobby of the Waldorf-Astoria, of the Sands, the Fontainebleau, to a table at the Copa. And I'd marched alone. Worse. Often to black derision. But had I done "enough"?

You always have choices: your commitment versus your fear. And as no two things are equal, one outweighs the other. My fear was there: "Why am I doing this, man? I'm scared." But the guy in your heart says, "You've got to do it because otherwise what is your life all about, and all the things you would like to stand for, plus what you already stand for? You've got your own children now . . ."

When I got back from the theater that night May said, "I spoke to Shirley and she says that George isn't going."

"Darling, in its simplest and *only* form, I have to go, I have to be there. A lot of black, and white, performers have said, 'I'm not going. I'll give you my money, you've got my heart, but I can't go down there. I can't deal with it.' Others, like Marlon and Shelley and Sidney and Harry and I, feel 'I have no choice. I have to go.' I don't blame George at all. There's nothing he could accomplish by going there. Just another body. But I don't have his anonymity."

We left New York for the airport early in the morning in my car—Hilly, his girl Sheila, Murphy, Joe Grant, Herb Seeger, who'd worked for me as a security man, and Billy Rowe, who had been Deputy Police Commissioner of New York. We were without luggage. Nothing to delay us getting in and out of Alabama. Sitting in a corner of the limousine, listening to the sirens of our police escort, imagining them in Selma, I remembered Dean Martin's joke when I got "roasted" on his NBC-TV show: "Sammy Davis, Jr., has proved that a black man can eat in a white restaurant, live in a white hotel, eat at a white lunch counter, and ride in a white ambulance."

The air was hot and heavy in Alabama and as we crossed the tarmac I recognized Bull Connor at the gate staring at us all.

Medgar Evers's brother was waiting for us with a Buick station wagon. He said, "Put Sammy in the middle," and I sat between Murphy and Joe Grant. As we drove toward Selma the radio was on and we listened to the news of our arrival. The broadcast signed off: "This is ABC, the *white* news."

A bus took us all to where the march was to begin. The streets were barricaded with wooden horses. We walked. Not aggressively. Solemnly. Martin Luther King, Bob Abernathy, Harry, Shelley, Leonard Bernstein, Hilly, his girl. Whites, blacks. Three thousand of us.

On both sides of the small-town-looking street stood the local people glaring at us, resenting us, angry, fear in their eyes. There were no jeers, no insults, they watched us in silence, despising us. The National Guardsmen, local boys, there to protect us, were little comfort. My stomach, my arms trembled. My legs were weakened and I walked heavily. But I was glad I was there. Those who watched us walking across their city recognized that our presence was causing cameras and printing presses to record what was happening, to bring our protest to tens of millions of other Americans. And they saw an era fading, a way of life coming to a close.

MY CHILDREN were in the backyard playing on a jungle gym I'd bought them at F. A. O. Schwarz. It was noon, I'd had breakfast, and I was free until four o'clock. Then I had an interview with Gary Moore over at CBS radio and at six dinner at Sardi's with an AP feature writer. I was ecstatic to be lounging around my house doing nothing for a few hours. May and I went into the living room and I read the theater section of the *Times* while she gazed out the window at New York's version of a blue sky. "Sharley Brown?" I looked up. "Let's make a picnic basket, take the kids and find a woods somewhere and rough it for lunch."

I was in my town house, wearing a Sulka robe, holding a Steuben glass filled with bourbon and Coke. "Darling, rough it? You know what's my idea of roughing it? When Murphy's not here and I've got to make my own drink. Also, there's not enough time."

"Okay, okay. It was just a thought." She picked up the newspaper. "Anyway, it's sure nice to have a few hours together."

At 3:30 I was dressed and ready to go down to CBS. "Got the cast party tonight, darling. I'll be home a little latish." She kissed me goodbye and nodded, sadly. Her expression stayed with me on the ride downtown. Yet the parties and the bowling really did show in the performance.

IT WAS A crisp, wintry Sunday-in-New York morning and as I was settling into the Sunday *Times* I heard "Sammy, we've got the whole day free, let's take the kids to the zoo."

"May, I can't walk in Central Park *by myself*, let alone with you and the kids. It'll be a crowd scene with autographs and staring, and you're not going to enjoy that, and the kids aren't going to enjoy it. And possibly it's dangerous. Not that I'm sorry to miss going to the zoo to have a million laughs staring at animals."

She was conciliatory but determined. "I accept the fact that you're famous. But it doesn't have to be Central Park. Some fathers take their children camping, they make tree houses for them, they play ball with them. Mark would love to have a catch with you right here in our backyard."

"Then somebody will have to teach me how to have a catch. I never played ball. When I was Mark's age I was sitting around Green Rooms playing pinochle. And my son will not enjoy me making an ass of myself in front of him. The fun is when Daddy is better than you are. In this family Daddy sings 'Birth of the Blues' and he stars on Broadway and he's as good a father in his way as the guy next door is in his."

"Just because you're a father doesn't mean that you're a *good* father. It takes effort . . ."

"Stop! Time out! I don't need a lecture." I was more outraged every moment. "What am I, some kind of an ogre? I don't beat my kids, they're not starving in a ghetto someplace. So what if I *can't* walk in the park with them? And know now: I'm *never* going to build a tree house for them. I *hate* outdoorsy and woodsy things. I don't know how to do them. Does that make me Jack the fucking Ripper?"

I ran out of the house and slammed the door behind me. When I returned May was feeding the kids and we didn't talk much, nor did we as we dressed for the evening. Judy Garland was in town to play the Palace and I'd invited her over for Sunday supper and she brought her daughter, Liza Minnelli.

As the evening went on Judy started singing and Liza joined her, her voice and confidence blooming. Then Leonard Bernstein played the piano for Adolph Green, who sang some of the songs he and Betty Comden had written with Lenny for *On the Town*. Jule Styne played and Adolph and Betty sang songs they had written for *Bells Are Ringing*. I performed for them, inventing some new Charlie Chaplin pieces, trying to do things I didn't do commercially. It was a wonderful show business evening.

I walked over to May, wanting to share it with her. She was with Amy Greene. "Y'know what I was thinking?" I said. "Why don't we do a weekly 'Sunday at Sammy's'?"

"Why don't we talk about that?" she said. She didn't like the idea. She didn't like it *a lot!*

When everyone had left, we busied ourselves emptying ashtrays, taking the used glasses to the kitchen. She wasn't in any more of a hurry to talk than I was. But finally we'd run out of stalls, we'd gone upstairs, and we were alone in our room getting ready for bed. I said, "May?" She looked at me. Not angry. Sad. "Didn't you enjoy this evening at all?"

She shook her head and her lovely hair swung back and forth and I remembered the first night I had taken her home, to Malibu, with the moonlight shining on it. I could never have imagined we'd ever have a hard moment between us. I still couldn't. Yet she was close to tears and I didn't know how to turn them off. Neither hers nor my own, the dry ones that I could feel in my chest, constricting my throat.

"Darling, can't you get a kick out of the people that were here? An appreciation of what it means that they would come to my home?"

"Sammy, I love you but I hate our life." She was startled by the force of her own words. "To be very honest with you, I don't care about a big limousine or push-button windows or famous people singing in my living room. I'm sorry"—she began weeping—"but I just can't help that. I understand that it pleases you . . . but I'd rather have spent your night off alone with you. I don't want Judy

Garland. I want my marriage, my husband and my children . . .
I'm . . . lonely . . ."

I held her in my arms, stroking her hair, wanting her to feel all
the love I had for her, not understanding her loneliness but blindly
trying to help her across that unhappy wasteland.

I GOT UP at noon. May had left for the park with the children. I
went downtown to my office. Shirley Rhodes was at her desk staring
at a pile of my bills she had to pay. I was earning around $20,000
a week from *Golden Boy* but I was still splitting it three ways with
Will Mastin and my father, so she had a net of around $7,000 a
week to work with. Shirley was plump and adorable, but she wasn't
feeling very adorable that morning.

Playing it cute-face, I asked, "What street can I walk down
today?"

She looked at me beadily. "I think you should stay off the streets
altogether."

"Shirl, there's something I've gotta do."

"I'll draw you a map." Taking a sheet of paper, she crisscrossed
streets and avenues. "This is Forty-second Street and this is Fifty-
seventh Street and here's Broadway and there's Park Avenue." She
put an X at Forty-seventh and Madison, where Lefcourt's shoe
store was. "Don't go there, 'cause I can't pay them now." She made
an X at Fifth Avenue and Fiftieth. "And don't go past Dunhill's,
'cause they called me this morning." She made an X at Fifth and
Fifty-seventh. "Stay away from Tiffany's, 'cause that's so hot a hand
may reach out and grab you." She X'd out Gucci and Saks, then
brushed the pencil past Fifty-second and Fifth. "You're safe here.
I paid Cartier last week."

I browsed through the novelty items for ladies, gold bobby pins,
combs and brushes, a swizzle stick. I chose a simple six-carat sol-
itaire set in platinum with diamond baguettes surrounding it.

May handed it back to me.

"Don't you even want to try it on?"

"Sammy, you know what I want, and if you can't give it to me,
then at least don't give me what I don't want. Please return it and
save the money."

I guess I had known in my heart that a piece of jewelry wasn't
the answer, but I had the show and benefits and a record session
to think about. I'd have to work it out some other time.

At the end of that week an adorable infant, Jeffrey, came to us from the agency in L.A. Now we were a family of five. Or they were a family of four, plus me as the absentee father. I was leaving for the theater when I passed the living room and saw my children playing together and I felt overwhelming love and protectiveness, like I could sing both choruses of "Soliloquy" from *Carousel*. I looked at May, so caring, so devoted to them. She had no makeup on, she was wearing a shapeless cotton housedress and a pair of greenish-blue rubber thongs. She had not lost her great figure but she sure wasn't going out of her way to show it to me.

I sat in an easy chair in the living room and watched her with the children. When she looked over at me I asked, "May . . . ? Whatever happened to the Mary Movie Star that I married?"

She shrugged happily. "I couldn't care less about being in pictures. I'd rather be plain Mrs. Sharley Brown."

May had not understood and I didn't press the point. I stood up. "Listen, will you come by the dressing room tonight? In something a little svelte and sophisticated? I'll send the car for you at eleven. We can have supper at '21.' Or how about that Italian place you like, Orsini's?"

"The fact is, Sammy, I'm pooped. If I stay up till four in the morning, how can I take care of Jeff at six-thirty?"

I couldn't let the children see the sudden anger I felt. Smiling, modulating my voice, I asked, "How about taking care of your husband? I thought you were lonely! How about letting Lessie Lee Jackson take care of Jeff in the morning?"

She stood up and walked me out of the room to the door, whispering, "I thought it was understood that I was not going to have someone else bringing up our children."

WE WERE putting out lights, locking the front and back doors, getting ready to go upstairs, when Sy Marsh called me from the Coast. "Sweetheart! We've hit the jackpot! I have a firm offer from NBC for a full network series, an intimate variety show. They'll schedule taping so that you can do your Wednesday matinee. My only question is, with *Golden Boy* and everything, can you physically handle it?"

May looked at me with amazement growing to fury. "You haven't had one hour a week for the children with only the show to do. And benefits. And interviews. Now you're taking on a TV series? You might as well live in a hotel between the studio and the theater."

"Darling, I can't give up the prestige of my own network show."

"Sammy, I can't take this lifestyle anymore."

I went over to the bar to make myself a drink, as a prop, to give myself time to understand what she was saying. I sat down on the couch beside her and asked, "You say you don't want this lifestyle?"

"I've told you that. I don't enjoy the rewards of your celebrity. I hate this extravagant way we live. I was happy with our first apartment. I feel like I'm in your way. I think I'd like to take the kids and go back to California until you finish up with the show. I'm sick of pushing them on you. And to be honest, I can't stand to hear myself whining 'I want to see my husband.' I'd almost rather learn to live without him."

I felt hot and sick and I knew categorically that the last thing in the world I wanted was for May to go away from me with our children. Zoooom! and I saw that I had been risking everything we'd fought so hard for. I had to dig deep for breath. I took her hands in mine. "Darling, don't go. I love you and I love our children. Please stay. I'll cancel the TV series. Screw it. No more press, no more interviews. At least, the absolute minimum. I'll do my show eight times a week, we'll have every day until I go to the theater and all day Sunday. What the fuck, I'll even learn to go on a picnic . . ." The tears were flooding down her face, but she was smiling and her forehead had a smoothness and serenity I hadn't seen on it in years. "Oh, thank God, Sharley Brown . . ." and she put her arms around me. "But I won't ask you to go on a picnic."

"Why not? I'll go to Abercrombie and Fitch and we'll get the best picnic baskets I can charge." She looked at me to see if I was kidding. I really was. But oh was I glad to have her in my arms, and grateful that somehow, something had turned on a beacon before the ships had passed. I held her, appreciating being able to feel her warmth, shuddering at the insanity of almost losing her.

I called Sy. "Babe, I'm sorry about this but please tell the guys at NBC thank you but I can't do the series."

"You're putting me on."

"No. I hardly know my own kids. And I can't fix that by taking on more work."

"Sweetheart, I agree with you. I've got kids too. I . . . well, you just surprised me . . ."

When Hilly came into my dressing room I told him, "Tell our press guys not to schedule me for anything that we can't absolutely do without."

He blinked and shook his head, like he'd been struck. "Sam, that's not possible. We need constant promotion."

"Don't fight me on this, Hilly. Please! I've done the *Life* thing, we've had a *Saturday Evening Post* story, I've got a book on the best-seller lists, I've done every radio and TV interview. Now I've got to make time for my family."

I did whatever benefits I already had scheduled and then I was "not available" and I settled into a quiet married life.

Trying to think of things the children might enjoy, I remembered how I used to like Horn and Hardart's Automats, putting the nickels into the slots and taking the sandwiches out of the little windows.

I realized that exposing us to the public as a family had its risks for the kids, but I had to remember the overprotection by my father and Will. The fact was that my children were certain to run into racial problems. Someday, somewhere, somebody was going to call names or make jokes. As it was unavoidable, then how much better if I were there to buffer the shock.

Jeff was still too young, but the four of us went to the Automat on Fifty-seventh Street near Sixth Avenue. I had the car leave us off half a block away. We didn't need the scene of a limo pulling up to a cafeteria. Trying not to make a three-act play out of being there, I sat down at a corner table in the back and let the kids and May do the shopping. I watched the double takes as people saw these two black children with this very white woman, but nobody got out of line.

As we walked up the block toward the car Tracey was hanging on my arm. Mark said, "Dad, that was fun."

At home May hugged me. "I think you're great, Sharley Brown, the way you're *trying* with the kids, thinking up things to do. Kids can tell the difference."

ONE OF the gypsies stuck her head into the dressing room. "Sammy? Someone said you're not coming bowling tonight!"

"Can't, babe. But the team still stands. We're leading the league."

She shrugged, making a face like bowling-schmowling, and I

heard her in the hall: "He's *not* coming. Let's go to Downey's instead."

I WAS IN bed having coffee, giving myself the luxury of waking up gradually, first my heart, then my brain. Ah, good morning, Legs and Arms . . . Fingers.

Tracey came in and climbed into bed with me.

May was trying on clothes, a sexy silver lamé dress she'd just bought because she knew I'd like to see her in it. We had an after-theater supper date that evening, just the two of us, to go to Orsini's. The telephone rang and Lessie Lee ambled in. "It's Frank Sinatra, Mr. Davis. You in?"

"Whaddya say, Smokey? Listen, is this show *Golden Boy* any fuckin' good? I've got some tickets here for tonight."

"You're in town? Francis, that's great!"

"Now don't get nervous tonight because there's a pro in the audience. After the show we'll go to Jilly's joint. Catch you later, Charley."

I got busy stirring my coffee.

May asked, "What did he say?"

"He's coming to the show tonight."

After a few minutes she said, "Sammy, if Frank wants to go out after the show tonight, I understand we should go with him. He *is* your friend."

We were at a table for eight in the back of Jilly's, a small bar and restaurant on West Fifty-second Street, drinking, eating Chinese food. Frank was not married or going with anyone in particular and he had a few girls with him. May was ravishing in her silver dress, seated between two men who couldn't have been very interesting to her, but she was being charming, trying to add something to the conversation. At around two-thirty I told Frank, "Matinee tomorrow," and we said our goodbyes.

In the car home I told May I appreciated the way she'd handled the evening. She said, "Thank *you* for ending it when you did. I know you wanted to stay up all night with Frank."

"No, I didn't." I heard myself say it and wasn't sure of the truth myself. Yes, I *had* wanted to stay up with Frank. But I had also wanted to not want to stay up. What I wanted was to want to go to bed at a normal hour and keep my wife and children happy.

Before putting the light out we looked through the newspapers.

"Do you want to see something beautiful, Sharley Brown?" She handed me Earl Wilson's column in the *Post*, which said, "Night owl Sammy Davis, Jr., is now a domestic animal. Rushes home after the show to be with Beautiful Wife, May Britt, and to kiss their three children good night." She was beaming.

I felt odd, uncomfortable, like it wasn't really about me.

When I got up at noon Lessie Lee brought in my tomato juice and coffee. I went downstairs and walked over to the bar doing hangover patter. "A little taste for the face, a little toddy for the body." I poured a vodka and Coke and turned around. "Just to get the old heart pumpin'." May was not smiling. "What's wrong?"

"Nothing."

"Are you upset because I didn't get up earlier to play with Mark and Tracey?"

"No. You need your sleep, God knows."

But she was not happy with me. "Look, I can't do a congressional investigation, because I'm not a congressman, so will you please just tell me what's bugging you?"

"It's not bugging me. Well . . . I *would* like to have a simple mother-and-father conversation. What is your feeling about the children always seeing their father with a glass of booze in his hand? At any hour. Morning, noon . . ."

I sat down. *That* I never would have thought of. For as long as I could remember, a glass was a natural extension of my hand. "Darling, have they ever seen me stagger? Have I ever gotten out of line with them? Or with you in front of them? Have they ever seen me bombed and bringing six chicks home to ball?"

"No . . ."

"Then that's my opinion of it." I took a sip. "I'm not a 'social drinker.' I don't see why someone has to wait until five-thirty in the afternoon to drink if he wants one earlier. 'Ah, the sun is finally over the mizzenmast, I'll have a salty dog,' and he topples over from wanting it all day long. Forget it. When you see me staggering in front of the kids, then you can ask me again."

Tracey, Mark, and Jeff were sitting on the floor watching a Steve McQueen Western. I joined them as Mark hooted, "Wow! Lookit the way he rides. Turns that horse on a dime. Dad, do you know Steve McQueen?"

"Yes, son, you met him at our house when you were a baby. But that particular shot happens to have been done by a stuntman. I was there the day they shot it."

Steve was good on a horse but no better than I was. Maybe not as good. When Mel Tormé started me doing quick-draw with single-action Colt .45s, I'd met Arvo Arjala, who made all my holsters. He'd worked me past being a good "show business" gunslinger into being really good. At the same time I'd asked him to help me get the right riding lessons and I'd worked at it. I put in hundreds of hours preparing for what I hoped would be the first Negro cowboy film, which I did finally make for Dick Powell on the *Zane Grey Theater*.

"Mark, listen, would you like to go horseback riding with me? I'll teach you."

I had my blue jeans and Western boots but I ordered the car for ten o'clock and Mark and I went down to Miller's and we got him fitted out with cute cowboy boots, jeans, a plaid shirt, and I flipped a Western hat onto his head.

We went to a stable on West Sixty-seventh Street. The riders were dressed as in *The Philadelphia Story*. It wasn't a "stable," it was a "riding academy," and the horses had English saddles. I asked, "Don't you have a horse with a Western rig?"

"No, sir, Mr. Davis. But you'll get used to this after a while. Just hang on to him with your knees."

I didn't want to get used to anything in front of my son. But I couldn't back out. Thank God I hadn't boasted how good I was, planning to let him see for himself. I felt like I was sitting on a rail, holding on to the saddle, which I knew was wrong to do, but the alternative was to fall on my ass. It would be dangerous for me to teach Mark, as I'd told him I would. I asked, "Can we get an instructor for my son?"

By six o'clock that evening my thighs were so stiff I could hardly move my legs except spastically. Me! A dancer, starring on Broadway. I hadn't been spectacular with my son and I'd fucked up with my show.

THREE OF the girl dancers gave two weeks' notice. They were going to new shows. Without me pulling the kids together I noticed a lack of the cohesion they'd had before. Enough so that the audience wouldn't feel the same intensity, the wave of emotion that their oneness had previously projected.

Hilly came backstage. "Sam, the competition's getting all the press, Zero Mostel, Bob Preston . . . new shows opening every day. And your sudden drop out of the public eye is showing." He laid out some accounting papers. "Here are the comparative figures of daily advance sales now, against a month ago. By not promoting us on the talk shows and keeping the name in the papers as a reminder, *Golden Boy* is selling tickets on the reviews, advertising, and word of mouth, but we're missing that little x percent extra which we used to have—and it was the perfume on the gorgeous lady."

The difference was significant. I also recognized that my responsibility went beyond appearing onstage eight times a week. The producer and backers had a right to expect me to use all my weight to make it as profitable as I could. And for the last month and a half they hadn't been getting all that they were buying.

"Sam, I don't want to press but I've got a strong request for lunch tomorrow with Maurice Zolotow for a piece for the Sunday *Times* . . ."

"I can't, Hilly, I'm taking my children to the circus." I was embarrassed by my own words.

I bought the kids cotton candy and all the circus toys and junk foods and I tried to enjoy the show, but I was irreversibly tuned in to everyone around us. When I heard "Look . . . look," which was normal for any celebrity, I automatically wondered what they meant. Even when people didn't say anything I could hear them looking. By the time the circus was over I was fatigued. My shoulder and neck muscles had been tensed for too long. As we left Madison Square Garden, I told May, "Drop me off at the theater. I'm going to take a nap in the dressing room." And I did, but it wasn't enough and I did a sluggish performance that night, half a beat below my normal.

Being in public with May and the children was too heavy. I bought games for us to play at home. I tried Monopoly, which I liked, but they were too young. Darts. Shuffleboard.

It wasn't the best use of me. I wasn't anything special as a father. But that wasn't serious. I loved them and they knew it. The danger was that I was not being the best Sammy Davis, Jr., I knew how to be.

As I read the newspapers and watched the television news and talk shows, I saw that my image was changing or fading. For "Sammy" to be in a town and not be in the middle of what's happening was a contradiction in style. Earl Wilson had said it, I was developing the domesticated animal image, which was great for Perry Como but not for "Sammy" the saloon singer, the legend of perpetual motion, the swinger, the boozer, and "Wowowoweee-wow, it's a party!" Aside from *Golden Boy* I had to be looking ahead to when I got back to Vegas and Tahoe. One of the reasons for taking a break from clubs was to be missed—not forgotten.

When I got to the theater there was a sign posted on the bulletin board: "Birthday party for Lola. Tonight. Everybody welcome. Love, Hilly."

I was making up when Hilly came by. "Sam? It would mean a lot to the kids if you'd show up tonight." He was looking at me through the mirror and his face was a lot more serious than a birthday party.

"I'll be there, babe."

I called Sy Marsh and asked him to try to revive NBC's interest in me for a series or for anything constructive. "Get me back into the business, baby. And hurry." Then after the show that night I went home and sat downstairs in the living room with May. The kids were asleep, the house was quiet, and I tried to explain it. "Trying to change my lifestyle wasn't a good idea. I used to be an original. Then I stopped being a good Sammy Davis and I was just ordinary as an 'around the house with the kids' and 'he's taking them to the circus' kind of a father. I got where I am by single-mindedness, by one hundred percent involvement: I ate, talked, breathed, slept, lived show business. Then I started phoning it in. I became a part-time Sammy Davis, Jr. It was insanity. Fortunately, temporary.

"For me to try to be something I'm not, to go with society's image or your image of how a father and a husband should look and act would eventually be a disaster. I can't afford it profession-ally. Right now I have to work. There's no level road in show business. It tilts up or it tilts down. So I have to grow while the opportunities present themselves."

174

She had been listening attentively. "I've always understood your need to be the biggest and the best."

"May, it's not a matter of being the biggest and the best. It's not the disease of ambition, to get there and accomplish it, to be Mr. Versatility, Mr. Everything. No. It's the fear of *losing* success. To let the high ground I'm standing on slide out from under me. And as I explained to you when we were first married, when the ground goes out from under 'Sammy Davis, Jr.,' it's not the same as it would be for 'May Britt.' "

"I understand that perfectly. But if you're now going to do a TV series plus *Golden Boy* it means we'll never see you at all. So it's goodbye family life."

"Not entirely, and not forever. We'll do the best we can. But I cannot let anything get in the way of 'Sammy Davis, Jr.'—not me, the person—I mean the figure SD, Jr. He is what makes everything happen. I'm not going to get trapped in a false sense of my importance to you and to the children. If Tracey and Mark and Jeff and May have to wait awhile till they have hang-out time with me, then that's how it has to be, because 'Sammy Davis, Jr.,' comes before anyone. If what *I* personally want doesn't work for *him*, if I want to play golf but he thinks he should play a benefit, then we play the benefit. He comes first. Period."

We looked at each other in silence, in fatigue.

I touched her arm. "Darling, I tried. I really wanted it to work. But it couldn't work."

"I know you did, Sharley Brown." She wiped her eyes. "I know you did."

On January 7, 1966, I hosted the first *Sammy Davis Jr. Show* on NBC with my guests Elizabeth Taylor and Richard Burton.

When we'd recorded the original-cast album of *Golden Boy* my voice had been so bad that a year later when it had unexplainably straightened itself out and I was wailing, Hilly said, "Reprise is willing to rerecord the album."

I told May. "It's incredible. To get a second shot. We're doing it next Sunday at noon. Why don't you come down about two, after we're past the rehearsing and we go for takes?"

"I can't, Sammy. I'm taking Mark and Tracey to Westchester. A birthday party for a boy in Mark's class."

"You booked up Sunday? My day off?"

She looked at me as if she was making up her mind whether or not to say it. "But it isn't, is it? Next week it's the record session. Last Sunday it was the Friars' Roast, the Sunday before . . ."

"Okay, okay . . . anyway, come and bring the kids."

"I can't, Sammy. They're looking forward to this party."

"Darling, there are thirty-three kids in that class, that's thirty-three birthday parties. They can miss one. Send regrets and a little present." She was shaking her head. What kind of values did she have? "May! I am rerecording the original-cast album of a major Broadway musical. In twenty years our sons and daughter will hear this album being played and they'll be able to remember that they were there, they saw their father doing it."

"I'd like to, Sammy, but I can't. Children have to be able to count on things."

Sy CALLED. "Sweetheart, I've got a real off-the-wall thing here. There's a feature film they're going to shoot in New York, *A Man Called Adam*, and they've got Frank Sinatra, Jr., Mel Tormé, and Peter Lawford co-starring, with Louis Armstrong in a cameo. I told them you haven't got time to breathe but they insisted I call you."

"Babe, I'm available. I'm not needed for the bulk of the TV rehearsals. I've got hours free every day."

After the first day's shooting, when I rushed home to change clothes for the theater I started to tell May, "I did this good scene with Frank Jr. . . ." But I stopped. I had the sudden realization that she would find my enthusiasm offensive.

I was back in the daily papers. They marveled: "Nobody in history has ever starred in a Broadway musical, taped a TV series, and shot a movie all at the same time." I was hot again. Every move I made turned up the three cherries on the slot machine. The recognition, the career building, the money.

And the excuse not to go home. Not the least bit the latter. When I went home I wanted to be so tired, so drained that conversation was impossible. Day by day the chasm between us had widened from bickering to silence. We came and went, pursuing separate lives, I with my work, May with the children. We hardly exchanged a word, for fear, I think, of the dangerous wrong words. So we exchanged only pleasantries. We had become a family of strangers.

I came home late after the show and a benefit and for the hundredth time we stared at each other in silence.

May was in bed reading. She didn't tell me where she had taken the children that afternoon.

I undressed. I didn't tell her that the rehearsal for the TV show got a standing ovation from the stagehands.

May didn't tell me that Tracey was getting her new teeth.

I didn't tell May that I was doing *Mike Wallace* tomorrow and why not come to the studio.

May didn't tell me that Mark had fallen off his bike and skinned his knee and she'd taken him to the doctor for an anti-tetanus shot.

We had long ago stopped saying "I love you," but we didn't tell each other *anything* anymore. I wanted to say and to hear all of those things. But I was afraid of being taken over by them.

From the outside it looked like I was skiing down the Alps without the sticks, and everybody was going, "Look at him . . . he can do it . . . it's miraculous . . ." But inside I was going, "Oh, shit . . . ," waiting to fall, to crash, to have half of my life say goodbye and walk away from me.

The very things that motivate you in the beginning and allow you to get there can be so destructive if you permit them to take over your life. But the car I was driving had only one gear: forward. It didn't even have neutral.

I got home so tired one night that I didn't make it upstairs and fell asleep on the couch in the living room. When I woke up, May brought me some juice and coffee.

"Good morning," she said.

"Good morning," I replied.

"The weather's not so good today."

"Yes. But the weatherman said it may clear up."

When you exchange only pleasantries they stop being pleasant.

I think she waited until I was fully awake before she said, "What's the point in this, Sammy? It's only getting worse. We've been through too much together to let ourselves end up disliking each other. I think it's better to walk away from it."

Funny how you can love somebody so much when you don't want to, when you know it's useless. But what did love have to do with living?

I said, "I really can't believe this is happening."

"Neither can I."

"It's not what I want, May."

"It's not what I want either."

"I never intended to say I was going back to my career alone. I meant with you and for you . . ."

But there we were, two people who loved each other, being severed by priorities that didn't mesh.

She began crying and her voice was pinched by tears. "I know that I can never replace Judy Garland and Liza and Frank, or when the curtain goes up and the lights go on."

"You shouldn't have had to."

Nodding her head, her hair moving like a curtain in front of her thoughts, she said, "I know that. I know that I should be able to live with you *and* with all that stuff, but I don't like it, I *really* don't like the life of Charley Show Biz . . ."

"Then why did you marry me?"

She looked up. "I fell in love with you."

"But that *was* me. It *is* me, it will always *be* me."

Again she was nodding her head as if waiting for her sobs to stop so she could speak.

I took her in my arms and we held each other, not as husband and wife anymore, but as friends now, friends who shared a mutual loss.

Maybe if we were angry it would have been easier, less sad.

ON THE morning they were leaving I stayed in bed, pretending to sleep, while May and the children did their last-minute packing. I couldn't have handled a long goodbye.

"Mom." I heard Tracey's voice. "Should we wake Dad or just kiss him while he's sleeping?"

I said, "I'm up," and I put on a robe.

It was a drizzly New York morning as I stood in the doorway watching May and Tracey and Mark and Jeff get in the back of my car with Lessie Lee. The doors closed and the car with the license plate SAMMY started moving away. As it neared the corner I walked out onto the sidewalk and waved goodbye, holding on to them for a moment longer, but as I did it occurred to me that maybe nobody was looking back. Then, thank God, I saw Mark's and Tracey's faces appear in the oval-shaped rear window, waving goodbye to me.

15

THE HOUSE WAS emptier than empty, quieter than silent, as though everyone but me had evaporated. May's clothes closet contained only the hangers on which I could visualize the dresses I had liked to see her in. The children's rooms showed no sign that they'd ever been there. Not a toy. Even the wastebaskets were empty. Through the back door I could see the jungle gym and their seesaw in the yard. Looking away from them, I thought: *They really left me. With all my glitter, with all that I could give them, they preferred not to be with me.*

My driver returned from the airport and handed me a small red knitted mitten. "I found this in the car, Mr. D." I took it from him. Why would a child leave something behind like this? Was it to maintain contact with me? Or was she angry and throwing it away, breaking with me? I held it against my face. It had Tracey's clean soapy smell.

What did I give this up for? Isn't this what life is about? To have a wife you love. And children you love, and you take care of them and show them how to survive in the world . . . you try to guide them over the bumps you've had without them getting the bruises. And you have a little fun together. And you get older and you die, but something of you is left behind, the good of you. And they remember that and miss you for it.

It seemed that I *had* made a deal with the devil after all. Irrevocable now because I'd gotten my part. And for that the kids would be all right. They'd have money. And they had a good mother. And one day we'd get our time together and we'd have a relationship. Or if not, then I'd lose. And I'd accept the loss. I wasn't a victim. I had made a choice.

I heard someone at the front door and Murphy Bennett walked in, perturbed. "Sammy, the door was open. You've gotta be more careful. They'll rob you blind."

"Ain't nothin' left worth taking, babe."

He knew me well enough to ignore the melodramatic line. Looking at my hand, he asked, "What've you got there?"

"It's my daughter's glove, Murphy. It's all I have left of her. Do you mind?"

"No, Sammy. I'm glad you've got that much."

I glared at him. "What does *that* mean?"

He began fumphering. "Well, only that . . . you're such a big star that you didn't have time for your wife or your kids . . . that's natural in show business . . . so it's nice that at least you've got a mitten."

Whenever something was really eating at me Murphy found a way to divert my thoughts, even, and often, if it meant getting me furious at him. I was grateful to him for getting me over the morbid moment. He always did. But I played my role, shaking my fist at him. "One of these days you're going to push me too far."

If I'd written a script in which "the wife walks out" I'd have had the "swinger" turn his house into a Playboy mansion, so that when you turned on a faucet out came twenty naked chicks. But it didn't play that way in life. I had no desire to celebrate failure. I was lonely for people I hadn't enjoyed when they were there, when I'd had no room for them in my life.

After two years of *Golden Boy* I had nothing more to accomplish on that stage, nothing more to do in New York. I needed to get back into my own world of different shows every night, in different cities, to different people. I gave Hilly an option on me for a year in something else and he posted the show's closing notice.

May had taken the children to California, to the Selznick house with the push-button windows she had never liked. And she called regularly to keep me posted.

I asked, "Has the split been tough on the kids?"

"No, they're fine. That you're not here all the time is as natural to them as another child's father who was always around. We got lucky there. With a nine-to-five father he stamps out the door and 'Daddy's gone' and life is different, but this never happened with us. You were always packing and leaving for Vegas or Tahoe, or going to the theater or sleeping because you were exhausted . . ."

I knew that she hadn't meant for it to hurt. On the contrary, she was the mother hen relieved to say that the kids were not suffering. I went upstairs and got into a hot tub. As I was shaving I thought: *You can't get them back. You've made a choice, paid a price. But let it not be in vain. Let it not be for nothing that you gave up your family.*

That night I did *Golden Boy* for the last time, I went back to that empty house for the last time, and in the morning I woke up on the couch in the living room for the last time.

OPENING in Vegas for the first time since the divorce, we were sold out in advance for every show, but what was waiting for me out there? How were they feeling about me? You never know with the public. If many of them hadn't liked an interracial marriage, how would they react to the divorce? Well, if they were going to start off hating me, they weren't going to leave there like that, because if I had to stay on all night, if I had to sing every song, do every joke, every trick that I knew, if I had to push my heart and soul through the space between us, they were going to like me.

Singing "What Kind of Fool Am I?" I saw them looking at each other, nudging, and I knew they were whispering, "He's singing about his wife, about May Britt." I felt warmth, support. They cared about me, and knew about my life, so that a simple ballad became a point-of-view song. They read drama into it, drama that I would never go for deliberately. It had happened to Frank. During the breakup with Ava he'd sing, "I could have told you she'd hurt you . . ." and people would think: He's singing about her. But the fact is, it was a song written by two guys in the Brill Building. They'd had an idea and they'd expressed it in thirty-two bars of words and music. They didn't say, "Hey, Frank, how do you feel about Ava? We want to write this song, 'One for my baby and one more for the road . . .' " Everyone forgets it was written for Fred Astaire to do in a bar in *The Sky's the Limit* because Joan Leslie had left him.

But I didn't want my audiences to see me as the brokenhearted husband. After Frank had split with Ava Gardner he'd done "The Loser" as well as anyone would ever do it. Further, it wasn't me, it would have been a lie, because I'd caused the break and to capitalize on it would be cheap theatrics, a breaking of faith with the people who had made me, the only people I had left.

THERE WAS little partying. I was looking after business, literally thinking about my shows while I was sleeping. George Rhodes supported me with a telepathy that had developed over the years. I never said, "When I do this, then you'll know I want . . ." It came with time, with thousands of shows. When we'd get to a town George would rehearse the orchestra, making sure they knew twenty-five of my numbers. I didn't have to show up except for a sound check. I'd sing a song or two to hear if the sound system was balanced the way I wanted it. Before each show George came into my dressing room and showed me our song book and I'd say, "Let's do these four," and we opened with those. Nothing else was programmed. From then on it was up for grabs, depending on what I felt the audience wanted.

There is no way I can explain the analyzing of an audience. Osmosis. It's a feeling, almost spiritual. I leave out a certain song because I don't think the audience wants to hear it. Don't put a blue in there. Put a green in there. In almost every show, I do a medley of the Tony Newley and Leslie Bricusse songs I brought back to America from London in 1960: "What Kind of Fool Am I?" "Gonna Build a Mountain," "Evie," and "Talk to the Animals." Sometimes I'll do the medley early—they want to hear those songs, let me get them out of the way early—then I'll do pop things, then obscure things. Sometimes they couldn't care less if I get to "What Kind of Fool Am I?" or "Hey There" or "This Is My Beloved." Not every audience wants to hear them. Sometimes you've got a jazz audience, they want it to cook. Or you've got a show audience, a talk audience, or an audience that involves all of those things. How I recognize them is uncanny. Blindfolded, I hit it ninety-nine percent of the time.

George and I had developed our own language. When I tell the audience, "Ladies and gentlemen, there's a group of songs that I brought back from England . . ." he knows I want the medley, and while I'm talking to give him time, he tells it to our lead trumpet, Fip Ricard, who tells it to the saxophones, who tell it to the trombones, and it spreads across to the piano, the strings, and the drums. Each number has its own natural introduction: "Ladies and gentlemen, in 1940 the late Jerome Kern wrote . . ." and George tells the orchestra to open to "All the Things You Are."

George was big and he walked slow. His firm step and my bung-achungabung-chung worked beautifully together. I needled him onstage: "Anytime you're ready, George. Don't speed now." We were the tortoise and the hare. This little guy, me, flying all over the place, and this big guy, George, steady, reliable, standing back there, digging the performance and going, "Yeahhhh."

Much of what I could do on the stage came from how comfortable I could feel musically. I could move my shoulder and he'd know I'm not going to do that number. When I'd say, "Y'know, ladies and gentlemen . . ." George would think: He's going to change it.

I'm the only performer around who changes the show every performance. At the beginning, the first time I asked for a number they hadn't rehearsed, George said to me, "It'll take a little time before we can find that music," and I joked with it: "We'll now do six bars of 'The Search.' " Today while they're looking for a song I'll tell the audience, "If you could get up close you'd hear them saying, 'Why can't the li'l bugger do the show he rehearsed?' "

I try for a 110 percent show every night, which is why I carry a full rhythm section, my own piano, drums, guitar, and bass plus a lead trumpet. The local musicians—it doesn't matter who's performing, be it Frank or Liza Minnelli—are going to get lackadaisical sometimes, so I can't rely on them. I depend on my own guys. They take off like a rocket and the rest of the orchestra has no choice but to keep up with them. Fip, as leader of the trumpet section, is actually leading the whole horn section, trombone, saxophone . . . the leadership comes from the lead trumpet, he's the loudest. And he has a cohesion with the lead sax and trombone players. They are responsible for setting the lead for their people. If they have no choice but to keep up with Fip, then their guys have no choice but to keep up with them.

Still, there are shows when the orchestra will dog it and I have to pick them up, keep them listening, involved. I keep thinking of things to break them up. I'm performing as much for the musicians as for the audience. I need them to like the show and keep attentive to it, wondering: What's he going to do tonight? I don't want them to turn their music to "the next number," then sit there sipping coffee or chatting back there while I'm talking to the audience. At times, after we've gotten past the first few nights, George has to admonish them: "Talkin' back there." I want them listening, thinking: What's he gonna do next? I switch the numbers around and it keeps them on their toes: "He don't know what he's gonna call for, so I can't go in there and sleep. He's liable to call, 'Make up something.' Then in the middle of that he may say, 'No, let's not do that.' " I don't let them sit there and yawn and wait to go home. I'm playing to *two* audiences, the one behind me and the one out front. When the show is over I always talk to the orchestra and almost always I can say, "Good show. Thank you."

I can't see the people out front. The lights cover them after the first three or four rows. But I feel them, I hear them . . . from the back of the room I can hear. I don't look at them, even those first few rows, because if you see an attractive chick down there and you start doing the show for her, then you lose everybody else.

George's additional value to me was in writing arrangements. I can't write doodly squat on paper but I'll get an idea and hum it into a tape recorder and then George can write it, but the concept has to come from me. There are fine performers who have teams of people who do everything for them—the writers, the choreographer, the director, musicians. But I have to do it myself. No writer knows my audience like I do, and what they will accept from me humor-wise. I've had writer friends come back after a show and say, "That line about such and such, that's not a funny line, how come you get a big laugh on it?"

Like nobody ever said to me, "Hey, you should wear six rings, maybe create a thing about the jewelry." It just happened. I was wearing a diamond pinky ring, which is what Frank always wears; then a friend of mine in Europe gave me a big ring with his family crest and told me, "Wear it on your index finger." Looked great. It harked back to Henry VIII. The ring on my pointing finger, because of the crest and everything, seemed like "Behead him." Then I thought: I need a ring for the middle finger, and another one for here. Get outta here. How dare you be so bodacious? No, it's a giggle. They'll laugh when they see rings on all of my fingers.

It grew to both hands, bracelet, necklace, lapel pin, and everything short of earrings. And I got humor out of it, like "I don't know what Washington, D.C.'s doing for the old folks but I've got *my* social security." From there it went to other people doing jokes about my jewelry, as they'd done about my being Jewish . . . wearing tight pants . . . none of which was planned, like "Hey, I'll do this and they'll talk about me."

I WAS PLAYING bid whist in the dressing room between shows with John Hopkins. The phone rang. Murphy held his hand over the mouthpiece and whispered, "It's the head of the Civil Rights Commission of Nevada."

"So? What're you whispering about?"

"Maybe you've been revoked and you're not black anymore."

"Oh, get outta here." It was Bob Bailey, a man I'd known since before the time when there were any thoughts of civil rights in Las Vegas. He wanted to meet with me and his directors. "Sam, we've been talking with the hotels for years, asking for jobs, but they aren't budging. If they don't make a move in two more weeks, we're going to picket and bring it into national focus. You'll still be playing here then, so we want you to be prepared."

I spoke to Jack Entratter. "You're going to get picketed and it's going to be very embarrassing, because I'm going to be on the picket line." He sat forward like his tooth had been attached to a door that had just been slammed. "Right, Jack. I'm not going to, quote, be in a hospital recuperating from mild pneumonia and exhaustion, end quote. I'll be right out front, walking back and forth."

"What should we do?" Jack asked.

"Like I said two years ago, meet them halfway. Hire some bell-men, waiters. You don't have to start with managers. But get some black people being seen working here. And gambling here. No-body's saying take out an ad in *Ebony* magazine: 'You're Welcome at the Sands.' But if the security guys don't turn purple every time they see a black cat at the door it'll be a step forward. And tell your people to serve them. I mean tomorrow. Not in 'we'll think about it' time, because that'll be too late. Tomorrow."

"The other hotels aren't going to like me, but you've got my word on it."

I looked at him with all the affection you can feel for a man who steps into your fight and says, "They'll have to hit me too." I hesitated, not wanting to push too far, yet it had to be done. "Jack, speaking of the other hotels, what do you think I can do about them?"

"The Hotel Board is having its monthly meeting tomorrow. Come and speak to the guys."

The presidents and owners of the seven Strip hotels met in a boardroom at the Sands. One of the owners smirked: "On what grounds are they going to picket us? They have nothing to do with us. They don't work for us. Our own people are happy, well paid. Nobody's on strike. We'll kick their asses into the fuckin' desert. They can't picket shit."

"Sir," I said, "they can and they will picket all the hotels where there are no black people working. It is no longer legally possible to ignore twenty percent of America's citizens when you employ people."

He grunted, "Some fuckin' free country we've got."

They looked at me and then at each other, a handful of powerful men unwilling to accept that a way of life was changing, yet knowing that it was, that history was being made, that an ocean of people was no longer lapping at a fortress wall but that the civil rights movement had gained momentum and, like a tidal wave, it was going to climb right over the wall.

Leaving the meeting, walking toward the casino, Jack put his arm on my shoulder. "I'm moving on it." In the lobby we saw the only black employee of the Sands Hotel, a bellman. "He's a bright kid," Jack said. "He goes to the front desk end of this week and we'll start training him. And we've hired ten waiters."

"Jack, over in Westside they've got some pretty classy blackjack dealers."

He nodded. "I'll ask Carl Cohen to go over and look at them." He smiled at me. "Tomorrow."

Weeks later when the NAACP picketed Las Vegas they did not picket the Sands. They did not exempt the Sands because I was playing there but because Jack had moved before the others.

I TOOK A week off because I had committed to be present at a rally in Tougaloo, Mississippi. The rally was to be the starting point for a march to Jackson, the state capital, with James Meredith, who'd been shot and wounded a few weeks earlier. There were going to be thousands of students from Tougaloo College, SNCC workers, militants, middle-of-the-road workers, and dozens of theatrical people who were committed to civil rights, as well as every racial leader from Martin Luther King down. I'd promised Harry and Sidney and the black leaders that I'd be a part of the program.

It was the first time in years that I'd returned to L.A. without a house or a family to go to, but I wanted to see my children, so I checked into the Century Plaza. Mark and Tracey looked wonderful, they were going to school in Beverly Hills. Jeff would be starting in another year. When May and I were alone I asked, "How are they doing in school? Any problems?"

"No, racially it's fine. The only thing is that Tracey can't understand why we live in a house that's so much grander than what her friends have."

The showplace Selznick mansion was, I agreed, wrong for them. May had fallen in love with a smaller, homier place on Angelo Drive. I agreed to buy it for her and keep the big house for myself. May wanted to do her own housekeeping, so after Lessie Lee had helped her with the move she would come back and look after my place for me. Angelo Drive was close enough so that when I was home the kids could ride over on their bikes.

I was having dinner at Matty's with Peter Lawford. He got a telephone call at the table, then handed me the phone. "A friend of yours wants to talk to you."

It was Bobby Kennedy. "I've got bad news, Sam. They're waiting for you in Mississippi, in Tougaloo. Don't go down there. They're out to get you and I can't protect you."

"But, Robert, I'm committed."

"I'm telling you *don't go*. Pull out of this one. Of all the celebrities who'll be there, the word is out: 'Get Sammy Davis, Jr.' I have no power to help you, but if you insist on going I'll speak to somebody over at Justice and ask them to try to have some agents keep an eye on you."

I'd chartered a Lear jet to take us there from Los Angeles: Rafer Johnson, Tony Franciosa and Marlon Brando, Murphy, Joe Grant, and myself. As we were getting ready to land I stood up in the center of the plane and announced, "After the rally is over and we meet at the reverend's house, or whoever the host and hostess are, I'm having a cup of coffee, but the second the amenities are over I am leaving. They've arranged rooms for us in people's houses but I ain't staying overnight."

Marlon said, "I'll be staying on in Tougaloo. I have to meet with the chancellor tomorrow." Marlon was in civil rights down to his toenails, full commitment. Not for self-aggrandizement, but from a profound belief in the right of it. Some people were in it because it was the popular thing at that moment. But you couldn't say, "There's Marlon Brando, he's doing this to promote his picture." Civil rights wasn't *that* popular.

I said, "You do what you have to do, Marlon, but if we get away with this evening, I will not be there tomorrow."

Rafer said, "I'm coming back with you."

Tony Franciosa said, "I'll stay." He had a romantic, gazing-at-the-future look in his eyes. "I want to get the feeling of what's happening, I want to see these grounds where history is being made."

"Babe, that's beautiful, but I am going back on the plane tonight. We'll do whatever we have to do, but then I'm getting out."

When we were on the ground I told the pilots, two California guys, "Don't let nobody on this plane. Not to clean it up, nothing. You do whatever has to be done. 'Cause they don't like you guys for bringing us any more than they like us."

"We know exactly what you mean, Mr. Davis. We'll never be far from the plane."

Walking toward the small airport, Murphy at my side, I was thinking: *I should have listened to Bobby. I'm down here in the bowels of the South. Somebody's gonna shoot me. Nobody can stop them.* And I didn't feel better when, as we drove to the college, I saw a sign saying "Hanging Road."

There were twenty thousand people gathered at the college, it was night, there were floodlights, cameras shooting from the trees, NBC was doing a live coverage.

As the speeches went on, Martin Luther King hugged me. "I got you to Mississippi. Sam, I knew I'd get you down here."

"Yeah . . . you got me here to Mississippi. I love you, Martin, you are my spiritual leader, but you have gone too far. Frankly, I am scared!"

Harry and Sidney were near us. They were like great black knights. "Don't worry about anything, Sam, we're here, we'll protect you."

All they had was the spirit in their hearts. I said, "You fuckin' crazy! They could kill you too. Don't you know that?"

Harry said, "Well, we'll talk about it tomorrow."

I guffawed. "Unless you comin' back to L.A. with me you ain't talking to me about nothin' tomorrow, 'cept by phone. *Long-distance!*"

My role was to do a few songs and then introduce Martin. The program went off without a hitch, no thanks to the police, who were standing there listlessly. We had only a few dozen black security people without weapons, college kids who were giving their bodies in service.

As we left the podium Martin said, "I'll meet you at the reverend's house. We've got to talk you into staying over . . ."

"Martin, I love you, but I am not going to be in Mississippi tomorrow."

He laughed. "Oh, you down here now, we got you here at last . . ."

"You just want to see me laid out here dead someplace."

"Nobody's gonna bother you. You're too little."

Harry touched my shoulder to get my attention. "Make sure we all leave in a group."

I asked, "What do we need that for?"

"Well, that way we protect each other."

"I thought you said there was nothing to be worried about."

"Well, just in case . . ."

We traveled together to the reverend's house and we were all seated in his living room, having a cup of coffee, when one of the sisters of the church said to his wife, "Ohhh, Hazel, look where Mr. Davis is sitting. That's right by the window where . . . Oh, you got the pane fixed . . ."

My coffee cup rattled on the saucer. "What pane?"

"The windowpane. That's where they threw the firebomb in."

I got up and sat across the room against the wall. Tony heard that, he'd seen the rednecks and the attitudes. He moved to my side. "Don't leave without me."

"Aren't you staying?"

"I just remembered I think I'm due at the studio . . ."

We both started laughing. The underlying tension made it even funnier. Sidney, Harry, Marlon, the leadership, they still had things to do, but we'd done ours.

THE DODGERS were playing at home. Mark and Tracey would love to see them, so I pulled some strings and got a great infield box. I called May to make arrangements.

"Oh, Sammy, that's great. They'll love it."

"Have them ready at eleven and I'll take them to lunch on the way."

Frank called. "Come down to the Springs for a long weekend, Smokey. We'll sit around the pool and watch the Bums. I've also got some more crummy Rat Pack scripts we can get sick over together. I'll send the plane to Burbank for you." As we talked I could imagine May's face; hear her telling me, "Children have to be able to count on things."

Well, they can count on their food, their clothes, their house, their school, and when they really need me. And they can count on having my box behind first base to sit in at the ball game, but they do not need me to be there to buy them ice cream. And I could hear her say, *You haven't changed.* And I snapped, *No, I haven't changed. And I haven't changed color either.*

I knew that Charley Next Door would have said, "Thanks, Frank, but I'm with my children," except that Frank Sinatra wouldn't be calling Charley Fucking Next Door and the Springs was where it was happening for me and that's where I should be and wanted to be.

I was not going to call May and get involved with that kind of a conversation. Instead I called Mark. "I can't make it tomorrow, but you've still got my box, and Sy and Molly can take you. It'll be more fun, they'll bring their kids . . ."

It didn't mean that someday I wouldn't love to take Mark and Tracey and Jeff to a ball game and yell and scream and have a beer . . . but I had other priorities.

Natalie Wood and R. J. Wagner were at Burbank waiting for Frank's plane and we flew down together. Frank was at the airport with the station wagon and there was a second car for the luggage. "Dinner's at nine, we'll meet for drinks around eight o'clock. I'm cooking." He's a good cook. Anything Italian. Basically a man's-kind-of-food cook: steaks, chops, a roast. He knows his kitchen well and he's got a good touch with pasta, a delicate touch with sauces.

Frank's home is on the golf course, and he has a lot of security, a whole wall around the house. The main building can seat sixty for dinner in the dining room, or it can be cut down with panels. That building also contains his private areas, bedrooms, dressing rooms, and steam rooms. Then there's the large building he put up for the Kennedys, and four guest bungalows. The one I stayed in had two bedrooms, large living room, full kitchen with a stocked refrigerator and bar, coffee available at all times, and personalized matches: "Smokey."

I bathed leisurely, using a mix of Lactopine, Hermès, and Au Sauvage, and at around five to eight walked into his living room and Frank was waiting for us. There was no wandering in and "Hey, where is everybody?" He was always waiting for his guests. "Let's have a taste," and he made drinks. Jimmy Stewart was there for the weekend, Jimmy Van Heusen came over for dinner from his own house at the Springs, and we sat up all night boozing, talking about the business, and enjoying each other.

Somebody said, "The Rat Pack should make another picture."

Frank made a face. "So what else is new? I've got four scripts for us on my desk but nobody's come up with anything we haven't already done."

In the morning, which was around two in the afternoon, we sat around boozing and watching the Dodgers game on television. The camera landed on my box and I saw Mark and Tracey. They were having a good time. And I was where I should be. But I wasn't much of a father. No buts . . . fuck it.

ONE OF THE columns wrote, "Is SD, Jr., torching for May Britt? His current dinner date is look-alike Jean Seberg."

Jean was one of the sponsors of the Black Panthers. There was a Hollywood contingent that gave money to the Panthers and she was intensely involved. I didn't start dating her because she looked like May, nor did I think she did other than being very white and blonde, but if that's what they wanted to think, I was not sorry to be getting back a little he's-a-bachelor attention, the swinger image which served me.

I went with Jean to a meeting and I saw Ron Karenga there. He was the most feared as well as the most respected civil rights activist in L.A. He was a super-militant, scary, dark glasses, bald head, Fu Manchu mustache, ominous-looking.

The militants in CORE and SNCC and the Panthers as well as the middle-of-the-road groups and leaders—Martin, Jesse Jackson, the NAACP, and the Urban League—were working to arrive at the same place, but they were on parallel lines, and without contact they were wasting effort. They needed a conduit, somebody to make linkage so there could be a cross-action. I told Karenga, "I'd like to meet with you. Talk a bit."

Unsmiling: "If you're sincere, meet me by yourself." He gave me an address on Central Avenue in L.A. just this side of Watts.

I rented an anonymous-looking Chevy and drove it myself, through parts of L.A. where I'd have been afraid to walk if I wasn't known. As I neared the address I began to doubt that the meeting was a good idea. It was a restaurant with vinyl tables. He was sitting in the back with three of his guys. Oh, great. But *I* had to come alone. The mothers were sitting there with "do's" out to here and beards and black glasses. I'm not talking about shades, I mean *black* glasses.

"Hi, Ron. Guys." Nobody's smiling. Nobody's talking. Grim. They don't stand up to greet me. They don't invite me to sit down. "Well . . . guess I'll pull this chair over . . ."

I can't even be sure they're looking at me, because you can't see an eyeball through those black glasses. These cats were scaring the life out of me. *Why do I do this? Why did I put myself on the line? I ain't comin' here no more. I ain't havin' another meeting.* Meanwhile, I was there and I couldn't just keep playing their game. "Hey, brothers, you think I'm scared of you?"

They nodded.

"Well . . . you right *there*." I grinned.

No response. "And you're not our brother."

Karenga said, "Mr. Davis, what is it you want?"

I thought that my presence had been saying, "I'm black too, let me in, it's cold out there all alone." I wanted to be called "brother." But their attitude hardened my fears into anger. "A bit of courtesy would be nice. I did not barge in here. Yes, I wanted to meet you. But you did agree, you gave me this address. I didn't stumble in here on my way home."

Karenga removed his glasses. "You're entirely right." As he spoke I heard an educated man. He extended his hand to me. "If we may, let's start again."

I said, "I just want to help in my way, what you're doing in your way, once I understand something about how you work."

"What don't you understand?"

"Well, bullshit aside, what's it for? This intimidation. Why scare everyone to death? What does it get you?"

The man sitting to Karenga's right, a lieutenant, said, "Fear is a necessary commodity, Mr. Davis. Far too little has happened, and far too little is going to happen until white people are afraid of black people for a while."

Ron Karenga said, "You know very well that many white leaders won't talk to a reasonable man like Dr. King. You also know that he has been holding back the forces of violence, almost single-handedly preventing riots, pleading with young blacks to pray in and kneel in, and yet some redneck police threw him into jail. In his own state! So there are a lot of us who feel that white people need to see militants with our do's and our black glasses and shaved skulls and guns and they need to hear us shouting 'Kill whitey' so they may be shaken up enough to appreciate the alternative, to think: Hold on. Let's get that nice peaceful man out of jail and see what we can arrive at."

I said, "I understand what you're saying but I worry it might boomerang. I know a lot of white people who are sincere about integration and equality. I'd hate to see them scared away, to lose their goodwill."

Karenga was shaking his shaved skull. "Job equality, housing equality, educational equality will never come to us from sincerity, because they sincerely don't want to give it to us. It's costly. They don't want to give up their job advantages. Et cetera, et cetera! Labor didn't make its gains on goodwill. Only the threat of a strike, or violence, or a riot brought management to the table to talk. So we intimidate."

"But why intimidate *me?*" I rubbed my face with my hand. "This don't exactly come off, y'know. I'm not Al Jolson."

"But you ain't black either," the lieutenant said.

I would have laughed but for the tragedy I read into the statement. "I've met some people who disagree with you."

He insisted, "In the vernacular, 'you *is* black, but you don't *be* black.' You married a white woman. You live in a white community. You're publicly associated only with white friends. And you work almost exclusively in white, even Jim Crow towns."

I almost said that it was none of their fucking business how I lived, but as I had gone there to understand them I had to let them understand me too. I said, "I married the woman I loved. Period. Okay?" They nodded. "I live in the best house that I have the money to buy. I was born in Harlem and I lived in enough second-rate hotels and boardinghouses so that now that I can afford it there ain't no first class that's first-classy enough for me. Dig?"

They nodded, this time less reluctantly, and I had the feeling that they hadn't understood that I was born in Harlem, that they were so young as to have started knowing about me when I was landing in the papers with Marilyn Monroe and Kim Novak. Like they could have believed I had been born in Beverly Hills.

"As for working places like Las Vegas: nobody in Harlem and Watts has offered me a hundred thousand dollars a week."

Karenga's stone face began to soften, slightly. First at the eyes, then around the mouth. "Well . . . you right *there*."

We talked for two hours and we made dents in our ignorance of each other. When I'd walked in I'd seen black glasses on blank walls, and they'd seen black skin on a guy who lived with white people.

I said, "Jesse's coming into town next week. I'd love to see you guys get together . . ." Obviously Jesse Jackson couldn't be seen with Ron Karenga any more than Shimon Peres and Arafat could meet publicly. "I'd be delighted to give you my home. It's private, all the security you'd want. I really believe you guys have to finally get together. You can't be fighting the system and fighting each other . . ."

When they met a few weeks later I had the good feeling that I had done something more tangible than just another benefit, or being seen at a march.

As I STEPPED out of the El Al plane in Tel Aviv hundreds of Israelis in uniform began singing to me. They had a red carpet leading up the stairs to the plane, a military band was playing, and I was so touched that tears began in my heart, coursed through my chest, past my throat, and uncontainably poured out of my eyes. I knew exactly why I related so strongly to Israel. I had come to the land of the unwanted, as *I* had so often been, and they were reaching out to me.

Years before, I'd converted to Judaism, attracted by the affinity between the Jew and the Negro. The Jews had been oppressed for three thousand years instead of three hundred, but the rest was very much the same and I admired how they'd hung on to their beliefs, enduring the intolerance, the abuses against them because they were "different," time and again losing everything, but never their belief in themselves and in their right to have rights, asking nothing but for people to leave them alone.

I performed in the Mann Auditorium, a benefit for the wives of soldiers lost in the Six-Day War. In the front row were all the brass, and in the aisles, in wheelchairs, were boys without legs. I did the best show that I have ever done and as I closed I said, "I am going to sing a song because I am here in this place which it represents, this end of the search for all wandering persons," and I sang "Exodus." I don't know where my voice came from. I sang like a cantor in a temple. And because Israel was not just a physical place to me, but something spiritual which had permeated my being, despite my throat being constricted, despite my soul sobbing, a majestic voice that I cannot call my own rang out through the hall.

The reception was backstage. I had brought half a dozen of my fancy eye patches for Moshe Dayan, patches with rhinestones on them, and we were doing lines with each other like "I'm so glad we can see eye to eye . . . ."

At the hospitals I went from bed to bed, talking to these nineteen-year-olds, singing to them. One of them, wearing a bandage over one eye, told me, "I lost an eye like you did, and I was really scared, but since I heard you were here I've been thinking that you made it with only one eye, that maybe it isn't such a handicap, so why can't I?"

Topol was there. He played guitar and I sang, and we became friends. The wards were small, so they rolled the beds out onto the sidewalk, twenty or thirty wounded soldiers, and I performed for them in the streets. After a day in the hospitals I had to get out and walk off some of the tension. The Sephardic Jews are very dark. I'd see a couple of them and I'd nudge Murph. "Look at the brothers hangin' out on the corners. Just like in Harlem . . ." We laughed and we both began feeling better.

By the time we left I had four lucrative offers to come back to do a series of concerts. But I did not accept them. I would return to Israel as often as I could be useful, but I would not take money.

During the flight back I thought about the boy who'd lost an eye, and I remembered when I'd been in a hospital for a checkup and a nurse had asked me to go down the hall and talk to a basketball player who was going to have his eye removed. I knew that there was a connection between my having to lose my eye and helping these kids. And more. Why had God made me so that people sit up in hospitals to see me and I can make total strangers feel better? It was a power and there was an implicit responsibility to use it, to use it well. But why was I given this? Why me? Not just the talent to entertain but the drive to work as hard as I've worked. Why was I not made to cave in, accept anonymity, poverty, second best? They seemed to go together, the talent to make it and the need to make it, so that the hard work was the only road, and *not* to have done it would have been harder still. God put those pieces together. Why? I knew that I was never really going to get an answer but I also knew that I'd better be aware that whatever it was, and whyever it was, I dared not just keep that gift for myself, because there is no way it was meant for me alone.

16

THERE ARE CERTAIN romances that belong in certain cities, in a certain atmosphere, in a certain time. Some kinds of romance just don't travel well. You can't take them out of their natural sites and times and transplant them. But where they were born, you hear strings playing and it's sunny.

With Romy it was that way. In Paris we would laugh, we would giggle. There's something about staying up late in Paris, drinking French 75s, being upstairs at the Calvados, coming down to the bar after dinner and the cat's playing the piano late, it was like a movie. There'd be a little mist hanging in the air. We walked to the Champs-Elysées and had the car follow us . . . there was nobody on the streets . . . a little drizzle . . . we walked to the Faubourg St.-Honoré and window-shopped and I felt romantic. I had the impression that it was a moment to hang on to because this was as good as it was ever going to get. In Europe I felt total freedom to be with anyone. Romy and I could go anywhere we wished and nobody raised an eyebrow except to acknowledge that we were two celebrities. There was never any thought of marriage. That was neither her frame of mind nor mine. It was just two people who had met and enjoyed the existence of the other, of being together, at that moment.

I was playing the Olympia for the first time and I was the new, hot kid in town. The new kid had been doing these tricks for more than twenty years, they just hadn't seen them over there yet, and for those three weeks I owned Paris. I had met Porfirio Rubirosa through Frank in America. When I got to Paris we used to hang out at a little bar, the New Jimmy, which Régine was just starting.

Rubi was the most elegant man I've ever known. It was easy to understand why the daughter of a chief of state and the heiresses to two major American fortunes had married him. He was charming, erudite, amusing, attractive, and without a doubt the world's best-dressed man. I have always cared about clothes, and I will go to any length to look good. I have spent fortunes on shirts, shoes, suits, hats, jewelry, walking sticks, mink coats, and every possible accoutrement to make sure that even crossing a hotel lobby I look and feel at the top of my profession. But the way Rubirosa dressed made me feel as if I'd fallen off a garbage truck.

I was impressed with the man's knowledge. He could put a reading on anyone. He would just trim the fat off everything. People would come in and he'd go, "Bullshit artist." He had unerring instinct. And he knew how to live with nobility and royalty. "Give them the respect they deserve for their rank, then we're all equals."

For no reason I was aware of, in Paris I just wanted to get drunk. Rubi and his buddy Jaime de Mora from Spain, the man who'd given me my pointing-finger ring, were dangerous friends. They'd say, "Have another one," and I'd start in the morning with Rubi before lunch with the salty dog. Jaime would join us and we'd drink all day and night, ending up at the Calvados and be absolutely pissed, but in control—until I stood up. When you stand up whiskey starts finding every opening where a vein is. It's like there are little men inside you and you hear "Hey, there's a spot here, put whiskey in there. Fill that vein. Need more whiskey . . ." "Whiskey coming, whiskey coming . . ."

Sitting at the table, shooting it down, glass after glass, being very erudite. "Yes, of course, how charming . . . amusing . . ." I was being just ruly enough to be company, entertaining. "Okay, everybody want to leave? Well, how 'bout a nightcap at my place across the street? Wonderful! Murphy, Shirley, did you get the check? Wonderful, mahvelous . . ." Then I stand up and it was ". . . bluh . . . bluh . . . bluh . . . Mrphy . . . Mrvey . . . Jerleee . . . Jawwwrgge," and you start to slobber and you go from a sophisticate to a fucking drunkard.

I could see myself doing it. I was having an out-of-body experience. Like I was watching myself on a screen. It was raining, five in the morning, and they were taking me back to the George V. Hours ago they'd locked the side door of the Calvados. By 3 a.m. I'd blown off four girls, called them all kinds of names . . . people had been going "shhhhh" in the Calvados, which I "owned" at the time. I'm sitting there ranting, "Mbrh, Shwirtw, lezavunuvr dringggg . . . ?" and not making any sense at all except every other minute out comes a dirty word, clear as crystal, "FUCK" . . . with clarity. "Mrveybby, lezavagdtm . . . MOTHERFUCKER . . . Rubbbbibbbabbe . . ."

They finally got me to the door and Shirley says, "Upstairs. Get upstairs and get into your *bed!*"

I got her into focus. "You don't want me to have any fun, do you?"

"You drank up half of France. Get to your *bed!*"

"No, you don' wan' me to have any fun at all . . ."

CATHERINE Deneuve and I were seated together at several parties as dinner companions. I liked her, but Rubi said, "No-no-no-no-no-no! Romy. Romy for you." It was not a put-down of Deneuve. He just felt we had a different sense of humor, or any one of a thousand things. Mainly, he adored Romy.

Romy Schneider was a fiery, beautiful lady. Odile and Rubi introduced us. They had a party for me and there she was. Rubi had known we'd have a line of communication. We looked well together. We were both little. Romy only came up to my shoulders but she had such great carriage that you'd think she was five-eleven.

ODILE AND Rubi had a chic apartment in Paris and a wonderful three-story home outside the city. His memorabilia, his photographs with celebrated people boggled my mind. I knew everybody in the world. But he knew more and better. His and Odile's bedroom was on the second floor. On the third floor he had a gym with a standard-size boxing ring and he'd get into it every day with a fighter who came over and they'd spar. He worked out regularly and had a good body.

We'd party there and I'd leave at daybreak to go back to the George V, or the four of us would be dining in Paris and then drinking until it was light out and we saw people going to work.

As we parted he'd say, "Meet you at eleven o'clock. At the American Bar. There's this café on the Left Bank where I want to take you for lunch." I'd leave a wake-up call and I'd struggle to get myself together and when I got downstairs he was standing at the bar sipping a Ramos gin fizz like he'd gone to bed before the evening news. You never saw a red eye, never puffiness. Impeccably dressed, the brown tweed jacket with the patches on the elbows, gray trousers, paisley shirt, brown suede shoes, argyle socks, and you just wanted to say "Fuck it" and go back to your room, rip off your clothes, and give up. Hanging from the bar to support myself, I implored, "How do you do it?"

He explained reasonably: "Your profession is being an entertainer, mine is being a playboy."

"Have you ever worked, Rubi?" and he shrugged. "When would I have time to work?"

As we lunched he said, "There are some nice people you should meet." He mentioned some journalists, some social celebrities, among them Martine and Patrick Guerrand-Hermès and Yves Piaget. "These are good people. Don't waste yourself on shit." And he steered me away from others. I had a lot of people hitting on me. Some countess would say, "Come for the weekend," and Rubi would be in the background shaking his head like "That won't be good for you" or "You don't want to know them." He would never sit down and say, "Now, this is the reason why I said this." That wasn't his style. Sometimes there was a nod in the affirmative. But most of the time it was negative. Which is a sad commentary on people.

The day after I met Romy I asked Rubi, "Who's the best florist in Paris?"

"What are you going to send her?"

"Six dozen roses." He was looking negative. "*Twelve* dozen?"

"No-no-no-no-no-no-no! Just one yellow rose. And have someone bring it in with a bucket of champagne."

I'd been watching all these Europeans kissing women's hands, so at what seemed like the appropriate moment I gave it a shot. Rubi shook his head almost imperceptibly. Later, privately, he explained: "Kissing a lady's hand is done more with the eyes than the lips. If you are being polite to a lady, if, for example, she is somebody's mother, kiss her hand gently and keep your eyes on her hand. However, if she is somebody's ravishing daughter, then you should look her in the eyes as your head lowers to her hand. If she is one with whom you wish to sleep that very evening, then also look her in the eyes as your head comes back up. But never bend more than a little way. Always raise her hand to your lips."

When not being avuncular Rubi was a shit disturber. He loved to start arguments, get people fighting. "You know what Romy said about you? She doesn't like the grease in your hair. She'd like your hair to be very short."

Romy had a marvelous apartment that was a fifteen-minute drive from the George V. And the way they drive in Paris that's a long way out. I know because I walked it. We had an argument one night and I said, "Oh, yeah? Well, to hell with you." My whiskey told me, "Walk out and slam the door behind you. Show *her!*" One of those suave moves. I walked out into the darkness. She called after me, "Let me ring for a cab."

"No-no-no-no. I'll find my way." And there I was by myself, in the dark on the outskirts of Paris. Never walk out of a place at night in Paris or anywhere without the car waiting. Do it and you're alone. Only Fred Astaire can do that, with a cast of thousands.

We liked the Calvados, and we liked calvados. Toward the end of one evening she said something which made me suddenly realize: "Sometimes you've got no fucking sense of humor."

She glared at me. Lengthy silence. The evening was over. Going downstairs, I decided to kick her. It seemed to me, at that moment, that anybody with no sense of humor required a good kick in the ass. I missed her completely and my body followed my foot and rolled down to the bottom of the stairs. Being totally drunk, I didn't try to protect myself and didn't break anything. I just rolled to the bottom like a basketball. When I got there and the sound of my fall had subsided, I heard her laughing. I stared up at her. She laughed harder, till she was ringing.

Those three weeks with Romy were irreplaceable. I felt like we were living inside a marvelous romantic movie in which I was a duke or a prince and the world was mine. We were together at other times, in other places, but it was never so good. That first, wonderful time was a part of being in Paris, the fun of knowing Rubi, of not being stared at, of briefly being without complications, of being on the rebound and ready to be in love with her in that setting, at that moment.

IN LONDON every day was like going into Tiffany's or Cartier's, it was "What's going to happen today that's new and glittery and shiny and bubbly?" and push all the shit behind you, guilt from a failed marriage, three children with a sometime father, being broke, the wearisome fact of being black in a white world—push all that shit behind you, to be handled some other time.

I was appearing at the Palladium, and staying at the Mayfair Hotel, in the Maharajah Suite. After the show it was supper at the White Elephant or La Terrazza. Since I'd been going to England the Elephant was a home base. I was there almost every night with my British friends, actors, writers, and composers.

Most afternoons were devoted to styling myself for the act. I was getting my gear at Mr. Fish on the King's Road, where Mick got his stuff. Everything was one of a kind. I had the long coats, beaded jackets, bell-bottoms, big puffed sleeves, military braid, beads from Carnaby Street, and the paisley shirts. My Nehrus came from France. Onstage I was wearing skintight solid-color jumpsuits with low-slung belts that hit below the waist. I had one made by Cartier and another by Hermès and they were a glittering offset.

After I got off at the Palladium I hung out with Jimi Hendrix and Mama Cass. In London I was King of the Mountain in my sphere, and they were hot as a pistol. Mama Cass would smoke joints and take pills, that's all that was visible. She was giggly and fun, as opposed to someone who's svelte and great-looking and is getting hit on. Nobody was hitting on Mama Cass, so as a result she was the running buddy, that was her protective covering, to be laughs and fun so you always wanted her in your company. Jimi Hendrix was moody and impressed with self. He didn't show up except at the smaller gatherings. He'd have his own little group of flower kids around him, sitting in a ring at his feet, and he'd have his guitar and he'd be playing or listening to music, holding court. My London scene was: Mama, Jimi, Blood, Sweat and Tears, Evie and Leslie Bricusse, Anthony Newley, Georgia Brown, and the actors Olivier, O'Toole, Finney, Dudley Moore.

Roger Miller had written "England Swings Like a Pendulum

Do" and we went to his disco and it was the chicks with the micro-miniskirts and the leather dresses with cutouts at the waist and around the chest. Sundays at lunch we went to Alvaro's on the King's Road, Sibyl's, and it was loose, cats would be smoking shit, but you didn't see anything heavy. Even cocaine was hard to get there at the time. They'd bring in the Jamaica grass and that was supposedly very heavy. I was drinking. I'd take a few pokes of a joint and sit around and talk music.

The sound that was going on in England turned my head around professionally. It was good music, and I got especially hung up on what Blood, Sweat and Tears were doing. It was also the time of Jimmy Webb and "MacArthur Park." He'd hang with us a lot. Richard Harris had his big hit with "MacArthur Park." As I'm prone to do, I fell headlong into that "England sound," as I had with the "gear," and incorporated it all into my shows: the paisley shirts and beads, the whole Carnaby Street look; "Spinning Wheel," "You Make Me So Very Happy." That was what the sixties looked and sounded like to me.

While I was in London, an American magazine published a cartoon of a portly, elderly man bulging out of a jumpsuit and his matronly wife looking at him critically: ". . . because you're sixty-five, you're a meat packer, and you're *not* Sammy Davis, Jr."

I remembered a line that Robert Sylvester had written in the early fifties in the New York *Daily News* when we opened at Bill Miller's Riviera: "God made Sammy as ugly-looking as He could and then hit him in the face with a shovel." Fifteen years go by and suddenly I remember that. I hadn't been aware of hating it at the time, because the important part then was that it was a fantastic review of our act. But I guess it had cut deep for it to stick that long and I wondered if Sylvester had imagined how much those words could hurt. Probably not. Nor could that artist imagine how happy his cartoon was making me—the image which was what I'd have ordered.

I ran into Tom Jones during supper at the Elephant. I was going to be doing his TV special. We were a good personality combination; we'd do the bumps and grinds together. "I'd like you to sing 'Bojangles,' " he said.

"Mr. Bojangles" was written by Jerry Jeff Walker, who had a hit on it. Neil Diamond had a hit on it, and the Nitty Gritty Dirt Band had a hit on it. At the studio when Tom's manager brought up the subject I said, "I can't do that song. I hate it." I wanted nothing to do with it, with the character. It was the story of a dancer who became a drunk, a bum, and he died in jail. The name "Bojangles" had nothing to do with Bill "Bojangles" Robinson, who never went to jail, was never a drunk, retired rich, and died popular. The song spooked me. I had seen too many performers who'd slid from headlining to playing joints, then toilets, and finally beer halls and passing the hat, reduced to coming backstage to see the star, their pants pressed on a hot electric light bulb, but with frayed collars and cuffs, and asking, "C'n you lend me some money . . . for grits . . ." Now here comes a song about that kind of a man.

The song was my own nightmare. I was afraid that was how I was going to end. The juxtaposition of the front, the glamour— "He owns the *world*"—but in my mind I'm worried that twenty years from now I'll wind up with those frayed collars and cuffs. How not? How long before the road tilts downward and then there's nothing coming in to pay for it, to keep that ball rolling, to keep up the front?

"I don't want to touch that song." They kept insisting, so I said, "Tom, you sing it and I'll act it." And working with his choreographer, we devised a way that I could do movements to show the young guy at the beginning, lithe, a dandy—then, by the end, old and doddering, drunk and pathetic, while Tom was in a jail set, singing that song about him.

The first time we ran through it for the camera with lights and costumes the normally half-interested crew dropped their props, the cables, whatever they were holding, and applauded. The producers and director went bananas, coming out of the control room to rave about the number.

Tom said, "Sam, it's a natural. Sing it too. Take the whole number. Believe me, it's great."

As I'd finished the moves, playing this tragic, depressing, dead-legged old sot, I was more convinced than ever that I didn't want to get stuck with such a dramatic downer. My career, my mood was up here and the number was on the ground. No way was I going to be telling people, "Look, here's where I'm going, into the toilet." I walked away from the conversation. "I'm not singing that song."

At times I felt that I could live the rest of my life in London. Part of the charm of Europe is that once you are something special you remain something special, they want to come back and see you do what they've seen you do always. And they will make the effort to keep you alive commercially—design a new and fresh album cover, organize a tour of the provinces. Few American performers in America are "evergreens." You have your hot record, or you ride a new trend, but then the road changes and you're history: "It's over for him. Get somebody who's *now, today.*"

I would have loved the comfort of living in London, a town house in the Mayfair district, staffed, filled with the best, and a two-person elevator. If you wanted to come up to the music room you'd have to come up two at a time. That life would be like a permanent hot bath, but London was not where I could have made it as I had, it was not where everything was happening for me, so as much as I loved being there, I was glad when it was time to go home.

17

I WENT TO John F. Kennedy's gravesite at Arlington National Cemetery to pay my respects and I placed flowers at the eternal flame. Early in my run at the Shoreham I was invited out to Hickory Hill and it was a warm, family-style afternoon, with lunch served on the outdoor terrace, the kids falling out of trees, and a lot of good conversation, but nobody mentioned anything about Robert Kennedy running for President. The whole country was speculating about it but at the Kennedys' home, among friends, nothing.

After a few sets of tennis Bobby had gone into the house to shower. Looking for him, not familiar with the upstairs, I called out to him. A door opened, he stuck his head out and chanted, "Here come de Judge! Here come de Judge!" a catchphrase I'd been doing on *Laugh-In* with Rowan and Martin. It was invented by a comic called Pigmeat, but I did it on network television and it caught on and for about six months it was *the* catchphrase.

Bobby had changed clothes and was brushing his hair. I sat on the edge of the bathtub. "What are you going to do, Robert? Are you going to run?"

This was before the ground swell happened for Bobby. There was a lot of "Aw, the Kennedys . . . what do they want? A dynasty?"

"I don't know if I can get the nomination."

Disappointed, I said, "Well, if you decide to go for it, you know I'll be out there for you."

Ethel Kennedy came in to see the show with some girlfriends; Pat Kennedy came in a few times. One night Bobby and Ethel caught a late show and came backstage. I said, "Let's not go up to the suite, too many people and phones." I loved being with him and with Ethel. They were affectionate to each other, like two comfortable shoes together, not openly demonstrative but you knew this was as solid as rock. I also enjoyed being with them because Bobby was a marvelous listener.

Not satisfied with Eugene McCarthy as my presidential candidate, I said, "I'm sorry to be pushy but I really believe our country needs you. Are you going to run? Or what're you going to do now?"

Ethel said, "I wish he'd give you an answer, because he hasn't given me one yet."

"Come on, Robert. We'll all get on your bandwagon."

He half smiled. "Of the group I think you and Peter are the only ones who will. Frank and I still don't talk." Bobby had ordered a ham and cheese sandwich and a beer. He chewed slowly, took a sip of his beer, and as though thinking aloud, said, "It's such a tough race out there . . ."

"But come on, I can cover some bases for you . . ."

He had the habit of rubbing the front of his nose while you talked. He sat there listening to me throw out names I could get to help, rubbing a forefinger up and down the bridge of his nose. "I need some time, a little more time."

As I was checking out on my way to catch a plane to the Coast, Peter called and said, "Bobby's going to run." Then Bobby got on the line and confirmed it and I spoke with Ethel. "Sarge will be in touch with you."

Driving through Washington, passing Pennsylvania Avenue, I felt excited about helping to put another Kennedy, maybe even a better Kennedy into the White House.

It was announced a few days later, on March 16, 1968.

I HAD TO park on the street outside May's new house because the children's bikes were all over the driveway. There was a basketball hoop over the opened garage door and I noticed May's station wagon and visualized it filled with kids, going somewhere you take kids to. This was what she'd wanted. And I was happy that she had it.

May was in the kitchen giving Jeff his lunch. "Hello there," she called out to me, "we'll just be a little while." Tracey and Mark were in the backyard playing with an Erector Set and I sat down with them, thinking I could help make a skyscraper. The instructions said to take a wrench . . . I couldn't handle the wrench and a screwdriver together, I was inept. Worse, the kids were being polite about it, watching what I was doing, and smiling, politely.

I put down the wrench. "There's nothing I can do to impress you guys, right?"

Tracey giggled. "Try 'Birth of the Blues.' "

Mark picked it up. "Do some quick-draw, Dad."

My kids were ad-libbing with me.

I drove over to my house, into my circular driveway that didn't have any bikes in it. There was nothing to go into the house for. I continued around the driveway, out and over to the Factory, a disco that I had a piece of. I ran into a bunch of young actors I knew. One of them said to me, "Hey, man, there's a party, you wanta go?" Each of them had one fingernail painted red, an inside thing among Satanists to identify themselves to each other. I was curious. Evil fascinated me. I felt it lying in wait for me. And I wanted to taste it. I was ready to accept the wildness, the rolling in the gutter, and having to get up the next morning and wash myself clean. Whenever I had, being a bit of Dorian Gray, I'd looked at myself in the mirror and it was "Heh-heh, I got away with that. Now, what lies ahead tomorrow?"

The party was in a large, old house up in the hills and they were all wearing hoods or masks. They had a naked girl stretched out and chained to a red-velvet-covered altar.

I played it cool. "Hey, what is this?"

"We're Satanists."

"Oh, this is a coven . . ."

"Right. The chick's going to be sacrificed."

I'd read enough about it to know that they weren't Satanists, they were bullshit artists and they'd found an exotic way they could ball each other and have an orgy. And get stoned. It was all fun and games and dungeons and dragons and debauchery and as long as the chick was happy and wasn't really going to get anything sharper than a dildo stuck into her, I wasn't going to walk away from it.

One of the leaders of the group tilted his hood back to show me his face. It was a good friend of mine, Jay Sebring, my barber, who'd become famous in Hollywood. I'd always known Jay was a little weird. He had a dungeon in his house and he'd say, "You've got to come over, man, see what I got downstairs. I've got some real antique pieces."

"Yeah, Jay, I'll be over." Never. I never went there. But we were friends and often went to the same parties.

The following week I was playing San Francisco and I met Anton LaVey, the head of the Church of Satan, who warned me, "Don't get involved with this unless you really want to commit yourself to something."

"Oh, really?" First of all, I wanted to have every human experience, and secondly, all someone had to tell me was "Don't do it," so I had to do it. I came back from San Francisco with one fingernail painted red. It was weird and freaky. Notoriety, when it's a giggle, is fun. I enjoyed wearing the mysterious red fingernail. It was bodacious and shocking and I wanted people to know I could get away with it.

Murphy asked me, "What's the red fingernail?"

"Never mind."

I wore it every day, on the street, even on network television. Whoever didn't know what it meant didn't question it. Probably people thought: Here's a cat who wears beads, Nehrus, gold-embroidered dashikis. Why not one fingernail painted red?

Occasionally someone would understand and ask, "Are you into Satanism?" I played it misterioso. "Well, I've read about it . . ." It was a turn-on. The chicks loved it.

In my total, most swinging mood, in the back of my mind, no matter how gin-soaked or vodka-sopped it is, I always have an awareness of danger. I fought it with "I don't give a damn" bravado, wanting to see how far the rubber band could stretch, how much I could tempt fate, how close to the edge I could go and still come back . . . but something inside always told me, "Too far . . ." and I knew not to take that extra step.

One morning after a "coven" that wasn't quite fun and games, without anyone telling me to, I got some nail polish remover and I took off the red fingernail.

SEVERAL months earlier I had agreed to do a limited engagement of *Golden Boy* for Hilly in London. We were going to play a month in Chicago to iron out the problems, but we were rehearsing it in New York. I co-directed it, with Mike Toma, who had been our stage manager. With more than half of the original chorus kids back, and Lola Falana, and our bowling team all there, it was more like fun than work. On a Thursday which I will always remember to be April 4, 1968, we were onstage, loving the work, doing jokes, when Murphy came up to me. He was crying. "Dr. King . . ."

"Murphy, what is it?"

"They shot him. He's dead." He had meant it as a whisper but others heard it. I rushed to my dressing room and listened to the details being repeated on the radio. The kids in the cast had followed and were listening to it with me.

Turning it off, unable to stand hearing it repeated, I went back to the stage. Everybody was paralyzed. Then they started to react. One of the black actors said, "We should kill that motherfucker, we should kill all the white people . . ."

I snapped, "Who are you going to start with, the kids in the show?"

He stared at me, at the others. The black kids were glaring at the white kids. Half an hour earlier we'd been a family. Here are show people who've seen both sides of the racial thing, we're doing a show which is about race—if it can happen with people like this, people who've been brothers and sisters, then what's going to happen with the cats on the street, the brother on the corner in Harlem who's going to blame every white store owner?

I called NBC and got Johnny Carson on the line during his rehearsal. "I've got to come over and say something. New York's gonna blow up."

"You're right. It's happening all over the country."

I don't remember getting into my car, only arriving in it at NBC and going up to the sixth floor, thinking: *Don't preach, do it in Martin's name . . . remind them . . .* In the studio they were taping that evening's *Tonight* show but I was not kept waiting. Johnny introduced me, I walked on camera, and the taping resumed. "John, this is one time I'm going to dispense with the jokes and the songs. Ladies and gentlemen, today something tragic happened, a leader, a man who was my friend, was assassinated. The next seventy-two hours could mark the destiny of the next hundred years. I'm going to ask all good-thinking people, all the people that he tried to help, as well as all the people who marched in Selma, in Mississippi . . . if they would be kind enough to remember the man's *dream*, what he believed in, nonviolence. Please. We can't answer his assassination with violence. He had a dream! To destroy that would be the worst tribute we could pay him. So please . . . cool it, please, don't do anything! All my brothers and sisters out there: Don't do it . . . that isn't what the man was about . . ."

Billy Rowe, who'd gone with me to Selma, was waiting for me and we went to CBS and did the evening news, then ABC. I did the six o'clock news everywhere. As did every black performer people would listen to.

Then I went to Atlanta, to the Kings' house, and paid my respects to Coretta and the children. There was a cross section of people there, from the Vice President representing President Lyndon Johnson to senators, state governors . . . almost everyone there was a recognizable personality, yet everyone walked quietly in the shadow of the occasion.

Martin's father performed the funeral service at the Abyssinian Church. Thousands of people for whom there was no space in the church stood outside and listened to it over loudspeakers. During the eulogies I was thinking of the good times, the joy in the progress. Looking back brought the full-stomach feeling of achievement.

At the house there was a deep spiritual feeling, also blood-stopping sadness—everyone was aware of what Martin had accomplished and, tragically, but factually, that even his death would be a step forward with all those borderline people who would think: Hold it . . . that's too much. You don't kill such people.

Coretta was strong, gracious, going from person to person, thanking them for coming. Their children were brave. Martin's spirit was alive in that room. Andrew Young and Jesse and I were in a corner. We tried not to get mired in the tragedy we felt. We talked about the occasions when we'd all been together. Andrew said, "We have to continue what he stood for." "What're we going to do?" "We'll wait awhile, then all get back together and sit down and see what we have to do, which direction we can go in." "Yes," Jesse said, "they can kill the dreamer but not his dream."

WHEN I GOT back to New York, Sarge Shriver called. "Bobby said you want to help the campaign. We can meet at the Hotel Plaza, in the bar."

More than ever Robert Kennedy's presidency had urgency to me. Now Bobby was hope. If I were not already committed to a producer, investors, a large cast, and theaters in England and Chicago, I would have taken a few months off from performing and joined the Kennedy campaign full-time. I attended rallies, introducing him as I had done before. One evening we sat together and talked into the night, mostly about how to attract votes, but when we took a break for sandwiches he told me that he was aware of the risk of assassination, that he accepted it because of what he wanted to do for his country. And I, like everyone around him, was moved by his idealism to the point where I heard the drums, I heard the bugles, I saw the flag flying, and I believed—as I had never before believed in any political person—that marvelous things were coming, that Robert Kennedy was going to lead America into a new age in which all Americans would be free and rich and love each other.

CHICAGO WAS in the midst of the worst race riot in its history. Mayor Daley had instructed the police to shoot black looters. The civil rights movement was like dropping a piece of meat into hot fat . . . tssssssss. While the ghetto was burning we were fiddling with an interracial musical. Yet it was a bridge between two extremes of human non-understanding.

The Illinois and Indiana primaries were coming up and I spent every free hour campaigning for Bobby, often at fund-raising cocktail parties before the show. Essie and Irv Kupcinet gave one for Lakeshore Drive-type people with $500 to pay as entrance fees. I'd get up and say, "You know why you're all here . . . we need your money." It was very easy. They'd paid to get in and expected to give more. It wasn't fighting for your life like we did with civil rights rallies. We'd collect up to $50,000 plus the entrance charge.

Sarge Shriver would give me the list. "This is what you've got to do this week. Can you go to Northwestern on Sunday?" A faculty member would be having a rally or it would be a Students for Bobby Kennedy. Almost every afternoon I campaigned somewhere in Illinois and Indiana. I went out to the universities and talked about Bobby. I drew large crowds because my popularity was high and there was a known association with the Kennedys. The new young black voters were receptive to Bobby; his image with the ethnic groups in general was much stronger than John's had been; he had a deeper emotional key to the black people. I spoke to Bobby once or twice a week. He'd say, "Sam, you're doing a lot of good for us," and it was strength-giving.

At the University of Chicago one of the students stood up and asked me, "What about the Kennedys' involvement in South Africa?"

Talk about feeling hot and being brought to a dead stop. I said, "I don't know. I don't know what you're talking about."

"Why would you be with the Kennedys when Joseph Kennedy has been and still is involved with the government of South Africa?"

I listened while he did a dissertation with names of companies, dates of investment, and "exploitation of the black labor force." I admitted, "I did not know about that. But in any event that's his father. It has nothing to do with Bobby Kennedy."

"It's all the same money. Isn't it financing his campaign?"

He had me on the ropes. "I'm sorry, I'm talking about the man I know. You want to ask me questions about him? Fine."

Bobby called me that evening. "I understand you had a problem with one of the students this afternoon. Sorry you got roughed up. We should have warned you about that."

"It's true, right?"

"Well, Dad did some things that *now* we aren't too proud of."

THE DAILY papers, reporting the Chicago riots and beatings and arrests, with pictures of kids in physical and emotional agony, made me put down the paper at times to let my heart slow down and catch my breath. You can feel so bright, so tuned in, connected, potent, wise, but then you get cut down by wondering what you can actually do to alleviate the misery, the violence. I hardly knew about being black as they were black—the anonymity and despair, without the lifeline of talent and show business which I had.

I got Finis Henderson to take me to the black ghetto. As we walked he said, "Not that way. You can't walk there."

"Where can't I walk?"

"Down that street ahead of us. That's the Wall of Respect." He explained that the Panthers, the Keystone Rangers, and other ghetto gangs had established a spot past which nobody who was a part of the establishment could pass. "Don't feel badly, Sam. They wouldn't let Martin Luther King past there. Thought he was too Uncle Tom."

Martin Luther King an Uncle Tom? Talk about prejudice! And myself? I'd paid my dues with three broken noses and a lifetime of insisting on what I believed were my rights. Paid my dues? Hell, I'd earned a Life Membership. I didn't deserve to be an outsider. But I was. I was a member of the black race but not the black community.

A voice in my head said, "Fuck it, man, let 'em have their damned wall. It ain't your world." But another voice argued, "Don't believe that jive-ass. It *is* your world. It don't matter you livin' big, you *black*."

I told Finis, "I want to meet with the brothers . . . get to know them, let them get to know me. Not the leaders. I want to meet the kids on the street."

They came into the dressing room after the show. Four of them. Late teens, early twenties. When we were past the amenities I said, "Listen, I want to help. What are you trying to accomplish? Can you use some cash?"

They looked disgusted with me. "No, man. Givin' money don't mean shit. We can *steal* money. Steal the motherfuckin' money. We want your commitment. And we want it on a day-to-day basis."

"You got that. You've always had it. Listen, I marched in *Mississippi* in '66. *Alabama* in '65."

"Don't mean shit today. This is '68."

There was a time when you joined the NAACP and you paid $100 to be a Life Member and that was your commitment to race. But now, suddenly you're standing outside yourself, watching yourself walking along, and you believe you've done good work and you think: I'm a nice cat, and I'm walking down this road . . . and you look down and suddenly there's no road under you. You're hanging in air. Somebody put the road over *there*. And you hear "This is the road now, man. That road over there don't exist anymore." "But that's the way I always went." "No more. Road's over here now."

And the price to be on their new road was to be a part of what they were living through *then*. Wanting to help them tangibly was a frustration because there was no program, so they couldn't say, "This is what we want you to do." But they did want to know that

214

there was somebody in their corner who had strength, who would be supportive vocally and be there physically.

When they left I felt weakened by sadness, by my own impotence, and I thought: I should do my show, devote myself to helping Bobby get elected, and if that happens he would do more than a million hours of my rapping without direction. But that was "Let Charley do it."

Finis said, "The Commandos said they'll talk to you." They came to my hotel suite. They walked in angry.

"We don't like you," one of them said instead of hello. "You don't mean shit to us."

I understood that they were testing me. Was I tough? Strong? Or they had to show me how strong they were. I played along with them. "Then fuck you, man. Fuck you in the asshole. If you don't like me, then get the fuck outta my face."

"We don't need no nigguh lives with whitey . . ."

They didn't understand that I was thoroughly included in the hatred felt in Chicago for the blacks. During the show, sometimes I got booed from the audience and in the scene when the white girl refused me people would applaud. I had four security men, one private and three black Chicago Police Department officers, who were always assigned to me. But these cats didn't know about that, nor did I want them to if I was to give them any sense of support.

Another of them was staring at me, his neck craned forward, peering into my face. I looked at him, giving him the opening he needed. He shrugged. "You don't *look* white."

I don't need this, I don't want this, it's a bore, a useless bore. But then that other voice said, *No. You can't dump it. You might be of some help. You could be a conduit. To get some of the things told.*

"Okay," I said, "we can sit here for another hour and you can do numbers on my nose, and I can say 'Fuck you' right back, but then in a few weeks I pack my bags and I'm gone. I'll be in England. That's so far away they don't even know what chitlins is. But you gonna still be right here. Now you can use me while you got me, or you can waste me while you got me."

We started rapping. In reality everything about their lives was a problem. They had no homes, few jobs, and they had a major alienation between them and the white power structure even before the riots had begun. It was the cause of the riots.

"Well, now that we burned down the shit we been livin' in, what we want is for you to go tell 'em t'build first-class apartment buildings for us like they got over on Southshore Drive."

"Wait, wait, wait, hold it," I said. "You ain't never gonna get that. And I ain't gonna *do* that. Them cats on Southshore earned their bread and they saved their bread and that's what you gotta do if you wanta live like that."

"Save money? Shee-uht! We don't even have a Rexall in the neighborhood. How come we can't get a Safeway over there?"

I said, "Because the man ain't gonna come and build a thing for you motherfuckers to burn down again. He ain't just gonna keep buildin' up stuff. And we burnin' it down."

"Well . . . you right there . . ."

"So don't even ask about that stuff. There's certain things we can ask. I'll ask *for* you. But the man ain't stupid. I'll put you together with him . . ."

"We don't wanta meet with the motherfuckers."

"Okay, don't meet with them." I mentioned the name of the publisher of a major black newspaper. "Let me get you with him."

"Shee-uht. Ain't meetin' with no jive-ass motherfucker."

We had all gone from Negroes to blacks but there still wasn't black unity. There was no trust among blacks. I used to say onstage, "For all my brothers and sisters . . . and my cousins . . ." There was a *need* for "brother," for the black handshake, the locked thumbs. It was a search for trust, identity. You had to know: "Yeah, we're all in this boat together."

BOBBY WON the Indiana primary over Eugene McCarthy. It broke my heart that I couldn't campaign for him in California, my stronghold, but I was going to be in London doing *Golden Boy*.

On the day we were leaving I called to say goodbye and Bobby said, "I'm sorry you can't be with us to the end. If we're lucky enough to win, it won't seem right you not being there."

"That's awfully sweet of you to say. But I'll call you. And Peter'll call me and let me know what's going on."

18

I SAW THIS wild-looking chick in a long white evening dress, high in front, low in back, with ruffles. She was at our opening-night party in London. Her face and the shape of her head made her resemble Queen Nefertiti. I grabbed Shirley Rhodes. "Who's that girl?"

She looked at me like I was nuts. "That's your sister in the play. Altovise Gore."

"Alto doesn't look like *that!*" The part of my sister called for a nondescript girl with a dowdy hairdo who wears an apron-covered housedress because she's always in the kitchen.

Altovise was playing the role which Janet DuBois had played in the original cast. During rehearsals and in Chicago she'd come to the theater looking like the other gypsies, blue jeans, leotard. I respected Alto as a dancer. Few of the kids had her full classical, full jazz training.

I went over to her. "Let's go to my place and have a nightcap."

"Thanks. I don't drink. And we've got a show to do tomorrow." I liked her teeth. She gave me a shot with her elbow and laughed. "Tonight was just the opening."

"Hey, yoo-hoo, I'm in the show too, remember? And I'm not asking you to come up and drink a case of whiskey. Let's just get to know each other. And incidentally, I'm not Jack the Raper, you'll be able to leave when you want to."

"That's not what I've heard. They call you 'the Carpenter,' 'cause you nail every girl you meet."

"Get outta here."

I opened the door to the penthouse at the Playboy Club and let her walk ahead of me into a 280-degree view of London at night. It had the desired effect. "Heyyyyy! Oh wow! My God, this must cost a fortune."

"Not a cent. It's Hugh Hefner's and he's loaned it to me for the run of the play."

She had big, gorgeous eyes but they were like hubcaps now. "Right in the middle of London." She was nodding her head. "This is how a star *should* live."

Then, just the two of us sitting on a couch with that panorama of London before us, I got more of a turn-on looking at her. "How come you didn't try out for the original show in New York?"

"I was working down the street from you. *High Spirits*. I tried out for the London company because I wanted to get over to Europe and I needed someone to pay for my ticket."

"I think I'd rather have heard that the show excited you as a performer."

"It does now." She smiled and it was like fireworks.

"You're making a comeback."

She told me she was rooming in a house in Kensington with an older couple. "It's picturesque. You have to put ten shillings in the meter to keep the heat on."

"Kensington! That's a commute."

"I love it. I take the double-decker bus back or get into the tubes after the show. It's no problem, 'cause I don't hang out. I'm going with a fella in New York—he's studying to be a doctor."

She had studied with Katherine Dunham and gone to the High School of Performing Arts and Hunter College and was into theater and ballet and modern dance. She had a sort of worldly innocence, yet an acute Broadway theater awareness. She knew nothing about the early black show business that I knew, and hardly anything about modern Las Vegas. She wasn't in variety, she was in theater, but that she knew.

It seemed like no time at all had passed when suddenly she pointed toward the window. "Oh! Daylight. Dressed like *this* on the bus?"

"I'll have them call a car and I'll lend you some clothes." I gave her one of my Turnbull and Asser shirts, which was long enough to cover a pair of my pants which wouldn't zip up around her. She struggled into them, worrying, "Nobody's going to believe that we were up till this hour just talking."

Looking at her body, neither did I. That evening she brought my pants back to the theater. "I'd like to keep the shirt. It's beautiful."

I invited her to move in with Lola, who had a suite two floors down with an extra bedroom and didn't mind. Altovise and I flirted but we didn't date. She had her guy in New York and I was busy with Lola, who'd become known as "the Girl in the Golden Pants," plus I had a whole lot of London chicks who'd been waiting for me since the last time.

Outside the *Golden Boy* world I had my "upper social group," my pals at the Elephant, and my "lower social group," the rockers— Jimi Hendrix, Mama Cass, the new musical groups, guys from the Stones. They were the wild scene in London and we cooked.

I was still floating under about a bottle of vodka when I felt Murphy pushing my shoulder. "Sammy . . . wake up . . . Sammy . . . it's important . . ." I heard him crying. "It was just on television that Bobby Kennedy was shot. In L.A., just after he won the primary . . ."

Sitting up in bed, staring at the screen, waiting for a news report to come on, I was unwilling, unable to accept it. I could still hear Bobby saying, "I have to take my chances on being killed like Jack . . ."

The phone rang. Murphy handed it to me. "It's Peter."

I was afraid to take it. I didn't want to hear that from someone I had to believe. Peter was almost incoherent. "It's over. It's over, Charley. We'll let you know what we're going to do, but it's over."

He called back within minutes, more pulled together. "Sam. We need a favor. The press will be calling you, they know the relationship. We don't want it known until tomorrow that Bobby is dead. That'll give Ethel time to speak to the kids."

"Of course, Peter. And when you think it's the right moment, tell Ethel that I'm not calling her, 'cause she doesn't need that, but I'm thinking of her. Just remind her that Bobby is with God. Maybe He knew Bobby was too good for this shit down here."

I sat back in bed dreading the television reports, yet unable not to watch them. "He's obviously been seriously injured but we haven't any details yet. Senator Kennedy had just won forty-six percent of the vote in the California primary and was on his way to the pressroom via a backstairs pantry where the would-be assassin was lying in wait. The senator had just addressed an assemblage of his campaign workers, acknowledging his California victory, thanking them for their help. He said, 'I think we can end the division in the United States, the violence . . .' and he was shot within five minutes afterward."

I had to work that night as if Bobby were still alive. Then I went back to my apartment and watched television, listening to them say, "He's holding on . . ." I stared mesmerized by the ghastly front pages of the London newspapers, all with the same photograph of Bobby in the hotel corridor. A head wound. Like John. How were the family and our society going to survive this? Assassinations. Was it now worth our lives to be disagreed with? I was unable to stop thinking: Martin, John, Bobby. All the hope was being wiped out. With each one it seemed like another piece of you got broken off. Martin's death had been so bad, such a setback. But Bobby's might have been worse. Whereas Martin pulled us together and knocked on the door for us, Bobby had been close to becoming the man who could open that door. And he would have.

I CALLED MAY. "With the kids on summer vacation they could come over and spend a few weeks with me."

"I was going to take them up to Tahoe, to get out of this pollution, but London would be fabulous. I think Jeff is still too young, but it would be great for Mark and Tracey to be with their father, to see a different country."

When their plane landed the British customs people told them that I was waiting outside, and they cleared them fast. I kissed them both and hugged them close to me. In the car I said, "I love you guys and I'm so glad you're here. I miss you when I don't see you. I'm sorry that we don't all live together."

"That's okay, Dad," Tracey said. "We see more of you this way than we used to."

"Okay, here's the scam. We get to the hotel and we call room service and order whatever you want to eat. Tonight you go to sleep early and catch up after your trip, while I go to work. Then tomorrow we'll look around London; watch them change the guard at Buckingham Palace in the morning, then you'll come to the matinee . . ."

They were sleeping by the time I left for the theater. I went back right after the show in case they woke up. I brought some people with me and we were having a pleasant, quiet rap session, with the music going, but low, nice. The door from the bedrooms opened and I saw Tracey in her pajamas, looking at us. As I introduced her around the room I felt her drawing back each time it was a woman. The chicks upset her. Naturally. Here was her father, but not her mother, and a lot of other women. I saw the mistake and would not make it again.

I woke up at noon and realized I'd forgotten to leave a wake-up. Forgotten, hell! The way I was drinking I was lucky I'd remembered the bed. Since Bobby had been killed, more often than not I was waking up on the couch still dressed. I was grateful that some instinct had made me get to bed so the kids wouldn't come out and find me couched out in the living room like a derelict.

I put on a robe and went to look for them. They were dressed to see London. "I'm sorry, guys. I overslept. Have you had breakfast?"

Mark said, "Yeah, Dad. We called room service."

Tracey gave me a look and I saw May glowering at me. "It's time for *lunch* now, Dad."

"You're right. Listen, we'll catch the changing of the guard tomorrow. They do it every day. I'll dress fast and we'll get over to the White Elephant. It's a great restaurant and we can have lunch before the show." My voice was booming and cheerful. I was accustomed to feeling terrible every morning, but trying to conceal it from the kids made it worse.

That night I cooled it with the booze. But then I couldn't sleep. The more I lay in bed, the wider awake I became. I knew I'd be up until daylight and be a basket case for the performance. I made a drink and called Lola and Altovise to come up and keep me company and we watched television.

Tracey came into the living room, took one look at the three of us sitting together, and ran back to her bedroom. I went after her. She was biting her lip, trying not to cry. "I want to go home. You've got no time for me. I want to go back to my mom."

I got angry. "Well, if you want to go back, then go back."

Mark didn't say anything. I turned on him. "What about you? Far be it from me to keep anyone here against his will."

"Okay, Dad."

"Okay what? Are you staying or going?"

"I'm fine. I'll stay."

In the morning I was waiting for them to wake up. I ordered breakfast for them and sat at the table while we waited for it to come up. "Look, Trace, I was very wrong last night. I had no reason to get mad at you. I'm sorry and if you'll change your mind I really want to have you stay."

Looking at her lower lip quivering, I started crying. I took her in my arms. We were at peace but she still wanted to get back to her mother and I didn't blame her. Mark said, "Dad, I'd stay with you, but I don't think I should let Tracey go back by herself." I hugged him. I felt that I didn't deserve either of them.

I BEGAN hanging out mostly with my "lower social group" and got deeply into drinking and partying. I'd smoke some shit and take a hit and always I had a bottomless glass of vodka and Coke, anything to not feel anything. The partying was mostly at my place. These kids would come up and take their clothes off and sit around nude. There was some sex going on, switching partners, group sex, it was there to be had if you wanted it, any kind, any way. It was free-form, and when living got too depressing, hanging out with a group like that got your mind off it, for that moment at least it fogged your brain and you didn't feel so bad. Sex wasn't the point, though. *You didn't want to be alone.* Two or three people would get into bed with you and you'd fall asleep. You had physical companionship, that's what you needed, a quiet, friendly body lying next to you, and you'd sleep.

One morning I was standing on the balcony thinking that I'd gotten my mind off everything, but now the new day had drawn the curtains back and the sadness was still there. I smelled something cooking. I went to the kitchen. Altovise had come up and was there fixing eggs and bacon. "You haven't been eating, so you'd better have a little something . . ."

Altovise attracted me strongly, too strongly. She was too good-looking, too wholesome, fun, easy to be with. Too potentially habit-forming. I hadn't given up my wife and three children to fall into that lifestyle again. Get outta here! I was back and swinging again and there were only three people in this world who counted: Sammy, Davis, and Junior.

WE WERE in the middle of Act Two when I saw a man stand up in mid-theater and come walking down the aisle straight for me. He reached the edge of the stage and then climbed the few steps to get up from the audience. He walked straight toward me on the stage, put his hand in his pocket, and served me with a summons.

In the dressing room Murphy's face crinkled with sympathy. "Sammy, that's embarrassing, in front of your audience, to have a process server climb onto the stage . . ."

"Murph, it happened, it's over, it's past. Forget it. I'll call Harrah's . . . ask 'em to advance me a hundred grand . . . pay off the London shops . . ."

"But maybe it's time to change the spending a little bit, just for your image. We could work out an economy plan . . ."

"Sure, I'll walk around in last year's clothes. And I'll fire the musicians. Better still, I won't pay your salary."

"I'll take a cut, Sammy. A big one. Anything to help you straighten out."

How can you figure life, or plan it? You need a dresser, someone to pack and unpack and look after your clothes, so you hire a man, the years go by, and he's your best friend, your confidant. He signs my autograph, carries my jewelry and my money. Nobody in the world knows who I want to talk to and what I want and don't want as well as Murphy. Murphy's spent more time with me than with his wife. And he's got six grandchildren.

Now he was staring at me, pleading with me to cut his salary and straighten out. I couldn't stand it. I waved my hands in the air and shouted, "I've got no time for this, man, I don't want to know about it! I'll work and I'll pay off everything and fuck it, let's have a party."

19

I PLAYED A six-week tour of Europe and took Altovise and four other dynamite chicks from *Golden Boy* with me. Altovise was the mistress of ceremonies, she introduced me, and during my act she'd come on and hand me a drink, light my cigarettes, the girls would dance around me and do jealousy bits over me. From the audience it looked like I was traveling with my personal harem. When we got back to the States the girls continued traveling with me; it was a new look to the act and the raised eyebrows were good for business.

I think that so much emotion had racked my mind and body through the past year that what I wanted was either to get drunk and blur the pain of loss, to simply not feel anything, or to exaggerate life enough so that through the numbness you could feel and enjoy something, almost like sprinkling monosodium glutamate on your emotional system.

In Vegas there were three incredible chicks I was seeing, all featured in different hotel shows. They were with me one night in my place at the Sands. Just the four of us. As dawn was breaking, we were resting, drinking, having a couple of hits, and I was thinking, *This is the perfect lifestyle. Not only the physical joy of it but the kick of "He lives with three women." Talk about swinger images.* I said, "Y'know what would be wild? You move in here with me and we live together, we run together. We have an exclusive commitment to each other. And we keep it within the confines of us four, absolute fidelity, none of us goes outside of this."

They moved their stuff over to my place by noon that day. On our first night "at home" after our shows I said, "Hey, why don't you chicks ball and I'll just sit here and watch." You can get off on just the idea of the control you have with that. The off-the-wall physical delight of it was wild, sexually stimulating in the extreme. They went at it and I loved seeing it happen, I felt privileged to be watching those beautiful things going on, but after an hour or so I began waiting for them to pause so I could join them. I waited. And I waited. And I had the distinct impression that they were happy without me.

As I got into bed, by myself, with the three of them still together, I wondered: Have they fallen in love with each other and I'm out?

The next night I stayed away from the suite. When I got home they were each sleeping in their own rooms. I figured that if they weren't together, then maybe I'd been wrong. After a while I slipped out of bed and into one of their rooms.

In the morning, still half asleep, I got "Hey, how come you didn't visit *me* last night?"

It doesn't work because everybody gets jealous. You cannot eliminate the evil of jealousy. Plus, the commitment. I had a tough enough time committed to one woman, let alone three. It was impossible. These weren't little groupies that I was feeding. They were gorgeous, successful women. Always packing up and moving as I was, it couldn't last more than two weeks. Fortunately, it wasn't intended to.

That whole segment of my life was an effort to blot out reality, to prove I was a swinger, the life of the party. But the physical part of it, most orgies and things that you go to, I have found, most of it is sad . . . most of the games people play is like taking off the comedy mask and underneath it you see the sad mask.

All that wildness, all those laughs were like the shining silver and gold paper on packages, but there was nothing inside.

Only one promise fulfilled itself: when I walked onstage. That was like walking into a friendly home . . . like I could smell the food cooking. The feeling was so precious, so dear that you could wear it. I hated to leave that warmth. But finally, when the applause stopped and the curtain fell and the lights went on, when the people went out to gamble and there were only empty tables with empty glasses, what could I do then? So I tried not to let them leave. I stretched shows from an hour and ten to an hour and thirty, even forty.

I was playing Harrah's in Lake Tahoe. The house didn't like the long shows, not for the cliché reason of getting the people out to the tables, but because they needed the time to break the room down and turn it around for the next show. When I stayed on too long the next audience was kept waiting outside. But there were nights I couldn't bring myself to break away from all that love coming at me.

I had my own Keno runner there. When you're spending five or ten thousand a day on Keno they give you your own runner. Great-looking chick, short skirt, long legs. I overdosed on every excess that fame or money could provide. I *felt* like a superstar. And I had all the cliché loneliness that goes with it, that *had* to go with it, but that didn't matter. The customers were standing in line to see me every night. That was reality.

May brought the children up for a visit and I took them to dinner in the hotel's Summit Room, which has a dramatic view of the lake. Tahoe is six thousand feet high and she had always loved the clear air there. She gazed out at the lake and the woods. "This is where kids should be living. Not in that phony Beverly Hills–movie star atmosphere. That's a shitty place for kids to grow up." She asked, "How would you feel if I looked around for a house and we moved up here?"

Her face and the children all came into focus, like a portrait of wholesomeness. Of course neither she nor they belonged in that atmosphere of "my daddy's over the title" and "my Rolls is shinier than yours." Beverly Hills is great if you're in the business but if you're not it's an oppressive golden ghetto. I said, "Whatever you think is best for them."

That night I called May from the dressing room before the second show. I knew she'd be in their suite putting the kids to sleep. "How about you? Don't you think you might get lonely up here? I mean, how many single guys are you going to run into living in Lake Tahoe?"

"I don't know. But it *would* be great for the kids." Then: "What about you, Sharley Brown? Are you happy?"

"The career is cooking, things couldn't be better."

"I know *that*. I meant your private life."

"May, we discussed that years ago . . . This is what I have to do. I've made my bed . . ." and at least there were a dozen chicks in it.

My suitcases and trunks went out early in the morning to Vegas by truck. Murphy had all the small pieces, my jewelry, the carry-ons. Holmes Hendricksen and Doug Bushousen, Bill Harrah's one and two men in entertainment, were waiting for me in the living room of my suite. They were unlikely people for me to feel so close to—Doug the outdoors guy who loved hunting and fishing, Holmes the conservative businessman, totally foreign to everything I was—yet we had a kinship. For a few weeks a year they were my family. I got out quickly. I'd said too many goodbyes to say goodbye.

The hotel limos drove us to the Lake Tahoe airport. Because we were flying in one of the Harrah's jets we didn't have to drive an hour down the mountain to Reno. The cars brought us onto the tarmac and up to the plane. I'd brought Shirley and George and Murphy and the girls with me. The Harrah's stewardess handed me a Bloody Mary. Flying private was a joy. No rushing to get there on time, it goes when you're ready. No check-in, no cats you don't know sitting around you . . . Yeah, if you're gonna be a star, be a star!

I WARNED myself: *You're not close enough to bankruptcy? You need to buy a private jet to get you there faster?* I was in Las Vegas inspecting Kirk Kerkorian's Lockheed Lodestar. It was for sale or lease. It seated twelve luxuriously. I was visualizing my name and caricature painted on the nose and the tail. The salesman told me how much it would cost to buy, but it was so many millions of dollars more than I had that I asked, "What would it cost to lease and operate this?"

"The overhead would average five thousand dollars a week, which would cover the pilot, copilot, hotels for them, servicing, insurance, fuel, airport landing and parking fees . . ."

Hell, I could give up Keno and have a private jet! What's five grand? I average a hundred thousand a week, I'm constantly losing time waiting around airports, plus don't forget the cost of all those first-class air tickets. I could bring the family with me; George and Shirley; Murph; Rice, my security man; even a couple chicks; save all that money and still have all the luxury in the world . . . I caught myself smiling at the salesman and the other voice in my head started in: *"You wanta put the stew in, stupid? Now shake the man's hand, say thank you, and let's get outta here."*

I went back to my suite at the Sands and paced the living room. *"You're not seriously still considering this???"* . . . *"Well, it would be a wonderful image."* . . . *"Get outta here! This isn't just self-destruct at Cartier. This is no swimming pool. It's the whole ocean. Five thousand a week, he says. But there's fifty-two of them in every year. Kirk Kerkorian's getting rid of it and he owns MGM, for God's sake!!! Now forget this insanity."*

I CALLED Sy. "Listen, why don't you and Molly come down for the weekend? I'll send my plane."

May and the children had moved to Tahoe. I told her, "Anytime you want to come down to Vegas or L.A. with the kids, or swing over to San Francisco for some shopping, just call me and you can use the plane."

It was time to discontinue the girls in the act. I do a single and once around was just right for the change. I finished it off gloriously. I had the plane fly Altovise home to New York.

A FEW DAYS into my run at the O'Keefe Center the kids I was hanging out with in Toronto brought me some brownies. I thought: *Hey, nice.* I was having coffee before the show and I had a brownie. I didn't know it had marijuana baked into it.

I did my opening number and as they were applauding I thought: *What a great crowd!* As they quieted down I said, "Thank you, ladies and gentlemen, you've been a most gracious audience. Thank you, and good night."

Going off, as I passed George he hissed, "Where you going?"

"To the dressing room, babe." *Damn! He's not only slow, he's dumb!*

He called after me, "You only did one number. You just came out here."

When I was in the wings and saw everybody gaping at me I realized George had been right. But it was too late to go back. What could I do? "Ha-ha-ha-ha, folks. April Fool." Also, I didn't feel so good. I needed some lay-down. I flopped onto the couch in the dressing room. Blowing a performance was hardly big time. And if I hadn't been running with those kids it wouldn't have happened. Nobody was feeding pot to Murphy, or to George and Shirley. I remembered that if you smoke pot and you drink something warm it straightens you out, so I told Murph, "Get me some hot soup, babe."

Wrong! It crossed my eyes! I learned the hard way that, unlike *smoking* marijuana, when you *eat* it something hot in your stomach gets you higher. I slept for twelve hours. Then I woke up and saw the front pages of the morning papers: "Angry Crowd Demands Money Back," "Sammy's Swan Song," "Poor Sammy One Song."

I played the last few nights to full houses, killing myself to do 120 percent shows, and I left the stage in glory every night, but nobody mentioned a return engagement. At the O'Keefe Center, if you're going to fuck up, do it right. They've never had me back since.

I'D LOOKED forward to getting back to L.A., where I had a week free, and I'd enjoyed planning parties at the house, being around town, in the hub. But my first day back I felt awful and slept around the clock. When I woke up, Lessie Lee made me a steak but I couldn't eat it.

"You wanta aig?" I shook my head. She eyed me bleakly. "Well, if you cain't eat by now, then you better get y'self a doctor."

Gerald Blankfort made a house call and took some tests. "Your liver enzymes are elevated. Also, I don't like the looks of your throat. Those polyps and your chain-smoking don't have a good future together." For the first time, someone explained to me how vocal cords work: "They rub together and they become callused, they develop nodes, and the hot smoke and nicotine will cause them to stay inflamed. Those nodes can turn into cancer. You have to give up smoking for your throat and drinking for your liver."

"I'm sorry, but this is not a moment in my life when I've got the desire to give up smoking. I enjoy smoking. And I'm not too worried about the polyps. I had them in *Golden Boy* and the doctors said the same thing and three months later I was singing better than ever."

"At least cut the drinking."

"Gerry, there is no way I can give up boozing. Not just for the pleasure. It's part of the image. The audience expects it. Take away my drinking jokes and that's seven minutes out of the act. And frankly, I just can't walk on the stage without having something to lean on. I always have, and I always will. I'm locked into it."

He wasn't pleased. "I think it's urgent that you recognize the fact that drinking has hurt you already and it's going to get worse. At least get off the treadmill where alcohol is a habit, a prop, and consequently a daily need. Like right this second, at noon. Sammy, you've got a good life . . ."

"Get outta here." Part of my life was fun, the professional part, often that was a *lot* of fun. But on a personal level most of it was very sad. I could remember saying, "Oh, fuck it . . ." a thousand times and never finishing the sentence.

ROMAN Polansky and his wife, Sharon, gave me a welcome-to-London party. I was there to shoot *One More Time*, a sequel to *Salt and Pepper*, with Peter and with Jerry Lewis directing. I had known Sharon Tate and Roman for a long time. They invited Peter and Jerry and our mutual friends to their flat. Later, after Jerry and the other "straights" had left, we had a little grass, a little coke, booze, fun and giggles.

I called Roman the next day. "Hey, what a ball we had last night. Till when are you guys here?" He said, "Sharon's going back tomorrow. The baby is almost due. I'll join her in a few weeks," and we agreed to get together around the end of the week.

The massacre happened three days later. The killers had tortured Sharon, then hung her upside down and cut the baby out of her womb. The London newspapers were filled with the devastation at her house in L.A., the slaughter of her, Jay Sebring, Abigail Folger, and others I used to run with. Everyone there had at one time or another been into Satanism or, like myself, had dabbled around the edges of it for sexual kicks. Hanging Sharon upside down to torture and kill her was highly ritualistic.

Two nights later the LaBiancas were wiped out. Nobody in Beverly Hills or Hollywood felt safe, and again it had the markings of the occult.

Peter and I were sharing a house on location, and as we read the stories and watched the TV news reports, he said, "We probably would have been there." That was our crowd. I knew that had I been in L.A. and there was a party at Sharon's I'd have been there. But something had saved me. The evil had missed me. But how close I'd come.

Work was the great lifesaver. You'd go to bed because in the morning you had to go back to work. You're on location, doing a comedy. You couldn't allow yourself the luxury of moroseness, of being down. But it was there, and though you fought it off, piling up sandbags to keep it back, at night it broke through and poured all over you.

BY THE TIME I got back to L.A. it was known that the killers had been the Charles Manson family. Friends of mine in the Police Department told me that Manson intended to kill two or three well-known black people and I was on his list. I hired a twenty-four-hour guard service.

Joe Grant, who'd started with me as a chauffeur–security man in *Golden Boy*, was running our office. Rice didn't want to travel anymore, so in London I'd used a free-lance security man, Brian Dellow, a white Englishman who looked like a business executive. I got on the phone and offered him all the money he wanted to leave London and come with me full-time. I trusted and liked Brian, which was important, because I planned to have him with me everywhere I went.

Then Jimi Hendrix died of an overdose in London. I had been with him two days before. It staggered me: while I was over there Sharon and Jay had gotten it here, then I got back here and Jimi died there. Six people I knew in that group had overdosed. The fear had always been getting busted by the police. Now, it seemed, *God* was busting these people.

I knew that I'd been pushing my luck at everything, stretching the rubber band financially, drugs, debauchery. Ten million dollars after I'd become a star I was deeply in debt. Okay, I'd been able to call Harrah's and get a hundred-thousand advance and pay off everybody in London, and I'd called the Sands and gotten another hundred-thousand advance to pay off everybody in New York, and more for Beverly Hills, but when was this going to end? I was almost forty-five years old. I had more clothes than I had closets, more cars than garage space, more jewelry, more everything if it could be bought on credit . . . but no money.

I offered Sy Marsh fifty percent of all my earnings to become my manager. "All I want is to get out of debt. We'll form a corporation, 'Sy and I.' I'll take care of the show and you'll take care of the business. I'm not looking to see how much money I can accumulate. I'm not interested in having them read big numbers over my grave when I die: 'Sammy Davis left . . .' I want to take care of my family, I want to go everywhere first-class and not be afraid to walk into a store or a hotel and have them say I owe them money." We were in my living room in Beverly Hills. "But you should know that straightening me out is a major challenge. There may be a lien on this room we're sitting in. Or if it hasn't got a lien on it, it's about to light up and say 'Tilt' because I honestly don't remember if somebody paid the bank or not. Now, that's assholian and I want to correct it, permanently. I owe a lot of clubs and my weekly overhead is $25,000 whether I work or not. I carry eighteen people. I've got three children and I have alimony. I've still got a three-way deal with the Will Mastin Trio. My father I'll always take care of, but Will's a rich man and I won't feel like an ingrate if at this point we speak to him about a settlement."

Sy paced the room. "It excites me. We could go into production, real estate . . . the potential is tremendous. But for me, from the point of view of security, if I stay with the Morris office, with retirement and stock I'll leave there a millionaire. Still, this could be thrilling. I want to discuss it with Molly first. Assuming she agrees, and I believe she will, if you'll let me do it my way I think I can accomplish what you're looking for."

"You'll have absolute autonomy. This will be the only ship that has two captains. One says, 'Good evening, ladies and gentlemen,' the other one handles the business."

He was involved already. "If we could maintain a reasonable control over your expenditures, we could build something, because as heavy as your debts are, your earnings are still greater."

"Sy, you decide what I can afford to spend and I'll stick to it. No charge accounts, nothing but what we agree on."

"How much do you spend now? Pocket money?"

"I draw $500,000 a year for fun and games." He sat down. "Sy, I earn a couple or three million a year, so I figured I was entitled to spend that, but if you think I'm out of line, I'll cut it."

SY AND I opened an office on Sunset Boulevard. I was playing Boston when he called. "Sammy, did you ever hear of some people in Chicago called the Commandos? And something called Sammy Davis Jr. Liquors?"

"Sure, babe, why?"

"Well, I got a call a week ago from someone saying, 'Listen, man, we need money.' I told him I didn't know anything about it, that I'd speak to you."

"Babe, the Commandos are some good cats I met in Chicago. They needed something to keep them off the streets, so I helped them to open a liquor store."

"And it's got your name on it?"

"Yeah . . . I think it has."

"Well, I just got another call ten minutes ago, and this 'good cat' said, 'Listen, motherfucker, you didn't call back, we're gonna come out and kill you, you white motherfucker.' Sammy, how much have you given them?"

"I don't know, maybe twenty, thirty thousand."

"Sweetheart, anybody who can lose that kind of money in a liquor store is a genius. We have to get out of it. Look," he said, "this is the beginning, so naturally cutting away the fat is painful . . ."

I knew he had more bad news. "What's up, babe?"

"Well . . . your plane has to go. It's a major drain."

"But it's a tax write-off . . ."

"The bottom line is it's costing you a quarter of a million a year after taxes."

". . . and my name on it . . . it's a wonderful image . . ."

"It *was!*"

"Okay, you're captain of the business. But it's complicated."

"Why? I've been reading the contract. It's a simple rental against purchase. We're only on the hook for this quarter."

"But there was a letter agreement besides the contract."

"A letter agreement? Where is it?"

"In one of my suitcases, I guess. But it says that if we don't buy the plane there's a quarter-million-dollar penalty, which is what they figure it takes to repaint, refurbish, redo the engines . . ."

There was a long silence at the other end, like the start of an ulcer. "Well . . . it still has to go. There's no way to survive it.

We'll pay it off somehow . . ." His voice came over stronger. "Listen, sweetheart, hang in, we're making progress."

Staying out of the shops wasn't easy, they were my natural playgrounds, but every time I felt like I needed a new watch I called Sy and he told me the right time.

I was playing the Deauville in Miami Beach but we talked every day. He said, "I've been thinking about things for you to earn dough without having to say 'Good evening, ladies and gentlemen.' Real estate and production have to wait till we accumulate some cash. But how's this for a 'gimme'? Alka-Seltzer wants you to do their commercials. One day's work a year for $250,000. Great exposure too, television, lots of print media. We can choose our day next month. Shooting will start at 8 a.m."

"Baby, my eye doesn't open that early."

"Sweetheart, if you were making a movie you'd be up earlier, every day for a month. Do it. This is a great deal. We're getting off the ground . . ."

I'D FINISHED the second show and was thinking about going to sleep when I got back to my suite, which was filled with my usual party crowd. The music was going, I had tables of Chinese food from room service and a waiter working the bar. Automatically I looked through the group to find the chick who interested me.

I went into my bedroom, took off a very expensive Piaget and put on a Cartier tank watch that I wouldn't miss, and went out to the living room. I sat down next to the chick and started in with the jokes. I got up and brought her a drink. At the right moment I said, "I've got a little present for you," and I took the watch off my wrist and put it on hers. She was enjoying the attention and I was being pretty fucking charming for that hour in the morning.

People were beginning to say "Good night" and go home. I could see them glancing at us and I knew they'd be saying, "They were getting ready to get into it when we left."

Daylight was coming in the window, we were still doing the waltz, and all I wanted was to go to sleep. I heard myself saying what I'd said a hundred times like this before. "Hey, can I see you tomorrow?"

I woke up at noon on the couch. I'd been running nonstop for three years since the divorce and partying had become a bore.

The phone rang. It was Sidney Poitier. He was in Nassau and when I said I was closing Miami the next day and had two weeks off, he said, "Then come on down here and get some rest. Q's down here. Bring George and Shirley. Bring a date. I'll charter a boat and we'll cruise and I can show you the Bahamas."

Ideal. Two weeks of sun and rest with George and Shirley and Sidney and Quincy Jones and their wives. Occasionally, in California, I'd chartered Duke Wayne's boat and I loved that life of bathing suits, sunshine, rest, booze, taking it easy. I thought of Altovise though I'd been trying hard not to. I asked Shirley, "Call and see if she can spend a week or two with me."

We sent her a plane ticket to Miami, then I had a seaplane fly her out to where we were anchored. It was a wonderful, lazy kind of a trip, lying in the sun, humming gently on piña coladas, quiet dinners, and easy conversations. Altovise was enjoying it all, being flown from Miami to the Bahamas in a seaplane, being my date, getting to know Sidney and Quincy, having a valid professional appreciation of Quincy's music, telling Sidney, "I loved you in *The Defiant Ones.*"

I enjoyed the fact that she was impressed and didn't take celebrities like "So what else is new?" She didn't have May's "I couldn't care less" attitude. She was taller than me, but she had a wild, full, in-shape body.

We were stretched out on deck chairs enjoying the sun. She said, "I used to watch you at the bowling alley Thursday nights. You were the only one who had your own bowling ball, and you didn't carry it yourself, you had a guy who brought it in and took it away. I thought: That's big."

The two weeks went by very fast, getting on and off the boat, giggles, silliness: "Shall we shower on the boat?" "Thanks, I'll just wash ashore." Walking down a street in Nassau, slipping away from the others to a restaurant, the fun of being by ourselves, all part of a normalcy I don't generally have.

It was 1970. I was turning forty-five and I had no complaints career-wise, I was cooking. But being with Altovise pointed up my continuing ache for a companion, someone to enjoy things with, to be amused by things that were our things and that we got a kick out of. Yet I feared threatening the image, diluting the oneness.

We were standing at the rail of the boat on our last evening when she said, "Did you ever wonder: Where did the waves go? They were here this afternoon, until an hour ago, now it's smooth as glass . . ."

She was describing my life. The turmoil, the running, now this period of calm that I liked so much, that felt so good. Moonbeams were lighting her face, her arms. Her wrist was bare and I imagined myself putting a diamond bracelet around it. Black skin is a great base for diamonds. That other voice in my head heard it. *"You must be losing yo' mind! Get this chick back on the plane to New York!"*

"Listen," I suggested, "my partner and I are taking over the old Cocoanut Grove at the Ambassador in L.A. We're going to operate it as Sammy Davis' Now Grove. How about coming back into the act and opening it with me?"

Then, when I took the act on the road, Altovise and I started dating seriously. Introducing her to a friend, I said, "This is my old lady." She beamed and waggled her head in wonderment. "When I was a kid going to professional school, you were the one we all talked about . . . Sammy Davis, Jr. . . . Now you're my guy."

I felt great affection for her, very protective of her. She was full of enthusiasm for life and she was great, great fun; unspoiled, thoroughly natural. She enjoyed my show business friends and they enjoyed her and I admired how in L.A. she'd easily coped with the uncomfortable spot of being the outsider meeting all the lifelong buddies.

I kept thinking how much fun it would be to take this child so steeped in innocence and expose her to my world, the dark side and the light side. I had the feeling that with her I could get myself on the road to a straighter, more productive life. And above all, I believed that I could marry her because she would enjoy being a part of my life without resistance to the way I had to live it.

I took Tracey and Mark and Jeff horseback riding at a ranch in the Valley, then that evening they came to my house for dinner with me and Altovise. When she excused herself from the room I told the kids, "I want you to know I'm going to get married to that lady. I haven't asked her yet. She doesn't know. I wanted to tell you first."

Tracey asked, "Can we tell Mom?"

"Of course tell your mom. She'll understand and she'll explain it to you."

I WAS SITTING with Altovise on the plane from Los Angeles to Newark en route to the Latin Casino outside of Philadelphia. We were laughing and giggling as usual, and I said, "Y'know what I love about you? You're the quintessence of fun." Taking her hand in mine, I said, "I'd love for us to spend the rest of our lives together."

She nodded dreamily, as though she were watching a movie and enjoying the love story, not realizing I was talking about real life.

"Altovise! I'm proposing! Would you like to marry me?"

She sat forward. She smiled like Roman candles. "You mean *us?* Yes. I'd love to be married to you."

I told her, "But no children." She was disappointed. "Darling, I've got three great kids whom I've neglected. Badly. I won't do that to any more. I know my limitations and they stop short of being a father."

"Maybe you'll change your mind."

"Know now: I won't."

"But you love your kids. I've seen you with them and you seemed like a good father."

"I'm not. Believe me. Taking my kids for a day here and a weekend there for an aggregate of maybe five weeks a year does not make me into Robert Young."

I wanted to explain my thinking on the marriage that I had in mind. "What I'd like for us to do is to be married but remain independent individuals. Married physically, but single mentally. I know that's a contradiction. People are either married or single. Well, I've been both and neither of them is perfect, so I'd like to try something else."

"You mean you want to be married but you also want to fool around?"

"It isn't the physical thing with the broads. What I *don't* want is to say 'I do' and automatically I disappear from the scene and someone asks, 'Whatever happened to Sammy Davis, Jr.?' and they say, 'Oh, he got married, you don't see him around much anymore.' I want to have a great married life with you but I want us to keep out front, in focus. I can't afford to lose that. I want us to have an open marriage. Naturally, neither of us does anything to offend the other. But we'd both have the freedom to have our lifestyles, we can each have our indiscretions, but no major infidelity, nothing to get divorced over. I want the legal thing of it, and I want you to be obligated to me, and me to you, but not too much too suddenly."

I called Carl Barry, the comedian, who lived in Philadelphia, and he arranged the license and we signed the papers, but we didn't have a date set. I didn't want a "wedding" with her parents flying in and my parents flying in and a best man and maid of honor . . . too much commitment to conventional marriage.

One morning, I was supposed to play golf but it was raining. I was drinking coffee and looking out the window. It was a steady, nice, springtime, green-making rain. What I wanted to do most in the world was get married to Altovise. I did the Mike Douglas show that morning and as we left the studio I told her, "Let's do it today. You'd make me proud if you'd become my wife." We were married in the Philadelphia courthouse at 5 p.m. As we left, there was just a bit more than a heavy mist in the air. I took her arm. "Let's walk in the rain," and it was refreshing and clean and it felt like a good beginning.

When we got to Rittenhouse Square and we passed Nan Duskin's I bought her a long, black-diamond mink coat and she put it on over her jeans, which were tucked into high boots.

Unable to take her eyes off herself in the coat, she said, "I worry that because I'm younger than you people are going to say I married you for your money."

"Don't worry about it. I *have* no money." She laughed. She was a great laugher. She sounded like ten bars of Beethoven. "It's true. And I probably won't have any, to speak of, for another two years. But after you're married to me for a while you'll stop worrying what people say because you'll find out they'll say *anything*."

It was exciting to see what happened to her when she slipped on the coat. All that money might smother or dominate another woman, but Altovise wore it like a star.

"You've got talent," I said.

She giggled. "To wear mink?"

"That too. But I meant for being the wife I've always wanted, the wife I need. I don't want a 'gypsy' or 'a nice little housewife' that comes to parties with me once in a while and they say, 'That's Sammy's wife, whatshername,' and she never has an identity. I want you to become a personality in your own right so that when we arrive somewhere it's 'Hey, there's Sammy and Altovise.' "

Happy, a bit self-conscious, she swirled the coat around her, then sidled up to me and, opening the coat, closed it around me. Being taller than me, she spoke through the neck opening, like into a funnel. "Aren't you worried I might upstage you?"

I got out of the coat and smiled, pleased with her. "Definitely try to upstage me. 'Cause you ain't never going to be able to do it."

"You mean no matter how hard I try I'm never going to hear 'Hey, it's Altovise and her husband, whatshisname'?"

"Only from yo' mummy an' yo' daddy. But seriously, why should it be necessary to out-glitz each other? What about: we're in our car arriving at a premiere and the fans look inside and they scream, 'Hey, it's Sammy and Altovise' or 'It's Altovise and Sammy'? Let's develop a combination of two individual personalities!"

20

A REAL ESTATE broker showed Altovise and me some properties in Beverly Hills. It was a great September day, top-down weather. We saw a house that I knew well, Tony Newley and Joan Collins had bought it from Janet Leigh and Tony Curtis and it could be made into exactly what I wanted. "If we knock down that wall and that one and make a living room—den out of almost this whole downstairs, and use the upstairs bedrooms as guest rooms, then over there we could custom-build our own section . . ."

Sy looked ill as I told him. "Sammy, you've got a mansion, we're just beginning to get solvent."

"Please, Sy, I want to develop a real home with Altovise. The Newley house has the land we need. Bear with me on this."

"You've got it, sweetheart . . . you work too hard and you make too much money for me to deprive you of something you want. I can't say no to you."

I knew that because he admired me as a performer I could run circles around him, and I knew I had to be careful not to take advantage of that power.

When it was signed and sealed, Alto and I stood in the driveway that I had first driven into over twenty years earlier and I told her, "It's a coincidence, but when I was just making it, in the fifties, Janet Leigh and Tony Curtis were already movie stars and this was their house. Jeff Chandler was living then, and he, Janet and Tony, and I were buddies, *good* buddies. Except they were all big stars and I was a little black kid, with some talent and one record, 'Hey

There.' I always wondered what it must feel like to be stars like they were, to have a house like this . . ."

We selected an architect and a decorator. The construction was going to take several months, so we moved into a suite at the Ambassador Hotel.

Mary Benny called. "Jack and I would love to have you and your bride come to dinner on Thursday."

Altovise panicked. "*Jack Benny!* And *Mary Livingstone!*"

"Darling, relax, they're friends."

"*Your* friends, but they don't know *me*."

"They'll love you because *I* love you, so you open with kings."

"What should I wear?"

"You don't want to blend in like just another wife in a designer dress from Rodeo Drive. Let's keep your own free and youthful style. Be an original. I think you should wear hot pants."

"No, Sammy . . . please, these are older people, they'll think I'm a tramp."

"Not if *I* wear them too. We'll go in matching tuxedo-style hot pants. Trust me. It'll be a giggle."

Sy Devore made them for us and we tried them on together. I looked nice, normal. But she looked like fire alarms going off.

Milton Berle was standing near the front door at the Bennys'. "How does an old Jew like you get such a gorgeous young wife?"

Lucille Ball came straight over as we walked in, threw her arms around Altovise, kissed her, and said, "We're going to be friends, I hope."

Lucy and Gary are lifelong friends and I love them. She's the mother hen of all time. "What are you doing? Where are you going? How come you're not . . . ?" Gary and I go back to when he was the comic on the bill.

Mary and Jack did it for Alto in their way, with all the warmth in the world. All of that level of Hollywood society was there, George and Gracie, Mary and Swifty Lazar, the Nivens, Loretta Young, Georgie and Ricardo Montalban, and Frank, whom she already knew. Around forty people.

I had planned to stay close to her to give her support over the first few hours of meeting people whose faces and voices she had grown up with. But Lucy and Polly Bergen took her around the house to show her Jack's small bedroom next to Mary's large one, then brought her into conversation groups, and she was swinging without me; she was laughing, they were all laughing, she'd won everybody over.

In the car I squeezed her hand. "I was proud of you."

She was high on success, rattling on. "Lucy said I should call her and that when you're out of town I should hang out with her and Gary."

"Well, do it. They're wonderful people."

"And Janet Leigh said she wants to propose me for SHARE? Isn't that a charity?"

"Yes, for retarded children. A serious charity. You should join SHARE. Those women are your peers in this town. And you'd be the first black woman ever to be a member."

"Sammy, I'm a gypsy, not a charity woman."

"Don't be scared. Do it."

"How do you know I'm scared?"

"*I'd* be if I were you."

In our suite at the Ambassador she said, "You're going to think I'm so square it's embarrassing but I've *got* to call my father and tell him I met Charlie Bronson and Edward G. Robinson."

I hugged her. I was so pleased that there was no tug-of-war, that my wife was made happy by what I was able to give her. I said, "Darling, enjoy it, keep a little of the stardust. Maintain that wonder, that naïveté. Keep 'the little girl looking into the candy store.' I'm not saying that everything should be 'Oh, it's a movie star . . . eek!' But I want to always be excited that Mary and Jack Benny invite me to dinner, that I can talk to Fred Astaire. I love that I heard Judy Garland sing with Liza. Savor the moments that are warm and special and giggly. Keep yourself vulnerable to them."

It was fun for me to introduce her to this life which she'd never thought of or dreamed of having. I gave her her first car, a Rolls-Royce with her own license plate, ALTOVISE. She drove it in a circle around the Ambassador's driveway. Breathlessly she got out and hugged me and kissed me, and grabbed my buns. "Y'wanta fool around a little, honey?" and she ran upstairs to tell her mother in New York.

I hadn't anticipated the Daddy Warbucks syndrome, the pleasure derived from being able to give her expensive things. I could never get that with May. If I had put May's name on her license plate it would have embarrassed her. And so would a Rolls. She preferred a station wagon with the kids piled in. May's values were what the world considered better. But Altovise enjoyed and adapted to *my* values.

I loved the image of her shopping on Rodeo or going to lunch at the Bistro Garden, arriving with the right equipment. Granted that status symbols are out of all proportion in Beverly Hills, that it shouldn't be that way—but it *is*, and if she was going to become a part of the Beverly Hills world, then I was delighted that I could provide the right wardrobe and props, and that Alto was tickled to be given them.

I was on the Johnny Carson show and I mentioned "my wife Altovise . . ."

He gave me a look. "Anchovies?"

"Get outta here, John. Alto-vise . . . it means high view." I liked talking about her. No black performer ever before had gotten on television and talked about his wife. Yet everybody knows that Bob Hope's wife is Dolores.

I DROPPED in on our office, a suite of four rooms on Sunset Boulevard in Hollywood. Sy said, "It bugs me that we aren't making any money in the record business." He got up from his desk and was pacing around the office and I thought he was too high-energy to be held down by a desk, he should just have a portable phone. "Sweetheart, we should get away from Reprise–Warner Bros. and go with the best. I had a talk with Berry Gordy and he was very excited by the idea. He said, 'It would be great to have the world's number one recording company, which is black, sign the number one entertainer in the world, who also is black."

Berry's Motown label was releasing people like the Supremes and the Temptations. He practically owned the top of the charts. We had a press conference to announce that I had signed with Motown, and Berry said, "I believe I can make Sammy Davis the world's biggest recording star." I set aside two weeks for the record sessions and we made two albums. Then they released the first album and it did nothing. Maybe the best stuff was on the second album.

JACK ENTRATTER had died. The Sands had become a Howard Hughes hotel, although HH remained the town's Invisible Man. After the opening one of his guys came back and said, "Mr. H.

wanted you to know that he snuck in last night and saw the show from the back and thought you were great."

Altovise came down for the weekend with fabric swatches and about a hundred pounds of wood samples for the floors and marble for our bathroom and filled me in on the progress. "Lots of hammering and sawing and dust. I love it."

Driving to the opening of a new shopping mall, she turned on the radio. "I keep listening . . . when's the second album coming out?"

"Great question."

Sy went over to see Berry Gordy. "When are you going to release the next album?"

Berry began hedging. "Well, my men out in the field don't think he's got the Motown sound."

"Certainly he hasn't. Sammy sings ballads."

"I'm sorry, but it turns out that it's not the material we're capable of releasing successfully."

Sy reported it to me by phone, spluttering angrily, disbelieving. But I could easily believe it. Ballad singers were in trouble, with few exceptions. The money was so great in rock 'n' roll that the record companies weren't bothering to promote and distribute a ballad singer because the stores wouldn't give us shelf space. *But* why hadn't Motown thought of that before taking bows with the press, investing a half million dollars in two albums, and wasting a lot of my time?

Sy was thinking out loud. "Berry Gordy's not going to want people to think that he lost Sammy Davis. Hang on, sweetheart, we're not going to leave there with nothing."

He went to see Berry and said, "I, Sy Marsh, not Sammy Davis, but I personally am going to tell the press that Sammy went with Berry Gordy in good faith, that he recorded two full albums of material which you selected, and now half of all that artistic effort will not be released because Berry Gordy later decided that 'this is not the Motown sound,' like Berry Gordy had never heard Sammy Davis, Jr.'s sound."

"Sy, why would you do something like that?"

"Or you can give me all the unreleased material, all the tapes, and I won't even announce that we severed the relationship. We'll just ease out of it."

"Sy! We're talking a quarter-million-dollar investment."

"*You* are talking investment in tapes that are worthless to you. *I* am talking about the world's greatest entertainer who worked for nothing for two solid weeks. He could have made nearly half a million in Vegas in that time. Instead he made records you're not going to release."

Berry called Sy in a few days. "Draw up the papers. You get all the material and you're out quietly."

In the meanwhile Sy was in touch with Mike Curb, who was the new "hottest record producer in town" and had just been made president of MGM Records. Sy confided to him, "We're under contract to Motown but it's the wrong operation for Sammy. If you'd be interested I'll get out of the Motown deal."

"I'm more than interested. I definitely want Sammy Davis."

Sy flew down to Vegas to tell me. I hated the idea. "Mike Curb? That cat's square, white bread."

He shrugged off what I said. "What's the difference? The important thing is that when I negotiate the contract I'll make a deal with MGM to release our Motown tapes for just a distribution fee. They'll do it 'cause they've got no investment to make back. Which means that instead of a five percent royalty, sweetheart, we'll get sixty percent." He returned to L.A. and called me the next day, gleeful. "Sweetheart, I made the release deal for the tapes, and with the lion's share like we've got, if the album does anything at all we'll make like three million on it. And they're excited about you coming in to record. In fact, Mike's got a single that he did an instrumental on with the Mike Curb Congregation. He said, 'If Sammy would put his voice on it I think it would be great.' He says you've got the youth and exactly the right cuteness about you."

"What's the name of it?"

" 'The Candy Man.' "

"*What?* 'The *Candy* Man'?"

"Something like that. Tony Newley and Leslie Bricusse wrote it for a movie with Disney or something."

"I've heard the song. It's horrible. It's a timmy-two-shoes, it's white bread, cutems, there's no romance. Blechhh!"

Sy was getting nervous. "Sweetheart, please—don't make waves. The important thing is that they release your Motown album. You've got to record with Mike Curb's Congregation. You've got to do 'The Candy Man.' "

"Get outta here. Can you imagine me, a swinger, a cat that's done everything ninety-two times around the pike, and I'm gonna sing to kids? Like I'm Julie Andrews? Who's gonna buy this? It's stupid. Blechhhh, blechhhh, blechhhh."

He placated: "Who cares nobody'll buy it? The important thing is don't rock the boat so they release the stuff we've got from Motown. That album is gonna buy us an office building that we'll live on for the rest of our lives."

I hated it but I agreed. When I got back to L.A., Sy went with me to the MGM recording session. I looked at the lead sheet for 'The Candy Man,' forced a smile at everybody, and we did it in one take. I went into the control room to listen to the playback. It was icky cute. I glared at Sy. He smiled back like "So what?"

Mike Curb said, "Sammy, could you put in a couple of di-ah-do-ah's . . . ?"

"A couple of what?"

"Just some ad-libbing in the middle . . . 'cause I have to bring in the Congregation behind you."

I smiled like sugar, like a candy man, and I went out to the studio and did it again, this time with some di-ah-do-ah's. Then I listened to the playback. Mike Curb was looking delighted. I elbowed Sy and hissed, "This record is going straight into the toilet. Not just around the rim, but into the bowl, and it may just pull my whole career down with it."

"Sweetheart . . . so you invested a little time . . . mainly what we want is for them to release . . ."

"Okay, Sy, we've done it . . . you've had it your way."

WE WERE moving into our new house the day before my birthday. Our two acres were surrounded by an iron fence and I'd hired a squad of five guards to patrol the grounds twenty-four hours a day. As I waited for the guard to open the gate I held my wife's hand, glad for the opportunity to linger outside thinking: *My God, how far from Harlem, the cold, the garbage in the courtyard . . . how far from Westside, Southside, and wrong side.*

Altovise guided me through the house. The floors of the living room, dining room, and entrance hall were beautifully polished wood. The living room–den had a cozy sunken conversation pit, and the bar had comfortable swivel armchairs. Four sets of French doors opened into the garden. She said, "It's ideal for entertaining:

a lawn party, or something indoor-outdoor, or just for having the buddies over." Our projection room was built behind the living room and the screen was concealed by a four-panel mural. The hallway leading to our bedroom, with floor-to-ceiling bookshelves, had separate guest bathrooms for men and women. Our "closet" was a duplex pair of rooms. Alto was leading me around like we were on a treasure hunt. "Honey, remember how you liked the way Bill Harrah kept his sunglasses? Well, I borrowed the idea for you." And she showed me my collection of sunglasses on display racks like in optometrist shops. Upstairs in the foyer between the guest rooms she'd put my pool table and hung my gun collection on the walls around it. And half a floor below our bedroom she'd built an office for me with shelves for all my record albums and videotapes, and closets built for my cameras. In our bedroom the television set was hung just right for watching in bed.

I put my arms around her. "I love it all. And I love the lady who got it all done and is going to share and enjoy it with me."

In the morning the guard at the front gate called in. "Mr. D., there's a truck here and the driver says he's got your birthday present from Howard Hughes."

The men brought in a pair of new 35mm motion picture projectors. I called Virgil, my own projectionist, and had him come over to supervise the installation. When he saw the Italian projectors he got me aside. "Mr. D., these are the best machines in existence. Better than any head of a studio has in his home and better than any in the screening rooms at the studios. They'd cost around $250,000 if there were any around to buy."

I was stunned. Anything new had to be better than my old projectors, which were "breakdown of the art," but it was like when you think you've got a nice car and a serious collector sees it and says, "My God, you've got the XCLM II Mercedes . . ."

Alto and I had coffee sitting at the bar, looking through the wall of French doors opening onto our backyard and pool area. I opened a cigarette box. It was empty. I said, "This is not a Giacometti sculpture, so it had better function." There were three lighters on the bar. All dry. "Darling, I'll really appreciate it if you'll see to it that somebody keeps the cigarette lighters filled. There's nothing chic about a gold lighter that doesn't make flame." I softened it. "This is our home, let's always have ample supplies of mixed nuts, cigarettes, plenty of soft drinks. There's no reason for us *ever* to run out of *any* of the staples that we enjoy. Please keep us stocked on everything. I appreciate the monumental job you've done. I'm an ass to be demanding. I just want our home to be comfortable, luxurious."

"Don't apologize. You're right. And I want to learn." She pushed out a smile. "But I've got to admit that with my father being a career man in the Navy our home life didn't have much to do with maintaining 35mm movie projectors."

Late that week I got a call from Sy Marsh. "Uhhh, sweetheart, about your wife . . . she's a chip off the old block. I'm sending a messenger over with an envelope to show you what I mean."

The envelope contained a bill from Sey-Co, a gourmet shop in Beverly Hills. It was long and itemized: cases of caviar, gourmet potato chips, mixed nuts, pistachios, blanched almonds. $5,200.

I found Altovise and waved the bill at her. *"What is this, please?"* Not noticing the fire coming out of my nostrils, she showed me a closet overflowing with bar supplies and half a refrigerator of caviar. "You said never run out. I've also got three cases of lighter fuel."

She was in my league. I was almost proud of her.

I was opening in Tahoe in three days. The separation of marriage and career was working. We had a routine: I went ahead and, with the freedom to be single-minded, I got the openings and their peripheral chores behind me. Then Alto came down and we enjoyed the rest of the engagements together. I said, "I feel sorry to leave you behind, alone."

"Frankly, I need the time at home to get ready for the annual SHARE party. I'm on the Invitation Committee and we've got a lot of work to do . . ." She smiled happily. "You were right. I love working for SHARE. Besides, who's alone? I've got Lessie Lee and five security men. And I've got my lighters to keep filled."

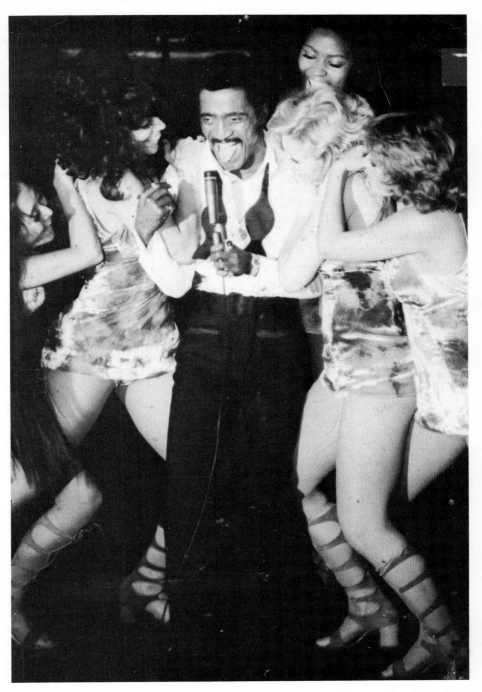

If you want to get known as a swinger you hire five sexy chicks and let them fight over you onstage and for the cameras. That's publicity, man. But you don't swing where you sleep.

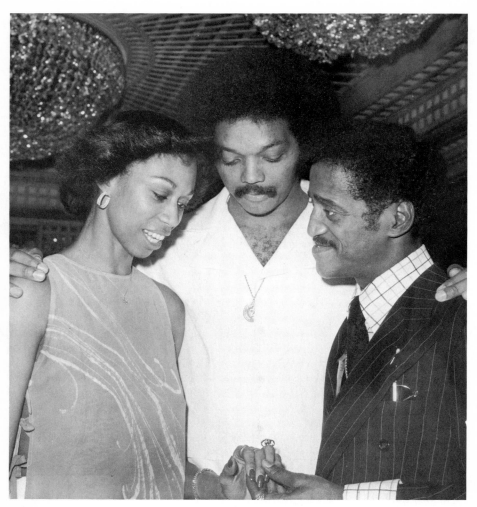

When Altovise and I were married, there were no friends or family present. After a few years, we decided to get our families and friends together, and Jesse Jackson tied the knot a bit tighter.

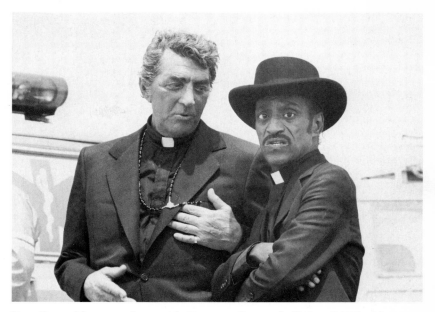

Burt Reynolds teamed me with Dean in *Cannonball Run* (1981). I knew it wouldn't bring me to the Academy Awards, but I needed to hit the big screen for impact, exposure. It doesn't matter that you're averaging $200,000 a week in Vegas and at Harrah's. Those places are wonderful but insular. Now, after fifty years in show business, what the kids say when they come up to me on the street is: "You were in *Cannonball*." That's the power of the big screen.

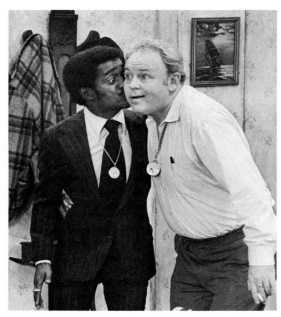

The longest laugh in the history of *All in the Family*

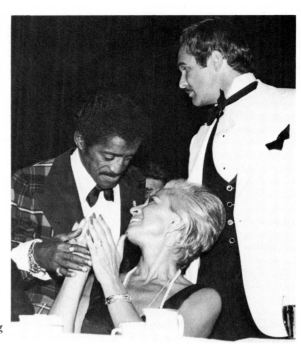

When Dinah Shore was going
with Burt Reynolds

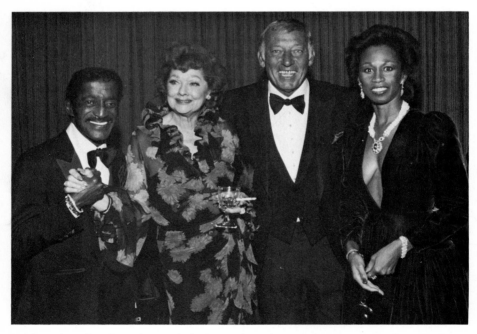

Lifelong friends. I love them. She's that matriarch type. "What are you doing? Where
are you going? How come you're not . . . ?" The mother hen of all time. Her husband,
Gary Morton, and I go back to when he was the comic on the bill.

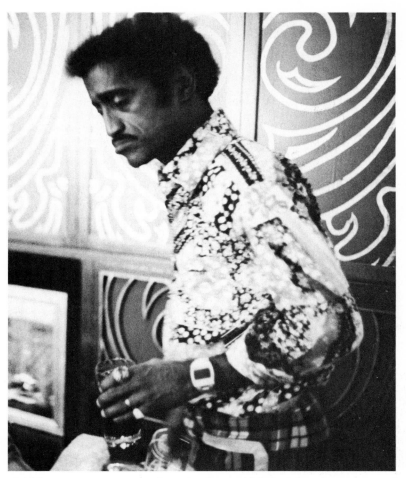

If I'd known I was going to live this long, I'd have taken better care of myself.

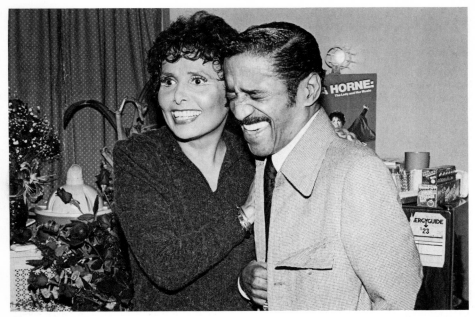

In the old days we were all thrown together in the one hotel where black performers were allowed to stay in Miami or Vegas: Lena, Nat "King" Cole, Billy Eckstine, Sarah Vaughn, Pearl Bailey, Count Basie, Duke Ellington. And it was fun—we couldn't wait to finish work and rush back to the hotel and have laughs. Now that we can stay where we work, we're all spread out and hardly see each other. Though I love the luxury of the Waldorf Towers, room service there doesn't do soul food.

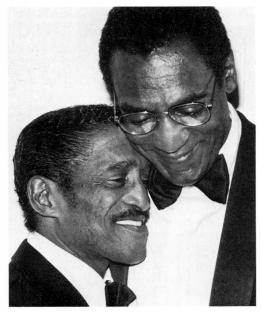

We've been friends since before *I Spy*, back when Bill was playing coffeehouses. And though he's a lot richer and more famous, he's still the same dear man, with the same warm heart.

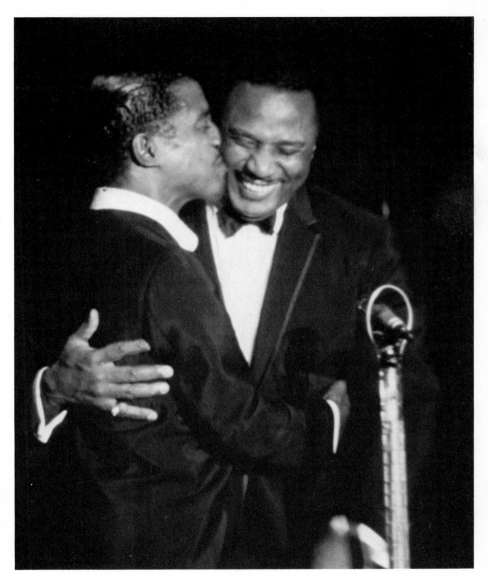

George was my conductor, my friend, my brother, my heart, my skin.

Portrait of a One-Man Show

I used to be rather impressed with myself for carrying thirteen people plus containerizing and shipping 6,500 pounds of equipment and personal effects, including my kitchen utensils and spices, from city to city. Then Michael Jackson went on tour with 100,000 pounds of equipment and a staff and tech crew of 150 people, among them two hairdressers and two chefs. And he only eats two carrots for breakfast and doesn't eat at all on Tuesdays.

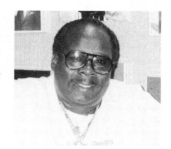

Earl Jolly Brown,
stage manager

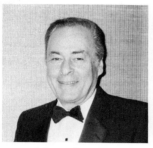

Morty Stevens

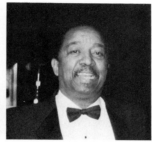

Fip Ricard, *lead trumpet*

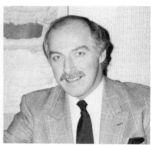

Brian Dellow, *security*

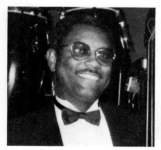

James Leary, *bass*

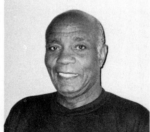

Bernard Wilson, *dresser*

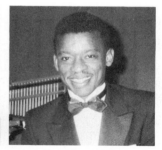

Clayton Cameron, *drums*

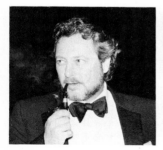

George Genna, *pianist*

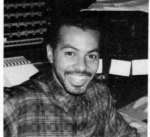

Dino Meminger,
lighting director

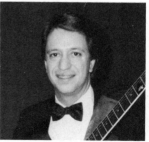

Frank Accardo, *guitarist*

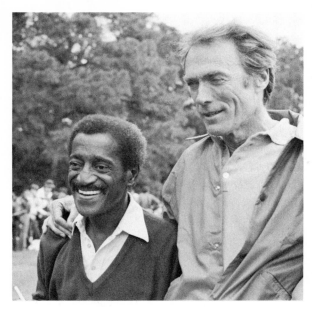

We've been friends for over thirty years: I taught him how to draw a gun. Clint reminisces: "Remember when we used to come by your house every Sunday, before I got *Rawhide*, and Rosa B. [my grandmother] would cook up a lot of stuff? That was the one good meal we looked forward to every week."

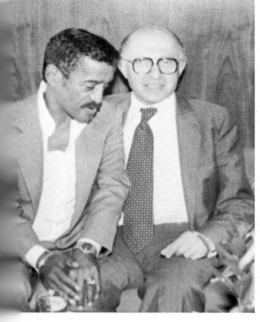

Menachem Begin invited me to his office. He was a nice, little Jewish man. "Sammy, would you like something to drink?"

I said, "Thank you, Mr. Prime Minister."

He asked, "Would you like a glass of tea?"

"Sir," I replied, "are you sure you're not from the Bronx?"

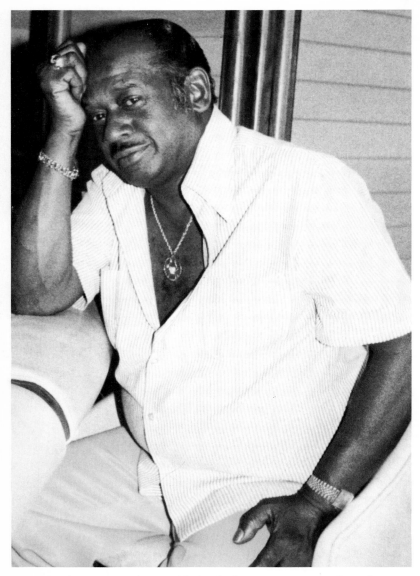

Once, in the sixties, when we'd checked into my suite at the Eden Roc Hotel in Miami Beach, I found Murphy sitting on a chair in the living room, crying. He tried to smile. "I know I look foolish, Sammy, it's just that I never thought I'd see the day I'd walk in the front door of a Miami Beach hotel. When I gave the bellmen the tip"—his eyes flooded with tears again—"they said, 'Thank you, sir.'"

I see too little of friends like Michael Caine, Lionel Blair, Albert Finney, Peter O'Toole, Richard Harris, Leslie Bricusse, Yves Piaget, Martine and Patrick Guerrand-Hermès, and so many others that I love. With an ocean between you and your European pals, you have to keep them in your heart.

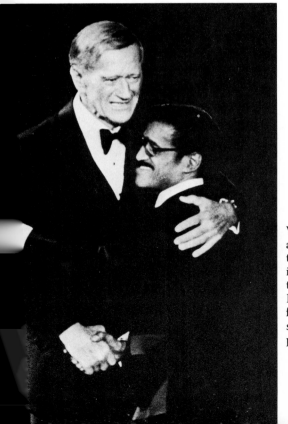

When there finally was a role calling for a Negro cowboy, John Wayne gave me the hat he'd worn in *Stagecoach* for luck in playing it. He said, "I didn't let my kids touch this Stetson. It's very dear to me. But I guess you'll be able to find a home for it." Duke Wayne was politically a conservative but he was not a racist. I'm proud to have had his friendship.

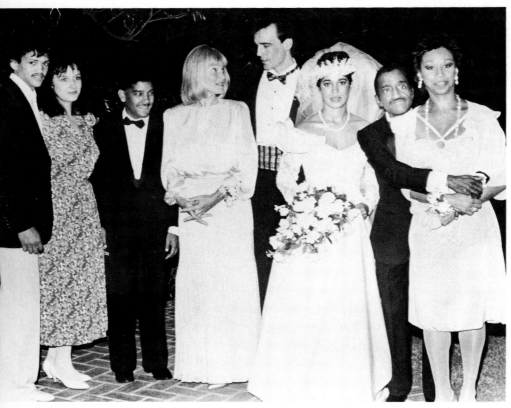

Following Tracey and Guy's wedding ceremony. L–R: My son Mark and my daughter-in-law Jane; my son Jeff; May; my new son-in-law Guy Garner and Tracey, his new wife; Altovise. A lot has changed since my marriage to Tracey's mother a quarter century ago.

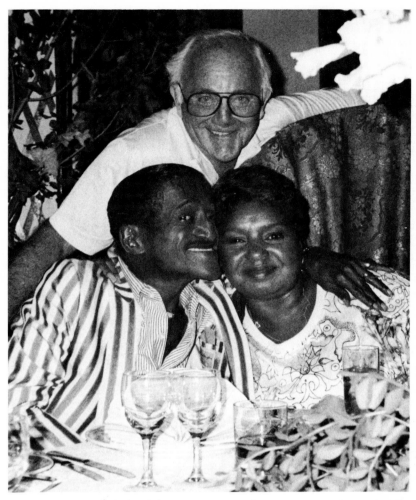

Celebrating Shirley's birthday in Monte Carlo in 1988. Another of God's marvelous coincidences: Ben Garfinkel, standing behind us, was one of my closest friends and my running buddy. Several years after George died, Shirley and Ben started dating.

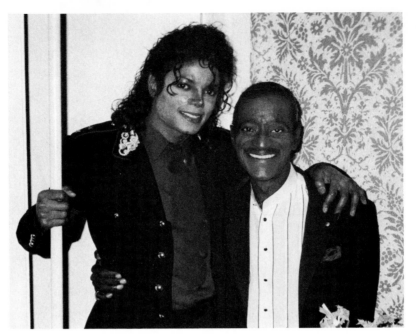

Michael used to come by my house—"Can I borrow some of your tapes, Mr. D.?" And he'd go to my library and take what he wanted of the shows I'd done. Visiting me in Monte Carlo in July of '88, he said, "Y'know, I stole some moves from you, the attitudes."

I'd known that. It's terribly flattering for the young to feel that way about you. Especially Michael, who I think is the ultimate professional. A lot of young performers have become multimillionaires on ten big records, but they still don't know how to bow and get themselves off a stage. Everything Michael does on a stage, though, is exactly right.

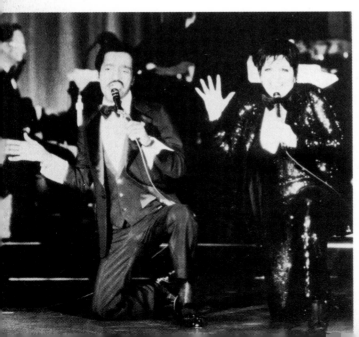

When Liza was a child, she used to sit on my lap and call me Uncle Sammy.

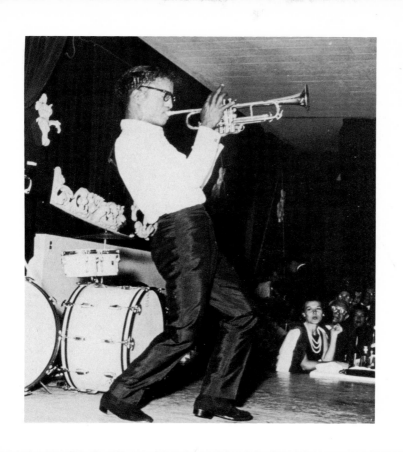

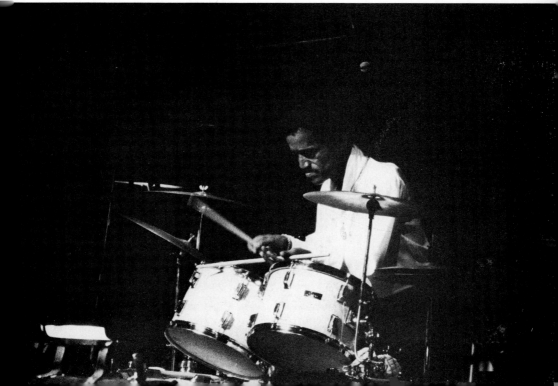

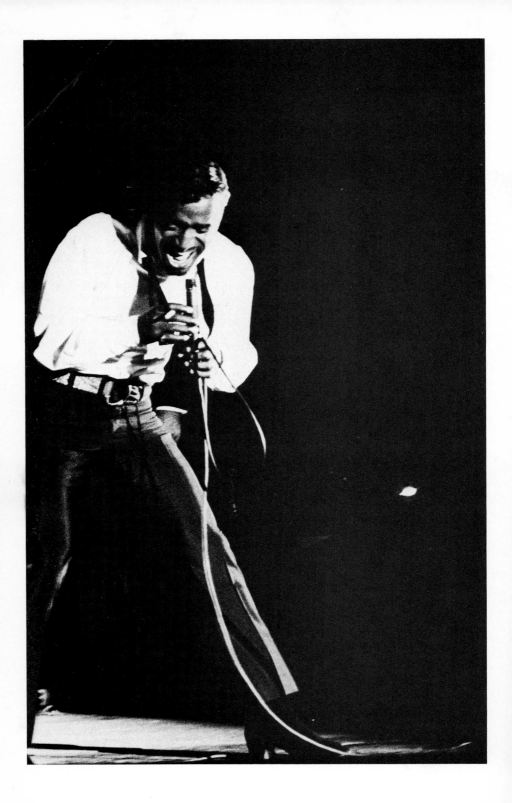

21

ALTOVISE CAME into the bedroom and made signs for me to pick up the phone. "The White House is calling."

It was Bob Brown, one of the founders of the Southern Christian Leadership Conference, who'd worked with Martin Luther King. "I'm coming out," he said. "I need to talk to you." I knew that he'd left his business in North Carolina and was working for President Nixon in Washington.

Altovise and Bob and I sat in the living room. "Sammy, the President has spoken highly of you and he wants your help with some of our programs. *I* want your help. I'd like to get you involved, I'd like to see you do some meaningful kind of things, bigger than anything which we as private citizens can do. We have an opportunity to better the lives of many people around this country. We've got Jim Brown with us, and we've got James Brown, we've got good people, but the President wants you. From time to time he asks me, 'How's Sammy doing? Do you think he'd help us with this?' He asked me to tell you that he wants you to be a member of the National Advisory Council on Economic Opportunity."

I was astounded. "Bob, I'm a Democrat. I'm strongly associated with the Kennedys, with Democratic goals."

"Understood, but don't close the door on Nixon. Use his power to accomplish the things you and I believe in. Accept the post on Ec-Op. Later, if you feel he should be re-elected, then become a Democrat for Nixon. Or if you don't believe in him, then walk away. But won't it be better to judge him by your own experience

249

firsthand? That's what I did and I say that he feels a commitment to causes you and I believe in. If I'm not right, then why has he got *me* there? The Nixon White House has more black people in high positions than any President has ever had, including JFK."

We saw him to his car. "Think seriously about this, Sammy. I'll be in touch." Alto and I went into the house, to the bar for a nightcap. I said, "I believe Bob Brown. Trouble is, Jim Brown and the others can do it, but if *I* make a move ten guys'll be writing, 'Sammy wants to be Ambassador to Watts.' I'll be seen as an opportunist. There ain't nobody gonna understand me going over to Nixon."

"Why not get a sounding? Call someone you trust."

"You're right." What a pleasure it was to bounce thoughts off someone I could trust about things that mattered to me. And get good answers. "So you're not just another pretty face, great ass and legs, eh?"

I got Jesse Jackson on the phone and he said, "I'm not a Nixonite, but there's no question that he's carrying on the civil rights programs, he's not scrapping them like he could have." I spoke to others within the civil rights structure, leaders of the NAACP and the Urban League, and the consensus was positive. "If we could get you in there, to have the President's ear . . . we could get some things done."

Upon arrival in Washington I went to the cemetery to put down flowers and pay my respects to John F. Kennedy and to Bobby. Then I went to the White House to be present for the signing of my appointment to the Council on Economic Opportunity. President Nixon walked around his desk in the Oval Office to greet me. "Sammy, I'm grateful for the assistance you're going to give us." He signed a certificate appointing me and he gave me the pen with which he had signed it.

Excited by the potential of what I could do, I called Harry for some constructive goals I could work toward. He was out of town. I left a message for him to call me at home. I left a message for Sidney Poitier too.

At my first monthly board meeting we talked about the disenfranchisement of the blacks in America, the unemployment of black teenagers, and the drug problem. Proportionately more black people were arrested and harassed over drugs than white people. Even in minor neighborhood disorders it was "We've got no time. Lock 'em up and let the judge straighten 'em out," and suddenly a family man is in jail for three or four years before his trial comes up. We got the Justice Department to look into it.

While I was in town I called Ethel to say hello, to ask about the children. "Mrs. Kennedy isn't in at this moment, but if I can have your number she'll get back to you."

The days and evenings were filled with meetings. Only when I returned a few weeks later did I realize that I hadn't yet spoken to Ethel.

"One moment, please. Who may I say is calling?"

"Sammy Davis, Jr."

She was out. She would get back to me.

But she didn't. I tried once again. Blank wall. Silence.

Nor had Harry called me back as he always had. Nor Sidney. All of the liberal Democrats, people who had marched for what we all believed in—when I went to work for Nixon they stopped talking to me. Nobody said, "Hey, give me a reason . . ."

During the next six months I was in Washington often. I always went to John's and Bobby's graves. But I didn't call Ethel again. It was an ache. I thought she was wrong, I thought Harry and Sidney were wrong. But I could get sick over it and weep for cherished relationships I'd lost, or I could do what I had to do and say "Fuck it," and kid myself that I meant it.

Before going to my meetings with black businessmen and senators I always started with Bob Brown for a briefing in his office in the Executive Office Building within the White House complex. Bob had four secretaries there, plus three staff people working in the White House. He was not just a conduit on the black situation, he was there on all levels. With all of John Kennedy's liberalism never did he have a black man anywhere near as close to him as Robert Brown was to Richard Nixon.

On the day Mahalia Jackson died I was playing Las Vegas and I got a phone call from Bob. "Sammy, would you go to Mahalia's funeral in an official capacity representing the President?" I told him that it would be a great honor, but I had to be back in Vegas that same evening. "No problem. I'll lay on an Air Force plane to pick you up and bring you back."

As I stood at her grave, watching the coffin being lowered, I was thinking: *Mahalia . . . you know all those times we thought: Hell, it ain't never gonna get better . . . Well, sister, who do you think sent me here to pay his respects?*

I KEPT hearing about black kids getting busted in Vietnam for smoking a joint. Of all the GIs over there in the drug rehab hospitals, the majority were black. It was out of kilter. Blacks are a minority. And when I was in San Francisco at Haight-Ashbury there were more white kids than black kids taking LSD and smoking joints. Yet in Vietnam black kids were getting bad discharges for minor abuse, while whites who'd been caught with the same thing were getting off clean. It was causing riots on military bases and on ships. I asked Bob, "Does the President know about this?"

He called me back. "The President asks if you'll go to Vietnam for him, be his eyes and ears and report back to him."

I flew to Washington and Bob and I met with Dr. Jaffe, the head of the President's drug commission, who explained: "The problem lies in the quality of the military in charge there. Vietnam is not a top job, so the assignment does not go to the best people. Like in the embassy jobs: leave London and Paris and the rest of the assignments are bummers. The officers in command there are older men at the ends of their careers. A joint to them is 'dope.' One of them once said to me, 'Those niggers're all dope fiends.' The bigotry is incredible. Chappy James told me, 'There are Army officers in Vietnam who still don't believe black people can fly an airplane.' Their prejudices are damaging these kids' careers and their future lives. If you were to go over there . . ."

"Just give me time to put a show together. While I'm there I'd like to do something for the guys."

Dr. Jaffe said, "I'll send my top people to help you, but it's not going to be pretty for you. The kids are going to think you're a jive-assed motherfucking Uncle Tom coming in . . ."

This was a white man telling me that.

WE FLEW in an Army C-50 with no windows, a heavy transport that usually carried jeeps, like an empty garage, with benches along the sides, no insulation, eating TV dinners on a rough and rainy night: Altovise, the girls who would dance with her, George and Shirley, my musicians, twenty-five of us. I brought everyone except Murphy. I didn't feel he could handle it.

252

We landed in the daytime and were put up in a house that was on a level with officers' quarters. Two Vietnamese women, mama-sans, took care of it for us. That evening we met with the officers at a dinner. They served fried chicken.

The next day, arriving at a detoxification center, I was stunned to see barbed wire surrounding it and watchtowers with armed guards looking down, like Sing Sing. I walked in and most of the forty or fifty inmates, sixty percent of them black, were sitting in rows glaring at me. I kept my smile going. "Hi, guys."

"Motherfucker, whut you doin' here?"

"I wanta find out why you're in here. How they're treating you. You've gotta fill me in."

"Shit, we don't have t'fill no muh'fuckin' jive-ass in on nothin'. The white man sent you over here, he musta told you what happened."

Despite having been warned, it shook me. "No, you've got it wrong, I came over thinking I could do some good."

"Aaagh, bullshit! You here t'use us for a TV special. T'do *yourself* some good." He turned to one of the officers who'd brought me there. "We have t'listen t'this?" Another sneered at me: "Man, what the fuck you know about it? You walk in here with all these motherfuckin' officers, we don't know them, they white. You come in wrong from the git-go."

It was scary, a *mano a mano*, with attitude toward attitude. I wasn't "Sammy," a brother, I was establishment. I'm black and I'm sent there by the white President? Get outta here! They trusted me like they would have trusted Bob Hope if he'd come in talking about drugs.

I put up my hands. "Wait a minute, wait a minute. Just 'cause I don't say, 'Fuck you, motherfuckers,' and because I care, doesn't make me part of the establishment—but incidentally, I *am* part of the establishment, the good part that cares what's happening to you . . ."

"Fuck it, man. Fuck it. Shit. He's bullshitting."

"Okay, but give me a fucking shot at it. If I don't accomplish anything, then you can just go back, or sit here, or whatever you gotta do, and say, 'Look how right we was, he *is* a jive-ass motherfucker.' "

I was wringing wet and beginning to feel that I wasn't going to make it, that this was a loser. I turned to the first guy. "If I'm taping a TV show to take back and get rich on, then where's the fuckin' cameras? In my bad eye? And *you* tell *me* why I'm here at the ass end of the fuckin' world 'steada bein' with ten chicks in Vegas and makin' a hundred grand a week. Like, I'm shrewd, I've got me this snappy jeep to ride 'round in over here 'steada my shitty ol' Rolls-Royce and Caddy convertible . . ." I had their attention and I didn't let go. "Look, man, I've been in the Army. Not as bad as Vietnam is now to you. But it was fucking lousy then for me. I was in the first integrated regiment in the U.S. Army. How'd you like to sleep with twenty-eight rednecks hatin' your ass? You think that ain't payin' your dues?"

It registered. "Hey, man . . . so then what the fuck *are* you doin' here?"

"Tryin' to help. Paying back. God gave me a lot. More than anyone has the right to hope for. Maybe He wants me to use it to help some guys He couldn't get around to. Whatever His reason, He gave me the President's ear. And when I go back and tell Mr. Nixon what it's like here, maybe he'll do something about it . . ."

"And maybe he won't."

"That's no worse than where you are now. At least I'm going to try."

He stared at me, absorbing it. He nodded. A smile began shining up his eyes. "Yeah, man. Okay. Fuckin' right." The rest of them had quieted down. "Whaddya wanna know, bro'?"

I nodded. "Thanks. I want to understand what's going on. Let me communicate it to the top. What can I tell them?"

"You saw the barbed wire? You saw the gun towers? You wanta know why I'm in this *medical facility*? I been here in Nam six months. Killed guys. That's my job. Almost *got* killed. That's my job too. Came in from the fire base. Five bucks to a mamasan, got me a joint and a hit of coke. Urinalysis. Bam. Addict. Get his black ass out on a DD."

Again, once past the hard exterior I heard them crying for help. One of the others asked, "You here to fight drug abuse?"

"I'm here to fight the abuse of *you* . . ." I saw suspicious eyes looking at me, not disbelieving so much as nonbelieving. "I want to hear what's going on, and I can't promise anything except that it will get on the desk of the right people. I promise you I will beg them to take the barbed wire down. And the gun towers. Those fuckers are coming down."

A boy with a sweet face that looked like it must hurt him to act tough asked, "You ever take drugs?"

"Yes."

They murmured surprise that I'd admitted it. "Whaddya think about drugs?"

"I think it's shit, man. And I don't mean that in the modern terminology. I think it's pure shit because it fucks you up. If there was a way you could do it that wouldn't mess up your learning, your thinking abilities, and it wouldn't hurt other people, then, man, I'd get stoned every day. But I know it's got to do all that. Nobody gonna beat that. Whatever problem you're fighting by taking a joint or havin' a hit, whatever, when you get off your high the problem is still there . . . and sometimes it's gotten bigger 'cause you've wasted a week, month, maybe two or three years being stoned, out of it, and you've given your problem time to grow. Plus you sure as hell ain't got no money left. Look, right here. You're in a rehab 'steada on your way back home . . ."

I'd done this before at drug abuse centers I'd visited in the States. My hope was that maybe some kid would think: Hey, Sammy's pretty hip, if he can't handle it . . . I could give them personal testimony: "Fucked me up. I went onstage stoned, feelin' good! Sang one song and walked off. Thought I'd done the whole show."

From then on I got rid of the officers. One of Dr. Jaffe's men, a civilian, always accompanied me. I said, "This man sitting here, he's not an officer but he's from the top and he's gonna tell them the truth."

It was the mamasans who were bringing in the cocaine. The American Military Police couldn't search the Vietnamese women. They'd sell little vials for five dollars. Pure. You'd twist the tobacco out of a cigarette and pour the hit in there, twist it and light it. The cats would get stoned on that. And with pure cocaine! Hooked.

I did four big shows on a stage with a full band at Danang and a few others for twelve or fourteen thousand soldiers. Altovise was mistress of ceremonies for those shows. She came out in hot pants. Cats went crazy! I had to fight for my life to get their attention. "Hey! You gotta ease up on my *wife*. That ain't my old lady, that's my wife, *man*. Don't let me come out here and have to cut some- body . . ." And the rapport was building.

Night and day cars took us off to the planes or to helicopters. The musicians and others who did only some of the shows went by bus or truck. I went by plane so I could sleep an hour more because I was doing them all. Mostly I was performing near fire bases, a hundred, two hundred soldiers, sometimes only fifty or seventy-five. I'd take four or five people with me and we'd get there and an NCO would say, "You do the show here, in this round area," and he'd point to a few square yards of ground, my stage. A few hundred yards away the enemy was fighting. A cat would warn me, "Don't sing too loud, Charlie can hear you." Often I'd take only a guitar player with me and there'd be only ten or twenty guys and I'd sit on the ground and sing to them and then we'd rap for a while till the shooting started.

A week before I left, a group of NCOs invited me for a meal. "When you came here and you did the first show we'd already decided against you. We came in mad. If you'd have come over here and been shooting a TV special or some of that bullshit, bringing one nigger over here to impress us, if you'd done that kinda show, which we thought you were going to do—and waved the flag at us—we were gonna walk, en masse. But now you've got us, if there's anything we can do . . ."

THE WHITE HOUSE

April 4, 1972

Dear Sammy,

From the glowing reports which I have received your recent tour of our military bases in Vietnam and Hawaii was an outstanding success. Realizing the many demands on your time I want you to know how much I appreciate your willingness to undertake such an extensive trip. My sentiments are undoubtedly shared by all our servicemen who were privileged to meet you.

Sincerely,
Richard Nixon

Bob's voice boomed with excitement over the telephone. "The Man wants to see you. He wants to have lunch with you. Are you available Thursday? You've got an opportunity. You've got carte blanche to go in there and talk to him, to say anything you want and have the President of the United States listening to you. Use your shot to make long strides forward."

The President put his hand on my shoulder as we walked into his dining room. "It was a good trip, Sammy. I've heard wonderful reports about it, you've made a lot of friends. And you'll be happy to know that the barbed wire is coming down."

As lunch was served he was warmly social for about ten minutes, then guided me onto what I was there for. "How can I do some good racially? Where is the help needed? In what form?"

I spoke to him about education. I also asked if he was aware that federal monies were rarely available to black small businessmen as they were to white. At that time no proportion of loans had to go to minorities as it does today.

There was a dinner being held in Washington that month by the Negro Republicans. No American President had ever attended their dinner. I asked President Nixon if he would come as a speaker. He said, "I have some close people delegated to attend. I respect the Negro Republicans, I know they influence the black voters . . ." He hesitated. "Incidentally, it *is* okay to say black?"

"Yes, Mr. President, we say black now. Negro and colored are not in use."

He had a notepad and he wrote, "Black is preferred, colored is not," and he asked, "How did that happen?"

I told him about James Brown's song. "It's all changed around, sir. In the old days it was 'If you're white you're right, if you're brown stick aroun', but if you're black you're in back.' When I was growing up, nobody wanted to be called black. Everyone wanted to be called colored. Today 'colored' is an insult to the young kid on the street. He wants to be proud of his blackness."

We returned to the subject of the dinner. "Sir, your presence there would lend great credence to your support of the programs that interest them. *I* know firsthand you're behind them, and I'll gladly do an hour telling them for you, but your appearance, even briefly, would say it better."

"Let me check my schedule. I'll try."

As the dinner began there had been no official acceptance or turndown by the President. It was a mixed crowd racially and politically. Every prestigious civil rights leader was present. Among them were the Democrats for Nixon, plus Democrats who were not for Nixon, and important black military, like General Chappy James. Bob came over to my seat. "The President has a very tight evening. He's got two speeches he's been committed to all year."

I was disappointed. But I kicked myself, mentally: Don't do an ego thing. You're a star, but he's the leader of the whole free world. Stop pouting. If he couldn't make it, then he couldn't make it.

An hour into the evening Bob came over to me, trying to contain his excitement, "The Man's on his way over. You pulled off a coup."

I was on the dais, I'd already performed, when there was a perceptible change in the level of conversation. Suddenly everyone's attention was drawn to one spot, and then here comes the President. The band played "Hail to the Chief," everybody stood and cheered, he shook hands with people as he walked through the room. Coming to me, he stopped, hugged me, and continued to the center of the dais, to the speaker's position.

"Sammy told me I had to be here."

It got a big, warm laugh—especially from me—and then he made a relatively long speech, six or seven minutes, ending, "I would love to stay here, but I've got commitments and I just wanted to come by and let you know . . ." He went out as he'd come in, shaking hands, surrounded by the Secret Service agents.

Jesse looked at me from his seat on the dais and nodded, like "Not bad, old buddy. That was a good move."

IF BOBBY were living I would have worked for him to become President. Now I believed it urgent that Nixon remain in office to continue the programs which I had seen being implemented and taking shape. There was no selling necessary in campaigning for Nixon. I would simply attend Republican affairs. I'd be in a town and the man there would call and say, "Sam, we're having a fund-raising cocktail party, will you come by?" "Of course I will," and I would go by, bringing Altovise whenever she was with me, and socialize. Sometimes it was "Sam, will you sing a song?" "Yes, of course." Just as in the Kennedy campaign, they came in expecting to contribute. But I didn't have to explain Richard Nixon, the incumbent President, as I often had tried to sell Bobby.

What I had to explain was me. But none of the Kennedy people ever asked me. They just slid the doors closed on a lot of once good relationships. It's a sorrow, and a piece of your heart goes with it, there's a dull area in your emotions, a sense of loss for all that time you spent building a friendship. Many a night I lay in my bed and wept, or shouted, "Why can't I keep my friends? Why don't my other friends talk up for me?" But crybaby shit'll get you nothing.

Then after a few weeks of "Why?" finally I got around to "I did what I had to do." If I'd done something wrong I'd take my lumps for it. I always have. But to be shunned? I didn't give drugs to children or give away America's secrets.

The only person who asked me "Why?" was Shirley MacLaine. She made a special trip to see me in Las Vegas, she came back to the dressing room, waited till the others had left, then closed the door and asked, "Sam, why did you do this thing? I don't care what anybody else says. I want to hear you."

"Because Nixon has the power and the desire to do things I believe in. I'm not looking to be Ambassador to Nairobi, Shirley. He can't give me a job. I make more money in one week than he makes in a year. I'm just trying to do some good."

"It's just such a shock. Don't you know all of the things this man does not stand for? All of the things you have stood for, and fought for. He's diametrically opposed to all that. He doesn't believe in the things you believe in . . ."

"Shirley, I'm interested in what he *does* believe in. I know that when I told him that kids in detox centers were herded behind barbed wire and machine guns, they came down. Gone. Everything I know about Richard Nixon, not what I *hear*, but what I *know*, is positive. And I've got to be telling you the truth, that I believe deeply in what this man is doing for black people, because what could I be getting out of it that would be worth all the friends I've lost?"

We talked until three or four in the morning. She said, "I think you're wrong but I had to come out and talk to you."

I admired her for that. Sandy Vanocur was the one other person who asked me the same thing, in Washington. "I don't want to put it on the air, Sammy, it's not that, I just want to know . . ."

MGM RECORDS had released my Motown album and "The Candy Man" as a single. "The Candy Man" appeared on the charts at number 56.

Sy got a call from Berry Gordy. "Sy, I see you're with MGM and I also see that you're on the charts." Loving it, playing it cool,

Sy almost yawned. "Yeah, Berry. First record we release and we're on the charts."

Next week *Billboard* came out: 34 on the charts.

Berry Gordy called Sy. "I see your record's moving up."

Next week: 21 on the charts.

Sy and I were in a limo going to an airport and the driver put the radio on. "The Candy Man . . . he can . . ."

It was incredible, absurd, ridiculous—but a fact. Who can figure it? Go explain my career! I can name ten songs I recorded that I'd have bet my house would be hits. But: toilet! Now, the one record I resisted, the one record in my life that I *least* expected . . .

It went to number 1.

Berry Gordy called Sy. "I'm just on your phone to admit to you that we blew it."

"The Candy Man" was the biggest single of the year, and by far the biggest single I had ever had. With a five percent royalty I made half a million dollars.

There are a lot of regional hits, or national hits. Hits in the South, or hits in Australia, or London, but rarely does a record become an international hit. In the middle of the discotheque craze people all over the world were hearing "Who can take the sunrise, put it in a jar?. . . the Candy Man can . . ." People were going, "What's happening with the music business?"

We were in another limo, en route to another airport. I asked Sy, "What about the Motown album?"

"It's a collector's item."

I got the drift. "But there aren't many collectors?"

He groaned like a man who had just lost three million dollars. "Right, sweetheart."

I had also begun singing "Mr. Bojangles" and though I hadn't recorded it I couldn't finish a show without the audience screaming, "Do 'Bojangles' . . ."

We stopped at a light and some kids looked into the car, idly at first, then they saw me and got hysterical. "It's the Candy Man!!!"

As we pulled away I marveled: The two songs that I wanted nothing to do with, the two signature things which everybody associates with me—I backed into them both. Which shows that you can be in this business fifty years and you still don't know anything about it. So let's never pat ourselves on the back that we've got all them theatrical smarts. I ignored "The Candy Man." I had nothing to do with its popularity. Did I go on Carson and sing it? Did I call William B. and say, "Do me a favor"? Did I do *anything* to build on this and say this will be my "Some of These Days," my "Over the Rainbow," my "Rockabye"? No!! As with "Bojangles," I backed into it. So go out there and play it by ear, but leave a lot of room for the people to discover something you're doing. Because it's the people who lay it on you.

THE 1972 Republican National Convention was scheduled to be held in Miami. Bob Brown called. "The President would like you to be involved. We'd like you to head up a big show at Marine Stadium, where there's going to be a Young Voters for Nixon rally, the new eighteen- to twenty-one-year-old, first-time-out voters. It's scheduled for the night when the President should receive the nomination by acclamation. For your information, normally the President would not make an appearance anywhere until he goes to the floor of the convention and accepts the nomination, but he indicated to me that if you do a show he will appear to speak."

"FOUR MORE YEARS . . . FOUR MORE YEARS . . . FOUR MORE YEARS . . ." The kids were growing hoarse from shouting it . . . the stadium overflowed with young people involved in politics for the first time in their lives. Borne on their enthusiasm, I worked onstage for two hours looking out at thousands of banners and campaign hats and buttons and flags.

I was about to introduce another rock group when a Secret Service agent, holding a walkie-talkie, came over to me. "Sammy, the President is arriving." From the stage I could see a group of bodies moving like a train along the side of the stadium, the President surrounded by an escort of Secret Service, moving quickly through the screaming crowd.

The kids out front were politically tuned in enough to know that it was completely unheard of for him to appear there that evening, so when I announced, "Ladies and gentlemen, Young Voters, the President of the United States," it was pandemonium.

The President did not hurry to quiet the Young Voters, he let them go on screaming, chanting "FOUR MORE YEARS . . . FOUR MORE YEARS . . ." Finally he raised his hands for silence.

"Sammy Davis . . . all of those who have entertained here so splendidly at this program, I understand earlier, and to all of you who are attending this Young Voters rally . . . as I was driving over here from my home in Key Biscayne, the thought occurred to me that this is one of those moments in history that has never happened before and it will never happen again. I do not mean by that that I have not been nominated before. As a matter of fact, I was nominated in 1952 and 1956 for Vice President and I have twice had the honor of being nominated for President and tonight makes it the third time. And now to put all this in the historical context: all of you know that this is the first time in the hundred and ninety-five years of the history of America that young voters eighteen to twenty-one are going to participate in the election decision, and I believe that it is particularly appropriate that the first appearance of the President of the United States after his nomination be made before first voters . . ."

"FOUR MORE YEARS . . . FOUR MORE YEARS . . . FOUR MORE YEARS . . ."

"As I was coming in I was stopped by one of the fine commentators for the ABC network and he asked me . . . what was going to happen to the youth vote? He said he was beginning to wonder if I had concluded that the estimates that the youth vote was just automatically going to go over to our opponents might be a little high. I can say this. I want to give you an answer that I want you to think about a bit. I don't think that the youth vote is in anybody's pocket, I don't think it ever will be, I think young people are going to vote for what they believe in, they're going to be independent. I think the young people of America are going to listen to both candidates. They're casting their first votes, they want it to be a good vote. We've got just as good a shot at it as the other side. And we're going to get it with your help."

"FOUR MORE YEARS . . . FOUR MORE YEARS . . . FOUR MORE YEARS . . ."

"I want to express appreciation to all of the celebrities—that's the word we use for them—for Sammy Davis, Jr., and the marvelous groups that you've been hearing here . . . and I want to ask all of you to realize what it means to them to be here.

"Now, my business is the business of politics. It's a very honored business. I hope lots of you get into it, maybe full-time. But I want you to know that when you're in politics you assume—you have to under our system—that what you're trying to do is get somewhat more than half the vote, and the other man or woman, as the case might be, will get somewhat less than half.

"Now, in show business, which is Sammy Davis, Jr.'s business and the business of others who are here, they are not trying to get half, they're trying to please everybody, and so you see when somebody in show business comes and participates in a political rally he or she is doing something that is a very great personal sacrifice and even a personal risk.

"I heard on Monday night one of the commentators question Sammy Davis, Jr., when he was sitting there with Mrs. Nixon in the presidential box, and point out what I had known and what Sammy Davis of course strictly agreed with, that he had been a very enthusiastic supporter of President Kennedy when we ran against each other in 1960 . . . and when the commentator said, 'What is your reaction, Sammy, to the fact that many people who have been your friends and your supporters, perhaps many who think you're great in show business, think maybe that you've turned against them? And that you've done so . . . you've sort of sold out . . . because you were invited to the White House to see the President.'

"Well, let me give you the answer: You aren't going to buy Sammy Davis, Jr., by inviting him to the White House. You buy him by doing something for America."

So touched, so overwhelmed by the realization that my problems were on the President's mind, that he was taking an occasion to try to overcome them for me, I walked up from behind him and put my arms around him, hugged him, and stepped back. There was applause and then he continued.

"When Sammy and I and his wife were chatting the other day I want you to know it was one of the most moving experiences for me and I hope it was for him. We talked about our backgrounds. We both came from rather poor families, and we both have done rather well . . ."

Cheers . . . laughter . . .

". . . and I know Sammy, who's a member of the other party, I didn't know when I talked to him what he would be doing in this election campaign, but I do know this . . . I want to make this pledge to Sammy, and to everybody here, whether you be white or black or young or old: I believe in the American dream, Sammy Davis believes in it, we believe in it because we've seen it come true in our own lives, but I can assure you, my friends, that the American dream can't be fully realized until every person in this country has an equal chance to see it come true in his life.

"Today, I pledge to you, we have worked toward that goal for the past four years, we are going to work toward it for the next four years.

"I want you to know that we're grateful to the celebrities who have stuck their necks out, taking the chance, as they have, that they might lose some support because they realize that it is important to get into a campaign that affects their future and the future of their country, and the future of their children.

"I'd like to close on one note about you. This is your first election campaign. It will not be your last. I know that many of you will go into public service, I hope all of you will continue to participate in politics. As you go along some of you will go into business, some of you may go into show business, some of you may go into some other kind of activities where somebody's going to come up to you one election year and say, 'Stay out of this campaign,' because you might risk some money, you might risk some customers or clients, whatever the case might be, and I just want to urge you, don't ever do that, because what you do for America is more important than anything you do for yourself."

THAT NIGHT we had the late news on and Altovise exclaimed, "Hey, look at that . . ." A shot of me hugging the President. "That's my husband up there with the Prez." The morning papers across the country carried the picture on the front pages. Then it was in the newsmagazines and the angry comments started coming in. More than a few people felt that I, a black man, had done a bad thing by hugging the President of the United States. The White House was receiving calls from Republican campaign fund supporters threatening cutoffs. Nobody liked it. The Democrats who had seen me with Bobby and John were angry all along that I had gone to a Republican, and the hug was a catalyst. Bill Gibson's wife wrote me a scathing letter telling me she never wanted to see me again, that I was an embarrassment. The black press excoriated me. "Sammy sold us out."

Altovise was frightened by the scorching hostility from our own people. I tried to comfort her. "Darling, those cats don't have the facts. You know what the leaders, people like Jesse, said." I gave her the W. C. Fields reading: "Tut-tut, m'dear, it's just a minor kidney blow in the fifteen-rounder of life."

"It's not funny, Sammy. These are black people and they're mad at you."

"They shouldn't be. They shouldn't be standin' on the corner with their lips akimbo saying, 'He sho' let us down.' No way! I didn't do anything to hurt the black people or the black movement. On the contrary. But they're looking at me like I slapped my mama. Some of my former best friends are such 'liberals' that they won't even speak to me because they disagree with me politically. What's the next degree of taking exception? To shoot me like Bobby and Jack and Martin?"

"Should I dump Nixon? Should I tell him, 'Thanks, but call off the Justice Department, tell 'em to forget helping the black cats who got busted, they *prefer* to stay in jail'? Should I tell him to put the barbed wire back up?"

I received a 17 × 20 copy of the photograph, inscribed: "To Sammy Davis, Jr. With grateful appreciation for helping to make the 1972 convention a great success. Richard Nixon." With it was a letter addressed to "Hon. Sammy Davis, Jr."

THE WHITE HOUSE

September 14, 1972

Dear Sammy,

Since the enclosed captured a good deal of the spirit and enthusiasm of the rally and received such wide coverage in the press, I thought you might like to have a copy as a memento. Many thanks to you and Altovise for the great job you both did in helping to make the convention the success it was.

With warmest personal regards,

Sincerely,
Richard Nixon

I was appointed to the board of UNICEF and I went to Europe to do shows in Holland, Germany, Sweden, and England. We spent a few days in Paris and on the plane back to England I told Sy, "I need a check for $25,000 for Jesse Jackson. I'm flying direct London–Chicago to appear at a fund-raiser for PUSH."

"Sammy, please, you just gave him $25,000 for Operation Breadbasket. Plus you're flying in there to perform."

"It's called PUSH now and they need money. I won't appear without kicking in. That would be like 'I want all you cats who make two hundred bucks a week to contribute but I'm a star, so all I gotta do is sing.' "

Operation PUSH was a mix of various programs—get-out-and-vote, educational, anti-drug—but principally to excel, pull yourself up by yourself, man, don't wait for the white community to do it. Jesse was always begging, "Sam, we need funds . . ." That's no pleasure. I admired him for doing it and I could never turn him down.

Sy was shaking his head. "The problem is, we don't have it."

"Find it. Get it from one of the clubs, a hotel."

"I hate to do that. Then you'll be working for nothing, and if we get a better offer we can't take it."

"Sy, I want to do this."

He despaired. "At least Cartier and Chanel give us charge accounts. How can Jesse expect money you don't have?"

"That's *my* problem. It's not his fault I'm broke."

We stayed overnight in London and were about to leave our suite for the airport when Sy burst in. "Sweetheart, listen, I just got a call from Paris. Chevalier fell out in Deauville and they're desperate for tonight. We could get fifty grand easy for an hour's work. Seventy-five if I squeeze."

"Babe, you know I can't, that I'm scheduled for PUSH. They're expecting me."

Sy appealed to the ceiling, both arms in the air. "I'm going bananas!" He turned to me, softly, reasonably. "Sammy, that's a benefit. Send them the money. Jesse'll understand."

"Babe, if it were just Jesse, he *would* understand. But it's not. It's all them cats on the corner who've been told, 'Sammy's coming.' I can't disappoint the brothers, Sy. That's it!"

Alto and I flew directly to Chicago with George and my rhythm section. Backstage at the stadium I gave Jesse the check. There were about seven thousand people out front.

As I hit center stage smiling, there was a loud booing from the right-hand corner of the stadium. It struck me as with physical force, knocking the wind out of me. It grew louder. I wanted to run off the stage, get away from there, but Jesse's arm was around my shoulder and I heard him reprimanding the audience: "Brothers . . . if it wasn't for people like Sammy Davis you wouldn't be here, we wouldn't have PUSH today. Now, I expected some foolish people were going to react like this because the man hugged the President of the United States. So what? Look at what this gigantic little man has committed himself to over all these years . . ."

The words blurred in my ears as memory of the booing poured in and out of my head. Tears were coming down my face. Jesse tightened his hand on my shoulder. Jesse is very large. My head came up to his chest. He held on to me. I looked at him, wordlessly imploring: *Let go of me. I want to leave.* But he held me there by physical force, wordlessly imploring: *I understand what you're feeling, but stay!*

Then I heard him saying, "I'm going to ask our brother Sammy to sing something, and if anybody doesn't like it, then get up and leave." He didn't understand. I couldn't have spoken, let alone sung. He waited a moment, staring the crowd down. Nobody moved. He turned to me. "I want you to sing 'I've Got to Be Me.' "

I couldn't run, I couldn't stay. I didn't know what to do. The music began and somehow my voice came out and I sang "I've Got to Be Me," and by the end of it they were on their feet and cheering.

But the booing stayed with me. I heard it over the sound of traffic driving toward the airport, over the engines of the plane that was bringing me to Las Vegas. Because I'd been in Europe for UNICEF since the election, I was not aware of how heavily my people were against me. I was ignorant of what was being said on the street or I would have protected myself, I'd have called Jesse: "Sorry, I can't make it. I'll send a check."

In Vegas, as we walked through the airport, the skycaps, brothers who'd always waved and shouted, "My man," "Sammy," turned the other way as I went by. I wanted to shout, "What the fuck did I do? *My* kids don't need the Negro College Fund. *I* don't need to get sprung from jail. So why would I be doing it if I wasn't buying some good for us all?" And I wanted to cry.

There were black clerks working at the front desk of the Sands.

As I walked through the lobby I saw a young black couple lounging on stools in front of a dollar slot machine, her feeding, him pulling, laughing, giggling, having fun. She saw me and tugged at her husband's arm. He looked around at me, then turned away harshly, pointedly.

I thought, *you wouldn't be standing where you are if not for me* . . . And again I wanted to cry.

THERE WERE no black faces in my audience. In recent years I'd been getting a good proportion of black people, but I'd stopped watching that, taking it for granted because I was breaking attendance records—the Nixon people loved me and that was ninety percent of America—but now there were none of my people out there.

Murphy was flicking glances at me in the dressing room, as if he wanted to tell me something but couldn't. I walked over to him. "Murph, what's wrong? Lay it on me. It can't possibly hurt me as much as it's hurting you not to tell me."

"I hate telling you this, Sammy, but I know you'd want to know. Last night George was having a drink in some bar across town with the musicians and he heard a guy talking about you. George was just sitting there and drinking and this guy didn't know who he was and he said, 'That little nigger ain't nothin' but a jive-assed motherfucker!' Well, George raised his hand till the guy noticed him, then real quiet, like George talks, he said, 'If you say one more word about him, you gonna have to *kill* me.' And the guy went, 'What . . . what . . . what???' And George said, 'I know what that man is. I know how many times he's fucked up. But the good he's done . . . Hell, nigger, you wouldn't even be walkin' these streets without that man and what he's contributed, and you stand up here bad-mouthin' him and don't even know him . . . Do you *know* Sammy Davis, Jr.?'

" 'No, I don't know him but I read about him . . .'

" 'Then shut your motherfuckin' mouth 'fore I kill you.' "

When George came in I said, "I hear you're goin' around attacking people in bars."

It embarrassed him. "Well . . . he didn't know what he was talking about . . . You'd do it for me." He grabbed me up and hugged me. "I love you, you li'l nigger, y'know that? I *love* you."

Johnny Johnson, the owner of Johnson Publications and publisher of *Ebony* and *Jet*, called me. "I'm sorry about what people are saying, but the brothers on the corner don't know. I say you're with the right man. So what if he's a Republican? You can butter bread with either side of the knife."

But how could I have lost so many friends—white and black—by being with the man who got the most votes of anyone in the history of the White House?

I ran into James Brown, the number one soul brother. He was also working for Nixon. "Whew," he said, "you're taking a lot of heat. I never got it this way."

Again I saw that another black artist could do something unpopular and it was more or less accepted, but our people put me in a special place. By their definition I had let them down. In their minds there were certain things I could do, certain rules I could break. I married a white woman and I hardly got any heat. But by going with a Republican President I had broken faith with my people. I couldn't reach them and tell them about the results we'd had, and the tangible reason to hope for more. I couldn't explain, and I didn't want to. But it was a body blow, a senses-stunning, throbbing pain. Maybe it was the Lord's way of saying, "Don't ever take the warmth, the devotion of those people for granted."

I had been controversial all my life but at no time did surviving pain make the next time hurt less. Yes, I had learned that I would survive it. But it hurt.

BOB BROWN called. "The President said, 'I'd like to arrange for Sammy to entertain at the White House.'"

"I'd be thrilled. I've always wanted to."

"You're joking! I thought that you'd entertained there a number of times."

He was thinking of the Kennedys. "Never."

Bob said, "I need you here in Washington for three days running if possible, to have some meetings, first with me and some others, and then with the President, a private, one-hour breakfast meeting. Just you and the President. And the President would like you to stay at the White House. You and Mrs. Davis, and whomever you need with you."

Richard Nixon showed us to the guest rooms, which were on

the same floor as his own quarters. "I wanted the pleasure of having Sammy Davis, Jr., stay at the White House. No black man has slept here since 1914 when Booker T. Washington was a guest of Woodrow Wilson."

When we were alone Altovise and I sat down and we didn't say anything as we looked at each other, realizing it was a fact: we were living in the White House; the President of the United States had shown us to our room. I could not think of a word to say that would not have been corny or that could begin to describe what I felt. Nor could Altovise. We must have sat there for half an hour without speaking.

I stood in the wings and listened to the President introduce the members of the Cabinet, the Senate, and the Apollo 17 astronauts. "I want to welcome you here at this first evening at the White House in the year 1973 . . . I think that all of us realize that the flights to the moon, the landings on the moon were perhaps the best illustration of what we like to think is the American can-do spirit, and for that reason I think it is fittingly appropriate that our special guest tonight is one who exemplifies that can-do spirit. We all know about his records, his motion pictures, and his personal appearances around the country, and we also know about his best-selling book, which is entitled appropriately *Yes I Can*.

"When we think of Sammy Davis, Jr., we remember that he began as a relatively poor boy, we remember too that he overcame the poverty and the prejudice and went clear to the top because he had that spirit of 'Yes I Can.' Tonight, as I think about how appropriately to present him here in the White House to this distinguished audience, I think we could refer to him as our Golden Boy, we could refer to him as our Candy Man, we could refer to him as our Mr. Wonderful, but I think what he would like more than anything else, this man who demonstrated that he could make the American dream come true with his own life, that he would like to be introduced as I introduce him to you now: Mr. Sammy Davis, Jr., a great American."

My music came up, the President took his seat in the audience, and I had to try to be worthy of that introduction. "Thank you, Mr. President. Mrs. Nixon, distinguished guests, may I say how very honored I am to be here tonight to try to entertain you. I've been in show business over forty years. I have never done a tougher show than the one I'm about to do tonight.

270

". . . Under normal circumstances, ladies and gentlemen, if I'm working in a nightclub or giving a concert I usually build my show. You start off with something amusing and hope that it builds to a climax. I have not had as many hits as people would have you believe. I've only had a couple and I'm going to do one of them to open the show. Under normal circumstances I wait until later, hoping someone will say, 'Isn't he ever going to do it?' but I ain't taking no chances. I'm opening with the heavyweights. Because as we used to say on the corner, this is about as far uptown as I'm ever going to get."

I sang "The Candy Man," "I've Got to Be Me," and I closed with "Mr. Bojangles." The President and Mrs. Nixon were standing, applauding me. Everyone was.

I changed from one dinner suit to another and went out to the ballroom, to the receiving line, and Altovise and I stood with the Nixons saying good evening to the senators and their wives, the astronauts, to the Cabinet members. The President whispered, "When you want me to cut this off, let me know." Then we were seated at a table with the Nixons. I saw Shirley and George on the dance floor, dipping. I was trying to reach them: *You're dipping? Nobody dips anymore. Aahhh, go ahead, you're dancing in the White House, do what you want, have some fun. Dip.*

The President asked Altovise to dance and I watched my wife dancing with the President. I asked Mrs. Nixon, "May I have the honor?" and then I was dancing with the First Lady, in the White House.

Senators and their wives came over to our table to say hello. Supreme Court justices, statesmen, the people who ran the country visited to say something nice to me and my wife. The President recalled our first meeting: "When I was a senator from California I went with Pat to the Copacabana, where you were appearing with the Will Mastin Trio, and they informed me at the door that it was sold out, there was no room at all. I asked if it was possible to get word to Mr. Davis that Senator Nixon, a fan of his, would love to be able to see him. You pulled some strings and we sat at your table at the ringside and there was so little room that you performed on top of the piano." At two o'clock the President nudged me. "Whenever you want to leave, don't stand on protocol, we're going to have breakfast together."

When we'd said good night I thought I'd step into the kitchen and say hello to the cooks and the brothers who worked there. I knew very well that Milton Berle did not feel he had to say hello to the Jewish employees everywhere. Yet I wanted to take a bow with the brothers. I wanted them to be proud of where I'd gotten. They were having a late snack. I said, "I see you got a Virginia ham over there. Brother, can I have me a little sandwich upstairs? I missed dinner, I couldn't eat before the show." A beautiful tray was sent up.

I went to sleep trying to feel having made it on a social level with the President of the United States, having sat up and talked to him until two in the morning—going to bed then only because the next day we had to be up for a ten o'clock breakfast. I could not fit it into my mind. In less than a lifetime: Mama's place in Harlem . . . "Those niggers out there are assigned to this company. I'm gonna stick 'em down there" . . . "Nervy nigger wanted a room" . . . my father and Will and I sleeping on the floor . . . the day I couldn't rent a house in the Hollywood Hills . . . being sent to the delivery entrance at River House. Then, somewhere along the way, without my being aware of it or knowing when, I had escaped.

At 10 a.m. the President and Mrs. Nixon were waiting for us in the President's study. We had a cup of coffee together, then Mrs. Nixon took Altovise to her quarters, where they would have breakfast, and the President and I went into his dining room. Following Bob's advice, I had a list: again, education in the ghettos, black businesses, the Negro College Fund and black colleges in general. They had never had support from any administration, ever. I asked for funding wherever possible, but also for the administration's arm-around-the-shoulder to facilitate network public service announcements, which the FCC could do, so that private donors would be encouraged to make endowments. The President was inquisitive, and there was a constant exchange.

BOB CALLED me in L.A. "The President talked about you at the prayer breakfast. He came over and shook my hand and told me I'd done a good job. He said how much he enjoyed the show but, more important, how much he enjoyed the breakfast.

"Sammy, you are as close to Nixon, in terms of being able to influence his thoughts, as any black man has ever been to a President. I can't think of any man he holds in higher esteem, white or black. We stood there for about five minutes just talking about you. The Man said, 'Sammy is one of the great living Americans.' He has said that many a time. 'Our friend Sammy, he could make it anywhere. It wouldn't matter what color he was, or what he wanted to do. With his intelligence he could make it at anything, anywhere in the world.' There is almost no limit to what may accrue to black people as a result of this."

It was nice to hear, and I appreciated it, but I couldn't help thinking: *As long as God lets me keep my talent.* Forget intelligence, forget sophistication, forget the friends I'd made along the way. All I really had was my talent. Without that I wouldn't be welcome at the White House, I wouldn't be able to help anybody, not even myself. If God ever took away my talent I would be a nigger again.

22

FUCKING youth freaks. We were in bed watching a rock-'n'-roll show with all these great-looking young kids on roller skates, break-dancing, young skin, young stomachs, young arms, and young legs . . . good music. Young music. I snapped it off.

"Hey! I was enjoying that."

"Sure. My child bride *would*."

She stared at me from her side of the bed.

"Fucking youth freaks. Dumb fucking assholes. Fuck! Fuck!" I turned it back on and gazed at the young dancers. How easily they moved.

Altovise was thinking, biting her upper lip under her lower lip. "Sammy, do you think you're going through the male menopause?"

"You must be losing your meno-fucking-mind." But she was right. I hated the sight of fifty. I had this carved-in-granite image: the finger-snapping, perpetual motion, tight-pants swinger. But was there anything more depressing than an aging swinger? And how could there be an old Sammy Davis, Jr.? She was holding a copy of *People* magazine with some juvenile on the cover. He'd been in high school yesterday. I fumed. "The whole thing on youth. You pick up a magazine and after thirty you're out of it. Every advertisement. Kids."

She put the magazine out of my sight. "I won't have it around anymore."

I was not going to answer that. Certainly not say thank you. I needed air. "You're in my space. I can't deal with it."

"With what?"

"With anything." I glared at her. "And what are we doing in bed at midnight like a couple of geriatrics?"

"But you said you were tired . . ."

"Fuck tired." I bolted out of bed. "I'm going where there's some action." I called out over my shoulder, "You've got fifteen minutes if you want to join me."

As I shaved I looked in the mirror and saw my father's face on my body. *Black guys don't show their age. Bullshit!* I was shaving two and three times a day because it was coming in gray. I could touch up the hair on my head, but there was nothing you could do with a new growth of beard every few hours. And as much as I hated looking at fifty, I detested the cliché of hating it. I pulled on a pair of tight-fitting chocolate-brown leather pants, a silk shirt, and alligator boots. I stepped out of the house, studied my cars, and got into my new Corvette. Altovise came running out behind me.

As we drove down to Sunset, she tried to console me. "Being fifty the way you're fifty is no big deal. Really, it's not old."

"Darling, not for people who wear normal clothes and do normal work. On them it can even look good . . . a little mature, distinguished, but on Sammy Davis, Jr., it's death. I painted myself into a corner with 'Where does he get all the energy?' the avant-garde clothes, the tight pants, jump suits, the whole glitz trip. But do you think a fifty-year-old should be dancing around on a stage in tight pants? Even if the glitz is pretty damned good, isn't it anachronistic? But that's what I am, tight pants and glitz, and I can't suddenly turn into Fred Astaire. They won't buy it from me."

We went to the Comedy Store, a club on Sunset. I felt like some laughs to take my mind off myself. Comics, white and black, who looked like they were wearing their first long pants were getting up and the first words they said were "Bullshit, mother-fuckers . . ." Without even "Good evening." The language, on a stage, made me feel like a hundred. I remembered Will Mastin telling me not to do impressions of white people because the audience would think I was making fun of them. Now here was this black cat calling them motherfuckers and getting belly laughs.

He put up his hands for quiet. "Motherfuckers . . . let's cool it with laughs for a sec 'cause there's a gentleman who has done me the honor of sitting in my audience. I have idolized him since I was a child when he was already a great star. This magnificent artist is a dinosaur, the last of his kind, his generation, the end of an era, the golden days of show business. He was learning our trade in vaudeville—yeah, motherfuckers, vaudeville! You're too young to remember it, by the time you were born it had died. He's the dean of show business, his name belongs on the Roll of Honor along with Al Jolson . . ."

I stood up. "I'm sorry to interrupt, but my funeral's in half an hour." The audience applauded and I walked to the stage. I hugged the asshole who'd done my eulogy and I addressed the audience. "I want to say something. Our friend here was right about one thing, I've been in show business for forty-seven years"—applause—"and it was a very different show business than you have today. I've always wanted to say something but I've never had the opportunity which the young performers of today take for granted. I have had the honor to have played for royalty and Presidents—and now I thank you for this wonderful opportunity to finally realize my great ambition, which is . . . to stand on a stage and be able to say 'Bullshit! Bullshit, motherfuckers!' "

We drove over to the Factory. The valet-parking kid looked too young to have a driver's license. He was gazing at my Corvette. "Wow, when'd you get it, Mr. D.?"

"I'm Sammy, babe, and it came in this week. I always have the first one every year."

As we walked into the room I felt a hand rubbing my buns. I turned around and it was a wild-looking chick. She was a little stoned, enough so she didn't let go of me. She squeezed. "Feelin' *good*, Sammy."

We sat with some kid actors. They were smoking joints and taking hits right there at the table. It was so crowded that nobody could see what anybody else was doing. They offered it around and I took a few hits. I told them, "Come on by the house tomorrow after midnight and see a movie and have something to make you feel good . . ."

I'D SEEN THE bowl in the window of a silver shop in Beverly Hills, a small bowl with a lid. It had probably been made for a man to store his snuff. It was perfect for cocaine. Nothing spectacular, not a bowl bowl, like for winning Wimbledon. It was not even large enough for soup, it was small, it could hold four vials of cocaine, and I'd bought little spoons like you use for salt, and people could dip in. It was an amenity, how to be a proper host today, like you wouldn't have a bar without scotch. Almost any movie you could name at the time had a budget for drugs, ten grand or so a week, which went under "Miscellaneous," to keep the actors going. I filled the bowl and put it next to the mixed nuts.

Everybody was happy, spread around the living room, six or eight of them in the conversation pit, another six or eight on the couch near the windows, and some more at the bar with me. Listening to conversation, I lined up a hit. I don't mean to say I was sniffing up half of Peru, in truth I wasn't a heavy hitter. I was a social drugger. I liked the scene. Even the asinine banter: "What do you propose, for my nose?" But for feeling good I preferred booze, from the taste and effect down to just the pleasure of holding the glass in my hand.

Jack Haley, Jr., was with me. He and Liza Minnelli were lifelong friends of mine and hang-out buddies. I was his best man at their wedding, and Altovise had been the matron of honor. I took my hit and waited for the feeling of well-being to settle onto me. I smiled at Jack. "Nice. But I'm still waiting to get high on this shit. For me, throw all the coke in the ocean, just give me three fingers of vodka." Jack raised his glass in agreement. Yet coke was "today." Booze was Bogey and yesteryear and "the older generation." I wished I didn't like it so much.

It was a good evening. I enjoyed sitting behind the bar. I liked the way I looked, the kids all thought my house was fantastic, I was providing good booze, wine, coke, whatever anyone wanted. We showed a new PG movie and then I ran an X-rated and by five they had all straggled out. I could have gotten laid five times just with lifestyle fans.

When everybody was gone and Alto and I were in bed she leaned over. "Honey? Sweetie?" I waited. Whenever she called me "Honey? Sweetie?" trouble was on its way. "Listen, I know what you want and so I've gotta tell you something. We have to remove the mirror from behind the bar or you can't sit there. I mean with people. 'Cause from out front your bald spot shines like the moon."

DRESSING FOR the evening, Alto said, "I love having the projection room, being able to show new movies."

I was thrilled to hear it, to be able to give it to her. I wished I could buy her one piece of jewelry that would cost like four million dollars. The kind that would cost $100,000 just to have a paste copy made of it. The kind of a stone that has a name, like the Hope Diamond. I'd love to give her "the Altovise Emerald." I wished I could say, "Any shopping that you want to do, darling, Neiman-Marcus, Saks, Giorgio, wherever on Rodeo, every time you want to buy something, just go and buy it." I wished I could give her four years like that, let her just go crazy for four years.

I kissed her on the cheek. "Actually, we've got the Last Stage-coach to Dodge. It's probably the last projection room that will ever be built in this town, because unless you're a movie producer, who needs one?"

I too liked seeing first-run films at home, and I enjoyed having our friends come to the house and be able to see them, but with the big television screens and videotape it was no longer a "necessary luxury."

While Virgil was setting up a second film I got up from my pit and went to the bar to remake my drink and I saw a kid filling his coke bottle from my bowl.

I sat down next to Jack Haley. "Did you see that? A druggie bag?"

Jack was studying my head. "How come you started putting the grease on your hair again? I liked it dry. It looked good."

I leaned toward him. "For your ears only: slicking it down covers the thin spot in back."

He waved away my tonsorial problem. "I saw Frank and Dean over at the Friars' last night."

That was strange. Frank always called when he was in town. Unless something was wrong.

Putting out her night-table light, Altovise commented, "Strange about Frank being in town and not calling you."

I snapped, "It's not strange. We're grown men, we're not tied by a cord. Obviously he's busy with other things." I put on my earphones and turned back to the television I was watching. I'd begun using earphones to watch TV so that Alto could sleep, but they served nicely to block out things I didn't want to listen to.

But it *was* strange. Frank's history with other people is when he didn't like something they did, then they didn't exist anymore. Just suddenly he's in town and they'd get no call. There was a blank space where that body used to stand. But in my case, as in the early sixties when he worked the Fontainebleau and I was playing next door at the Eden Roc and he was burned up over something I'd said on the Jack Eigen show, he'd made a point of getting the word to me. Now, nothing. I knew it was not over Nixon, because I'd seen him since then.

WE WERE in Vegas, in the suite, having supper. Altovise asked, "Honey? Sweetie? Do you think you might ever change your mind about having children?"

I pushed my steak away and put my napkin on the table. "Does that answer your stupid question?"

"What's stupid about it?"

"Because they'd be like my grandchildren. And I'm not ready for grandchildren. Far from ready."

May called from Lake Tahoe. "The kids have two weeks off from school and if you'd like to have them visit you for a week . . ."

"No!" I wasn't ready for my children either. I needed to hit all the parties. "I'm going to be very busy in L.A. I'll take them to Hawaii for Easter, but next week is out. Impossible. Forget it . . ."

"Okay, okay, holy mackerel, it was just an idea."

She was right, I'd gotten hysterical. I changed the subject. "Listen, I hear you've been going with the same guy quite a lot. Anything serious?"

"It's serious but we're not going to get married."

"May, if you love the guy, marry him. Listen, neither of us are spring chickens . . ."

She laughed. "I know that, but I don't want to remarry, not while the kids are still young and with me."

"Don't they like him?"

"They all get along very well. But another father would complicate their lives. No. I'm totally set as a mother now. And I'm happy about it. The most fun in the world is weekends when we pile into the station wagon and go off to the interstate basketball games. Mark is very, very good, but Tracey has star quality on the court, she's really a talented athlete."

"Well, that's great and I'm proud of them. But you're not going to have them with you forever. They're going to get married and what are you going to do?"

"I don't know. But I'll try to do it gracefully."

SUZANNE Pleshette and Tommy Gallagher had a costume party when we got back to L.A. and I went in tight black leather and Altovise went as Purity. *Deep Throat* had just been released and was playing at the Pussycat Theater on Santa Monica. People were talking about it, they wanted to see it, but the Pussycat was not a place you went to. And a porn film like *Deep Throat* was not something you could order from the studios.

I told Altovise, "Let's rent the Pussycat for a few hours one night, have it cleaned up, keep the popcorn stand open, and invite all these straight people here to go see *Deep Throat*. It would be marvelously decadent to have them all sitting there seeing that big thing on the screen and then take them to the Bistro for a foie gras and Château Margaux kind of supper."

We invited Suzanne and Tommy, the Berles, Dick and Dolly Martin, Steve and Eydie, Lucy and Gary Morton, Ben and Jackie Garfinkel, Sy and Molly, Shirley MacLaine—people who would never go to the Pussycat. I took them over in limos, which was safer than leaving your expensive paint job parked in that neighborhood.

I was intrigued by the porn world and wanted to meet Linda Lovelace, so I called her and got friendly with her and her husband, Chuck Traynor. I also became close to Marilyn Chambers. When Linda and Chuck divorced he and Marilyn got married in my suite in Vegas and I was their best man. I met most of the kids who were making the porn films in L.A. They'd come to my shows and the cats in the band would say, "Hey, isn't that . . . ?" and I'd say, "Yeah," and they'd start grinning. "Go *ahead*, Sam. My *man*." And I liked it, having everyone thinking that there wasn't a porn star on the screen that I hadn't partied with or didn't know—clutching on for dear life to the image of swinger.

As IF IT wasn't bad enough to have a sledgehammer hangover, the headache woke me up. Altovise was still sleeping. I felt pressure on my ears. I'd fallen asleep with the earphones on. I looked at my watch. Noon. I put on a robe and dragged myself toward the kitchen. I needed some coffee. What I really needed was to sit under a vodka waterfall.

Scotty, the captain of our guards, was leaving the kitchen with a mug of coffee. "Thanks, Mrs. Jackson." Lessie Lee had a pot of my Kona coffee ready. I leered at her. "Mrs. Jackson, eh? I knew you fifteen years ago when you was young and cute and 'Lessie Lee' 'steada old and dignified and 'Mrs. Jackson.' " I got a chuckle out of her and went into the breakfast room. I liked sitting there, having coffee, talking to no one, and looking out at my cars. I always left the Rolls and the Ferrari up there, with the Corvette in the center. I got more pleasure out of looking at them than driving them. I didn't put fifty miles a year on a car. I occasionally drove into Beverly Hills, but for hotels and restaurants it was more convenient to use a limousine service.

There were a couple of cars that weren't mine. Nor did I recognize them. It was too early for people to be doing drop-ins. How'd they get in here anyway? I was dying to go to my bar and make a vodka and Coke but I didn't want to have to talk to people now. I went into the kitchen. "Lessie Lee, ask Scotty why he let people in here this early."

She was giving me that blank look, through those big glasses. "Ain't that those cars come in today. It's that they didn't go out last night."

Leftovers. Like popcorn on couches, empty coke vials, used glasses, the smell of last night's smoke. None of those things belonged on a sunny morning. "Where are they?" She thumbed upstairs, toward my guest rooms. "Get someone to do some cleaning up there, make some noise . . ."

I slipped into my bar to make a drink. Three more were passed out in my pit. I went back to the breakfast room, closed the door, and sat where I could see and not be seen. I sent the vacuum cleaner into the living room too. In a while they came out, cats and chicks that I hardly knew.

Altovise came in. She was not smiling. "What are we doing having strange kids waking up all over our home?"

"Terrible."

Her voice softened. "Sammy . . . this way of life that we're living lately—it's not making you any younger."

On the contrary, I was exhausted, grateful that I didn't have to work for a couple of days. On Thursday I was starting a new Las Vegas career at Caesars Palace. With Jack Entratter gone Sy had found us dealing with people who talked about "the bottom line" and wanted to cut me to $75,000. Las Vegas had become computerized. I'd have stayed on at the Sands for Jack for nothing, but if I'm going to be working for a computer, then I'd better get every dime I'm entitled to, because the second those long lines of people aren't there to see me the computer'll shout, "String 'im up."

The guys at Caesars offered me anything I wanted. I'd lingered on at the Sands for another year before making the break, remembering Jack's kindnesses, his help in opening doors, the hilarious days when we'd shot *Ocean's Eleven* and the Clan was born. But Jack was dead, and with him ended the era of the individual owner, someone you could talk to. I left the Sands and all its good memories. I signed with Caesars for my top Vegas money, $175,000 for a six-day week, and I had to be in shape to justify that money. At $175,000 a week there's no room for "He wasn't cooking tonight."

ON OPENING night at Caesars I had only been dancing for three minutes but my legs kept getting heavier, my breathing was visible, I could hardly conceal from the audience that I was puffing and panting. I knew I couldn't get through the full seven or eight minutes that I usually did. From strenuous tap dancing I switched to a soft-shoe. Holding the mike by the cord, I lowered it to the floor close to my feet, and I did some semi-dancing. The audience of fourteen hundred people, fooled by the change of pace, thought they were seeing something extraordinary and they watched as I rested but looked like I was dancing. When I'd caught my breath I ended by going back to the taps on my shoes and beating out: boom diddy boom boom . . . boom boom!—doing a total of four minutes instead of seven. I hated fooling them, but what choice did I have? "Sorry, folks, but I'm getting too old to entertain you." Then get off the stage! But I couldn't afford to do that.

In the dressing room I put five sugars into a cup of coffee and dropped into a chair. Age. Dissipation. Leaning on talent. It was showing. You can't be my kind of an entertainer, at my age, and run yourself stupid partying and boozing and drugging. I used to be able to do it. But I couldn't anymore.

Altovise came backstage with her mother, and my mother, and Shirley Phillips, her mother's close friend. I'd introduced my mother-in-law from the stage. The ladies were all "It was the greatest thing I've ever seen . . ." but Altovise was giving me a funny look. She gestured to the makeup room. "Can I talk to you real private?"

"No."

"Well, can I tell you something in your ear?"

I gave her mother the Jack Benny poker face. "I might just let you take her back and age her for another five years."

Alto sat next to me on the couch, cupped my ear with her hands, and whispered, "Was my old man feeling a little down during the dance number? Nobody'd notice it but me, but you didn't have your razzle-dazzle."

"Get outta here." *And don't call me your "old man."* She was looking at me sympathetically. I pushed her away. She laughed and bounced onto her feet. I was beginning to feel our twenty-year difference.

The sugar in my coffee was working. I took a handful of gum drops to keep the energy level up. "If you ladies will be so kind as to excuse me, I'll be right back." I beckoned to Brian and we went out front to the shopping arcade, the Appian Way, to the fur shop, where I'd noticed luxurious pieces just waiting for a high roller to come in with his girl to celebrate. We returned to the dressing room wheeling a clothing rack. I presented Mrs. Gore with a chinchilla jacket. "Just a little kiss from your son-in-law." I'd bought Mrs. Phillips a fox cape, and my mother a mink jacket.

Altovise was dumbstruck. I turned on her. "Are you waiting to be tossed a fish or do you always sit around with your mouth open?" I looked smugly into her eyes. *You wanta talk about razzle-dazzle?*

I WAS IN the casino, playing blackjack, not because I felt like gambling but because it was good publicity. People love to say, "Jerry Lewis took over from the dealer," or "My God, I saw Sammy Davis playing with hundred-dollar chips," and it's a reminder that you're there.

I saw Jilly Rizzo. He was watching the action but I had the feeling he'd been waiting for me to see him. I gathered up my chips and we went over to the Garden Room and ordered a drink. I asked, "How's Francis?"

"He's at the Springs. The word's out you're doin' great business. That's a bitch in this mothery stadium."

"Yeah, it's going great. Funny, I haven't spoken to Frank in a while . . . He was in L.A. a few weeks ago, wasn't he?"

"He was there."

"I heard."

Jilly dropped the mask. "Sam, you and me been friends a long time and maybe you wanta know that probably why Frank hasn't called is he hears that you're into this coke crap and he says, 'If Sammy's into that, then I don't want to be around him. And I don't want him around me.' "

The one thing I didn't want to hear was that Frank was upset. It winded me. God knows, I could understand it. But I said, "If he wants it that way, then fuck it. I'm not twenty years old anymore, Jilly. It's not like the old days with fingernails in the mouth and 'Oh God, Frank didn't call today!' I'm living my life . . ."

"Sure, Sam. You're doin' business is what counts."

In the dressing room I looked at a framed picture someone had taken of us at the Villa Capri, years before. I hadn't known it was being taken. I'd been sitting on a stool looking down at Frank and the shot of my face caught the love and admiration I always felt for him. Frank sent me a print inscribed: "The same goes for me, Sam. Francis."

That he was disappointed in me was an ache around my heart. Frank had an influence on me that no one else could have had. When I was a teenager I used to make Frank Sinatra scrapbooks. He'd always been my idol and I'd said it publicly and I'd tried to *be* him, professionally to emulate him, and personally trying to be a swinger, to do the kind of things he did: give me all that, send for this, buy all that, expensive gifts to strangers for a gesture . . . all that stuff is Sinatra. The attitude, the cockiness was Sinatra. Black people weren't cocky in those days. I could never describe what the Capitol Theater date with him meant to me, bringing my grandmother there, his putting his arm around me, telling me, "You should sing . . ." So twenty-five years later to hear he was disappointed in me was a misery. Especially as I knew that as he said it he also said, or would have said, "Keep an eye on him.

Don't let him get into any trouble. I'm never going to speak to the little cocksucker again but don't ever let him get in trouble. And don't *you* call him a little cocksucker."

Why couldn't I call him and say, "Frank, if it means that much to you, then it's history, I'll never touch it again"? But I couldn't let someone else dictate my life.

PLAYING Caesars was a mistake. The room was too big. I was a hero for filling the place, but it couldn't last, and then it would be "Sammy isn't making it." To fill that room six days a week, two shows a night, with fourteen hundred people, you need a hot record, or a TV series. Or you should have a major divorce. Or be a man just turned into a girl. But a performer like myself should play small rooms. Five hundred seats. Fill that twice a night at $25 per head for two drinks and you're not exactly out of the business. But at Caesars I had to attract fourteen hundred people for every show.

Fortunately I was getting a lot of repeat business. That is key. And the locals. If they come to see you on a Monday or a Tuesday, their night off, and you've been playing that town for years, it's a big compliment. More important, if you *don't* have the local people in your corner, forget it. Out! 'Cause there isn't anybody else going to be there on Monday and Tuesday.

You've also got to have the cabdrivers in your corner, and the guys who drive the hotel limos that pick up the high rollers. These are the first people that most of the Las Vegas visitors speak to, and when they asked, "Who's in town?" I wanted them to hear "Catch Sammy at Caesars, he's swingin'!" So I gave a party for all the cabdrivers in Las Vegas. It started at 3 a.m. I did a show and gave them all the steaks and booze they liked.

Sy called from L.A., distraught. "I can rationalize the cabdrivers. Clever. Good promotion." His voice was vibrating. "But I've got a bill here for sixty thousand from the fur shop at Caesars. It's a mistake, isn't it . . . ?"

I thought: *Yes, it was a mistake. But the bill is right.*

"Please, Sammy, tell me you didn't buy Altovise another mink coat."

"No, I didn't. I bought one for her mother, my mother, and a friend of her mother."

"Wh . . . wh . . . why?"

"Another magnificent gesture."

"Sammy . . . sweetheart . . . you're almost fifty, which is young if you have money, but it's old if you're broke. I have nightmares that something happens to you, an accident or you get sick and you can't work for a year . . ."

Like it hadn't occurred to me. My plain cold fear was of being cut down by age: "Sammy Davis can't do it anymore."

". . . what happens to you? Who picks up the mortgage on your house, the bank loans . . ."

Then I would be "Mr. Bojangles," the character in the song, bottoming out. Onstage I began dropping numbers that spooked me, starting with that one. If the audience didn't demand it I didn't sing it. More than ever I feared it. I stopped doing "If I Never Sing Another Song," a Matt Monroe number about a superstar who says that if he never sings another song, it's okay, because he's tasted everything that fame could bring. Well, if you're still on top of the heap, then you can sing that song. But if your voice is getting rough, if you're dragging through performances where you used to fly, if in your mind you're playing the lounges, then don't sing "If I Never Sing Another Song." Dump it before they start thinking: Yeah, he may never sing much again . . .

I WAS VOTED "Entertainer of the Year" by my fellow members of the American Guild of Variety Artists, for the fourth consecutive year. The awards ceremony, held at Caesars, was attended by all the main-room stars, the lounge performers and opening acts in town, and many who came in to lend their presence to the awarding of the Georgie, for George M. Cohan, our highest honor for live performance.

Accepting it, I told them how honored and grateful I felt, but the inside joke would have been: *I wish I were alive to see this.* It was almost a posthumous award, because "Sammy Davis, Jr.," was dying. He could no longer unfailingly deliver the performance which had made him.

In a short speech I disqualified myself from it for the next year, to be gracious, and also perhaps because, knowing the shape I was in, I didn't imagine I could win it a fifth time. For the moment only I knew it—like a beautiful yacht looks fine from outside, but

286

if you're inside, down below, and you can feel the water coming in, you know it's sinking.

To show everybody I was still a superstar I gave a party for the entire city of Las Vegas. I invited every performer from every hotel in town to have steaks and champagne. I stayed for half an hour. It cost me fifty thousand dollars.

Altovise had come back for the awards ceremony and stayed for the last week in Vegas. Elvis was in town and we hung out one night, Elvis, Altovise, myself, and his bodyguard. We got into his limousine, my limo followed us, and we hit all the joints, being superstars. Elvis had on a short cape with the high collar, dark glasses, and he had Altovise by the arm and we were running, covering all the lounges, and people were saying, "Look . . . Elvis and Sammy . . ." But what were they seeing? Elvis was troubled and puffy in the face and the contrast was so great from when I had first seen him at the Hilton, when I heard Space Odyssey and he'd walked out and you heard dong, ta dong, dong dong, dong . . . and he was in shape and he wore the skintight clothes and women were going crazy and men were going, "Yeah . . . he's something!" He'd looked like ice cream and cake then.

And me? I couldn't stand to think about it.

THE HARRAH's plane picked me up in Vegas and took us to Reno, where I began a four-week run from which I'd segue into Harrah's Lake Tahoe for another three weeks, seven weeks without a day off.

Every night, an hour before show time, I called the maître d' and I heard "We're sold out, Sammy, we'll turn away fifty or sixty, both shows." But it was frightening. I was a dancer who couldn't dance anymore, an aging legend of youth and motion. Okay, I was still at the top club, still headlining, but tomorrow, next week, next month, one night I wouldn't be able to make sparks and the people would think: He's not so great anymore, and they'd stop standing in line for me.

I did all the off-the-wall things I could think of. I tried to come alive with the clothes, the jumpsuits, the leather pants, diamond rings on every finger, even his-and-her wigs with Altovise. Brilliant. I spend a lifetime making myself recognizable, then I put on a wig to look like my wife. Desperation was my producer. What I was really saying was: "Will somebody help me, please? I'm losing it . . ."

It wasn't coming naturally to me as it always had, it wasn't by osmosis anymore, I was trying to kill the ball, and when they applauded or laughed I was relieved, and I did another song, another joke, waiting for failure, waiting for the song that gets polite applause, for the joke they don't think is funny . . . but then I'd get the strong applause, the big laugh, and the feeling of relief was a euphoria that lasted a few seconds but then dropped me lower each time because I wasn't sure if I could do it again and, exhausted, I had to climb back up, I had to do it, make it, they were expecting me to be a star, they were waiting for me to be a star, they had paid their money and they were entitled to be watching the best.

On Fridays and Saturdays the third show didn't start till two-thirty in the morning. I played those shows to a thousand people and didn't get off until five or five-thirty. The sun was always coming up as I went to my suite, relieved, fatigued by fear. Whereas previously something had lived and breathed between me and the audience, now I couldn't wait for the shows to be over, to be free of the suspense. As always, I escaped into debauchery and alcohol to forget that the magic was waning, that the image was fading because I was fading and I didn't know how to get young again.

The party was already underway with all the kids from the other shows. Room service had set up steam tables with the Chinese food, and the bartender was taking care of people. Joe Conforti, a longtime friend who owned the Mustang Ranch, the biggest whorehouse in Nevada, where prostitution is legal, always brought over eight or a dozen of the most beautiful, the wildest girls. I never had to call Joe. He'd always come by to say hello and bring girls with him. "They're yours, all yours. The car will wait for them till you're finished." I usually had my own, but nobody at my parties was ever lonely or in need of a drink. I was depressed to remember that only ten years earlier I was shooting *Ocean's Eleven* and head-lining at the Sands with Frank and Dean, boozing, partying, staying up all night, feeling great, and performing at my peak. I wouldn't accept that I couldn't do it anymore. So I did it harder, later, and we kept partying till we dropped at nine or nine-thirty in the morning.

I woke up at two o'clock in the afternoon and tried to drag myself out of the booze and after-the-party stupor. My head and my throat ached. Lately my body had been threatening: "If you do that, then I ain't goin' nowhere tomorrow, I ain't gettin' up," and it was finally making good on the threat. I knew I couldn't go on that night. I got Murphy on the phone. "Call Dougie and tell him I've got a touch of flu."

Doug knew that the touch of flu was the suiteful of kids and the nonstop partying, but he said, "I'll have to get a substitute for a few days. We can't go dark. I'm going to call the hangar and send the plane to Burbank. I'll tell the pilot that he may be picking somebody up, and he may not. Then I'll get on the phone and start looking. Can you help me with anybody?" I called some friends—Alan King, Don Rickles, Bill Cosby, Liza Minnelli. Liza was available.

As eight o'clock arrived and I was having a drink in my living room instead of being where I should have been, I understood that I was self-destructing. And at the same time I was relieved not to have to face the audience, suffer another test.

ON OPENING night in Tahoe the party started in the dressing room and I carried my glass from the party onto the stage. I was about ten minutes past the opening numbers when a joke didn't get a laugh. The first few rows were just sitting there looking at me. Not a reaction. To a really funny line. I went back to the piano to get a cigarette and whispered to George, "What a stiff crowd! If that didn't turn 'em on, then they've got no switches."

His voice was flat. "They laughed the first time you said it."

Repeating a joke? My God, it was bad enough when I couldn't go on. But to appear on the stage drunk . . . to have them leave there and remember me making drunken mistakes. That was death. I dug down and started working. I pulled out everything I knew how to do, stuff I hadn't done in years, the quick-draw tricks, the drums, impressions. When the curtain fell I had been on for two hours and I had done a hell of a show.

George walked past me without speaking and went to his dressing room. He was never effusive with praise. When I'd done a great show, as I came off the stage his idea of a compliment was to hit me on my ass and keep walking. But this was ridiculous.

I looked into his dressing room. He was taking off his coat. "You don't want to say, 'Nice show, Sam,' or 'Well, you saved that one'?"

He was unsmiling. "You saved it."

Doug and Holmes came in. Doug looked at his watch. I groaned. "You're not really going to do that cliché with me."

"I was trying to be polite and not ask 'What the fuck was that all about?' "

"Babe, I started off drunk . . ."

Murphy picked up the ringing telephone. I heard him telling Sy that I was busy, that we'd call back. But apparently Sy was insisting.

He sounded out of breath. "Sammy, I need to get with you about the IRS. They insist that we make a commitment and stick to it or they're going to do a thing called 'piercing the veil,' which means going after us personally even though the debt is corporate."

"I don't want to hear about it. Handle it. That's *your* job. I've got the shows to worry about," and I hung up.

I needed to rest. It was a Saturday and I had two more shows. I told Doug and Holmes, "I'm sorry I ran over . . ."

Doug was studying me. "You're looking awful. Partying till nine in the morning . . . you're killing yourself. I've got an idea. I'm going camping in Alaska next month. Come with me. It's a complete change of lifestyle. We'll live in a Winnebago but we can take nights out where the trailer can't go and camp out in tents, rough it . . ."

"Camping in Alaska? In tents? You crazy? My idea of roughing it is when room service is slow. No color television. Me and Alaska? Camping? Get outta here!"

He smiled, not really amused. "Okay. But why don't you skip the party tonight and then tomorrow let's go riding, or golf, get some air, take advantage of this weather."

I hadn't noticed. All I'd been seeing was fog. "That's closer, Doug. Thanks. I'll call you when I get up."

Closing the door to my makeup room, I called Sy. "Babe, explain something to me. How can I be broke and owe the IRS? I never stop working. I just made three hundred thousand for two weeks in Vegas. I'm in the middle of seven straight weeks for Harrah's at one-fifty, which is over a million dollars for this date alone."

"Sammy, for openers, you *earned* but did not *receive* three hundred thousand dollars at Caesars because when we signed that contract we took an advance of two-fifty to pay off Kirk Kerkorian for the plane. The fifty that was left was used up by the Las Vegas party. And before either of us wakes up every Friday morning twenty-five grand is spent. In fact, sweetheart, we're running behind so badly that today I had to ask Molly to go to our savings account and make us a loan to pay salaries. Your mother called today. If her check is a day late she's on the phone, collect, 'Where's my money?' I also had a call from May. She says you told her you'd give the school ten grand for a new roof."

"Babe, the people on the school board read all the big numbers— 'He makes $150,000 a week'—so how can I tell them, 'No, I won't give you ten grand'?"

"Look, I'm a father, I understand you can't embarrass your kids. But it was five grand three months ago, another ten before that— you've practically built that school. Sam, if you're going to survive, there's an accumulation of fat we have to trim from our weekly overhead, like your father's cars. Sure, it pleases him to have two Cadillacs, but that second car which he never drives costs you two thousand a year in insurance."

"Baby, he's an old man, he's out of show business, if it makes him happy for two grand . . ."

"I know, pal, I know. But you're almost fifty. I ask you again: What happens on the day you get sick and can't sing 'The Candy Man'? Who's going to take care of *you?*"

I WAS IN Washington for a meeting of the Equal Opportunity board. The Nixons were in San Clemente but the President had said, "Ask Sammy to stay at the White House," like a friend saying, "We're going to be out of town but use the house," and they had sent a presidential car to the airport.

The guards at the gates of the White House saluted and waved me through. I told the driver, "Wait." I knew the face of one of the guards, a master sergeant, around my age, but I couldn't place it. I looked at him, trying to remember, not wanting to be rude, a big deal arriving at the White House. He looked away from my eyes.

I rolled down the window. "Excuse me, but don't we know each other?"

"No, sir. Not that I know, sir."

He was lying. He was looking past me instead of at me, trying to show no recognition . . . and then I remembered him, that's how he'd looked through me a lifetime ago, in the Army, Harcourt, the man I'd knocked down and who'd told me, "But you're still a nigger."

He was standing at attention. On his shirt I saw his name tag, "Harcourt."

"I'm sorry, Sergeant." I told the driver, "You can go now."

This time I was given the Lincoln Room. Walking into it, without the President, without Altovise, I was vulnerable to the ambiance of the man who had freed my people, and consequently myself, from slavery. Thanks to Sergeant Williams, I had read everything worth reading about Abraham Lincoln, and I was aware that he had not had any profound feelings of benefaction toward the black Americans, that in fact he had wanted to free the slaves and ship them away from the United States to some other land to set up shop for themselves. But whether he had backed into his place in history or not, still it was his signature on the Emancipation Proclamation, and if not for him I might really be "totin' dat barge" instead of just singing about it.

I felt drowsy as I climbed into Lincoln's extra-long bed. But I couldn't sleep. I slid deeper into bed, cold, praying for a cloud of sleep in which to escape from fear. I tried to be sensible: *Any black man who's sleeping in the White House, in Abraham Lincoln's bed, ought to be smart enough to enjoy it, appreciate the moment.* And I tried to. But then my thoughts fell back to the fact that I was losing whatever it was that had brought me there and I didn't know what to do about it.

AT CAESARS a lady at ringside smiled and, pointing at my stomach, cooed, "Look at his adorable little pot." I'd been getting that a lot lately and I always smiled back and patted it. But I hated it. It wasn't *me* to have a paunch. I didn't like to see my stomach pushing against my shirt. I stopped eating during the day. Nothing until after the second show. Maybe a cup of soup around five o'clock. My energy level was on the floor. I kept going on coffee with five sugars in it, and vodka with Coke, also for the sugar.

I'd wake up at noon, have coffee, make myself a drink, and I couldn't wait to get back into bed and rest, watching the daytime soap operas from twelve-thirty to four: *Ryan's Hope, One Life to Live, All My Children,* and *General Hospital.* I didn't have the energy for anything else.

Frank and I hadn't spoken in three years except for a few bump-ins with cold hellos. Since speaking with Jilly, I'd heard Frank had said, "If he's still into that drug shit I'll kill him."

He was following me into Caesars. A few nights before closing, Altovise came down from L.A. "I saw Barbara Sinatra at the Bistro Garden. She and I are taking you and Frank to dinner when they get here. Just the four of us."

"Alto, this isn't your territory . . ."

"Barbara decided it is. And I agree with her. You two guys love each other; you should talk even if only to call each other dirty names. So if you're going to be stubborn mules, then *somebody* has to have some sense."

I walked out onto the balcony. God knows, I yearned for what Frank and I had had. And the pity was, the kid and his idol were getting older and there was little time to waste.

They closed the Bacchanal Room for us. Altovise and I had just sat down when Barbara and Frank walked in. He kissed Alto. "Hi ya, Big Al." He looked at me and nodded. The four of us talked about nothing for about thirty seconds. Frank got up, tapped me on the arm, and we went to another booth.

"Sam, I'm so fuckin' disappointed in you, with that shit . . . You deserve better than that. You're the fuckin' greatest talent that ever lived. You going to let this shit destroy you? Give it up. Disassociate yourself from it. Dump it. You're breaking your friends' hearts, Sam. You're a superstar. Establishment. Isn't that sweet enough?" I nodded, feeling emotional that he would make this effort for me. At best it was uncomfortable for him. "Charley, we've never lied to each other."

"No, we haven't."

"Then if you say you're going to give it up, I know you will."

"I'll give it up, Frank."

His mouth and eyes broke into that smile that lights up the world. He said, "And if anybody ever hits you, Charley . . ." He was looking at me, waiting to see if I remembered.

I picked up a napkin and wiped my eyes. His voice carried me back almost thirty years. I remembered not only when he'd first said that to me but how much it had meant. And I could still hear him telling me, "You've got a friend for life." I hadn't understood then what that would mean, but he'd proven it in every way, at every opportunity. During three decades, around the hairpin turns, the icy horseshoe curves, across the rickety bridges, along all the highways of my youth, Frank had always been there for me.

We got up and joined the girls. Thank God for them. With their help it had taken us only three minutes to wipe away three wasted years.

23

WILL MASTIN lived to be a hundred years old. He died in July 1979. I flew from Lake Tahoe to Los Angeles for the funeral, but I did not go down the night before to see him in the chapel. He would not have wanted me to miss a performance. That dear old showman.

There was no part of my early life, from childhood until long after I'd become a star, in which I could not see Will's face. During the funeral my mind wandered through the early years: Will standing in the wings and making funny faces at me, three years old, in blackface with the big white lips, rolling my eyes and making funny faces back at him, mugging onstage; my first billing on a theater marquee, at the age of eight: "Will Mastin's Gang Featuring Little Sammy"; his teachings: "There's only two things to remember in show business: making an impression and leaving them with it. Do your best, Mose Gastin, but don't ever worry, 'cause whatever you do your daddy and me'll come on and it'll be okay." . . . "Sammy, that heckler made you give a bad performance, but now you'll never let yourself get thrown that way again. One thing you can't ever forget: if anybody out there gets to you, ignore him and wait till you can make a clean exit." . . . "Sammy, brush that hat till it gleams. And remember this like it's your bible: if there's one person or one thousand sitting out there, you gotta look as good and work as hard for that one man as you would for the one thousand. Never sluff off an audience. They paid their money and you owe them the best you got in you." . . . "You didn't have your flash tonight, Sammy. Now, I know you're troubling and you're worried about Big Sam, but you can't take any thoughts onstage with you except the show you're doing. We all have our troubles sometimes, Mose Gastin, but those people out front don't want to know 'em. No matter how bad you're hurting, leave your troubles here in the wings, and come on smiling."

Will did not give me my talent, or even understand what to do with it, but he started me on the road and he taught me everything he could, which was a lot. If there had not been a Will Mastin there might not have been a Sammy Davis, Jr.

I WOKE UP feeling stiff, my whole body aching. And angry at myself. Why would anyone sleep on a couch when he's got a king-sized bed in the Star Suite at Harrah's? Bombed was why. Smashed. To not have to look at myself. It had been daylight when the party ended.

I dragged myself to the bar and, ignoring the coffeepot, I poured a vodka and Coke. I pressed away a throb in my forehead and thought of a line in *The Fire Next Time*: "Rufus, this shit is got to stop." I sighed. *Yeah, Ruf, but not right now.*

I watched the soaps for three and a half hours. Then I still had to get through until eight-thirty in the evening. I would have liked to play golf but I had no energy for it. I didn't want to go shopping and get suicidally creative. And I didn't want to talk to anyone.

Murphy came into the bedroom and told me some friends of mine were coming to the dinner show. I said, "Call 'em back, babe. Tell them to catch the second. The dinner show's too quiet." Hogwash. Lately I hadn't been able to get myself up and cooking until the second, so I kidded myself that the dinner show customers wanted it quiet and easy.

The phone rang. The operator told me the name of the girl who was calling, one of the kids I'd partied with the night before. Kinky. She'd worn a white satin body stocking with the belt made out of handcuffs. "Hi, Sammy, are you ready for some more state-of-the-art sex?" She sounded so young, so energetic, and I felt so old and weary. "Thanks, darling, but I'm going to just hang in here and rest up for my shows."

"You can't do that. We're downstairs. We want to party . . ."

And then she hit me with the line from any one of a hundred teenage tits-and-ass movies: "I'm a party animal."

"I'm in a meeting, darling, call me in a few days," and I hung up.

I smelled food coming from the kitchen, on the second floor of the suite. I went up there. Louise, my Harrah's housekeeper, was stirring something in a pot. "Greens and ham hocks. In case you got hungry."

"Well, I don't feel hungry, but let me do some of that stirring." I sat on a stool in front of the stove and took the big wooden spoon she was using and I began stroking the food she had in the pot. I thought of my father cooking for us on the road in the thirties and forties, heating cans of baked beans on the engine of the old touring car that got us from town to town. In those days we didn't have fifty dollars we could call an old friend. Now I had a full kitchen in my hotel suite. But I still didn't have fifty dollars that I had gotten to know real well. Forget it, stir the food.

The front door opened downstairs. Murphy came in with Dino Meminger, my new lighting man. He was young, worked out every day, and wore great *Miami Vice* clothes. Murphy knocked on my bedroom door and called out, "Sammy . . ." From upstairs I heard him tell Dino, "Funny he'd go out without saying anything." It never occurred to them that I was up there in the kitchen, nor did I tell them.

That night I asked Brian to buy me some cookbooks and I read them until I fell asleep. I had a TV set installed in the kitchen so I could keep up with my soaps and the news while I cooked. Murphy brought in the groceries I'd ordered. I began lopping the heads off the carrots, slicing the onions, peeling the garlic cloves, and then I was stirring my own pot of greens and things, sitting there, soothed by it, lost in it, my mind only occasionally flicking onto subject matter I wanted to avoid: age, fatigue, money, failure . . . forget it, stir the food.

Murphy wiggled his nose. "Smells *good*. You gonna call me when it's ready? I'd like to eat something you've cooked."

"I'll give you an autographed picture. Out."

Cooking was a refuge from myself and my mistakes as well as from everyone else. I soaked an anchovy in milk, then put it in a hand towel and twisted it lightly, pressing out the milk, which took the salt with it. I didn't cook to eat, or to serve food to others. I tasted a spoonful of the sauce I was making. Not that it was *bad*. But I didn't need "Yeah, he's a great cook for a singer." I didn't need to give anyone something new to review, to dissect and analyze.

I settled comfortably into this kitchen solitude, talking to my pots while I cut up green peppers. "Yeah, don't worry, you'll get this just as soon as I'm finished cutting it up nice and small for you." Sometimes I'd hear myself or catch a mental picture of myself on a stool, stirring. I was not very glitzy. Stir the food.

THERE WERE poinsettia plants at the front entrance to the house, a Christmas tree in the foyer with presents around it and spilling into the living room. Altovise had put poinsettia plants everywhere: four in the living room, two in the kitchen, in the breakfast room, on the balcony overlooking the driveway, and rows of them lining the walk in the backyard.

After we'd had our hellos I said, "Darling, the house looks beautiful but for next year maybe let's be a little more subtle with the poinsettia plants. I mean, I like the Christmas season but let's not have people think this is Headquarters."

"Because you're Jewish?"

"No. Because it's too expensive."

I'd been guest of honor at a Dean Martin NBC-TV roast and Altovise and I were watching the tape. Phyllis Diller was saying, "Sammy's a man who's come up from the ghetto to become a great star, and he has everything that goes with it, like the mansion he lives in on the best street in Beverly Hills; he wears the best custom-made clothes, expensive jewelry, drives eight foreign cars. Sammy has earned his success. He just hasn't paid for it."

Altovise winced. "The whole country's going to hear that we're broke."

"Do you care?"

"Not about the whole country, but our friends, yes."

I remembered joking with her on a day that seemed a long time ago: "Don't worry what people say, because I *have* no money." But there had been an implicit promise that I would have and I'd let her down. "Then let's show them it's not true. Let's have a dinner party."

"But it *is* true."

"Darling, it's not *that* true that we can't afford a quiet dinner for twenty-five couples we care about. Nothing spectacular, just simple, nice."

"Do you think so?"

"Of course I do. We're like what Mike Todd meant when he said he was broke but not poor."

We started planning the party. "Lessie Lee can make some of her great legs of lamb . . ." I was rewarded by seeing Altovise get a lift out of it and we started making a list. When the list passed one hundred couples and there were still people we wanted to invite, I said, "Okay, instead of a sit-down dinner we'll give the first party of the 1980s. Call it 'the Decade Party.' Let's invite everybody we like. They won't all be able to come but it will be a nice card, like 'Happy 1980s.' "

A little 1980s card? They won't be able to come? *Everybody* accepted. They called from London and Paris to say they were going to fly over for it. The Bricusses, the Piagets, the Hermèses, the Rubirosas, ad infinitum. Then we added Infinitum and even *he* was coming!

Watching the news in the breakfast room, I heard Altovise saying goodbye to somebody at the front door. "That was the upholsterer." She poured a cup of coffee, sat down next to me, and showed me a swatch of black leather. "We can't have people over without redoing the bar chairs. They look terrible."

When I came back from lunch at the Daisy, Alto was standing on the back lawn with three men. I went into the breakfast room and waited for them to leave. "Darling, who was that?"

"Construction people the caterers sent."

"Construction?"

"Yes. In order to put up the tent which we have to have in case of bad weather, we need to have a platform, but because the lawn slants they have to put it in with steel girders in the ground."

"How much is that going to cost?"

"They're sending an estimate. But they said their crew would have to have the lawn to themselves for three days to install it."

"Darling, as of this moment, how much do you think we're in for?"

"I don't see how it can cost less than forty or forty-five thousand

dollars. Just the two bands, flowers, house polishing, valet parking
. . . and of course the four bar chairs, which are five thousand
alone, except they really don't count because we have to do them
anyway. That leaves the food and drinks . . ."

"Stop." I leaped to my feet. "It was a bad idea. But it's not too
late. We'll cancel. I'm calling it off. This show must *not* go on!"

"Honey, you're not serious."

"Serious? It could be terminal. The party's canceled."

"What'll we tell everyone?"

"Tell them that I'm an asshole, tell them that I owe the world,
that I have no money, that I'm getting old and I'm losing my talent."

WORKMEN were on the lawn in the center of the garden finishing
a floor mounted on steel girders they'd sunk into the ground. Guys
on stepladders were winding flowers around the tent poles. I went
into the bar to make a drink and got a look from the floor-polishing
crew. I went to the kitchen. Scotty was watching the security TV
monitors. "Here comes one of the caterers."

"*One* of the . . ."

Eddie Peterson, our friend and "house manager," looked at the
monitor. "It's Rent a Yenta with the turkey, roast beef, the classical
food. The second caterer is bringing the soul food at five o'clock."
He smiled. "That was a great idea you had, two caterers."

Yeah, back when we were thinking of Lessie Lee cooking for
twenty-five couples and I'd thought it would be a nice touch to
have soul food too. Through the window I saw a dozen or more
kids in white shirts and maroon pants. Eddie said, "We could only
get fifteen valet parkers. For four hundred people we really should
have more."

Altovise was in her dressing room posing for me in a gorgeous
shocking-pink, sparkling gown. "It's my first Galanos." She blew
a kiss at me. "You'd better start dressing."

The music was starting in the tent.

The cross section of faces was astonishing—directors, producers,
the sporting world people, and the superstars, the Old Guard and
the new hot kids, obscure white and black actors, the main meat-
and-potatoes television people. Loretta Young was at the bar in
deep conversation with Marilyn Chambers. Jack Haley, Jr., the
world's number one movie buff, grabbed my arm. "My God, Eddie

O'Brien! I haven't seen Edmund O'Brien since . . ." Altovise was like a fan at her own party. "Did you see June Haver and Fred MacMurray?"

I tried to enjoy the party but I would have hated myself if I could. It was 6 a.m. when everybody had gone home and Alto and I were sitting on our bed. She had tears in her eyes. "Sammy, I'm sorry . . ."

"It wasn't your fault and it was a nice evening, everybody enjoyed themselves."

"You didn't, and I didn't. And it was my fault. If I hadn't been so stupid about what people think . . ."

"Darling, you were only the shovel. I dug the hole. It was a mistake but it's past. Let's forget about it." But we couldn't. In Hollywood private parties get reviewed in the trades and the local columns. "The party of the century . . ." "Insiders say the SDJr. blast cost him $100,000." For days the flowers and telegrams kept coming in. Sy came up to the house. "It was a wild party." He was looking at me grimly. "Except the hangover's going to last a year. Thank God you're playing Vegas next week. The bills are all in . . ." I waited. "Seventy-five thousand."

We were silent for a moment, like allowing a poorly chewed hunk of food to work its way uncomfortably down to your stomach.

Sy was staring at me with curiosity. "Sammy, what was the motivation for that?"

"I didn't want people to think I'm broke."

IT WAS TIME to go on the road again but for the first time in my life I felt a tug to remain at home. The road had always been my home, where life was easiest, the dressing room and the stage where I had total control. But it was no longer controllable, and I dreaded going out there and facing that reality.

I opened a door to the backyard. I took off my loafers so I could feel my grass on my feet and I actively enjoyed walking on my two acres of Beverly Hills, one of the few enduring rewards for all that dancing, all that sweating, all those years of "Good evening, ladies and gentlemen . . ."

I walked around my house looking at memorabilia: a letter from Fred Astaire, the suit he'd worn in *The Band Wagon*, Leslie Caron's corset from *Gigi*, Jimmy Dean's red jacket from *Rebel Without a*

Cause, Marilyn Monroe's high heels, Gene Kelly's shoes, the hat John Wayne wore in forty-seven Westerns and his gun belt and six-shooter. I stopped and stared at the original art for the program cover of *Golden Boy*, a large painting of me as the fighter. God, I'd looked good then, fit, slim, hard.

Waiting for the limo to arrive to take me to the airport, I went into the men's guest bathroom and stared at the cartoon of the paunchy elderly man in the skintight jumpsuit and his wife looking at him critically: ". . . because you're sixty-five, you're a meat packer, and you're *not* Sammy Davis, Jr."

I saw myself in the mirror, in profile, in skintight jeans with a little middle-aged paunch, thinning hair turning gray but touched up. Past fifty and wearing skintight pants? Not even for the stage? Trying to hang on to a gone age. But it's gone and you can't do it anymore. You're the trumpet player trying to get that note that isn't there anymore. I looked again at the cartoon. *I* wasn't Sammy Davis, Jr., anymore either. I could have been the meat packer. Except he had money.

SY REACHED me in Tahoe before the first show. "They're going to take away our houses." His voice was tremulous through the phone from Los Angeles. "The lawyers can't hold them off anymore. They're threatening to put a lock on your house, and mine, and then sell them at a public auction if we don't come up with a million four and fast."

When we'd hung up, my chest felt like my heart was trying to break out of it. I thought of the kids and May. Thank God their house was in her name. Nauseated, I put my head below my knees. I lay down on the couch in the dressing room. I had to go on in thirty-five minutes. After a while I got up and sat at the makeup table, staring at the face that stared at me, neither recognizing the other. Bernard brought in my clothes and spread out the jewelry. I started selecting the rings, a necklace, a pin for the lapel of my jacket. I heard myself doing the joke about the jewelry: ". . . here's *my* social security," and I felt like a fraud. I took the flashy diamond pieces off. I could not go on and do that again, wearing all that money. In fact, I could not go on again at all. There was no way I could face people and be Little Mary Sunshine and make them laugh.

There was a knock on my dressing-room door and Bernard called, "Thirty minutes, Mr. D."

Thirty minutes, Mr. D.? Well, thirty minutes, Mr. D., to you! How about there ain't gonna be no thirty minutes, Mr. D.? No show at all, because Mr. D. ain't going to be here. You *do the show.* You *go out there and sing "Thirty minutes, Mr. D."*

I grabbed the phone and called Sy in Beverly Hills. "I'm finished, Sy. It's over. Atlas can't hold up the fuckin' world anymore. I'm disappearing, I'm getting out of the business. I've worked too long and I've failed."

Murphy gaped at me as I strode past yanking on a leather jacket. "Tell 'em don't worry the show's late, 'cause there ain't gonna *be* a show."

I was on the street, the big road in front of Harrah's. It was dark and I ran past the marquee with "SAMMY" on it. I was not going to die in my own bailiwick, drag all that glory through the gutter, tarnish the glitter that I had created, the single-name identity, "Sammy," "the world's greatest entertainer." "Isn't he adorable?" I'd never break their hearts and my own with ". . . it's embarrassing . . ." *Never. I'll leave "Sammy" behind, I won't take that down with me. Who says you have to stay in until you get beaten? I'll run away to London or Australia and hide there, do a radio or a TV show, play music halls. At least in America when someone asks whatever happened to Sammy Davis someone else will say, "I don't know, but he was great, wasn't he?"* As I ran I thought of the people back at the hotel waiting in line to see me, my audience. *Oh shit, why am I doing this? Will somebody please come and stop me, give me a face saver? I've got to get back and do my show!* . . . And I kept on running.

It was bizarre, running away from success while fearful of losing it, running away from a place where they treat me like the Pretender to the Throne. *Idiot! If you're going to run away, run away in Syracuse. Or in Cleveland, for God's sake. Or Buffalo.* The stupidity of it. Where was I going? In the dark. Without security. No money.

I heard someone pounding behind me. "Sam! . . . Sam . . ." It was Doug. Thank God. He was panting. "Hey! C'mon. Wait up for me . . ." I yelled over my shoulder, "I'm not coming back," and kept running, I didn't know how to stop myself, like I didn't know where the stop switch was. "Sam . . . you're going to give me a heart attack . . . I can't handle this." He'd found the switch. I'd come to love Doug. I stopped. He caught up with me and I threw my arms around him and I cried all the water of the dry tears I'd been shedding for weeks, months. Doug had his arm around my shoulder as we walked back to the hotel. I looked at his face. My emotion had spilled into his life and he was hurting for me.

When I came off after the show I called the house. Altovise was frightened. "Honey, I didn't want to upset you between shows but a car's been parked across from our entrance all day. Scotty says it has federal government license plates and the driver told him they're from Internal Revenue."

"I'm sorry, darling, there's a problem. I owe them a lot of money and they're talking about putting a lock on our house. Do me a favor. Don't go out."

"Y'mean I might not be able to get back in?"

"I don't know. But I'd like to feel that I can call you after each show and get a report that nothing's happened. I don't think they'll make a move to take a house if a lady's living in it. At least it would seem to be harder and give us time."

I sat down at the makeup table. I had to go on and do it again. For ten more days before I could get home. I'd had some new clothes planned for the second show. Halfway through I was going to quick-change into hot pants. With the high boots. No man had ever done it. My legs looked good. I liked the Three Musketeers-type shirt, blousy, with the big sleeves. It was comfortable having that fullness to conceal my pot. I did thirty minutes in a tux, then changed into the hot pants. My voice was good, breath control, everything worked.

Holmes and Doug were in the dressing room and I waited for compliments. "Your voice was good . . ." "Yeah, the show ran right on time, on the button . . ."

I said, "Hey, guys, I just did a really swinging show and I'm getting 'Your voice was good . . . show was on the button . . .'?"

There was a dead second or two. Holmes spoke uncomfortably. "Sammy, we're talent buyers, we don't presume to tell great artists what to do on the stage. We just buy what we think is right for our customers."

I could see Doug steeling himself to speak. "What Holmes means is, the show was great . . . *until* the little black Jew came out with his bathing suit on. After that it wasn't very good."

Holmes nodded sorrowfully. "You looked skinny, small, ridiculous."

Later I studied myself in the mirror. I turned away from what I saw. They were right. I had become a circus. It had developed into "What's he going to wear tonight?" Instead of "What songs is he going to sing?" it was "What tricks will he do?"

Sy had flown down. Sitting with me in my suite, he told me, "Apparently when the IRS read about 'the party of the century' it broke the camel's back. They've never been exactly understanding about someone paying twelve hundred dollars for a tuxedo and living on that scale, but the party nailed us." He showed me a résumé of the company's books, specifics on what I had known generally.

I looked up from the figures into the once confident face I had loved for so many years, the man I had always gone to when I was in trouble. "How did we get into this deep a problem, babe? How did we let it go this far?"

He shook his head miserably. "We couldn't pay the bills because we spent the cash."

I appreciated the "we." "You mean *I* spent the cash."

We sat together, suddenly with nothing to say to each other, the Brooklyn kid and the Harlem kid . . . we'd both come so far, but it was short of a win.

"Sam, I'm out of ideas. And I think I'm out of steam. If you'd like me to step down, I will."

"It wasn't your fault, babe. I was unmanageable." He'd gotten hold of a team of runaway horses that he'd caught in midstream and it was too much for him. But he was right, it had to end.

The ships were passing with a terrible loss for each of us. Though we'd remain friends it would never be the same. With Sy and Molly there'd been great love and affection, for many years, good years. I remembered one of our times in Paris. I'd seen a Cartier watch, heavy gold, one of a kind, a prototype, and I'd given it to Sy, engraved: "Till we die. Sam."

Sy stood up. I walked him to the door, then I went with him to the elevator, prolonging the goodbye. Neither one of us reached out to press the button for the elevator. But then the down bell rang, the doors opened. Sy hugged me. "Till we die, sweetheart."

THE CAR from the IRS was parked across the street from my house as Brian and I arrived from the airport. It was a Chevy. We were in a stretch limousine. I waved sickly.

When I'd offered Sy fifty percent of my earnings I'd looked upon him as salvation. But salvation had failed because it was fundamentally a wrong idea. I needed somebody to function for me, but this time *with* me. No more "You take care of the money and I'll take care of the show" and then I go off and spend all the money and expect it to work out. My talent for earning was easily outrun by my genius for spending. I just wished I'd understood this when I was young and strong.

Twelve years earlier, before Sy, I had asked Shirley to be my personal manager, mainly to handle the money and say no to me, but she didn't want the responsibility then. But she was ready for it now. I said, "There's just one condition. This is not a trial. It's forever. I'm too old to find a new Sy Marsh, a new Shirley Rhodes. I want you to make plans to move out here, buy a house in Beverly Hills, and base yourselves here permanently."

The wreckage was everywhere but the most pressure was from the IRS. If it had been during the Nixon days, or even the Kennedy days, I could have found a friend who'd have arranged for me to have a few months' breathing time. But I had nobody in Washington. I knew Gerald Ford but not to ask favors.

I told Shirley, "I have to meet the man in charge of my case, talk, work out a plan."

She made a negative face. "His name is Callahan. I've been told that he's the roughest agent in the world. You don't want to meet him."

"Shirley, look where I am *without* meeting him."

WAITING FOR him to arrive, I was aware that he was going to pass a uniformed guard, and he was going to see my cars in the driveway. I could hardly expect all that to provoke sympathy. It crossed my mind to hide the cars. But that would be bullshitting him and nothing good that I'd ever done had come out of dishonesty. All the mistakes I'd made had been the result of pretense, false pride.

306

I was standing at the front door when they arrived and introduced themselves as Charlie Callahan and Bill Byron. Two normal guys. It's a funny life. A couple of men called Charlie and Bill. Probably had wives and kids and stores they couldn't pay and they had to take away my home. I gestured for them to precede me into the house. "I know I should have dressed shabbily, with my arm in a sling maybe, because the fact is, I'm about to plead my case."

As I led them to the living room we passed the walls of book-shelves and Callahan asked, "Have you read all these books?"

"I've read ninety-five percent of them."

The wooden floors glowed richly from years of regular waxing. The music was on, softly. I'd been playing some light Tchaikovsky to quiet my nerves. I felt them looking at me with surprise, as if they'd expected to be walking into a disco.

Mr. Callahan was looking past me at the pictures on the wall of the bar: my children, Altovise, and a lot of friends most people wouldn't recognize, close friends like Ben and Jackie Garfinkel, Mark Nathanson, Steve Blauner, my publicists Arnold Lipsman and David Steinberg, Holmes and Doug, and my golf and drinking pals from Phoenix, Cathy and Jack Monday. Then he studied me as if trying to put me together with the "party guy" he'd watched cutting the fool on TV or in movies.

I said, "No one was to blame except me. I didn't find myself in Cartier because it was cold outside. My accountant didn't tell me I had to go in there and buy diamonds. No. *I* did it. All I'm hoping for is some breathing time. I haven't been on top of my business affairs until now; I'm what you could call thirty years late in learning how to do my checkbook. My immediate problem is that for me to go on the stage and to concentrate as I must in order to pull myself out of this is very difficult when during every performance I find myself wondering: Did they put a lock on my house?" I hesitated, not wanting to sound maudlin, yet wanting to say it all as I felt it. "Frankly, I'm too old to start again and accumulate what I have. This home, which is my major asset, if you'll give me the chance I'm hoping I can save it."

Mr. Callahan said, "I can let you have six months. After that it gets taken out of my hands. I certainly would not want to see you lose this fine home you have." He nodded. "I know very well you weren't born in it, nobody gave it to you."

Reality is never as bad as the nightmare, as the mental tortures we inflict on ourselves. "Thank you. The IRS will never have trouble with my case again. That's my personal commitment to you."

"Mr. Davis, I suggest that you make a substantial payment as a sign of intent. Fifty to a hundred thousand dollars would make a lot of character. Then follow it with a regular payment plan."

After I'd seen them to the door I fixed a large drink for myself and poured a glass of wine for Altovise. In the bedroom I sank onto the bed. I could feel and hear the blood racing through my head. When I had my wind back I called Shirley. "Okay, we've got a breather. But they need a show of good faith. I want to give them $200,000."

"We haven't got it. You'll have to go to Harrah's."

When we'd hung up I hesitated. Had I tapped that well too many times? It's not as if Bill Harrah was still living. He had the autonomy to do anything he wanted. Now that Holiday Inns owned Harrah's it was more difficult, more complicated, more people for Holmes and Doug to ask. And they were only too aware of my slowdown, the diminished energy level, and they knew that if I couldn't work I couldn't pay back. But I had put myself into a no-alternative position. I was getting old and about to lose my house.

I got Doug and Holmes on the line and told them the situation. "If it is convenient I would appreciate an advance of $200,000."

"Do you want it sent to the office or to the house?"

I handed Mr. Callahan my check for $200,000. "And I'm going to pay you off at the rate of $100,000 a week. I happen to have bookings that pay enough for me to turn over $100,000 a week to you for twelve weeks in a row and clean up this debt." I was aware that I could have paid it off slower, but I wanted to get it behind me.

"You're very lucky. Most people with a tax bill like yours never get even because it usually happens on the tail end of earning power."

I *was* lucky, provided I didn't get sick and could perform at the level I had to in order to keep those dates.

WITH SY NO longer booking me I signed with the Morris office and told them, "I need money. I'll do industrials, whatever, if the money is right and it doesn't hurt my meat-and-potatoes dates. I'll work seven days a week."

And I prayed that I'd find the strength to do it.

Paying off the government at that rate and putting aside future taxes on those earnings left little money to pay anyone else. Shirley got busy on the phone with all of those people with whom we had weekly and monthly bills outstanding. She talked to the butcher, the baker, the candlestick maker, which in this case was my camera store, Sy Devore my tailor, Nat Wise my shirtmaker, the Thunderbird Jewelers in Las Vegas, the Jewelry Factory in Tahoe, the California Jewelers in Beverly Hills, Cartier, Tiffany, Gucci, Dunhill's, the car people, flowers, groceries, laundry and dry cleaning, a one-million-dollar bank loan, everyone. She asked, "Go on hold for us, please? We're going to keep in touch. You'll get a small monthly check. We don't know how long it will take."

She told me, "They all said things like 'Tell Sam not to worry about it. Next year. Or the year after that.'" Then there was a wry look on her face. "You have got to laugh or life will chew you up. The only one to give us a problem is a drugstore over an $89 bill. All these others are cool in tens of thousands but this druggist was on the phone threatening: 'You owe us $89. I'm going to sue. I'm going to tell the *National Enquirer*.'"

I had a meeting of the family in the house—Altovise, Lessie Lee, Eddie. I said, "I'm in deep shit. We're broke. We've got to go into complete austerity. *And* we've got to keep it a major secret. Being poor is the one image that this business cannot stand."

We were in the breakfast room and through the window I could see my Rolls-Royce. It had cost $125,000. "Eddie, if we can get over $30,000 cash for that car, sell it and we can pay some bills faster." It was gone overnight. I did not sell Alto's cars or touch any of her things.

There were no more powers of attorney, no more signature machine. Never before had I asked where the money was going, not in twenty years in which I'd earned fifty million dollars. I hadn't wanted to face my mistakes and so I didn't find out if there were others. I remember a period in which I never asked the price of anything, thinking: It's not chic to ask prices. But what's really not chic is being an asshole.

TRACEY WAS graduating from high school in Lake Tahoe. May was still beautiful, carrying the years lightly. I sat with her in a rear corner of the auditorium. She whispered, "Tracey worried at first that you weren't going to come, and then when you said you would she worried that everybody would be staring at you and that all of her friends' thunder would be stolen."

I was dressed in a navy-blue pin-striped suit with a dark necktie. No jewelry. I was the only black father there, and the only Sammy Davis, Jr., but the rest of the parents played it the way I'd set it up, and we all paid attention to our kids.

Tracey's fears were natural, I supposed, what with my being famous, plus having publicly worn everything from hot pants to skintight jumpsuits. How could my teenage daughter know that even in his wildest days her father always had a gray flannel and a pin-striped suit and a little taste, even though it was usually his role to misplace it?

During the ceremony, watching Tracey, I didn't feel that I had wasted my own youth by never having a traditional one. It served to get me from there to here. I regretted only never feeling I had time to pause to appreciate and enjoy what I'd achieved before I'd begun to fear I was losing it.

Tracey looked so young, so innocent. I wondered why it was that God had made it so that I could not give my daughter the benefit of my mistakes and all they had taught me, all those years of experience, good and bad. Why did she have to go out and get there on her own and all I could give her was a car or a dress or a few dollars, things more common than a lesson in how not to hurt?

ALTOVISE WAS remaking old dresses and driving Lessie Lee out to the Farmers' Market for the shopping instead of just calling Jurgenson's and Phil's Fish, the expensive Beverly Hills grocery stores. She laughed. "People see me and Lessie Lee in my Rolls and they think the two maids are going out to do the marketing." If she was amused by it, I was not. I recognized that it wasn't hell on earth, that it was Beverly Hills austerity, luxurious stringency, but she hadn't married me to wake up in an austerity plan. When Shirley told me that we were beginning to see daylight, that we had our tax money set aside and debt payments going out on schedule, I told her that I wanted to buy Alto a necklace I'd seen at Gucci for $13,000.

"No!" She was furious. "What were you doing in Gucci in the first place? Stay out of the shops!"

"Well, you said we were coming along . . ."

"Sammy, prosperity is your enemy. If I tell you you've got ten dollars that's not busy, you've got to find some way to spend it. Why can't you just have money that's there, that you don't have to spend? I have to hide money from you so I can pay the bills.

"Your problem is that you've never had to pay the light bill every month, or the mortgage. Dad did it, or Rosa B., and later your office. You earned the money. But that's just numbers. You've never had the feeling of writing a check and paying a bill and seeing the balance diminish.

"If you get sick I think your attitude is: That's not my problem, that's Shirley's, or it was Sy's, *they* have to worry about that, not me. Wrong! You've got to work with me. I can't do it alone, saving pennies, cutting corners, and then you want to drop thirteen thousand at Gucci."

"I'm sorry. I know you're right."

"Sammy, God has picked you up in his arms for what might be the last time. Don't blow it."

I WAS AT the Friars' Club and I passed that room where they have the portraits of me and Frank and Dean and Joey Bishop. A young member came up to me and, glancing at the pictures, then back to me, said, "You're the only one who still looks like yourself."

Didn't he see my stomach? My hair? The face getting hollow? "Thanks, babe. Never more than three packs a day and one bottle of vodka," and I kept walking.

At home I studied myself in the mirror in profile. It wasn't me. It wasn't Sammy Davis, Jr. It was an impersonator who looked five months pregnant. My shirts, always slim and form-fitting, were about to split. I looked terrible. Yet I was down to one small meal a day.

That evening Elizabeth Taylor and Tony Gary and Richard Burton and his wife, Susie, had a quiet dinner with me and Altovise and we wound up sitting around our bar with the champagne flowing and Richard going on magnificently, and endless repertoire, hilariously told, with little asides to Elizabeth like "Darling, you remember when we . . ." and Susie sitting there being very gracious. It was an evening you wanted never to end but I started getting tired. It was only midnight, but I said, "Will you please go home? I'm starting to nod and I don't want to miss anything. Will you please come back another night?"

Elizabeth knew me from the old days when I outlasted everybody. "I don't believe, Samson, that you really said that. You saying good night to us?"

The next night Alto and I went to a party in Malibu. At dinner I whispered to her, "You sit here but I've got to go inside and take a lie-down." When I woke up, Linda Evans was on one side of me and another gorgeous girl on the other. I looked at these two incredible women: *Did I do something rude? Did I hump them? No, they've got their clothes on.* Then the girls "woke up" and I understood that they'd come in to do bits with me, that the joke had been: "He'll wake up and not remember what happened."

It was funny. But ominous. What was wrong with me that for two nights in a row I couldn't stay awake with people I enjoyed?

BERNARD WAS at the house and I was showing him what clothes I wanted to take on the road. I gave him the slacks and suits I'd had let out, the new blousy shirts, the stretch-out sweaters I'd bought. I hated having to warn the audiences that they were going to see "my little potbelly" as I took off my coat to do a number. I'd begun doing lines like "I'm a little chunky now . . ." and "Isn't he adorable this way? A little chubs?" I tried to comfort myself by thinking about movie stars, major performers, who had paunches. It still wasn't *me*.

And less and less did I *feel* like me. I was always dragging. In 1972 I'd had a PGA tournament named after me, the Sammy Davis Jr. Open, and I'd always played in it. This year they were making bets that I wouldn't get through four holes. They were wrong. I was planning to wait in the bar.

BILL COSBY and I had been friends going back to before *I Spy*, when he was working in the coffeehouses. We did a benefit somewhere, around 1980, we just bounced some lines off each other and the chemistry was right. We played some Harrah's dates and the rapport was positive between us, no upmanship, no "How many laughs is he getting?"

We opened at Caesars. Although sometimes it hurt me in the stomach to hit the big notes I absorbed the pain. I couldn't dance at all, and had stopped trying. I could do postures, like with Bojangles, but I was sluggish, stiff, leaden. So I talked a lot, and I got laughs, and I sang as best I could.

I began to feel Bill observing me, watching me. After an early show during our first week he came into my dressing room and looked pointedly at my stomach. "What the fuck is wrong with you?"

I sipped my vodka and Coke and patted my paunch. "Age, babe. I'm not fighting it. Grow old gracefully, they say."

"You're drinking all the time now." It was an accusation. That wonderful, caring face that looked like it had been run over by every kind of trouble and sadness in the world, but still remembered how to smile, was frowning. He said, "Whatever you're doing . . . don't end like this."

My CADDY held my drink while I was shooting. After we'd played three holes I told Doug, "I've had it. Bed." He said, "Let's have lunch." I patted my paunch. "Can't, babe. Gets me sluggish before the show." Also, I was too tired to sit at a table. I opened my portable bar and made myself another vodka and Coke for the car ride back to the hotel.

I lay down on my bed but couldn't sleep. I got up at five and ordered some soup. The vodka had half worn off and I felt like hell. I made myself another and sipped it as I walked to the dressing room.

I put on my makeup but I couldn't get myself together. Even on the worst nights the metamorphosis always set in as the hair got smoothed down and I picked out my clothes . . . but this time I looked at the table and I thought: *There's not a fucking piece of makeup here that can save this. Metamorphosis, where are you?* I couldn't imagine myself saying, "Good evening, ladies and gentlemen . . ." My feet were swollen to a quarter again their size, so I was going to go on in slippers. My skin was ashen. My stomach hurt and my jacket was pulling across my body.

I couldn't lift the show off the ground. I was trying with every trick I knew, everything that had ever worked for me, but I just couldn't excite them. As I got near a big note I knew I wasn't going to make it and so I climbed up under it and a woman called out, "You tried, Sammy. Don't worry about it." But I hadn't tried for it and taken a chance on missing. I'd settled for safe. And I didn't try for the next big note either. My stomach hurt too much. I was functioning at thirty percent. I couldn't sing, my timing was halting. I was embarrassed to be performing like this.

I'd done forty-five minutes when I stopped the music. "Ladies and gentlemen, this has not been a good performance and tonight I'm not capable of making it good, so I ask you to excuse me and accept my hospitality. You are all my guests." When the curtain closed I turned to the band. "God was right. He took Sundays off. He knew. Don't work on Sunday."

By the time I got to the dressing room Murphy had already heard about it. His eyes were blinking. "You picked up the tab for the whole room? For eight hundred people?"

Holmes came in. "Sammy, that wasn't necessary. The show wasn't that bad."

The bill came to $17,000. Within a few days it was in *Time*, *People*, and *Newsweek*. Normally I would have enjoyed seeing stories on my "magnificent gestures" but it only depressed me, reminding me of being inadequate on the stage, impotent in what had always been my kingdom.

I HAD A week off. I desperately needed a few days of bed rest before opening Reno. Doug called. "Holmes and I were wondering if you could get up here a few days early. There's a TV special, a syndicated show, *The Super Stars and Super Cars*, and it's featuring Bill's collection of old cars. We were hoping you'd narrate it . . ."

"Babe, count on it." There was no way I would ever turn down Doug and Holmes.

We had some people over the night before I was leaving, but I said good night early and went into my bedroom and lay down on the bed. I fell asleep still dressed. When I awoke, a little groggy, and tried to pull my pants off over my boots, sort of jumping out of the trouser leg, I tripped and fell, banging my ribs against the night table with a ghastly cracking sound.

When I awoke in the middle of the night it felt as if I had a flame against my ribs and I gasped.

"What's wrong?" Altovise jumped awake. I told her and she said, "I'll call Gerry Blankfort."

"Darling, I'll be fine. Just let me get some more sleep."

In the morning she pursued it. "You should have an X ray."

"Alto, the X ray will show I bruised my rib."

I did the TV show in Reno. On the day before opening at Harrah's the pain in my ribs had become unbearable. I had a salad-plate-sized black-and-blue mark and it hurt to breathe deeply. There was no way I could sing. I told Murph, "You'd better get me over to the hospital for some X rays . . . see what's wrong with these ribs. Maybe they can tape 'em or something." As I said it, I had a feeling that it wasn't going to be just a couple of X rays and tape up the ribs, that this time it was serious.

24

THE INTERNIST AT the Warsaw Medical Center in Reno told me, "You have a touch of jaundice, with overt signs of liver damage." He did the thumping thing and I could hear the difference in the sound when he was over my liver. He said, "That's all liquid. I think your liver has backed up on you."

The X rays showed that the ribs were not broken, but he called Gerald Blankfort. "He won't let me do any blood tests but you should know that his stomach is distended, the liver is enlarged. And there are some black marks on the X rays that I don't like. Shadows that reach down low, to the stomach."

Harrah's canceled the engagement and sent me to L.A. on the plane. Gerald was waiting for me when I checked into Cedars Sinai. Within an hour they had taken more X rays, and blood tests, and were giving me antibiotics.

In bed, waiting to hear what was wrong with me, I knew that I'd abused my body past where I could just dry out for a few days and bounce back like new. I wasn't new anymore. I was old and I was rotting away. God must have gotten tired of my bullshit, fed up with picking me up and giving me one more chance and one more chance. Instead He'd let me stay on a downward spiral professionally and physically. He'd let me destroy everything He'd given me, my health, my talent, my ability to perform, until I'd reached the bottom, sick, unfit to climb back up to that marvelous life He'd let me have. Finally I was Bojangles. I wasn't in jail but I was in a hospital decaying. And I'd done it myself. How was it possible to have feared ending this way and at the same time done everything to make it happen? Bill Cosby's voice resounded in my mind. "Don't end like this."

The next day there were more tests but nobody told me anything. Brian, Jolly, and Dino set up my suite with a VCR and a lot of my tapes. I hadn't asked for that. How did they know I was going to be here long enough to need my toys?

Shirley canceled all dates for the rest of November and December. "This way you've got no pressure on you to go back until you feel you're ready." She was bullshitting me. How do you cancel big-money dates unless you know something?

My children came by to see me. Covered by a sheet, my potbelly made me look like I was pregnant, while the rest of me was birdlike, and I knew I seemed shrunken, smaller than ever. Tracey and Mark and Jeff smiled at me with fragile, unconvincing cheerfulness, the way you smile at your father who's dying. George and Shirley and Steve and Eydie came up. Murphy hung around all day. Holmes and Doug came in from Tahoe and Reno. Brian, Jolly, and Dino, working eight-hour shifts around the clock sitting with me, took messages from all of the friends who called.

I'd fallen asleep and I had the dreamlike feeling of seeing myself looking down at me in the bed, an old man's face, contorted, unhappy. Then a tear dropped out of his eyes and I realized it was my father, that he'd come in while I was asleep. He tried to smile. "You're gonna be fine, Papa." He'd turned eighty. Lately I'd been doing lines with him like "Hey, Dad, I was just in Vegas and nobody sent you their regards." It broke him up. There isn't that much to laugh about when you're old and out of action and have Parkinson's disease. When you get old, people placate you but they don't do jokes with you. I was not going to change the relationship we'd always had. I was not going to do "Are you feeling okay, Dad? Sit here where it's warm . . ." On the contrary, when he was vague about something I'd say, "Of course you can't remember things, you're getting so old that all you can remember is the old days . . ." and he loved it. "Yeah, how 'bout that, Papa? But they're worth rememberin', weren't they?" But now I couldn't think of anything to kid him about. My brain wouldn't work. I couldn't even ad-lib with my father.

Gerald told me, "We'll have to lance your stomach. It has a

liquid lining. That's not a middle-aged pot you've got there, it's a reservoir, and we have to get that fluid out of there."

"An operation?"

"Not really. It will be done here in the room. We lance and drain it just like we would if it was a pus sore swollen up."

He brought in a specialist, the nurse gave me a local anesthetic, and they slipped the needle into my stomach. Always frightened to death of needles, now I welcomed anything that might help me. I sat on the edge of the bed, the doctor attached a plastic tube onto the needle, and liquid started dripping out. It filled three and a half quart jars. When the draining was over they took four stitches where the needle had been. The doctor sighed. "Thank God." He was looking at the liquid. It was as clear as water. "Had it been cloudy you'd be dying. It would have meant that the liquid was inside your stomach and then it would have been only a matter of time."

It was the first hopeful statement I'd heard in five days. "Then I'm okay?"

"You could be worse," Gerald said. "You can keep your liver in remission by not drinking, but once diseased it's diseased for life. It's not curable like an infection. Part of the liver is destroyed and there's no way of having that piece well again. I want to keep you here another few weeks. We've removed the liquid, and we've consulted as to anything further we should do—transpose veins away from the liver so we have better drainage, or whatever. The consensus is to do no more. Rest. And a strict regimen. No alcohol, no salt."

Alone, as I recalled the pain in my stomach when I went for the big notes, it was obvious now. My liver had become so enlarged that it was touching parts of my body that it normally wouldn't, like my ribs.

Altovise brought in a London newspaper. The headline was "SAMMY GIVES UP BOOZE."

My pot, my paunch, was almost all gone. The largest part of the puff had disappeared. It hadn't been middle age at all. No wonder it hadn't responded to dieting. It was all liquid bloat. "There's a period of time necessary for the rest," Gerald explained. "The walls of your stomach have to come back in. We can't tie it in the back, as it were.

"You've been lucky. When alcoholics reach this stage of liver disease, they most often go down, down, down. Further, you're not chemically dependent on alcohol. You haven't had a drink in twelve days, yet you've had no d.t.s, no shakes. All you have is a lifetime habit. But you can beat that. You're also lucky that you have longevity in your genes. You have a young mental attitude when you're happy, and you should be very happy because you've got great recuperative powers. But not another drop of alcohol. If you return to drinking you will die quickly. And painfully."

Altovise brought over a basket of chicken that Lessie Lee had made for me. Brian brought in Winchell's glazed doughnuts and Häagen-Dazs rum raisin. I couldn't look at any of it. I was hardly able to eat even my favorite foods, and my legs and arms looked like pipe stems. I felt too weak to step down from my bed and walk the few yards to the bathroom. Jolly or Brian or Dino had to pick me up and carry me there.

Shirley came in and sat by the side of my bed. "I told Holmes and Doug that I'd let them know if you could do New Year's Eve in Reno, then take a day off and start two weeks there."

I broke into a sweat. "Are you crazy? I have to be carried to the bathroom and you want me to come back and do the toughest show in the world? What's wrong with you?" I'd done the last four New Year's Eves there, in the Convention Center of the hotel, which seats two thousand people. It's the most important night of the year at a casino, maybe the one day when they can get even for the whole year. There's just one show, but it's got to be dynamite to attract all those high rollers. "What the hell's wrong with Holmes and Doug? They've seen me here, the shape I'm in. How can they think of it?"

"Maybe they thought it was a nice invitation," Shirley said quietly. "Yes, it's a tough show. But it's also a very important night for them. I don't think there's anything wrong with Holmes and Doug. I think they're saying, 'We're here for you, Sam.' The fact is, they need to attract high rollers; you play Harrah's quite a lot of weeks during the year and they'd be better off with somebody the people may not have seen so often." She stood up. "You don't have to give them an answer today. I'll get a bank loan to cover our overhead for the two months, and we'll catch up. Don't worry about it."

Falling back against the pillow, I couldn't imagine myself walking out of the hospital, let alone standing on a stage performing for two thousand people, doing jokes and love songs with a burned-out liver.

From my bed I could hear people talking in the living-room area, my father whispering, "I don't think Sammy can ever go back to work. I don't think he can make it." And Shirley answering, "Dad, he's *got* to make it. It's going to save his life. He's got to go back to work. Laying in bed, discouraged, getting weaker every day, he may die."

AT HOME Altovise took off my shoes and unbuttoned my shirt, and I lay on the bed letting myself be undressed like an invalid. I got under the covers and hid from everything for days. Finally, out of curiosity, I got up and tried on some clothes. My "paunch" wardrobe hung on me like bags. I was glad to have them taken in again. But my regular clothes were baggy too. I went back to bed, dizzy, sickened.

The next morning I forced myself up. I told Altovise, "C'mon, take a walk with me," and we left the bedroom and went into the living room. I sat down at the bar to rest. All the booze had been taken off the shelves. "Get outta here, Altovise! You're going to force me into being Ray Milland with three bottles of vodka hanging out the window."

"I thought the temptation . . ."

I took her hand. "Look, man, I appreciate the support you're giving me, but there ain't nobody can stop me from drinking except me. Or start me drinking except me. Don't worry about it. I'll miss booze. I'll miss it a lot. But as soon as you see a gallon of liquid drained out of your stomach you stop. I'm not ready to die. I can't afford it."

WHAT I learned from sobriety is that alcohol gives you infinite patience for stupidity. In the old days, which was until November 1983, when I got high enough everybody was groovy. I'd have enough booze in me and it would be "Yeah, lemme hear the rest of that." Sober up and your tolerance for nonsense goes right down the drain. You see and hear everything that you'd been able to avoid hearing before.

In a car to the Burbank airport en route to Reno, Murphy started telling me a joke. "These two black cats were in Miami . . ."

"Murph!!! I don't want to hear any jokes."

"I don't know why, Sammy. Why is it you don't like people to tell you jokes?"

"Because, for openers, I know every joke there is. Secondly, they're usually in bad taste. And third, people like you tell them very badly."

He looked away. "I'm sorry."

Hey, that was kinda sharp. I realized that I was nervous and wasn't able to hide it behind booze. "Oh, for God's sake, Murphy, tell the fucking joke."

"Well, there were these two black cats in Miami . . ."

The Harrah's stewardess had a Bloody Mary ready to hand me as I walked on. "Thanks, darling. I'm off booze." I gave her a can of strawberry Crush and a large plastic mug that I liked. "Just put these together with a lot of ice."

By the time we were in the air I was looking at Altovise, waiting for her to say, "That's the worst takeoff we've *ever* made!" But she was looking out the window, calm. Murphy was reading *People* magazine. Brian was absorbed in a newspaper. So was Dino. I looked at the impotent glass of Crush I was holding. It was a revelation how a few ounces of booze had always smoothed the bumps, the air pockets, but when you're straight, everything comes into focus. I'd been on a thousand flights until then and with a double Bloody Mary in my hand everything was cool up there. Now, with only a strawberry Crush, the pilots weren't flying nearly as well as they used to.

The plane hit an air pocket and dropped a thousand feet. I grabbed Altovise's arm. "This plane is going to go down. I know it."

Across from us Murphy said, "No, Sammy. It can't. I need three days' notice before I die."

I stared at him. "What are you talking about? God doesn't give people notice. He takes them when He wants them."

"I know that. Just the same I need three days' notice."

My nerves were raw. "Don't be ridiculous, Murph. Get your will taken care of and that's it. There ain't no notice. You can hide in the eye of a needle but He'll find you when He wants you."

Murphy was adamant. "I've done my will and I've left a letter about my funeral, but I still need three days' warning."

Damn, he could irritate me. "For God's sake, Murph, when it's time to go, why can't you just close your eyes and go, like everybody else?"

"Well, like now we're on our way to Reno. If I know I'm going to die I need time to get back to L.A. and go through my apartment and get rid of all those dirty magazines and videos. I don't want my kids going through my things and saying, 'Did Dad really read this junk?' "

"Murphy! How can you need three days for that? How much porno have you got?" A touch of smile flickered in his eyes. Despite myself I began to laugh . . . he'd done it again.

I'D GOTTEN to Reno a week ahead of time to acclimate but I went to bed and stayed there, frightened. Altovise, Shirley, Murphy, and the roadies were coming in and out of the room and doing jokes. They weren't saying anything funny, and I didn't do jokes back with them. I didn't need jokes. What I needed was to know how to stand on my feet without getting dizzy, how to be sparkly and graceful and sing like a person who isn't dying. I could hear Shirley in the living room pep-talking them: "We've all got to be *up* and keep *him* up. Don't let anything depress him. We've got to keep him up."

It was four days before New Year's Eve. I got out of bed. I had to move around a little, try to get my legs back. I went into the living room, to the bar, and fixed myself a glass of Crush with a lot of ice. All the roadies were sitting around watching me.

Altovise sighed. "My poor old man. He gets the male menopause and then they take away his booze."

"Fuck that male menopause shit."

"I'm sorry, honey."

"And fuck 'I'm sorry, honey.' "

Murphy muttered. "I can't stand it anymore. I'm going to put some vodka in his Crush."

I snapped at him, but I picked up the warning, that my crankiness was going past acceptable. I turned to Altovise, apologetically. "Don't feel sorry for me. They didn't take away my booze. I drank it all up. There ain't none left anymore in the whole world."

Back in bed I tried to imagine walking onstage without having that little taste in the wings, and then having a Crush instead of a vodka and Coke in the middle of the show. It wouldn't *look* like me. Part of the image was: boozer. They weren't going to see the Sammy they knew, and it wasn't like I had a new and better Sammy to offer. They had to be disappointed. I would have canceled if it wasn't Harrah's, with Holmes and Doug counting on me. And for myself. Though I'd become personally friendly with Dick Goeglein, president of Holiday Inns Gaming Division, and his wife, still Harrah's was a business and I had to come through on the stage.

On New Year's Eve day I went downstairs and did a sound check. I sat down and watched George rehearsing the band. Thank God for him.

At nine-thirty Bernard came into the dressing room. "Thirty minutes, Mr. D." And then it was show time. Leaning against a stool in the wings, I heard all the New Year's Eve sounds, bottles popping, noisemakers, a level of hilarity which tired me. Listening to the overture, I felt too weak to sing those songs.

I said, "Good evening, ladies and gentlemen," accepted their welcome, and then sat on a stool. I did forty-five minutes, all of it sitting down. I sang Bojangles from the stool without the physical moves. I didn't feel I could stand on my feet.

Doug said, "It wasn't one of your better shows. But it brought you back."

An hour later I got into bed and stayed there throughout the next day, not sleeping, just giving myself body rest, trying to save it up for the opening.

I used the stool for both shows, and the next night too. Toward the end of the first week I began feeling stronger on my feet, able to function. I missed the booze less, that little drink before I went onstage, but it was depressing to be cheating the audience out of the image they expected. By way of apology I held up my glass of Crush and ridiculed myself. "Look at this for the big swinger."

They applauded. It took me by surprise. Usually you bait them, you know what's going to get a hand, but this was a shock. As I looked out into the lights, the faces I could see were nodding at me, like "Yeah, you stopped boozing. Good on ya."

I went with it. "Frankly, I'm enjoying being straight. It's fun to wake up and know what I did the night before." They applauded.

But that time I expected it. Maybe they felt it was time for me to change. Maybe they were changing too. Whatever, it was working for me. They weren't disappointed in me. I said, "I'm pushing sixty. I've played Harrah's for twenty-five years and this year is the first time I've ever come onstage without a drink in me." More applause. "Of course, there's about three years of the twenty-five that I don't remember playing here." The laughter was filled with camaraderie. I said, "Oh? You noticed?" The warmth coming at me was like what you get in your living room with friends. They didn't feel that I had to give them perpetual motion, perpetual youth. It was "Yeah, Sam, we know you from the old days and we dig *you*, not the swinger, not the kid . . ." We were friends growing older together. They wanted what I *am*, not an imitation of what I'd been. In fact, for a fifty-year-old to be playing thirty was dishonest. Maybe that's why gradually I'd been so unhappy with my performances.

Doug was backstage every night, giving moral support. "The shows are better, you're better, you've got more energy. I'm fucking thrilled."

I had been wearing neckties onstage and halfway into my first number I always pulled the tie open, like "You ain't heard nothin' yet." I'd stolen that from Jolson thirty years ago and I suddenly saw it as not only corny but too theatrical, because it was not spontaneous as it was made to look, it was planned. I craved a higher level of ethics. I wanted to walk out pure. Tah-dah. Just a drumroll and the hands outstretched. That's what an entertainer comes from and I wanted that simplicity, that honesty with the audience. I cut out that piece of business. It was the start of a new level of honesty and rapport with the audience. I also stopped coming out with the jewelry on. It had been fun but when it becomes the takeover of what you are, then it's time to back away from it. And for simple showmanship you do not give the people exactly what they are expecting. They were delighted to see me come out clean of all the diamonds. On the other hand, you don't waste a good signature, so toward the close of the show, as I was singing "I've Got to Be Me," I started putting on the rings and it was a giggle because it showed that I was laughing at myself, not a "Hey, look at all this jewelry I've got!" And I'd do a line like "Do you recognize me now?"

I found that I needed solitude for a few hours before the shows. I needed to be alone to prepare. After returning from the edge of the abyss, each show was dear to me. I could no longer make them up as I went along. I owed more to my public and to myself than to walk on and hope for the best. There would be no more "Catch the second show" because I knew the first wouldn't be good enough. I didn't want to say that anymore. Catch any show you want. They all have to be good. Or else become a wastrel and don't give a shit and let's see where the money comes from then.

At four o'clock in the afternoon I went into my bedroom, cut the phone, and let myself come together mentally. Then around five o'clock I bathed and an hour later I had a tray brought in, a little soup, a small steak, and while I watched the television news I had my dinner alone and relaxed. I needed that time, to just sit, to tranquilize myself, to have my mind clear when I walked on. By seven o'clock I was in the dressing room putting my makeup on, charged up again, eager for the moment of getting out there with the audience.

Part of show business is magic. You don't know how it happens. You don't know what circumstances are the ones that affect you. It could be somebody saying hello as you walked down from your suite, or somebody coming to you with a piece of paper: "My grandmother loves you . . ." You don't know what that extra something is that makes you know they're with you, that puts that little straightener in your back and makes you know you can do it again.

25

THE DESERT INN wanted me to play eight weeks, four weeks at a crack, at $100,000 per week. It was a drop in price, but I was attracted to the show room, one of the last small Vegas rooms, a seven-hundred-seater. Weekends I could sell out anywhere, but I didn't want the pressure you feel at Caesars during the week, that only the pit is filled, which alone seats four hundred. Frank couldn't do it. He had left Caesars and gone to the new Nugget, which was downtown and where he had a marvelous seven-hundred-seater.

I had a good feeling about the Desert Inn, that I could create some excitement there.

Shirley was dubious. "Can you do four straight weeks?"

Without drinking, suddenly I got healthy and the energy level came back so strong that I could fly over buildings. "I wouldn't have dared try it a few years ago. But I never felt better than I feel now. Let's go for it. Tell them I'll do a one-man show. I don't want any opening act. Have them put that money into more musicians. I want a concert-sized orchestra."

Then, once having committed, I wondered: *Can I do it?* And why? Why put that extra pressure on myself? The answer rushed after the question: *Because I'm supposed to be the premier nightclub performer, the variety artist, the last of a breed. So I can't keep giving them yesterday. I have to keep growing, giving them something fresh, different.*

The marquee at the Desert Inn said, "Sammy, That's All." And I told them to eliminate the announcer saying, "Sammy Davis, Jr."

The audience knew who they'd come to see. I was in concert with a sixty-piece orchestra, in my best shape ever, and from opening night it was pure excitement.

In the middle of a dinner show I saw my tap shoes in the piano where they had always been. Impulsively I reached in and took them out, as though to fondle some favored memorabilia. The audience began applauding. I held the shoes in my hands. "It's been a long time since I felt I could use these. Maybe I'm not as old as I've been feeling."

They continued urging me on. Apprehensive, I needed a moment before I was prepared to commit myself to dancing. Audiences always enjoyed the sight of my yard-long shoehorn, which is a saber given to me by the Queen's Guards in London, made for me with a shoehorn at the tip by the Wilkinson Sword people. I held it up. "There's nothing in my contract that says I gotta bend down." As they laughed I lowered the shoehorn and slipped into my shoes. I flicked the taps a few beats to feel my legs. Okayyyy. The audience was applauding again, standing on their feet. I danced for them. I wished I could reach out and hug the whole room. I kept dancing, hugging them the only way I knew how.

The shows were fun again. I told Altovise, "I hate to admit how good I feel." With the surge in my energy level, and maybe the ability to think clearly, I could handle, or adjust to, my age and have fun with the change, settle into it instead of fighting it. I'd do "I've Got You Under My Skin" and get into the bumping and grinding and then "catch myself" and sort of apologize, "That's a little residue from the *old* days," and it got a tremendous laugh because the old customers remembered me that way.

How sweet it was to walk on after fifty-seven years of performing, do whatever your heart says is right, and feel the audience happy to go in any direction with you. When I was holding a big note I could feel them holding it with me, breathing with me, and then I saw some of them taking off their wristwatches so they wouldn't break them as they pounded their hands together telling me what they were feeling.

I drank Crush onstage and kidded myself: "I'm glad I gave up boozing. The only bad part is that when I wake up in the morning I know that this is as good as I'm gonna feel all day. Ain't gonna get no better."

I had no doubt that alcohol was poison for me, but I missed that marvelous little buzz. I'm not talking "Let's go get pissed," but that nice little glow, that cocktail that makes the whole system titillate, and you hear little voices: "Hello there, I'm awake, I'm alive. Remember me? I'm your heart." I missed the fun, the camaraderie of "Well, time for a little taste." And I missed a little of the devil-may-care, the scarf-over-the-shoulder.

Oh, did I envy those people who could still have that kick when they wanted it. I wanted to tell my children, "Respect it and you can enjoy it all your life. Abuse it and you'll go the last twenty years or more craving it, but you can't have any, 'cause if you do you'll die."

What I wanted now was solidity, reliability. I only had about two more mistakes left to me. When you're thirty-five and you own a piece of show business and you're doing *Ocean's Eleven*, you come up to bat fifteen times. So you strike out a few times. But when you're pushing sixty you're a designated hitter and every time you come up at bat you'd better do something. I didn't have hit movies, hit records, or a TV series going for me, I had to do it with performance, and with consistency. No more "Wasn't he great tonight?" No. He had to be "great" *every* night, twice a night, and it was not all from being talented and experienced. Much of it was in conditioning, being able to walk out there rested, together. I knew that if I dissipated, ate badly, missed getting the sleep I needed, the audience would feel "Gee, he's sluggish tonight." But if I was in training, if I went out there fresh, lean, with my fighting weight on, then it was a bout.

And it was exciting for George, it was the two of us out there doing it, like the old days. I'd come back to the dressing room and he'd be there ahead of me, and knowing I was going to walk in, he'd be telling Murph, "Damn, I thought I'd have to keep my arms in the air forever. Thought the li'l motherfucker was gonna stay on all night he was feelin' so good . . . Ooohh, here he is, shhhh, don't say anything . . ."

Without the obsession with youth and the swinger image, my mind was free for me to be a creative performer again, developing moments, an atmosphere, varying the texture of each show. I can sing the same songs but in different moods, so that the tapestry of it takes on a different hue, a different color. Sometimes it's bright and yellow, sometimes it's subdued. It shouldn't be just the cliché: "He never does two shows alike." The shows at the end of the week should be a collage.

Feeling my oats one night, I told the audience, "I'm going to tell you a story that ain't got no punch line but I think it's amusing." The story was about Fred Astaire and I'd intended it as a lead-in to my Astaire medley. The story is: Fred Astaire's house is across the road from mine, about four houses away, a few hundred yards. One day he was out on his terrace playing his music and I was on mine and I heard this music coming from his direction, great music, Jonah Jones kind of old-fashioned jazz, Billy Butterfield, that kind of thing. I thought: That's Astaire, and I knew he was on his deck listening to it. And I was on my wooden-floored veranda, also listening. When the record ended I stood up and tapped: "boom diddy boom boom . . ." and from across the road I heard him tap back: "boom, boom!"

Well, this long story died like a dog. Nobody even tittered. They just sat there looking at me. The guys in the band started to break up because I'd bombed. I turned to them. "Hey, I told the people it wasn't so funny . . ." I'd thought it was a wonderfully warm story but when the audience just looked at me and when that broke up the guys in the band, I said, "Okay, it's a dumb story. I never should have told it. I should have kept it just for the house. That's what I should have done. I knew it was going to die. I haven't the faintest idea why I did that. In fact, I felt myself sinking when I was in the middle of it, I was thinking: Nothing's going to save this. Do a tap dance, do some magic, fall down, *something!* . . . Why did I bring this up? I'm getting all this money, I've got diamonds from thumb to thumb . . . looking good . . . and I tell a stupid story like that . . ."

By then people were applauding. Yet the fact is that though it's a cute, charming story, it doesn't belong on the stage. I was trying to give the audience a little offstage picture, like "This is something you don't see all the time . . ." and into the toilet it went. Still, the failure had its value to me. It showed vulnerability: "Hey, not everything he says is slick and good . . . he's like me, he can fuck up." But being vulnerable is a two-way street: if they're tuned in enough to sympathize, to catch all the nuances, and to root for you, they're also able to catch even a hint of phoniness or "routine."

Most performers don't have that rapport with the audience. They aren't that honest with the audience, they hide behind a façade of perfection. They do it the same way every night, the same gesture, the same joke in the same place at every show, because that is their protection. It's all right to do that with a few numbers, as I do with my opening songs, but after that it's all ad-lib according to what I feel like doing and what I sense the audience feels like hearing. As a stage director will say, "Trust yourself. Use your instrument. Trust what God gave you." If you don't give yourself some stretching room, some freedom, you'll never find anything. You don't know you have the ability to be funny unless you try a line, you don't know if you can ad-lib if you're going to do the same jokes every night. There are lines I know are going to get a belly laugh but after a few shows I get sick of hearing myself say them and so I drop them. I forget them for three or four engagements, then when I bring them back in they're fresh for me. The one thing you don't want is that stale sound when you've done a line so much that you can't find a fresh approach to it. Drop it and you'll think of something else, you'll fill.

TRACEY AND her fiancé, Guy Aldo Garner, came to Vegas to spend Labor Day weekend with me and they stayed with me in my suite. Guy is a white Episcopalian. Tracey and he had dated for three years. I'd had a good chance to meet his family, who come from Redwood, California, understand his background, and learn that he was straight-arrow, possessing the strengths, character, and values which I always appreciated even if I didn't apply them to my own life. So, whatever color, he was the right young man. Nor did the religious difference matter, because though Tracey was brought up in Judaism and honors it she never followed the tenets of Judaism. That was her choice to make as she became an adult.

I liked Guy a lot, and I enjoyed them both. I didn't run from them, and they didn't run from me, and suddenly our relationship had quality. I cooked for them and we hung out together in the suite, talking and laughing. When she'd been an infant I used to hug Tracey and call her "princess of the world." Then there were the years when I had no time for her. Now I had all the time she would give me.

My suite had a swimming pool and I ordered a buffet breakfast put out for us by its side. We had a great morning and after we'd sat in the sun chatting for a while Tracey said, "We'll see you later, Dad. We're going to the hotel pool and use the floats."

It was 1987, nobody was going to bother them or stare them down or even take special notice that they were there, except for their friends who were waiting for them. It wasn't like 1960 was for May and for me. My mind knew that but my stomach still worked on reflexes. It probably would for the rest of my life. But fortunately not Tracey's. It wouldn't occur to her that a mixed couple might have trouble around the pool in Las Vegas, because they no longer did. She was a child of the civil rights movement that had caused this change.

"Change" was hardly the word to describe it. I thought that I had never in my life seen any era become ancient history as completely as the civil rights movement. There were no more militants, no more black glasses and "do's." The black leaders had gone to three-piece suits. Ron Karenga was wearing a tweed jacket and working as a professor of African Studies at a university in California. I had the off-the-wall feeling that if Kim Novak and I ran into each other and one of us said, "Let's have dinner," the joke line would have been: "But what's the fun of it? Nobody'll care."

I loved having my kids with me, but then, too quickly, it was Sunday afternoon and they said they had to pack. We were in the living room and they went upstairs.

For all of Tracey's life, when it had been time to part I'd said, "See you later. Bye." But I didn't want them to go. At sixty you begin thinking about the last years of your life and you know that you have no time to waste. I went upstairs. "Listen, if you don't have anything special planned, why don't you hang out with me for another day?"

Tracey looked up from the suitcase she'd been packing. Her face appeared startled, looking at me with a mixture of emotions. I knew that face when she was an infant, I remembered it smiling at me from her first bicycle, looking at me in London when she saw me with women she didn't know. I knew that little face in anger, dismay, eagerness, pleasure, a hundred ways, but I had never seen the smile I was looking at then. "Y'know, Dad? That's the first time in my life you ever said that." Tracey did not brush away the tears, she let me see them. They were a kiss, a hug that said, "I understand, Dad."

THE OLD-TIME excitement was back again at every performance. At that juncture in Vegas history, when everything was computerized, at a time when some performers were taping their numbers and mouthing them, phoning it in, I was ending the shows wailing, "If I Never Sing Another Song," hitting every note with clarity. And the customers were coming back to see me two and three times in a week.

Clint Eastwood came backstage and gestured me off into a corner, looking at me studiously, the serious actor. "Sam, what does it feel like to have all those people out there and everybody loves you?"

Looking into the face I'd known as a friend for over twenty years, suddenly, zoooom, I saw that face in the context of the number one box office star in the world but it occurred to me that he would never know that feeling. He gets it through his mail, through his millions of fans, he can walk along a street and stop traffic, all that, but not being a down-front performer he would never know the feeling of standing dead center on the stage in the spotlight, having that love come at you in waves that make you feel good-looking.

Frank came to Vegas to play the Nugget for the weekend and he called me and did mock angry: "What is this? Why don't you retire? This is no time to start doing one-man shows, for crying out loud. What am I supposed to do? Get rid of all the comics that go on with me? And all those musicians! You trying to support the union?" Then, jokes done, he leveled: "I hear the show's marvelous, just marvelous, and that your voice is in great condition. When am I going to see you?"

Saturday after the second show I met him in his dressing room. "C'mon," he said, "we don't want to go up to the suite." He turned to his security guys. "We'll go to the lounge." As we walked in he said, "I've never been here before." There was a little table that they kept reserved for him in case he ever came in. He said, "No, let's sit over here, up front."

A few minutes after we were seated a drunk started toward us, you could see him staggering. Frank said, "Here it comes. Oh hell, it's a white guy too."

I said, "Sure, *my* people can't get in this section."

"Damn! It's a white guy, it's a white guy."

His security guys let the man through and he signed the autograph. Despite a lot of bum raps in this kind of a situation, Frank recognizes what all performers recognize: If you don't want to sign it, don't go out there. If you're going from a restaurant to the car, you're not in public, you're on your way somewhere. Or if you get caught while you're eating, your security guys will say, "See him a little later." But if you're in a bar, sitting there in public, be gracious or don't go there.

When we were alone again Frank said, "The word is out on you," and he began nodding his head with pleasure. "You're having a renaissance. I couldn't be fucking happier. All the reports are magnificent."

A young cat with two wild-looking chicks walked by and Frank raised his eyebrows. "Cuff links." We sat there together quietly, each with our own thoughts. I looked at the kid with no envy. I'd been there. And it had been wonderful. But now, if ever I hear that old voice on my shoulder screaming, *Hey, let's go, let's do, grab that chick, it's a party, wheeeee* . . . I immediately hear the other voice warning, *Hold it! Two shows tomorrow.* There's no such thing as lowlifing until eight, nine in the morning and then doing two good ones. Even without drinking, for one night of my old-style wild partying into the sunrise I paid three or four days of catch-up before I felt normal again. By the grace of God I was still in the center arena, with all the lights on, and I understood what it took to keep me there.

It was getting late. I'd done two shows, I'd sat with my friend, and I was beginning to nod. I felt that at that hour there was nothing happening anywhere that interested me as much as my bed. The thought of it made me giddy. Bed, oh bed. Bed, bed, bed, soft bed.

Frank looked at his watch. It was four o'clock. He marveled: "I was up till six o'clock yesterday. I haven't done that in *years.*" We walked out of the lounge. "When you and Dean and I used to hang out till six and seven in the morning, then slept three hours and got up and shot a movie and did two shows every night, we felt okay and we looked great, but today you pay for it if you stay up till six." He put his arm around my shoulder. "It's twenty-five years later, Charley, twenty-five years . . . a quarter of a century . . ."

26

"CAN YOU STAND some good news?" Shirley asked. "If I tell you that you're solvent, can you live with that, or will you have to go out and spend it?"

We'd backed away from the edge of the cliff. From here on we could build security. No, I didn't have to go out and spend it. On the contrary. "Shirl, I can't go broke anymore. I've been broke too many times and come back. People are tired of that. *I'm* tired of it."

"Good. Then I can tell you that we're solidly in the black. We've paid off every penny to everybody. Every shop, every club, every bank. And we've got three months' cash on hand." She grinned. "Now do you understand why black is beautiful?" I just smiled at her. "And you've got a little portfolio of blue chips."

"Like what?"

"IBM, GE, Polaroid . . ."

Zoom! In the midst of my giddiness my mind went back forty years in time, riding on one word, Polaroid. I'd been in Miami playing the Beachcomber. Steve Lawrence was in the Army but he was down there doing a show. He came to my dressing room. I started taking some pictures and he said, "Hey, you've got the new Polaroid. I own stock in that company. You should buy some of that stock."

I was twenty years young. Or dumb. "Stock? What stock?"

"I bought it for two dollars a share."

"Two dollars? For a piece of paper?" But complete dumbness.

"Two dollars for a piece of paper? Stock? Market might crash . . . you're crazy, spend your money and have fun with it. Hell, nobody's gonna buy these cameras 'less they wanta take dirty pictures. That's the only reason I got this. To take pictures of chicks' tits." In those days you got photographs developed at the drugstore and if there was a nude shot on the roll and you went to collect your pictures, the druggist was waiting for you with the tight jaw and the steely eye that meant: "Degenerate!"

And now Shirley was telling me I was a Polaroid stockholder. "Listen, Shirl, call Steve and tell him thanks for the tip on Polaroid and that I've decided to go ahead and follow his advice."

I stopped watching the soap operas. With my new energy level and without the alcohol numbing my senses, I asked myself, "Three and a half hours of your life on *that* every day?" I'd been putting off business appointments. A guy would say, "Can I talk to you about a TV series?" which might earn ten million dollars and I'm telling him, "At four-thirty," after *General Hospital*. Madness.

My perfect day was to get offstage before two, in bed by four, awake by noon, be on the Desert Inn's golf course at one and back in my suite at four, cooking and watching television, listening to music, closed off from everybody, taking no calls, easing myself into the ritual before going downstairs at seven to prepare for the eight-thirty show.

I'd begun putting the dancing back into the act, gradually, soft shoe, then a little tap and building up to a solid ten-minute chunk. Not in ten years had I done a three-chorus dance. Now I was out there doing it twice a night. People were surprised. "I didn't know he could dance like that." "My God, sure, now I remember, that's how he started." Tap dancing was anachronistic, so it had a nostalgic charm. It was fun doing it, fun having people react to it, so I kept it in, dancing, dancing, dancing . . .

My left hip began bothering me during the Canon Sammy Davis Jr. Open in Hartford, Connecticut, but I decided I was going to play a full round. When I came up the fairway on the eighteenth hole there were twenty-five thousand people standing there applauding me, like I was nine under. The next day a Hartford newspaper's headline was "HE FINISHED 18" and there was a front-page picture of me, like I'd won the tournament. But in fact, by the fifteenth hole I'd begun sitting in the golf cart every moment I could.

The pain got worse while I was playing Atlantic City. The hotel doctor saw nothing serious—age, arthritis, or rheumatism—and I treated it with hot baths.

I'd signed to play the role of the Caterpillar in *Alice in Wonderland*, starring Carol Channing. When I showed up for rehearsals with Jillian Lynn, the choreographer, she said, "Why don't you work out a little bit? Warm up."

"Get outta here." I gave her a look and tapped, boom diddy boom boom—boom boom! "Ready."

Tap dancers never warmed up. Our kind of tap isn't a question of getting the whole body in different positions like Fred Astaire and Gene Kelly, who are "ballet tap dancers." Simple tap dancers don't move their bodies much, it's all legs, from the waist down.

"Okay, then," she said, "let's get to work," and we began two weeks of rehearsals, leaping here, leaping over there, jumping up, jumping off things. I hadn't done that kind of "movie dancing" in years and I loved it. In the middle of rehearsing a number I did a turn-around and felt a sharp pain in my hip. Jillian caught it. "What's the matter?" She scolded, "I told you to warm up."

I brushed it off. "The Candy Man is getting old, that's all." After rehearsal I drew myself the hottest tub I could stand and tried to soak away the soreness. What I needed was about four fingers of vodka. But that was out.

On the set the next day it hurt but I kept doing my number. Then, at the finish, a girl had to sit on the Caterpillar's knee. It was more pain than I could stand. My left leg simply failed to support me and I found myself sitting on the floor looking up at Jillian. Alarmed, she said, "You're not *this* old," and she helped me to my feet.

Gerald brought me to Eugene Harris, an orthopedic surgeon. After examination and X rays he said, "Let me show you something," and he put the pictures on a viewer. "That's your hip bone. The dark area is deterioration. Your hip bone is disintegrating."

"From what?" and my mind started churning: *All that bad I've done, it's catching up with me. If I hadn't been putting that shit up my nose I'd be all right.*

He asked, "How old are you?"

"Fifty-eight, nine."

"Look, Sammy, the calendar has been very active. Those pages have been falling off a lot and it's showing."

"What are you saying?"

"You're suffering from dancer's, or athlete's, degeneration. You've been using your bones and your sockets harder and for more time than they're made to withstand. Since you've laid off alcohol you've got the energy of a twenty-year-old and so you're dancing up a storm and you're paying for it. You're taking a sixty-year-old hip socket and grinding it hard twice a night. Take a piece of wood and do that for ten minutes a night for only a year and see what happens."

"If I slow down the dancing will it get better?"

"No, the damage is done. But you have a couple of choices. I recommend a hip replacement—that is, a replacement of the total hip joint with a metal or a plastic hip joint."

It ejected me from the chair. I saw myself doddering along the street with a cane. I'm looking at him like I'm Nureyev, like I move and jump, like dancing is my whole life and "What? I'll never do *Swan Lake* again?" But in fact I was a singer doing ten minutes of tap at most and sometimes just two choruses of "I'll Go My Way by Myself . . ." slow, easy. Dancing wasn't my act, it was just a little frosting. But I yelled at the man, "No, no, no! I ain't doing no cuttin'. No way."

He wasn't a snap-your-fingers, shoot-your-cuffs Hollywood guy. Patiently, he said, "You need something done, Sammy."

"What else you got?"

"We could do a reconstruction. We can rebuild that hip bone in there for you, we don't insert anything foreign into your leg, the complications are significantly less, the blood loss is less, but it's only a temporary correction. In its favor, it is not a bridge-burning procedure. Should it fail, then something else can be done. If successful, you'll get a year or a year and a half out of it, maybe two at best."

I couldn't stand it. Everything had been so positive. In a week I was beginning a two-week date at Caesars with Bill Cosby. Then back into the Desert Inn.

"Temporarily, hip reconstruction can take you out of pain and keep you off medication. When you decide to do it, plan on needing eight weeks to heal. You'll be on your back for six weeks. But eventually you'll have to have a hip replacement."

"Let's handle that when we come to it. We'll talk about it. Meanwhile I have a picture to finish."

"I'll give you a muscle relaxant, Motrin. I recommend that you eliminate all dancing. We'll keep an eye on this and hope to defer surgery."

Leaving there, I thought: *Surgery? Nobody's ever going to cut into my hip. I'm a song-and-dance man.* I didn't mention it to Altovise, or to Murphy or Shirley, or any of the roadies.

I got through the filming of *Alice in Wonderland,* amidst pain, but it was done.

THE ENGAGEMENT with Bill was so hot and the shows were so good that I didn't want to go out there without doing it to the nines. So I didn't allow myself to limp onstage. Limping is just an evasion of pain. And even though it hurt like hell I danced. When occasionally I couldn't hide the pain, I'd kid it: "Damn, if I'd known I was gonna live this long I'd have taken better care of myself." Offstage I explained it away as "dancer's hip" and I spent a lot of time in hot tubs.

As night after night we drew lines of people across the lobby of Caesars, turning away customers from that fourteen-hundred-seat room at every performance, I was nonplussed by what it was saying. We were two black guys onstage to entertain a predominantly white audience yet it was hard to remember the last time there'd been a hater in the audience. Only twenty or thirty years had passed, not very long for such massive social turn-around.

During a second show, I told the audience, "You're sympathetic to what's happened racially or you wouldn't be here. The changes were not made only by black people. On all those marches, all those sit-ins and pray-ins, we had a lot of white buddies by our sides. I know that some of you were there with us. I don't recognize your faces but I recognize your smiles and I understand the vibes I'm getting. So I'd like to give you an illustration of the change there has been in our country. In the 1920s there was a book named *Show Boat* written by Edna Ferber. It was made into a musical play and the lyrics were written by Oscar Hammerstein, a liberal-minded man who later wrote *South Pacific,* which had lyrics like 'You've got to be taught to hate and fear . . .' The score of *Show Boat* included the song 'Old Man River.' I'd like to sing it for you with the original lyric."

I sang, "Niggers all work on the Mississippi . . ." On the word "nigger" the audience gasped, there was an intake of breath and that look on their faces like "My God, that's right . . ." Even after a minute-and-a-half preamble to do a song that lasts three minutes they were shaken by my saying it onstage. Dramatically it was right, and socially it was appropriate for a black man to look around him and say, "It's not perfect yet, but yeah, it's getting better," as Martin Luther King had said in the sixties: "We ain't what we oughta be, we ain't what we wanta be, we ain't what we gonna be, but thank God we ain't what we was."

When we closed Caesars I went to New York to receive an award at a Police Athletic League dinner, and then to be present for some fund-raising functions of the Sammy Davis, Jr., Liver Institute. I carried a cane walking through airports, using it jauntily as I had for years when I didn't need one for support. I should have allowed myself to be rolled along those long walks in a wheelchair but I didn't want the press to start speculating, and with a one-month run at the Desert Inn ahead of me I didn't want the "family" on my back. The thought of operating on my leg was terrifying, yet at moments the pain was so great that I felt like shouting, "Cut the fucker off." At the PAL dinner I was barely able to stand to accept my award.

By the time I returned to the Desert Inn the first two weeks were sold out. Opening night was scheduled as a single show, at nine o'clock. George rehearsed the orchestra and at around 3 p.m. I got dressed to go over for a sound check.

My suite was in the Wimbledon building, a hundred yards from the stage entrance in the main building. Shirley and Murphy were with me when Brian came by to get me and we all went together. Helping myself along with a cane, I walked down the corridor to the entrance. Ten yards from the front door my boot heel caught in a bump in the carpet and I felt a jolt of pain burn across my hips and legs. Tears teemed out of my eyes. Sweat washed across my body. Shirley and Brian caught me before I fell and got me back to the suite. They put me on the bed and I realized: *I can't make it.*

"Murph, call Altovise . . . tell her to make arrangements with Dr. Harris. I can't beat this. I'll do the one show but I've gotta close tonight."

Brian came to get me at eight o'clock. He had a golf cart out front. The road was smooth, a perfect sidewalk between buildings, but every pebble we rolled over reverberated through my hip and leg. I lay down in the dressing room. Bernard came in with my clothes. "How you feelin', Mr. D.?" I felt too terrible to be ornery. I nodded. George came in. "You in trouble?" I nodded.

Walking toward the center of the stage, as I tried to accept the pain instead of the limp, I couldn't, it was too much. The audience could see it. I sang the opening medley standing in one place.

"Good evening, ladies and gentlemen, thank you for coming here this evening. This was supposed to be the start of a four-week engagement. But in fact this is opening night and it's also going to be closing night. I've got a hip that's been bothering me and I've got to go in and get it fixed. I've been putting it off. I'm not going to tell you I'm feeling great, but you were nice enough to come here and my voice is wonderful—if I do say it myself—so let me sing some songs for you. It will be a while before I'll be singing again." I sat on a stool and did fifty minutes that were, under the circumstances, a great show.

Holmes and Doug sent a Harrah's plane to take me into Burbank the following afternoon. From there we had a helicopter waiting to bring me to the Cedars Sinai landing pad. In the hospital, waiting for Gerry Blankfort, I was incredulous. *How can this be happening to me? It's not possible. I've survived the liver, survived the change of image. Now this! Eight weeks on my back. All I wanted was to work steady, accumulate a little money, but I'm not going to be able to.*

Around twenty families were dependent upon my generating income. Canceling the Desert Inn was a $400,000 loss. And if I had the operation I'd have to cancel an Australian tour scheduled for January and a number of American concerts, a cash loss totaling a million dollars.

Shirley said, "Don't worry about how long you're out. We've got the cash to take care of everything even if you don't sing 'Bojangles' for three months."

"Great. But what if the operation doesn't work? Then what?" Gerry came in. Cheerful. I glared at him. "If I'd stayed on booze I'd never have danced and I wouldn't be here in this hospital."

"And you'd have died from your liver."

"Maybe." He was accustomed to my abuse. "I'm scared, Gerry. Cat gonna cut into my hip? What if he misses? Cuts too deep and the whole fuckin' leg comes off?"

"Sammy, he's a professional, the best in the business."

"So am I, but I've bombed. What if *he* bombs? On *me!* How do they bill me in Vegas? 'Peg Leg'? No. I can't risk it. I'll take the pain, but I won't have to come on like a sideshow."

Obviously concerned for me, he said, "Listen, you're in a hospital. You've had to quit a four-week engagement. You did one show and almost couldn't do *that*. Stop kidding yourself, Sam, you've got to have an operation on your hip." He pulled a chair up to the bed. "You've beaten bigger things than this. The victories you've had were the *vis a tergo*, the force from behind that always urged you on. I don't know how much you'll be able to dance again if you do this operation. But I know that without it you won't even walk much."

After a while he got up. "I'll come see you tomorrow. Meanwhile, be nice to the nurses. You don't have to chase 'em, but you don't have to be sullen either."

I asked Dr. Harris, "Will I walk with a crutch? Tell me as much as I can understand. The more I know about it, the better."

"Normally, there's an eighty percent chance of success. However, with people over fifty there are variables. You may be able to walk but not move well, you may have a permanent limp. I can't tell you about dancers I've operated on, because I have *never* operated on a dancer. But I have had many athletes, professionals and serious amateurs, who've done this with the result of full movement, and been able to go back to their sport."

"When will we know if the operation's a success?"

"Immediately after I do it. But we won't know about the recuperation for one month. I don't take X rays until then, because they wouldn't mean anything. The operation is up to me. The recovery and recuperation are up to you. If you do all your stuff, then I'll be a hero. If you don't, then I'll be a son of a bitch, or incompetent, or whatever. Frankly, I hate working with celebrities."

I asked, "Is this what you'd call a major or a minor operation?"

"In orthopedics, what you're having done is a minor operation. But anytime a doctor puts a knife into a patient there is nothing minor about it. It shouldn't be to the doctor, and it certainly isn't to the patient."

It wasn't exactly the answer I'd been looking for, but I appreciated the attitude. They say tonsils and appendix are minor operations. Meanwhile, you cut skin and blood comes out.

I watched it being announced on the TV newscasts. Then the telegrams and flowers began arriving. In twenty-four hours I heard from almost everybody I had ever known, from as far away as military hospitals in Israel. And there were a lot of jokes. Bill Cosby sent me a brown leg. Milton Berle sent me a small crutch. Charles Nelson Reilly, who'd had a hip replacement, sent me a walker. They were funny and they helped. And of course I got more than one telegram saying, "Wouldn't you know that if Sammy Davis had an operation it would be hip?" My kids came up every day. President Reagan sent flowers with a little message: "Nancy and I wish you the very best." It made me cry.

Shirley MacLaine called every day and we're such old friends that I let on what I was feeling. "Trust in them, Sam. Let them take charge. Don't you try to guide it all the time."

Frank called, "Who's your doctor?"

"Eugene Harris, a great bone man."

"Let me write that down. Give me his name again . . ."

"Thanks, Frank, it's Eugene Harris, but really, don't bother checking him out, I already have."

". . . because I can get the guy from Switzerland who does all the skiers. I talked to him and I can send the plane for him tonight."

"Frank, the man is good."

"Harris . . . well, I'll get back to you." The attitude was: "Wait a minute, clear the decks, I'll bring my ship in." "But I've got a boat." "No, no, that's too small for you." He called back. "Harris checks out good. By the way, how are they treating you in that joint?" Frank hates Cedars Sinai though he's given millions to it. "If they aren't treating you right I'll send the plane, bring you right out here to the Springs, get this great orthopedic guy from Switzerland . . ."

I FELT MY body move and I knew they were putting me back in my bed. I reached down for my legs and felt them both there. As my vision returned I saw Dr. Harris and he said he was pleased, that now it was a matter of careful recovery.

The limo waited at the black iron gate in front of my house while Scotty drew it open for us to pass. Lately I'd enjoyed looking at it, at the guard who opened and closed it, appreciating the solidity, the security, the success. I waved hello without looking. Until then I'd been on a hospital high, the center of attraction, on the TV news, a million years away from "Good evening, ladies and gentlemen . . ." But now, at home, I was a giant step closer to that day.

My cars were parked where I liked them but I had trouble looking at them too, and the grass, the trees, the cared-for hedges and shrubbery. They were happiness, stardom, and I wasn't feeling like that.

Brian handed me my crutches and helped me through the front door. I turned left, toward my bedroom, noting that the floor had been polished for my return, there was a "Welcome Home" sign and balloons, and I continued hobbling to my room.

Altovise began undressing me, which I hated, but I couldn't do it myself. I lay there wondering what happens if I'm left with a bad limp. "Oh, there he is, the cripple." And then they don't want me at Harrah's or the Desert Inn after that one curiosity appearance. Or twice, to see if I fall down.

I had no buffers, no drugs, no whiskey, just reality. And reality is fear of the unknown waiting around the bend. I had a month of suspense, the month before they could take an X ray.

You go from new boy on the block to a star to a superstar. Those are plateaus you can see. Then there are invisible plateaus. When do you become the so firmly established superstar that nothing can take it away?

That's where I should be by now, but am I? What if I'm not and I go into the toilet? Could I learn to live with not being a star? Sammy Davis the guy, the man on the street. I'd always known that when I went out past my front gate I was "on," and I'd learned how to handle myself. But how do I walk down the street and know that nobody notices? Like every celebrity, I'd played the anonymity game, with the dark glasses, coat collar up, and hat over the eyes, like "Don't notice me, please." And thank God for the moment when I heard "Hey, Sam, what's with hiding under the hat?" What would it be like not to need a security man with me all the time? After almost sixty years of opening any door with my fame, what would it be like to wait in line, to be asked, "Do you have a reservation?"

You'd better be able to deal with it, because tomorrow all the cars and the guns could be gone, and you could be living on Fifth Street. But for the grace of God and your intelligence, which also you got by the grace of God, you would never have gotten to this level in the world.

Now, what if He wants to take it all away from me? Then it's square one again. I'm too old to go square one again. I don't want to go square one. Yet the reality is, anyone can go back there. Reality is a terrorist knocking at the door. I'm not armed. Helpless. Well, who is it out there? Guy with a mask over his face. He's come to knock my balance off.

Altovise was trying to get my attention. "You look so depressed, honey."

I looked away. *Well, I'm extremely sorry if I'm depressed. I'm depressed because I can't empty the fucking bar out. I had just gotten that balance going and I was in business. And then the hip happened and knocked that balance off.*

"Honey, would you like anything?"

That was my support system standing there and I loved her and wanted to be nice to her, but I snarled, "Would I like anything? I'd like my career back. Leave me alone, is what I'd like."

In a few minutes she returned to the bedroom smiling, handing me an envelope which had just arrived in the mail.

THE WHITE HOUSE

December 2, 1985

Dear Sammy,

Nancy and I understand that Altovise has planned a wonderful surprise birthday party for you. We send our warmest congratulations and our special hope that you are well along the road to recovery from your recent surgery.

If this occasion brings about some reflection on your part you should have a fine time musing over the fullness of your life. From childhood on you have been a dynamic force in the entertainment industry. Whether it be singing, dancing, or acting, you have done it with rare talent and dazzling energy. You have given audiences some of the finest performances they have ever seen. So, when you think about your accomplishments, don't forget all those fans—including Nancy and me—who are captivated and delighted by "Mr. Entertainment."

Happy birthday, Sammy, and may God bless and keep you.

Sincerely,
Ronald Reagan

I looked again at the words "dynamic," "dazzling," "Mr. Entertainment."

"You'll feel better when you're working again, honey."

"Brilliant! Even assuming I can work at all, what am I going to look like? Okay, we now know that I don't have to be perpetual motion. But neither am I Rudy Vallee. The Sammy Davis they know comes out and says, 'Hey, look out,' and goes 'bungachung-abung chung . . .' and grooves and kicks and *does* it. That's the me that I created. Now, how do I do those moves? *Moves?* How about can I stand on my feet for an hour and ten minutes? Forget dancing and moving. Can I just physically support myself on my feet for over an hour? Try it. You're healthy. Stand over there for an hour and ten. And when you're dying to sit down, then bust your hip and try it."

Despite all the luxury around me the depression just sank in. Lying there, my livelihood on the line, I wondered: *Who really cares? Who isn't here only to make a buck out of me? Or because of the glitter? Who'd hang in if I had to go back to being an opening act?*

I lay in bed watching the people around me—Altovise, Shirley, Lessie Lee, Murphy, Eddie, all looking worried. *But is it for me? Or 'cause the fucking breadwinner is going out the window . . . the meal ticket . . . that's what worries them . . . not how I'm feeling.*

They'd come in, cute, cheer-him-up, "How's you today?"

What the fuck do you care?

"Boss, is there anything I can do for you?"

Get the fuck away, is what you can do. Leave me alone. Why do you have to ask nine times, "Is there anything I can do for you?"

Murphy was crying just for seeing me on my back. "Sammy, try to see the bright side. The doctor says you've passed the worst of it. There's a light at the end of the tunnel."

I attacked. "That's a cliché. And yeah, that light is a train coming straight at me. Which is a double fucking cliché."

His face was running with tears. I could see I was dragging everybody down with me but I didn't mind dragging everybody down. *Fuck it. I'm suffering, why can't everybody else suffer?*

"Mr. Davis, what're you gonna want for dinner? And when're you gonna want it?"

346

Hold it. Don't be sharp with Lessie. She's an old lady. Get rid of her nicely. "I'll have dinner at eight every night, in my bed, babe. Make me anything you want me to eat."

Altovise came in. "Richard Zanuck called and wanted to know how you're feeling."

"Tell him to go fuck himself that he's got a picture, that's how I'm feeling." She ran for cover. I broke myself up. I was aware that I'd said it to someone who I knew was not going to dial him back and say, "Mr. Zanuck, Sammy says to go fuck yourself that you've got a picture, that's how he's feeling."

Jack Haley, Jr., came in. "Hi."

"Go fuck yourself."

He turned around and walked out.

That's how you talk to one of your best friends?

Eddie came in. "I don't want to bug you but Mr. Sinatra's on the phone. Do you want to talk?"

"Of course I don't want to talk! To anybody. And of course I *will* talk to *him.*"

"With a capital H?"

"Get outta here."

Altovise was taking the brunt of it. Everybody else could joke and go home. But she was suffering. *Bullshit she's suffering! I'm the one who's lost his career! On a hummer! What about me? Fuck you, what about me?*

I didn't shave. I grew a beard. My hair was all messed up but I couldn't be bothered with it.

Shirley MacLaine kept calling. "Sam? It's bigmouth Shirley again."

"F'r chrissakes, what is it now?"

"I know you're not talking to anyone, I know you're in the shits, so shut up and listen. I know what you're worrying about. You think you're through. You think that maybe you won't be able to perform again, or that even if you can you won't be the same and they won't like you 'cause you're different, 'cause you're slower, but you're wrong, because you're overlooking the fact that you've got almost a sixty-year track record with those people."

"Shirl, you don't understand what the commitment is and how hard it is to meet it."

"Bullshit! You're just feeling sorry for yourself. Sam, the leg is no problem because you don't have to dance. You don't have the lead in *Giselle*. If you feel like patting your foot, do it. Or twisting a little. If not, then just stand there and let them love you."

"It's not that simple, Shirley. My obligation is, I don't want to limp on or limp off or limp around the stage. 'Here comes the guy with the cane.' I don't want the focus on 'Let's watch how he walks . . . look, he's moving without a cane . . .' "

"You're underestimating everybody, Sam. Yourself and the people out front. They'll be there and they won't be waiting for you to fall on your ass. And as for you, I've been around you enough to know that every time you're faced with adversity you've always come back twice as strong."

"Well, maybe I'm tired of coming back twice as strong, Shirley, maybe I'm fucking tired of making saves."

"Maybe you don't have any choice, Sam. Maybe it's God's way of saying, 'I've got another mountain I want you to climb, so get over it because the one after that is going to be dynamite.' You've always done it, Sammy, going back to when you lost your eye. I was there. That was a helluva clout. But you got up, and you made it. Whatever failure you've ever had you've been able to come back, rise up from the ashes . . . Everything that's ever happened to you that should have finished you, you've only gone on to be bigger . . ."

After we'd hung up I got onto my crutches and worked my way to the dining room to see if I could sit at the table. After a few seconds I was so weak I couldn't sit up. What should be easier than sitting? I tried to imagine myself on a stage. Forget about entertaining, forget about moving or even standing up for an hour and ten. Would I be able to sit on a stool?

That evening Lessie Lee asked, "Don't you want to come out of this bedroom and sit down at the dining table?"

"No, I don't want to sit down at the dining table."

Why wouldn't I let her know that I'd tried? Why did I have to always keep everybody off balance? I always had. It started as a defense. "No, I don't want to go to the fuckin' Stork Club." Of course I wanted to go there and to be able to tell my grandchildren that I'd seen the Stork Club, but I knew I couldn't get in, and who wanted to be mealymouthed? So fuck 'em, and it had become a personality trait.

Enough! Nobody ever said that life is supposed to be a smooth road. There's no way that life's supposed to be a freeway. You've got to hit some dirt roads, hit some rocky roads, detours. Sometimes when you're on that side road you have fun, you find a great diner and you go ". . . waaaaaggghh, this is fun!" or when you're bogged down in the mud you curse and yell and you want to lie down exhausted but after a little rest you know you better get yourself back on that highway. I watched them build this freeway, and helped build it a little myself, so I want to ride it to the end.

I shaved off two weeks of beard. I put the rag on my head to straighten my hair. Well, maybe I could slip on some pants. Suddenly I was dying for a break from pajamas and robe, pajamas and robe. I got my crutches and worked my way out to the breakfast nook.

Eddie saw me approaching. "Oh God! The ogre is out of his cage!" He did some funny lines with me and we laughed and then I went back to my room to rest.

Altovise put bells on my walker and on my crutches so they could hear me coming down the hall, like if they were talking about me, and I heard Eddie stage-whisper, "Careful! He's coming. It's either him or a fucking cow." I walked past them without making eye contact. I hated for Altovise to see me using the walker or crutches. I eased myself into a chair in the breakfast nook and took a look at the newspaper. There was a news photo of Mr. T. playing Santa Claus at the White House and Nancy Reagan sitting on his lap. It seemed like only a few years since the trauma when I hugged Richard Nixon. Every week I watched Benson kissing the ladies on network television, and nobody had a bad word to say. You think that's not progress from when they tried not to show my *GE Theater*? But phewwww, what a lot of heat we took to get here.

My thoughts went to Martin, as they so often did, and to Bobby. That whole period we went through. I don't know how our society survived it. The assassinations. How we withstood the total wrenchings of our modes, our types of lives, what we'd gone through! But we survived.

At one time in our lives it seemed that life was set, not success and failure, but "this is our lifestyle." Then it changed and it's over there now. When did bell-bottom trousers go out? With big buckles? When did you stop wearing beads? When was it no longer right to go, "Peace and love, man"? Kids kissing strangers. When did it start and when did it end? When did Haight-Ashbury and love beads turn into the haven of homosexuals?

Alto said, "Honey, now that you're up a little, can some of the people who care about you come over and visit?"

"All right . . ." and I had that stupid feeling of starting to feel better but not wanting to let anyone know, don't let them see me smiling. I found myself leaning on the cane a little more than absolutely necessary, dramatizing. I caught myself: "What are you doing, man? God catches you like this He'll say, 'Oh, you wanta playact? Okay, I'll give you something to playact about . . .'"

On December 8 I accepted the arrival of my sixtieth birthday with family and close friends at home. Milton Berle limped in on crutches to greet me on crutches. My father and Clint Eastwood and Danny Thomas and Jack Haley, Jr., and Steve and Eydie and all the buddies and family who were in town were there, and Altovise had Häagen-Dazs make a birthday-cake replica of my book, *Yes I Can*, which I guess was supposed to mean that I could beat this too.

Finally, the month was up and the X rays had been taken. Dr. Harris said, "It's coming along fine . . ."

God had wrapped His arms around me and was saying, "I'm not finished with you yet." He was letting me survive again.

". . . in another month you'll be walking without the crutches, but use a cane when you're in a crowd. It will work for you in keeping people away. They'll see you come in with a cane and they'll respect it. Don't baby your leg but don't overwork it either. If you've got a long walk, let them take you in a car or a golf cart. Don't be ashamed of it."

ALTO AND I sat in my office running tapes of *Sammy & Co.*, a talk and performance show I'd hosted in the seventies. I was hoping to learn something from my mistakes, which I was disappointed to see were legion. The reviewers had criticized me for doing phony breakups. It was painful reading it then, but fifteen years later I agreed with them. I saw the trap I'd fallen into. I love to laugh. Not just smile. Laughter. It's healthy. You will humor a joke, a piece of business, with a laugh, a breakup. Humoring a joke is George Burns taking the timing with his cigar before the punch line. But I overshot the road. I watched myself doing phony breakups, laughing too hard at things that weren't that funny, and laughing at things that weren't funny at all. It didn't engender laughter with the audience. People looked at each other. "Why is he laughing?"

I watched myself introducing guests. "My dear friend . . . a great talent . . ." I remembered reading that my introductions were too flowery. It was my vaudeville upbringing of giving another performer all the courtesy possible, verbally "carrying them on," but I belabored it. I'd resented reading it, but they'd been right.

Strange thing, videotape, sitting in a dark room and looking at the ghost of Christmas past. My youth was not attractive to me. I heard and saw myself enraptured by the sound of my voice. I'd thought: *What a wonderful thing to hear this articulate young kid on the stage, he's black, and speaks so well.* Fine, but I didn't have to go past Olivier.

By way of forgiving myself, I'd had no education, I was self-taught, I respected the value of words, of the resonant voice like Barrymore's. At Ciro's when Jerry Lewis told me, "You talk too English," I'd caught it but not enough. I was in love with the character, the elegance. Unfortunately, I wasn't born sixty years old. I had to work hard, fuck up a lot and consequently learn a lot.

Around December 20 I called Shirley. "Phone them in Australia and tell them we'll make the tour. I'll open in Sydney January 23. I'll work easy, no fast moves, but I'll sing and talk."

Once committed, I had to understand the performance I would be able to give. I know what I can wring out of an audience. I know I can pull their gut apart. One of my greatest assets is that I'm able to show my vulnerability . . . they can touch with that. But it's a fine line between drama and cheap theatrics. I love being theatrical. But I didn't want to use cheap theatrics. I didn't want to walk on the stage with a cane in my hand and go, "Good evening. Let us try and sing some songs for you." Not that the audience wouldn't love it. You talk about a standing ovation? If ever I walked on in Las Vegas with a cane and I just stood there and said, "Good evening, ladies and gentlemen," it would be screams. From the heart. From the soul. Pande-fucking-monium.

But that's Sophie Tucker being wheeled onstage in a hospital bed at the Latin Quarter in New York, with full makeup on: "I just had to come and let my fans know I love you." That's cheap theatrics. And the people loved it: "Who else but Sophie Tucker would have shown up?" "Such a pro!" Get outta here. Cheap theatricality. Of course I could do it, but that doesn't make it right.

Those were the thoughts. I wasn't whimpering, "My career is over." But I had to pull together all of the elements so that when they see the show they go, "Yeah! Go, babe!" Not "Ohhh, poor Sammy, he's out there, and trying . . ."

George called on the afternoon of Christmas Eve. "I hear we're goin' back."

"It's either a go-back or a go-'way."

"Then I'd better get onto those arrangements you wanted. How about if I come over tomorrow and we can run through them?" I got a powerful feeling of support from George, who had a house full of family yet was volunteering to work on Christmas.

In the middle of that night, at 3 a.m. on Christmas Day, the telephone rang. Altovise picked it up, then handed it to me. "It's Shirley."

"Yeah, Shirley?"

"He's gone."

I thought she meant that she and George had had an argument and he'd walked out.

She said, "He's gone. He had a heart attack."

"He's dead?"

"Yes."

As we walked in the front door I saw their Christmas tree with the unopened presents still under it. I put my arms around Shirley and we clung together. I could not grasp the feeling that he was dead. I had spoken with him only nine hours earlier about the music we were going to work on. Then a phone call later and he was gone. I'd never see him again. I'd never felt the pain of loss like that. My grandmother, Rosa B., was preambled by her age and illness. But George going suddenly left me with a gaping ache. Empty.

The suddenness! He was always there, a part of the success, and the failure. We could look at each other and there were a hundred words we could exchange without having to say them. We'd gone through every kind of up and down that people go through. Thirty years of walking onto a stage knowing George is there and because he is there the music will come in on time, it will be right, and I can concentrate on what I need to do. Thirty years of knowing if

I move a shoulder he reads it and tells the band what I want; if I forget a lyric he brings the band back again to where I got lost.

Fip Ricard, George's friend and our first trumpet for eighteen years, came in, dazed. I said, "I'm canceling all of our dates until further notice. I can't work. You can't work, Shirley. Fip can't work." They nodded weakly. I said, "I'll do the eulogy."

"No," Shirley said. "I don't think you've got the strength to rip yourself like that."

"You're right." The thought of it staggered me, but it had seemed the only thing to do. I called Jesse Jackson. He said, "I'll be there. I've got two speaking commitments that day but I'll work it out and I'll be there for George."

All the musicians arrived and dozens of George's friends. Shirley's doctor was among them. He said, "I'm going to give you some Valium to ease you over the next period."

"No," she said. "That stuff puts off reality, and I know I have to face this."

Lovingly we started joking about George, taking it from tragedy with what has always been the performer's saving grace, a sense of humor. I told them, "George didn't take no shit from nobody! The worst show of my life I did one night in Italy. When it was finally over we got into the car, me at the wheel, George next to me, and I started letting off steam. 'Motherfucker, you realize that they didn't even like "Birth of the Blues"? Goddammit, motherfucker, did you notice how they . . . ?' and I went on and on until finally George turned to me and said, 'You have called me motherfucker seventeen times. By actual count. Now, I ain't gonna be a motherfucker but two times more.' "

And we joked about him being slow-moving. "Somewhere, up there, he's saying, 'Wait a minute, I'll be there. Don't worry about it.' Walking slow. And St. Peter is impatient. 'Come on, George. Come on through the gates. Can't you walk faster?' 'I'll be there . . . Don't worry about it . . .' "

Shirley sighed. "Bobby Darin always wanted George . . ."

"Yeah, he got my conductor. If Jolson'll let him have him." And then everybody started to say a little line. "Damn, he left us down here in the shit and he up there . . ."

JESSE WAS eloquent, speaking of a lost friend. Seated on the dais, looking out at the church, which overflowed with more than a

353

thousand people, all friends or musical associates, I thought: This is the proof of what he accomplished, how good a person he was.

And then I was thinking of me, wondering what it would be like without him, how I would fill the gap of all that support, all that talent he'd contributed.

Shirley was receiving people at home after the cemetery but I was in a chronic state of tears. My leg was hurting but I didn't want to leave her even though she had hundreds of people going to the house. In the car leaving the cemetery she told me, "Don't come to the house. Go home. You're bleeding."

For days I lay in bed thinking: Maybe I was wrong, maybe God *is* finished with me, maybe it's His way of saying, "Get off the stage! How many warnings do you need? I hurt your hip. Now I've taken your conductor . . . Now get out of here."

Suspense was no friend of mine. I called Shirley. "How y'doin'?"

"Hangin' in."

"Me too. Look, I'm going to do Australia. I've got to find out if I can make it. I can't lay on this fuckin' bed looking at ghosts much longer. And I don't mean just George. I mean the ghost of me."

"Okay. I'll confirm our tour."

"No, Shirl, stay. Rest. I didn't mean for you to work."

"I've got to, Sammy. I've got to go everywhere we were together. I've got to see him there, and not see him there, and then maybe I'll be able to let him go."

WE HAD A meeting at the house, Altovise, Shirley, and Fip. I explained, "I don't want a conductor. I haven't got thirty years to teach that to somebody new. Nobody's going to replace George. If I bring somebody in, regardless of his ability he'll be an outsider and it would be too difficult for us all to relate to him. I'll set the tempos myself. Fip's family. Fip can rehearse the bands, and whatever else we need. When I do the medleys I'll call you down, Fip, to conduct. But stand to the side, please. I don't want anybody in the center in George's place."

Later, I told Altovise, "Australia's a long, hard trip . . . Stay here and be comfortable . . ."

"You don't want me there in case you fall on your ass, right?"

"Don't be ridiculous . . ." Why not admit it? "Exactly. I might fail and I wouldn't want you to see that."

"You think you really might?"

"Of course I might. Nobody can win all the races, forever."

I WAS ON an airplane for seventeen hours, without any alcohol, with a reconstructed hip that I shouldn't have been sitting on for an hour, let alone seventeen, on my way to do my first performance in two months. Since I was three years old no two-month period had ever passed in which I didn't perform. I lost my eye and I was back in six weeks.

The Sydney Hilton advertised it as "Sammy Davis Jnr.'s Return to Show Business." I went downstairs to watch Fip lead the band through my music. Shirley couldn't take it and left. Not seeing that big bear George, I too had to walk out and go upstairs and cry.

On opening night as I listened to the overture I looked through the curtain. People were standing up in the back and along the sides and I'd been told the room was packed with not only Australian press but English and American. I waited for my musical moment and I pushed myself into the longest walk I'd ever made.

"Good evening, ladies and . . ." I coughed and my voice closed. I tried to speak. Nothing. I whispered to the audience, over the mike, "My voice . . . it's gone." There was nothing else to say, they'd heard it go. I kept whispering, "Can you believe this? Here I've been worrying about my hip and my voice goes!"

I couldn't dance and I couldn't sing. Though I could be amusing, I had no delusions of being Milton Berle. I was helpless. This was the nightmare. It had come to pass.

My voice continued to eke out in a whisper, "Let me struggle through a couple of numbers, let's see what happens, see what I can do . . ." The voice came back and went away, came back and went away, like someone was turning my throat on and off.

I had stopped walking onstage with a cigarette in my hand because of a promise I'd made to the Heart Fund, but now I searched the ringside tables for a smoker. "Somebody give me a cigarette, please . . ." and I puffed and relaxed and semi-apologized: "I gave up drinking and drugs. Two out of three ain't *bad*." The voice came back a little, gravelly. "Actually, I went to a hypnotist to stop smoking but it didn't work. He was shining the light in the wrong eye."

I said, "I'd like . . . I'd like to do a show for you people who have paid your money . . ." They laughed sympathetically. I said, "A few years ago I was at Harrah's in Lake Tahoe, Nevada, and I did a show that was not up to my standards and so I picked up the tab for the entire room, and it cost me thousands of dollars, because I didn't want the audience to be disappointed. Now, you can imagine how I feel out here tonight, coming back to Australia, having been away for years, the press, the celebrities, all of you making me feel so at home, I walk onstage, I can't sing, I can't dance, I'm not feeling very funny . . . but I'm not pickin' up this tab! No more magnificent gestures . . . too expensive . . . can't afford that . . ." The laugh started in the back of the room and began to build. "No way," I said. "I'm going to buy you all some champagne . . . but then that's *it*, I ain't pickin' up this whole tab . . ."

Now I'm starting to get laughs, the show business is coming into play. *Yeah, you can work, you can do it . . . just keep dealing honestly with them.* There was a stool near the piano but I was still okay on my feet. I sang "Birth of the Blues" with cracks. I tried "What Kind of Fool Am I?" Ludicrous.

A man at ringside tried to help me. "Sam, do 'Bojangles.' "

I couldn't ignore it because he was right in front of me and his intention was kind. "I'm sorry, I can't do 'Bojangles' for you. My hip is still iffy. 'Bojangles' needs movement to the side and it's too difficult to even attempt. If I tried it you'd see a small Hershey bar stretched out on this stage." They laughed, they were with me. "But give me a rain check and the next time you see me I promise you I'll do it for you, 'cause this mother's gonna heal. I just need a little time." And the people applauded because it was honest. It was theatrical but an honest theatricality.

I did an hour and five with no dancing, no voice at all, and I left the stage with the people cheering. I'd sung horribly, I wasn't that funny, I'd done a poor show. But they knew that I hadn't lost it partying, that it was legitimate, and how hard it was.

The press came out with love letters: "The consummate showman . . ." With the tough Australian press it could have been: "How dare he get on the stage in that condition?" And they would not have been wrong. But they, like the audience, were giving me a pass, it was a Life Achievement award. All of the people who had put me there were saying, "Easy, relax, things'll work out, we'll wait."

I went to see Joan Sutherland's voice teacher, Dr. John Tonkin. He examined my throat and my chest. "You have no polyps, there's no redness down there. There's nothing wrong with your voice physically. You just lost your conductor and lifelong friend, you're tentative about your hip—it's all emotional. When you get the confidence back and when God decides you can sing again, you'll sing again."

I called Fip to bring up the song book and we went over my numbers and took out all the songs which I was not vocally capable of handling, the ones you can't con your way through with a lot of finger snapping. It didn't leave much. I don't have many easy songs.

I struggled through two shows the next night and the next few days singing songs for which I didn't have to sustain a note, like "Bye Bye Blackbird" and "Slow Boat to China," staccato with lots of rhythm. On closing night I still had no voice.

During rehearsal in Adelaide the music was too down-tempo. I called out, "George, will you . . ." I saw Fip staring at me and I heard my own voice. As I went to him I saw the tears in his eyes and I hugged him. "I'm sorry, babe. I'm sorry. You're doing the job. Doing it well."

As I walked into the dressing room Shirley was looking at me with compassion. I attacked her. "Why is there no food or coffee backstage for the musicians?" Instead of telling me to fuck off she looked at me, waiting for me to regain my sanity. I raised my voice. "Well, you can tell 'em that I'm not going out on that stage if there's no food here."

"Don't yell at me."

"I'm yelling at you."

"Okay, then yell at me. You happy?"

"Yeah." I looked at her helplessly and began crying. "I'm sorry. I'm crazy." We hugged and held on to each other.

"No. We're both going through the same thing." She gave me a pack of Kleenex. "We have to let him go. And it's not getting easier. In ten days we'll be home, where everything is familiar, the people, the grains in the wood on the stage, the stool George sat on. We're going to see him in every club, in every suite, the restaurants. We're going back to all those hundreds of places we've been with George and we're going to see him there . . ."

Through my tears I croaked, "An' I'm gonna say to him, 'How

come you get around so fast *now?* Every place we go you're sittin'
here waiting for us.' "

MY VOICE was better on opening night in Adelaide. By midweek
I turned to the band during the show. "Ohhhh, it's coming back."
And I started to stretch. Each show I began putting back numbers
which I had taken out. By the time I finished Adelaide it was almost
normal.

But always there was the awareness that George Rhodes wasn't
there. My right hand. My friend. Thirty years. I could feel him
there. I could hear his voice humming through the arrangements
he had written. I never stopped missing that wall that had always
been there, but I was careful to have strength around Shirley, and
that helped me. She was doing the same thing. She'd come into
the suite, Miss Bubbly, smiling, bouncing, "Good morning, all."
I played the grouch: "Here comes Miss Fuckin' Happy Toes. Take
a fuckin' hike."

At Melbourne, our last date, on opening night I walked out and
sang the first song and I heard the voice that I'd thought I'd never
hear again, clear, clean, and I looked at the audience and said,
"Ohhh, it's back. Ohhh, it is *back!*" and I wailed. I sang everything
I knew, going for the high notes and taking them from above, not
crawling up to them in hope, no, I attacked from the sky and I
never missed and to me it was like church bells ringing.

27

I ALWAYS THINK of Rubi when I'm in Paris. This time, coming out of the Plaza-Athénée at eleven in the morning with my son Jeff on my way to show him the Louvre, I thought: *Rubi, you wouldn't believe your old friend, the swinger.* It almost didn't seem like Paris without a hangover. Yet I was having fun there. I was finally grown-up enough for my teenage son.

We went to Cartier and Jeff chose a stainless-steel shockproof, waterproof watch for his fourteenth-birthday present. I was in France to do concerts in Marseilles and Deauville, a Red Cross benefit in Paris, and to play a week in Monaco. It was a sunny spring day and I wanted to take Jeff down the Seine. I told Murphy to speak to the hotel about renting a boat for eight or ten of us, with a picnic lunch.

When we got to the yacht basin I saw that they had hired us a boat that seats two hundred people. I'd been thinking of maybe a sixty-five-footer. "Murph, before we leave the dock, go ask the captain what this is costing me." He was back in a few minutes. "Not a cent. It's the hotel's gift."

They had it supplied with orange juice and champagne and a marvelous buffet. Here's six or seven of us and we've got this major yacht decked out for a large crowd. Shirley said, "You give a great party. You just don't invite enough people."

We cruised down the Seine, past the nude section, then the gay beaches, then the touristy section. Over by St.-Germain we saw the artists painting and sketching and Jeff was wildly photographing everything he saw. "Dad, I'm running out of film."

"Well, then don't take so many pictures."

"But I've never seen any of this before."

I turned to Murphy. "I've been coming to Paris since 1960 and until one party that Rubi gave on a boat I'd never seen the Seine. And I was so drunk I hardly saw it then."

On every boat that passed us they'd call out, "Sahmmmeee . . . Sahmmmeee." I didn't want to be upstaging Jeff's day, so we went inside for a while, but after five minutes, preferring the excitement, he said, "C'mon, Dad, let's go back up top."

It was fun for me to have French friends who had Jeff overnight to their château in Chantilly and took us to lunch with their son in the restaurant at the top of the Eiffel Tower.

My last date was in Monaco. I was there for six days, doing one show a night, staying at the Hôtel de Paris in the suite which I love on the second floor. Jeff met some girls from Dallas, Roger Moore's son was there, and they went discoing. Though we had Monaco security Dino was always there and he never looked like a bodyguard. It was twofold, protection for Jeff plus they were all having fun going to discos.

I'd finish the show and go up to the suite to go to bed when Jeff and the others were just getting ready to go out. "Okay, you got money?"

"Yeah, Dad, I've got money."

"Ten o'clock breakfast."

In the morning, at ten sharp, Jeff staggered into my suite, his eyes hanging down to his neck. He hadn't gotten back until daylight. Nobody else was even buzzing. "Gee, Dad, it was awesome last night." He flopped onto the couch.

He must have balled sixteen chicks.

"We danced till five o'clock."

"Would you care for some breakfast, son?"

"Oh no, Dad"—he looked queasy—"but I'm dying of thirst. I could use one of your Crushes."

As a hangover specialist, albeit retired, I suggested, "Get some orange juice and some ham and eggs and toast."

He shuddered. "Maybe later, Dad."

"What'd you drink last night?"

He shook his head in amazement. "I had two beers."

After a game try at eating he asked, "What're you going to do today, Dad?"

"I'm just going to sit out there on the terrace and read."

"Well, I think I'll go to my room," and he went back and slept.

I spent a quiet few hours, sorry that Altovise couldn't be with me, but she was in Japan in an official capacity as Ambassadress of Goodwill for the city of Los Angeles.

Jeff returned at three in the afternoon, a new man. Cooking! I said, "Put on a bathing suit and let's take a look at the beach."

All my guys were there and Jeff joined them going in and out of the water. I was having some Perrier and lemon when he came back. "Dad . . . down the beach . . . there are some girls laying there with only half their bathing suits on."

"Well, that's what they do in Europe, son. It's not like at home. Over here they go topless."

"Wheeeewww, Dad, oh boy. Look . . . one of the girls is waving at you."

I looked down the beach. "Those are the kids from the show."

A couple of them came over and I told them, "This is my son Jeff."

"Oh, sure, you introduced him from the stage last night." They were smiling at him, eyeing him.

I said, "Now don't go hittin' on my son. He's here to see some cultural things and you ain't included in cultural things."

The following day after his morning nap Jeff was back, in his bathing suit. "I think I'll take a swim."

"Okay, son. Go ahead . . . only keep in mind . . ." I'm thinking I'll be a great, modern father and tell him: *Look, son, "sophistication" is: you don't get an erection when you go to the beach in Monaco or Cannes. Even though you could, you don't. It's not the thing to do. You don't stare, but also you don't turn away. There's a whole technique to be learned in how to look at a woman who's got a great bust and she ain't got no top on her. You don't look here, or there, you're supposed to be sophisticated and not notice . . .*

"Yes, Dad?"

"Go on, son, and say hello to the girls, only don't stare at them."

He held up a pair of very dark sunglasses. "I'll wear my shades."

So they couldn't see him staring.

Culture shock. Overnight Jeff went from Monte Carlo with the sophisticated, topless European chicks to my golf tournament in Hartford, Connecticut, with Bermuda shorts and McDonald's. After about three days he asked, "You come here every year?"

"Yes. This is my tournament."

"I prefer Monaco and Paris."

TRACEY AND Guy were married in my home. Jesse Jackson performed the ceremony. Their marriage was both interracial and interreligious.

Later, during the reception at Nicky Blair's, I couldn't help observing the attitudes. It was: "Glad she's happy." "What a pretty girl." "Handsome boy."

Lord, what it took to get here! How many people had to suffer, how much crying and pain and hurt there had been, for this to happen!

I was tempted to take Tracey and Guy aside and tell them but there was no point to that. She knew, he knew, and thank God, the way society was now structured it was quite a way down on their list of worries.

I DIDN'T HATE being sixty as much as I had fifty. On the contrary, I loved it that Mark and his wife, Jane, had a baby and I was a grandfather. Tracey and Guy were happy. Jeff was doing great. And I was still in the business. What I'd hated, really, was the lack of time to do what I should have done by then. My fear had been to see the cat in the shroud going, "Pssst, come off the stage." Instead I was notified that I was to receive the Kennedy Center for the Performing Arts' Gold Medal for Lifetime Achievement.

The other recipients were Irving Berlin, who'd been unable to travel to Washington, Perry Como, Alwyn Nikolais, Bette Davis, and Nathan Milstein. Our medals were presented to us by the President of the United States.

There were a couple of moments with President and Mrs. Reagan when it was just eight people in the room and it was Ron and Nancy, if you will, but I couldn't get to that. Though I did jokes like "Look, when this is over we can do a few *GE Theaters*, a couple of *Death Valley Days*, and don't worry about your future, it's time to bring back the Westerns anyway," when I spoke to him it was "Mr. President."

And he laughed. "In about a year I'm going to be wondering what I'll be doing."

I had been much more formal with Richard Nixon, who did not have a Ronald Reagan sense of humor because he didn't have the theatrical background. With President Reagan show business gave us keys that opened up a lot of little doors. He had been twenty-five years in show business, more time than he had been in politics. Plus, when he was governor there were more than a few occasions when we'd be together at UJA functions or a benefit for the NAACP and in conversation I called him Ron. That was when Nancy and I started with the joke about being kissing cousins because of her name being Nancy Davis. But when he became President of the United States I forgot his first name.

On the flight back to Los Angeles, I sat with Altovise without speaking. When I arrived in L.A., I was going directly to Cedars Sinai to have the full hip replacement done. The hip reconstruction had been temporary, as Dr. Harris had said it would be. I got a year out of it before it started to bother me too much to live with. In the meantime two or three new processes had been developed which made it easier for me. There were choices: do you want it with cement or without cement, plastic or metal? My new hip was made of a new kind of steel, built to order for me because a standard size would have reached down to my knee. I had learned a lot since the first meeting with Eugene Harris and I didn't fear it medically or professionally.

More than half a century had been a lot of show business. If the end was coming soon, as surely it must, then I was, finally, ready. And I thought that when I go I'd like it if people think: Yeah, the little motherfucker was a great entertainer, and he did some good. Let that be the memory. Because the band plays on. As it should. I know that after I'm gone there'll be a dynamite kid saying, "Good evening, ladies and gentlemen . . ." and whatever I did on a stage he'll do it as well, maybe better—although in my heart I hope not, but . . . the band plays on.

28

WE WERE WEEKENDING with Frank and Barbara at the Springs because of Barbara's telethon for her complex at the Eisenhower Medical Center. Frank and Dean and I—the fun, the jokes, the camaraderie, the comfort of being together prompted me to say, "We've got to do something together again."

They looked at me like "Wonderful. What?"

"Okay, agreed, we've done it in films and nobody's come up with a new idea for us, so we forget a picture. But if we could recapture that excitement we had in Vegas in '60. We're all playing the Bally, there's no conflict . . ."

Frank said, "But there's a lot of people who never get to Vegas. I've been thinking about us doing a tour. We could get a train, live on it, each of us have a private car, plus a dining car and bar car . . . and go from town to town doing a whistle-stop tour, except they wouldn't be whistle stops, they'd be big cities which normally we don't get to: Houston, Pittsburgh, Bloomington, Detroit, Cleveland, Cincinnati . . ."

Dean groaned. "Why don't we find a good bar instead?"

"Let me think about it some more," Frank said.

Dean brightened. "The bar?"

Usually ideas which are exciting over a lazy weekend don't look so good the next day. But Frank called me at home on Tuesday. "Smokey, let's do it. It will be hard work but it could be exciting. And I think it would be great for Dean. Get him out. For that alone it would be worth doing." He was alluding to the death of Dean's son, Dean Paul, in a plane crash six months earlier.

A few weeks later there was a dinner at Frank's home in Beverly Hills. He took Dean and me off in a corner. "The train is out. It would have been fun and colorful, but it won't work logistically. We'd be traveling for a week to play two dates. We'd be carrying forty musicians and a tech crew of another twenty-five or thirty. Then I've got a staff of six, Dean's got two, and Sammy's got three. Besides ourselves that's eighty-one people. We can't afford to house and feed that many for almost a week between each performance. We'll have to fly. I'll use my plane and we can charter another G-2 for you guys."

The reason for the two planes was that though we're thought of as a "rat pack" the three of us have different habits. Dean and I like to be in a town the night before. I like to get a little feel of the atmosphere. When Frank plays Vegas he uses his plane to commute to his home in Palm Springs. His style is to arrive an hour before the performance, have his tea, do his makeup, then the show starts. When he leaves the stage he goes straight to the car and to wherever he's going, with the tuxedo on. Dean will dress up in his suite, come down, do the show, and go right back up to his suite. He never goes into his dressing room. If he does it will be to look at television and that will be it, but there are no pictures on the wall, no bar setup. I try to create a little theatrical atmosphere, homey. That's my focus. The theatricality of everything. I love the entertaining in the dressing room, friends coming back afterward. When Dean works Vegas he does only one show a night so that he can get to sleep early and be on the golf course in the morning.

The way Frank envisioned it we would play 15,000- or 20,000-seat indoor stadiums, and large theaters like the Music Hall in New York.

"You think we can draw that much?" Dean asked.

I said, "If they're not going to come and see us, then there is no show business."

From the beginning Dean had less enthusiasm for the tour than Frank and I. Losing Dean Paul had shattered him. They had been very close, and Dean Paul was a golden child, a near-professional-level tennis player, likable, a beautiful young man. Dean had continued playing Vegas as therapy, but that was completely different from what our tour would be. In Vegas he has his own audience and there's no travel involved. Being on the road would be stimulating because of the challenge of fresh and different audiences, but physically taxing. Dean certainly didn't need the money, because apart from being wealthy he lives humbly, dresses simply. When he plays Vegas he brings one tuxedo. He hangs it up and that's it. One shirt, one tuxedo. You go into his dressing room and there's nothing there, no makeup, nothing. He wears a pinky ring which Frank gave him and a watch which he himself designed. And that's it! It's a lifestyle not at all like Frank's and mine. I had learned from friends that Dean did not really want to do it, but we were all aware that much of the allure was the return of the Rat Pack thirty years later and he didn't want to let us down.

Frank was planning it for March of '88. "We should do about thirty cities, but in two parts. Let's work March and April, take a few months off to rest and play our Vegas dates, then go back for part two in September and October."

I told Shirley to start moving our Vegas and Harrah's engagements into the period between the tours.

"What are the financial arrangements?"

"We'll be on a percentage of the gross with Frank and Dean."

"What is the potential gross? And what will the percentage be?"

"I don't know."

"Can I call Frank's people and ask?"

"No. When he's got it worked out he'll tell us, and it will be right."

The hardheaded businesswoman in her didn't like it, but the woman who had been with me for thirty years and consequently understood Frank Sinatra nodded her head and got to work changing our dates around. When the details were available it was as I had known it would be, the percentages were right. And we were cutting up the whole cake, participating in all ancillary rights: souvenir programs, T-shirts, hats and jackets embroidered: "Frank, Dean, Sammy."

Although the news of the tour had long ago leaked out and had appeared in trade papers and columns, it was appropriate to announce it officially. We invited the press to Chasen's at noon. For a smile our plan was to arrive together at that hour in tuxedos and black tie. We met at Frank's house and drove over together.

As we walked in Frank put his hand on my shoulder. "You start it off, Sam." He was still highlighting me, putting me up front. We'd expected a good turnout but the crowd awaiting us was like for a major news event: all wire services, local newspapers, all TV networks and radio, major magazines, and the foreign press. We took our places on a dais and I started it off. "Ladies and gentlemen, we thank you for coming here today . . ."

From behind me I heard Dean's voice. "Is there any way we can call this whole thing off?"

When the laugh quieted I continued. "We want to officially announce that we're going to be 'Together Again,' the first time since Las Vegas in the sixties . . ."

Frank called out, "And definitely the last time."

A reporter asked, "Then this is not the first of an annual event?"

"Look," Frank explained, "Sammy is sixty-two, and he's the kid. I'm seventy-two and Dean is seventy. At our ages the only annual event you hope for is your birthday." He nodded for me to continue.

"We're very pleased to say that American Express is our sponsor and that Home Box Office will be taping one of the performances for emission subsequent to the tour . . ."

I heard Dean asking, "Doesn't he know any regular words?"

Frank explained, "Smokey talks a little English."

"He doesn't *look* English."

"He doesn't look Jewish either! Anyway, what he means is, after we've played all the live dates HBO'll air the tape."

Our chemistry and rapport was still what it had been and the reporters were enjoying it. The success of the Rat Pack or the Clan was due to the camaraderie, the three guys who work together and kid each other and love each other, so it's fun.

One of the European reporters got out of line and asked, "What about the book that woman wrote about you, Frank?"

The other press people waited for the explosion but Frank fielded it like an easy grounder. "We can talk about that some other time. Today we're here to announce the tour that kicks off in Oakland next month."

The atmosphere relaxed and someone asked, "Are you going to be doing the current kind of rock music?"

Frank said, "We're going to do the songs that people have known us for. We're not going out there to experiment." He grinned. "Maybe we can bring back good music."

A few weeks later Frank called. "Smokey, American Express is running an ad tomorrow in San Francisco for Oakland. They blocked out 7,500 tickets for their card members to call in for. The other 7,500 will go on sale later to the general public." He called back the next day at noon, elated. "Smoke, American Express sold out all 7,500 tickets in the first hour and a half." Day by day we were told Vancouver was sold out . . . Seattle . . . Bloomington . . . Detroit . . . Pittsburgh . . . Cincinnati . . . Cleveland . . . Washington, D.C. . . . Providence . . . New York City . . . all sold out within hours of going on sale. We were getting calls from London and Paris promoters for a European tour.

Frank told me, "The accountants say you should come out of this with from six to eight million dollars." I remembered Will Mastin saying, "Ain't nobody ever going to be bigger than Bill Robinson. He makes $5,000 a week."

The first two rehearsals were held at my house, talk sessions in which we and our producers sat around my bar, went over the general shape of the evening, and ran through some dialogue we'd had written. Our typical jokes: I'd say, "Frank, all kidding aside, we want you to know that we still think of you as the Chairman of the Board." And Dean would say, "Yeah, Frank. You're the chairman and we're bored." Or as Frank finished a song I would say over the mike from offstage, "It's wonderful that a man of that age can still sing like that." And Dean would agree: "But let's go out and help him before his oxygen runs out." The best of our humor would happen spontaneously in genuine ad-libs, but until we were onstage, relaxed and cooking, we needed a framework to begin with.

Barbara Sinatra's birthday fell in the middle of rehearsals and Frank gave a birthday dinner for twenty-five people at Chasen's. As we finished the main course Frank caught my attention and gestured for me to make a toast. I stood up. He groaned loudly. "Oh God, he's going to make a speech. Siddown, ya bum. Who needs ya?"

"Quiet, Frank. Shaddup."

Heckling, irreverence, but with the obvious affection. Much like it would be onstage during the tour.

The next day we were having a full physical rehearsal with our orchestra at Ren Mar Studios on North Cahuenga in Hollywood. A square-shaped structure had been erected: a duplicate of the stage we'd be performing on in Oakland and most of the other cities. It was an elevated stage, looking like a prizefight ring without the ropes. We needed to rehearse how we'd work and move around under theater-in-the-round conditions. I'd played theaters in the round and Frank had, but not Dean. Only in Chicago and at the Radio City Music Hall would we work with a proscenium.

The stage was lit, carpeted to avoid foot sounds, and had the same microphones, TelePrompTers, everything that we would have everywhere we'd play.

The orchestra brought in from New York was rehearsing under Morty Stevens. I enjoyed watching a fine conductor, seeing the control, watching the music appear to be coming out of his hands, the sounds of different instruments emerging each way he waves or points. I looked over at him, across the studio and through the years. Morty. We'd started in this business together in the early fifties. My father and Will Mastin and I were headlining Bill Miller's Riviera and between shows I'd gone down to the basement and I'd heard this kid noodling on a clarinet. I asked him, "Could you write an arrangement for me of 'Birth of the Blues.' I hummed what I had in mind and a few days later I liked what he gave me, not imagining that I'd be singing it that way for the next thirty years. He quit the Riviera and traveled with us as our conductor. After ten years or so he came to me, looking happy-sad. "CBS has offered me a great job. Apart from the money, it means I could stay home with Annie and the kids. I told them I couldn't leave you until you got somebody."

"Get outta here. Go tomorrow. Don't you dare risk a shot like that," and George Rhodes moved over from pianist to conductor.

Now Morty was head of music for CBS, conducting forty pieces for Frank, and Dean, and myself.

Shirley interrupted my reverie. "We've got a problem. That whole big orchestra the contractor hired does not have a single black musician. In 1988! That is *bad*. And we are going to be answering for that all across the country. I can't believe that Frank Sinatra is aware of this."

Frank came in carrying his music in an alligator schoolbag. Dean sat down with us at a table alongside the stage. He looked at Frank accusingly. "Everything I ate last night tasted like your finger. 'Hey, Dean, you should eat this . . .' and he poked his finger in it. " 'Here, eat these string beans, Dean, they're good for you.' " Dean shook his head. "I woke up this morning with your finger in my mouth." He was "on" for the stage managers and the tech crew who were milling around. He felt it his responsibility to be "Dean Martin." As the Clan we were expected to exist together in a constant state of clowning, drinking, and hip banter. In reality, I had my Crush, Dean and Frank had coffee, and we were all deeply concerned about what we were there for.

I said, "Frank, the contractor hired forty white musicians. The only blacks are my lead trumpet, drummer, and bass."

"Shit." He called over the contractor. "What the fuck is this snow-white orchestra? That stinks."

"But, Frank, it's too late to change 'em."

"Bullshit! I want at least thirty percent black musicians. Change 'em."

"That's expensive, Frank. We have to pay three weeks . . ."

"Pay what we have to. Fix it!"

WE FLEW into Oakland on Saturday afternoon before the Sunday performance. To my surprise Frank came with us a day ahead of his schedule. Hundreds of press and fans were there. We had nothing to say to the press until after the performance. Cars pulled up to the sides of our planes and we got away fast. The drive to our hotel took us past the Oakland Coliseum, where the marquee said, "Frank, Dean, Sammy. SOLD OUT." When we arrived at the Hyatt Regency we learned that there had been such an impossible volume of phone calls for each of us that the hotel and our security people had decided to deny that we were there. Anyone trying to reach us would have to know who we travel with and ask for them. The general attention we were getting, the press coverage, and advance ticket sales led us all to feel that we were going to make show business history.

There was a Saturday-night event at the stadium, so our stage, lights, and sound wouldn't be ready until 4 p.m. on Sunday. I woke up around noon. It was a clear, cool day, and I was excited, edgy but confident. I looked through the Sunday papers. Herb Caen's column brought me down a few thousand feet by asking what these old guys were trying to prove and why didn't we stay at home with our pipes and slippers and leave show business to the kids. But it was only an air pocket.

We went to the stadium for a sound check at five o'clock. The square stage stood in the center of fifteen thousand unoccupied seats, rising so high around us that the upper levels had giant television screens so the people up there could see the performers' faces. I had never played to that large a crowd in my life except at military bases, never to a paying audience. Ideally, Frank, Dean, and I play small rooms. We're saloon singers. Stadiums are rock-'n'-roll country.

Frank was staring at it too.

Dean asked, "Will someone tell me why we're here?"

I couldn't answer that, and Frank didn't either. We all had our lucrative casino dates in Vegas, Tahoe, Reno, and Atlantic City. Why were we putting it on the line again, exposing ourselves to ridicule?

I had a light dinner at five-thirty. Dressing to leave for the stadium at a quarter to seven, I watched the evening news, which led off with the presidential primaries, and then: "The Rat Pack is back, Frank Sinatra, Dean Martin, and Sammy Davis, Jr. . . ." and it went on for ten minutes, showing pictures of us together in the sixties, then a live pickup from the stadium, where a girl newscaster described the lines of fans that had been forming, the impossibility of buying a ticket. They were handling a theatrical performance as hard news.

Murphy had gone ahead of me to my dressing room at the Coliseum. The walls were hung with posters of *Ocean's Eleven* and *Robin and the Seven Hoods*, two of the five pictures we had made together in the sixties when the Clan and the Rat Pack had come into being.

I started doing my makeup. Morty came in dressed in his tux and new black silk shoes. "You're not very excited, are you?" I was looking pointedly at his feet. He blushed. "Who ever sees a conductor's shoes?"

I was strung too high to sit around the dressing room. The hall was jammed with all of our people, lighting men, sound men, musicians, dressers, everyone playing calm, professional, but the atmosphere pulsated with excitement. Beyond where we were standing there was a drone of voices from the stadium.

I looked in on Frank. Dean was sitting on a couch. Frank beckoned and we followed him out, past the people in the hall, to the point at which a curtain concealed the backstage from the stadium. Frank opened the curtain enough for us to look through. All of the seats which at five o'clock had been shining back in our eyes were occupied. He said, "Remember when we did the Summit at the Sands? With all the excitement of packing the place every night?" He looked at Dean. "Remember when you came running back all excited and said, 'The place is packed'?"

Dean had a how-could-I-have-been-so-dumb look on his face. "Of course we packed it. The joint could only seat four hundred people. And we were three big stars."

Frank said, "Tonight we will entertain more people in one show than we did during that entire run in Vegas."

THE SHOW was starting. Over the speaker in my dressing room I heard our overture and then Dean's music. I could picture him looking at the audience, laid back, playing the drunk, taking a sip from a glass, then asking his pianist, "How long have I been on?" I heard the sure laugh and him singing, "When it rains it always rains, bourbon from heaven . . ." to the tune of "Pennies from Heaven." When he finished it he asked, "Have I got time for one more?" and he sang, "When you're drinking, you get stinking . . . and the whole world smiles at you . . ."

I had about twenty minutes. I was going to follow Dean and do around thirty-five minutes. Frank would open the second half of the show and then the three of us would work together.

My hands were cold and dry. Unable to sit down and wait, I dressed and walked over to Frank's dressing room. He was in a robe, sitting on the couch, listening to Dean. He'd finished his next-to-last number and there was tremendous screaming and applause and you could tell that those fifteen thousand people were on their feet with excitement.

Frank stood up and as he put his hands on my shoulders I had the feeling that he'd had his arm around my shoulder since 1945 and he'd never taken it off in over forty years, except to push me ahead. I could remember his voice on a dozen occasions echoing back through the years, starting when we were a dance act, a flash act to open other people's shows, and he'd had us on the bill with him at the Capitol Theater in New York. "You should sing, Sam. Get yourself a style." . . . "No, Bing does not get third billing. It's me and Dean and Sam on top. Give Bing a box of his own. Sam gets billing over the title." . . . "Go ahead, Smokey, you introduce the next President."

When it was time for me to leave he said, "Give me something that's hard to follow, Charley."

I waited in the wings as Dean closed with "Volare."

I felt grateful for the fact of being there. After all the fears, after all the mistakes, still it wasn't ending for me as "Bojangles," there were no frayed cuffs and collar, I was not a disappointment to the friends, to the events, to the opportunities which had brought me to that moment in which fifteen thousand people were waiting for me. *Lord, thank you. For this, for the friends You've let me have, this wonderful life . . . I still don't know why You want me here, and I'm not asking anymore 'cause I know now You ain't never gonna tell me, but I hope I'm doing it the way You want me to . . .*

I heard them applauding Dean. I had a few seconds. The euphoria which had balmed my body, gentled my mind, began lifting, displaced by an awakening, as drastically different from moment to moment as when the earliest rays of morning sun first soften the darkness of night, then penetrate, crashing through, awakening everyone to the need to get up and get to work.

I felt that old, familiar hunger. For fifty years I'd stood in the wings of theaters and clubs and felt the need to please the people, to stay with them until they loved me. I felt that airiness in my chest that could only be filled by the people who were waiting for me. God had brought me to where I was standing. Now it was up to me. My hands and lips were dry. My mind flashed forward to the walk down the aisle, past the rows of people, then up three stairs to the stage.

I picked up the mike and I was aware of myself turning, facing the audience on all sides. Banks of blinding light poured down on me from every direction. Morty had begun my opening number, but the people were applauding, so he was vamping till I was ready. For as far as I could see before the lights dissolved everything into a platinum infinity, they were standing, applauding, smiling. I felt the clarity of mind that I wanted, the strength in my chest, my legs, my arms. The applause was pumping power into me. The music softened, the people were settling down.

I said, "Good evening, ladies and gentlemen . . ."

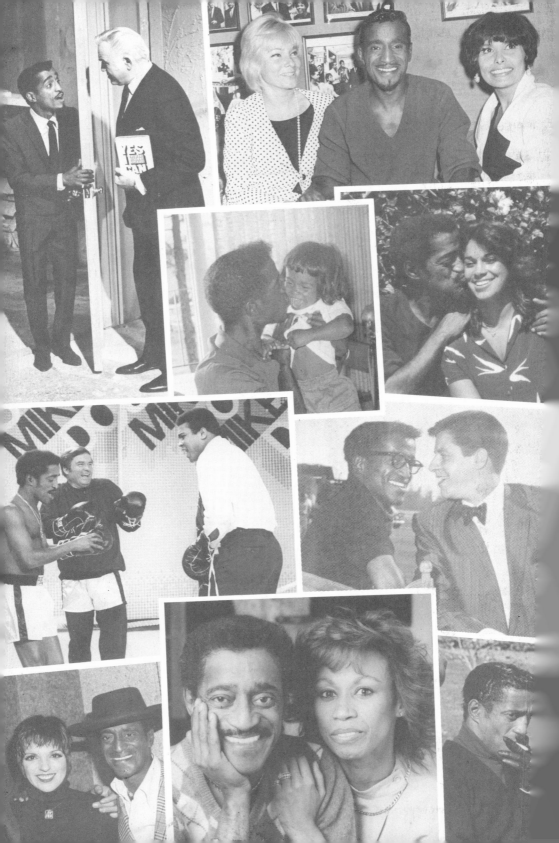